LEAD EXPOSURE AND CHILD DEVELOPMENT

An International Assessment

LEAD EXPOSURE AND CHILD DEVELOPMENT

An International Assessment

Edited by

M.A. Smith
Department of Child Psychiatry
Institute of Child Health
Hospital for Sick Children
Great Ormond Street, London, UK

L.D. Grant
Director, Environmental Criteria and Assessment Office
Office of Health and Environment Assessment
US Environmental Protection Agency
Research Triangle Park
NC 27711, USA

A.I. Sors
Commission of the European Communities
Directorate-General for Science, Research and Development
Environment Research Programme
Rue de la Loi 200
B-1049 Brussels, Belgium

Published for the Commission of the European Communities and the
US Environmental Protection Agency by

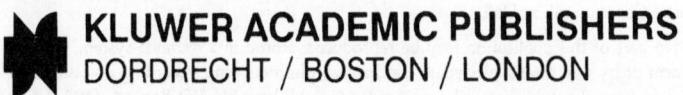 **KLUWER ACADEMIC PUBLISHERS**
DORDRECHT / BOSTON / LONDON

Distributors

for the United States and Canada: Kluwer Academic Publishers, PO Box 358, Accord Station, Hingham, MA 02018-0358, USA
for all other countries: Kluwer Academic Publishers Group, Distribution Center, PO Box 322, 3300 AH Dordrecht, The Netherlands

British Library Cataloguing in Publication Data

Lead exposure and child development.
  1. Healthy children. Effects of lead pollutants. Effects on health of children
  I. Smith, Marjorie A.   II. Grant, Lester D.   III. Sors, A.I.   IV. Commission of the European Communities   V. United States, Environmental Protection Agency
  613.1
  ISBN-13:978-94-010-6868-0   e-ISBN-13:978-94-009-0847-5
  DOI: 10.1007/978-94-009-0847-5

Library of Congress Cataloging-in-Publication Data

Lead exposure and child development : an international assessment /
  edited by M.A. Smith, L.D. Grant, and A.I. Sors.
      p. cm.
    "Published for the Commission of the European Communities and the US Environmental Protection Agency."
    Includes bibliographies and index.
    ISBN-13:978-94-010-6868-0 : £45.00 (U.K. : est.)
    1. Lead-poisoning in children — Congresses.   2. Child development — Congresses.   I. Smith, M.A. (Marjorie A.)   II. Grant, Lester D.   III. Sors, A.I. (Andrew I.)   IV. Commission of the European Communities.   V. United States. Environmental Protection Agency.
    [DNLM: 1. Child Development Disorders — chemically induced.   2. Environmental Exposure. 3. Lead Poisoning — in infancy & childhood. QV 292 L43035]
  RA1231.L4L378   1988
  362.1'989298 — dc19
  DNLM/DLC
  for Library of Congress   88-37512
                                                                                                CIP

Copyright

Publication No. EUR 11085 of the
Commission of the European Communities
Directorate-General Telecommunications, Information Industries and Innovation
Scientific and Technical Communication Unit

Published in the United Kingdom by Kluwer Academic Publishers, PO Box 55, Lancaster, UK.

Kluwer Academic Publishers BV incorporates the publishing programmes of D. Reidel, Martinus Nijhoff, Dr W. Junk and MTP Press.

Contents

CONTENTS

vii

Preface

This book arises out of a workshop on lead exposure and child development which was held at the University of Edinburgh on 8th–12th September 1986. It was organized jointly by the Commission of the European Communities (CEC) and the US Environmental Protection Agency (EPA), in association with the UK Department of the Environment and the Scottish Home and Health Department.

It brought together most of the internationally recognized groups working on the effects of lead exposure on child development including child psychologists, psychiatrists, neurologists, epidemiologists, toxicologists, statisticians, and medical practitioners. One of the unique features of the meeting was that it included workers from initially separate fields of lead research, in particular those undertaking studies in infants and in older children, and those carrying out behavioural research in animals, as well as those undertaking biochemical studies on mechanisms of lead effect.

The structure of this book reflects the main elements of the meeting. As such it includes three main sections. The first consists of two major state-of-the-art reviews, and two invited introductory papers. The reviews were prepared for the organizers of the conference by two of the Editors. The objectives were to assess critically the state of current knowledge in this field and to provide a scientific basis both for policy decisions and for further research. The review prepared by Marjorie Smith for the Commission of the European Communities focusses on methodological and design issues, and summarizes our present scientific knowledge in this area. Here, the emphasis is on cross-sectional epidemiological studies primarily carried out within the countries of the European Community. The review prepared by Lester Grant of the US Environmental Protection Agency reflects considerations of environmental policy, and reviews the studies particularly from the US perspective. It is recognized that there are some areas of overlap between these two reviews; however, it was considered useful to examine some key issues from two different perspectives.

The second and by far the largest part of this book includes papers containing presentations by the various invited groups on their findings. A substantial proportion of the work reported was carried out under contract to the CEC or to the EPA and other US-federal agencies, respectively. The presentations were organized under three headings: (1) Cross-sectional Epidemiological Studies of Children, (2) Pregnancy Outcome, Neonatal and Prospective Studies, and (3) Animal Studies and Mechanisms; these headings have been maintained in the present volume. The final short section is an attempt by the Editors to synthesize the main issues which were raised during the extensive discussion sessions at the end of the meeting. Based upon this, some general guidelines for the directions of future research are also suggested.

The organizers consider that their original objectives for the meeting and for the resulting book have been fully satisfied. The meeting provided a basis for a comprehensive assessment of the critical scientific issues, an extensive presentation and discussion of the latest original research findings, as well as important guidelines for policymakers. It should be noted that all three main sections of this book have been restructured as well as revised during the course of its preparation for publication. It is hoped that this final product represents a unique international assessment of the current knowledge in this field.

As joint organizers of this workshop, the Commission of the European Communities and the US Environmental Protection Agency are very pleased to have been able to collaborate in this important initiative. They also wish to acknowledge, with gratitude, the financial and administrative support of the UK Department of the Environment and the Scottish Home and Health Department, and the excellent local organization undertaken by Dr Mary Fulton and her colleagues of the Department of Community Medicine at the University of Edinburgh.

M.A. Smith
L.D. Grant
A.I. Sors

December 1988

Section 1

STATE-OF-THE-ART REVIEWS

1.1

The Effects of Low-level Lead Exposure on Children

M. SMITH

This review will aim to cover work on the possible neurological and behavioural effects of exposure to low levels of environmental lead which has been reported in the past 7 years. The review will be from a scientific viewpoint, thus it will not tackle the difficult problem of the policy implications which are attached to the findings, but will try to evaluate from a methodological and design viewpoint what is known as a result of the research carried out so far, and what we now need to know. The document is intended both as a description of the state of art, and as a guide to aid the interpretation and utilization of the results of existing research.

Because of the large number of studies which have been carried out in different countries it is not possible to review them all, and in choosing to include or exclude studies it is quite possible to bias the conclusions by omitting certain studies. This highlights one of the problems in interpreting the findings overall, and that is that apparently similar studies have different findings. The individual studies have not been reviewed in detail, but rather the aim has been to review across a number of studies in a comparative way, in terms of the methodology, the results, the interpretation which can be put on them, and the conclusions which can be drawn from them. Those studies which are reviewed are intended to be a representative sample, in order to allow examination of the possible reasons for conflicting results.

There are two main sections to this review. In the first section a number of methodological and theoretical issues of relevance to studies of low-level lead effects are reviewed. These include estimates of body lead and the correlations between different measures (discussed in greater detail in the introductory chapter by Mushak); outcome measures and issues pertaining to these; issues of design and sampling, including representativeness and bias in sampling; and the important issue of confounding variables and their control, and in particular the role of social disadvantage in the relationship between

Prepared for: Commission of European Communities, Directorate-General for Science, Research and Development, Environment Research Programme

lead uptake and outcome measures.

The second section concentrates on study results and current knowledge, and attempts to summarize what we 'know' as a result of research in relation to lead and intelligence, educational attainment, behaviour, and other psychometric measures. The contribution of animal studies, and studies with electrophysiological outcome measures, to current knowledge is assessed. The problems in interpreting the existing data are discussed in relation to some of the methodological issues described in the first section.

THEORETICAL AND METHODOLOGICAL ISSUES

The first results from epidemiological studies of children not exposed to a point source of lead were reported in 1979. Up to this time studies had been carried out around lead works, or on children identified by clinic screening programmes. The studies are described, in tabular form, in the review by Grant and Davis (this volume). Generally the children studied had moderately raised body-lead burdens (that is blood lead levels above about 30 μg/dl), but even at these levels there was little consensus on the significance results. Some studies found that children with moderately raised levels of lead performed significantly worse on psychometric tests (de la Burdé and Choate, 1972 and 1975; Perino and Ernhart, 1974), others found at least a tendency towards worse performance in the higher lead children (Ratcliffe, 1977; Kotok et al., 1977), and some (Lansdown et al., 1974; Baloh et al., 1975) found no such tendency, or even a reverse trend. Looked at as a group, the early clinic and smelter studies were characterized by a number of methodological weaknesses and design faults, and these make the interpretation of the results difficult, and may be responsible for the disparity in the results between different studies.

To summarize the main failings of the clinic and smelter studies:

1. Most of the studies were based on small numbers of children. This poses statistical power problems, as well as difficulties in interpreting any differences found.
2. In some studies there is a considerable loss between the numbers originally identified for the sample, and the numbers for whom results are presented. This is particularly pertinent where it is due to reasons such as children not attending for test sessions, as this can create a biased sample.
3. In several studies the choice of tests is inappropriate, or the standard of testing was poor. This includes the use of group screening tests, designed to screen for abnormalities, but relatively insensitive to small individual differences, or the use of results of tests which schools had carried out for their own purposes.
4. In some studies using blood lead as a measure of body burden there was a long period of time between when the blood was obtained, and when the psychometric tests were carried out. Since blood is a measure of body burden which reflects predominantly current exposure to lead, this can be relevant if exposure changes in some way. In some studies it was shown that in a number of children there was a considerable difference in their

4

blood lead between the time they were allocated to a lead group, and the time of testing, resulting in poor definition of group boundaries, with some actual overlap between the lead levels in the groups.

5. Some studies did not obtain any measure of body lead, or obtained a measure of body burden only in the 'exposed' group.

6. In some studies the high lead and control groups were selected by a different method, or from a different area, and both these approaches could result in bias. Equally, where the controls are selected from the same environment as high-lead children it is important to know why the groups have different body lead burdens.

7. The most important methodological shortcoming of all the early studies, is their failure to take adequate account of potentially confounding factors. Most of the studies matched, or controlled for, demographic variables such as sex, age and race, and some for additional variables such as pica or social class or socioeconomic status. However, considering the large number of other variables which are known to be associated with performance on psychometric tests, and with behaviour, and the large number of variables known to be pertinent to body lead measures, this is almost certainly not adequate, and can result in uncontrolled differences and biases.

Epidemiological studies have been marked by their identification of previous methodological failings, and by their attempts to overcome these. The attention to details of design and methodology is clearly of increasing relevance as the lead level of the population studied decreases, as any effects looked for would be expected to be smaller. At the same time, improvements in study design and methodology would be expected to reduce 'noise' from extraneous sources, and so enable any effects to be more clearly apparent.

The methodological and design issues are still of relevance today, as differences in design, or methodological variations or shortcomings, may be responsible for the differences in results between different studies. The methodological and design issues are discussed below, as well as some relevant theoretical points, while the problems they pose in interpretation are considered later.

Estimates of body lead

It is not proposed to discuss the characteristics and knowledge of different measures of body lead in any detail − that would be sufficient for a workshop in itself. Within this volume the subject is reviewed by Mushak, but the advantages and disadvantages of the different measures will be briefly discussed here, as these are relevant to the design and methodology, and more importantly to the interpretation, of studies of the effects of low levels of lead.

The problem in choosing a suitable measure is to select one which reflects as accurately as possible the amount of lead to which the body, or more precisely, the brain, has been exposed.

In reviewing the appropriateness of any measure, its suitability as an

5

indicator of exposure during the period of interest must be considered, as well as issues of availability of the sample, ease and ethical acceptability of collection, analytical problems, and the analytical reliability of the measure. Accurate assessment of lead status is crucial, since as lead occurs in trace amounts, an error of a few parts per million could result in a subject being assigned to the wrong lead status.

One problem (which will be discussed later) is that children are probably most vulnerable to lead when they are below the age of 3, but for psychometric reasons it is preferable to assess the performance and behaviour of children aged about 6 or older. This suggests that a measure which reflects the child's exposure history, particularly during the first few years of life, is the ideal one.

Lead is found in the body in the mineralized tissues such as bone and teeth, in the soft tissues, in blood, and in a number of blood constituents. It is also found in urine, and in hair. Most research studies have relied on blood or shed deciduous teeth as their measure of body lead, although some studies have used hair, either as the primary measure (Pueschel et al., 1972; Thatcher et al., 1983) or as a secondary measure (Vivoli et al., this volume; Winneke et al., 1985).

In studies of normal populations both blood and tooth lead measurements have been found to follow a log-normal distribution (Mahaffey, 1982; Winneke et al., 1983a).

Blood lead
Blood lead measures reflect predominantly current exposure to lead. The lead level in blood is in a dynamic equilibrium, which implies that with constant exposure it is relatively stable, and this has been shown to be the case in a small group of adults (Delves et al., 1984) but that it rapidly reflects changes in exposure, and takes some time to stabilize after a change in exposure. Blood lead levels in infants are much less stable with a correlation of between 0.1 and 0.2 in three blood samples taken during the first year of life (Rabinowitz et al., 1985), probably because, for developmental and behavioural reasons, their intake is not constant. However in older children much higher correlations ($r = 0.76$ and 0.74) over a 3- and a 5-year gap between samples, have been achieved (Winneke et al., this volume; Schroeder, this volume).

A single blood lead measure will not provide information on past exposure, or on peak exposure. It is not possible to know what the lead burden of a child was at age 3, from a blood sample taken when the child is aged 6 or 7. In order to have an accurate assessment of exposure over time repeat blood lead measurements are necessary, and these are being obtained in the longitudinal studies (e.g. McBride, 1985; Vimpani et al., 1985; Bornschein et al., 1985; Rabinowitz et al., this volume).

From a sampling point of view there are several disadvantages or constraints on the use of blood as an indicator. One is that the sample must be obtained by an invasive procedure, and is therefore classed as having more than minimal risk, and requiring strong justification if carried out on healthy children for research purposes (WHO/CIOMS, 1982). However, the work of Rodin (1983) indicates that adequate preparation, in particular the parents informing the child about the venepuncture procedure, can lessen the stress of the blood sampling. Smith (1985) has shown that, when adequately prepared, the large majority of school-age children show no negative effects of venepuncture (in many cases positive effects were reported).

Another potential disadvantage of using blood is that seasonal variations in mean lead level are reported (e.g. Angle and McIntire, 1979; Stark et al., 1982) which limits the time period during which sampling can be carried out. Blood obtained by venepuncture provides a better measure than samples obtained by finger-prick. There is an increased possibility of surface contamination in finger-prick samples, and this can lead to inaccurately high lead levels. It has also been reported that finger-prick samples can have artificially low levels, because of dilution with extracellular fluid from pressure around the puncture.

The use of blood as an indicator of body lead does not constrain the age of the sample studied. It also has the advantage of being an analytically reliable measure in a competent laboratory, with an error of measurement of about $2\,\mu g/dl$.

Lead can also be measured indirectly in blood by means of its inhibition of the activity of an enxyme, aminolaevulinic acid dehydratase (ALAD), which is involved in the haem synthesis pathway. ALAD is inhibited in an exponential fashion at blood levels from between 5 and $10\,\mu g/dl$ upwards (Berlin and Schaller, 1974).

Lead also has a toxic effect on the last step in the haem synthesis pathway, which is the insertion of iron into protoporphyrin to create haem. If the enzyme ferrochelatase, responsible for this change, is inhibited by lead, this fails to take place. The amount of protoporphyrin in the erythrocytes, called zinc-protoporphyrin or erythrocyte protoporphyrin (ZZP or EPP), can be used as a measure of this effect. However, it is a less useful measure in studies of the effects of low levels of lead exposure, as an increase in EPP may not be detected at blood levels below about $20\,\mu g/dl$ (Piomelli et al., 1982), although this threshold for the effect may vary with age (Succop et al.,this volume). Other factors, such as iron deficiency, can also cause an increase in EPP levels in the blood.

Tooth lead

Lead is stored in teeth in a similar way to lead in bone, reflecting cumulative exposure over time. Primary dentition has been shown to be a sensitive long-term store of lead, both for chronic and background exposure, with urban children having higher levels than rural children (Ewers et al., 1982), and for peak exposure, with teeth from lead-poisoned children having very much higher levels than those from children who have not been poisoned (de la Burdé and Shapiro, 1975). The use of teeth as a measure of body burden has the advantage that teeth are shed naturally, and so can be collected by non-invasive means. At the same time they have the disadvantage that tooth-shedding takes place only at certain ages, so that teeth can only be obtained during these periods.

It has been reported that there are systematic differences in the mean lead content of different types of teeth, with incisors having higher levels than

7

canines, and canines higher levels than molars (Mackie *et al.*, 1977), although not all studies have reported this difference (Fosse and Justesen, 1978). More recently one study has reported systematic differences between incisors from different jaws (i.e. upper or lower) with incisors from the upper jaw having significantly higher lead levels than incisors from the lower jaw (Smith *et al.*, 1983), and this may explain some of the differences which have been noted in pairs of teeth from the same child (Delves *et al.*, 1982).

Probably the main disadvantage of the use of teeth as measures of lead, although it is not one which affects any individual study, is the lack of comparability between laboratories in the types or parts of teeth analysed, and the analytical method. A tooth is not an homogeneous entity, and lead is not distributed evenly within it. Edmonds *et al.* (1978) studied the distribution of lead in human teeth using charged particle analysis. They found that the highest concentrations were always in the circumpulpal dentine, which is the strip 200–400 μm wide, around the pulp chamber. Lead levels in the pulpal dentine increase with age, whereas lead levels in enamel remained fairly constant. Dentine lead was found to be roughly equivalent to whole-tooth lead.

Some studies have analysed incisors and canines (Needleman *et al.*, 1979), some only incisors (Winneke, 1983; Vivoli *et al.*, this volume), and some have restricted the analysis to central incisors (Smith *et al.*, 1983). Some analyses have been of whole teeth (Moore *et al.*, 1978; Winneke, 1979; Smith *et al.*,1983; Vivoli *et al.*, this volume) while others have analysed a thin slice of tooth containing primary and secondary dentine (Needleman *et al.*, 1979) and others a sample containing only circumpulpal dentine (Grandjean *et al.*,1985). In this latter study a small number of pairs of (halved) tooth crowns was analysed, and these showed the upper/lower difference noted by Smith *et al.*, (1983), as did (although non-significantly) the analysis carried out on samples of circumpulpal dentine from the same lateral incisors. However, when the analysis was carried out on samples of circumpulpal dentine from the same paired central incisors, the difference in the eleven pairs of central incisors went in the opposite direction, and lower lead levels were found in the upper central incisors (Grandjean *et al.*,1985). The coefficient of variation was 45% for circumpulpal dentine samples, and 27% for whole-tooth lead levels, suggesting that where only one tooth is available whole-tooth analysis may be a more reliable measure.

It is likely that differences in lead levels in different types of teeth found in whole-tooth analysis, are in part due to the relative proportions of enamel, primary and secondary dentine in different teeth, but this does not explain why there should be a difference in samples of circumpulpal dentine from incisors in different jaws.

Methods of analysis also differ. The two analytical techniques most often employed are atomic absorption spectrometry and anodic stripping voltammetry. One inter-laboratory study using a (supposedly) homogenized tooth powder showed that the measurements obtained from different laboratories varied very significantly, with the results ranging from 4 to 15 μg/g (Stack and Delves, 1982). However, subsequently there has been a suggestion that the tooth powder was not adequately homogenized, and this could have been the cause of the poor comparative results.

The lack of comparability in the type or part of tooth analysed, differences in methods of analysis, and possible inter-laboratory differences make it impossible to know how lead levels from one study compare with those from another study, unless there is some secondary measure of lead burden available for at least part of the population.

Hair lead

Hair has the advantage that it is easy to collect by non-invasive means, and it can be collected at (almost) any age, so it does not restrict the age of the population sampled. It has the more major disadvantage of not being a very reliable measure. Hair lead measurements reflect exposure over a period of months, depending on how long the hair is, with the hair nearest to the scalp reflecting most recent exposure. It has been shown, in samples collected a standardized distance from the scalp, that hair lead concentrations can vary in different hairs from the same individual, and in hairs taken from different parts of the scalp. In individuals with similar exposure the lead content has been shown to vary with sex, the thickness and colour of the hair, with hair treatments such as bleaching and dyeing, and how often the hair is washed (Laker, 1982). Analytically too, hair causes problems, as it is difficult to remove surface contamination before analysis, without removing lead from within the hair.

Correlations between measures of blood lead and tooth lead

In animals dosed with controlled amounts of lead, correlations between averaged blood lead measures and levels of lead from extracted teeth, as high as 0.99 have been reported (Kaplan *et al.*, 1980). However, studies with children based on a single blood lead measure tend to report levels between 0.4 and 0.5 (Ewers *et al.*,1982; Smith *et al.*, 1983), with some studies reporting much lower non-significant correlations (Vivoli *et al.*, this volume). Since blood and tooth lead measures represent exposure over different time periods this modest correlation is not unexpected.

Correlations of blood lead with hair lead

Measures of hair lead and blood lead have been demonstrated to correlate moderately well ($r = 0.7-0.8$) in situations where the exposure is high and relatively constant; for example in occupationally exposed adults. In children exposed to lower environmental lead levels the correlations are much lower, at around 0.1–0.3.

What outcomes to measure?

The symptoms of lead poisoning have been known since antiquity, but these were clinical signs. There was no information on any preclinical signs which preceded poisoning. One of the problems facing early researchers in this area is that they were uncertain about the effects they were looking for. The work of Byers and Lord (1943) suggested a wide range of neurological after-effects of lead poisoning without acute encephalopathy. They followed up a group of twenty school-age children who had been hospitalized for lead poisoning and found that only one was making satisfactory progress at school. The others were described as showing a variety of symptoms including poor academic achievement, intellectual deficits, sensorimotor deficits, and behaviour disturbance. Later studies of children identified as having elevated lead levels, but without frank poisoning, were important in determining the areas of functioning which might be affected. On the whole the clinic and smelter studies, and many of the epidemiological studies, have used comprehensive batteries of tests, on the basis that since it is not known what effects are being looked for, the safest bet was to cover as many different areas of functioning as possible. Later studies have benefited from the findings of earlier ones, and have built on their experience, attempting to replicate results by using tests where effects have been noted, and in some cases dropping tests where no effects have been found. However there has been no clear model of the subclinical effects of lead to guide this choice.

In broad terms, the areas of functioning which have been included in test batteries for cross-sectional studies are intelligence, educational attainment, motor skills, reaction time (or more precisely, vigilance performance), and a number of different auditory and visuomotor tasks largely designed to access different aspects of memory and attention. In addition most research studies have included a measure of behaviour among their outcome measures. Not all test batteries, by any means, have included tests in all these areas, and different tests have been used to assess the 'same' skill in different batteries. This may be one reason why effects noted by one group may not be found by another team apparently assessing the same area of functioning.

Measures may be divided into those which are broad general measures covering a number of skills, and those in which the skill assessed is more focused and specific. Intelligence tests, as well as tests of reading, spelling and mathematics (which in psychological terms involve a large number of processes) would come into the first category, and tests such as a sentence repetition test or a vigilance test would come into the second category. The general measures cannot be said to be diagnostic, since they tap a number of areas of functioning, but they are useful precisely for this reason, and because they demonstrate the size, and functional significance, of any effect. Focused tests are included in test batteries for diagnostic reasons, to try to identify precisely which areas of performance are affected, for example whether deficits in attentional performance underlie any differences found in IQ tests.

Recently some research groups have obtained electroencephalography (EEG) measures. This highlights one relevant distinction, and that is the difference between measurable effects, and functional effects. If differences in EEG measurements are detected, the health or neurological significance of these is not known. For example, they could be a cause of a lower IQ, or a reflection of it (there are differences in the evoked potentials of normal and gifted children).

10

Children as a vulnerable population: age of testing

It is perhaps worth considering why studies of the effects of lead are carried out on children, and not on adults. In some ways a developing brain has been assumed to be less, rather than more, sensitive than an adult brain. It was a widely held belief that due to the greater plasticity in the organization of their nervous system, children's brains have a greater capacity to recover after physical trauma, than do adult brains (Levin *et al.*, 1982). However, children aged under 5 who suffer head injury, recover faster, but less completely, than older children (Rutter *et al.*, 1983). With respect to lead there are several other reasons for supposing that children, and particularly young children, are an especially vulnerable population. There is evidence that immature organs are most liable to damage at their time of most rapid growth, and this would mean that a child's brain was most vulnerable in the first 2 years of life (Dobbing and Smart, 1974). Young children have a faster metabolic rate, and therefore a greater daily intake of lead (through food), on a body-weight basis than either older children or adults. In addition to a higher intake, children also absorb more lead from the gut than do adults (Alexander *et al.*, 1973), and children under the age of 2 absorb very substantially more (Ziegler *et al.*, 1978). It has also been suggested that the blood–brain barrier in young children is less developed, which would result in a greater neurological vulnerability.

Young children, particularly those below the age of 3, are also at risk from their habits – the tendency to put non-food objects in their mouths, and to suck their thumbs or fingers. Blood lead measures in children exposed to particular sources of lead have been demonstrated to peak at around 2–3 years of age (HMSO, 1983), and this peak is also evident, although less marked, in populations of children not exposed to specific sources of lead (Mahaffey *et al.*, 1982).

The evidence suggests that children are most at risk, both from an intake and a neurological point of view, in the first 3 years of life. This would suggest that children in this age range should be studied to investigate the effects of lead. This is being done by the longitudinal prospective studies currently in progress, as they are assessing the status of children at 6-monthly, or annual intervals, from birth. The limitation is that measures of intelligence are not available for children below the age of 3 (and they are difficult to carry out on children younger than about 5). The measures which are available, such as the one most widely used, the Bayley Scales of Infant Development, are developmental scales, and have little predictive significance (Bayley, 1970; Rubin and Barlow, 1979). It is for this reason, and others such as the easier access to school-age children, and the much greater choice of psychometric instruments, that most cross-sectional studies have been of somewhat older children, usually aged 6 or older.

Intelligence tests

Tests of intelligence have been included in the test batteries of all epidemiological cross-sectional studies, with one exception. This is the cross-sectional study of McBride *et al.* (1982) where a picture vocabulary test was used as a measure of general cognitive ability. Most other studies have used

11

the Wechsler Intelligence Scale for Children – revised version (WISC-R) (Wechsler, 1974), or its translations. Two British studies (Harvey *et al.*, 1984; Fulton *et al.*, 1987) have used the British Ability Scales. The prospective studies where the children have reached the age of 3 have used the McCarthy scales (McBride *et al.*, this volume) or the Stanford Binet Intelligence Scale (Ernhart and Morrow-Tlucak, this volume).

There are advantages in many different studies using the same test, particularly when, like the WISC-R, it is also widely used outside the field of lead research. This means that it has a well documented validity and reliability. However, the advantages when the test is used outside America, where it was devised, might not be as great as they appear. A number of the verbal items from the WISC-R are culturally specific, and it is not clear how well these translate. Not all translations have been standardized in the appropriate country, for instance the WISC-R has been Anglicized for use in Britain, but never standardized in England. The WISC-R has been shown to be sensitive to a wide range of neurological insults (Bloom *et al.*, 1976; Schooler *et al.*, 1978) but also to social influences (Applebaum and Tuma, 1977).

Measures of educational attainment

A number of studies have included tests of reading, mathematics, or spelling abilities. Educational performance is clearly an outcome of importance as it reflects learning ability in normal circumstances, and over long periods of time. Tests of educational attainment, and particularly of reading ability, are highly correlated with IQ measures, so they do not provide an independent measure of an effect, but a further manifestation of its functional significance and an estimate of its magnitude. Tests of educational attainment are consistently sensitive to social indicators such as social class categorizations, or socioeconomic status.

The test batteries of Thatcher and Yule, and colleagues, included tests of reading, spelling and mathematics; Needleman, Smith, and Fulton and their colleagues included reading and maths tests, and Silva *et al.* (1984) included reading and spelling tests in their battery. However, there is no consistency in the tests used. All these studies used different tests, with the sole exception of Smith *et al.* (1983), and Fulton *et al.* (1987), who both used the British Ability Scales Word Reading test.

Other measures of cognitive or neurological performance

Early research results (Byers and Lord, 1943; Thurston *et al.*, 1955) were interpreted as demonstrating a defect in visuomotor coordination in children who had recovered from lead intoxication. De la Burdé and Choate (1972, 1975) reported differences in fine motor coordination in lead-exposed children.

Tests of visuospatial performance, auditory discrimination, gross or fine motor coordination, impulsivity or reflectivity, and attentional or vigilance performance, and reaction time, have been included in test batteries. In several cases the tests have been designed to test specific hypotheses about the primary processes, such as memory or attentional performance, which might be affected by lead, and which might underlie the differences noted in other more general tests.

12

The studies conforming to the protocol worked out at the WHO/CEC meeting in Dusseldorf (WHO, 1984), are recommended to include in their test battery: two tests of visuospatial and attentional skills (one a shape-copying task in normal and interference mode – the Bender Gestalt test, and a trail-making test); two tests of vigilance performance (one an automated reaction-time task, and the other a symbol-cancellation task); the Wiener reaction-time test; and tests of immediate and delayed memory.

It is often assumed that these more specific tests are independent of social and other influences, but this is not necessarily so, although the influences are not always the same ones. Waber et al. (1985) have demonstrated that aspects of neurological performance on a laterality task were related to social and economic status. Tests of specific skills are normally found to be correlated with measures of intelligence, and this suggests that where the tests are intended to be used diagnostically, intelligence should be controlled. A further disadvantage of some of the more specific measures is that they are often poorly validated (or not validated at all) and it is sometimes not clear what skill is actually being assessed. Standardization data and reliability data are not always available for specialized tests.

Measures of behaviour
Byers and Lord (1943) noted behaviour disturbance in the lead-poisoned children they followed up. The most significant finding from de la Burdé and Choate's follow-up study (1975), according to the authors, was the difference in behavioural ratings between the groups. A higher percentage of children in the exposed group was described by their teachers as hyperactive, impulsive and explosive, and having frequent temper tantrums. The other impetus to the inclusion of measures of behaviour, and more particularly, hyperactivity, in the outcome measures, comes from the work of David and colleagues (1972, 1977, 1983). Their approach has been different in that they have investigated hyperactive children, and then examined these children for evidence of increased lead burden. In 1972 David et al. reported increased blood lead levels in hyperactive children compared to non-hyperactive children of a similar background. As in the case of mental retardation, the higher lead levels may be secondary to the hyperactivity, rather than a cause of it.

Behaviour has been measured by direct observation in a controlled environment (Winneke, 1979; Harvey et al. 1984), or more economically by means of short forced-choice questionnaires (several studies, e.g. Yule et al., 1984; Hatzakis et al., 1985; Vivoli et al., this volume, have used the scale adapted by Needleman et al., 1979, or a modification of it); or standardized behavour rating scales completed by the mother or the teacher. The two standardized scales which have been most used are the Conners scales (Conners, 1969, 1973) and the Rutter Scale (Rutter, 1976). The longer the scale the more reliable it is likely to be, and summated scores or factor scores are likely to be more reliable than individual ratings, but practices and methods of factor analysis are also of relevance. In normal populations rarely occurring behaviours, although they may be of great significance, contribute too little to factor solutions, and so are eliminated.

The 'Needleman' questionnaire, which was adapted for use in a lead study,

13

from a longer behavioural assessment of known validity but designed for a different purpose, has been shown to be significantly related to measures of intelligence (Lansdown *et al.*, 1983). The standardized behaviour ratings, although validated as they stand, were designed for clinical purposes. The Rutter scales have been shown to be valid as screening instruments for the presence or absence of psychiatric disorder in children (Rutter, 1967), and the Conners scales have been demonstrated to be sensitive to drug-induced changes in behaviour over time, but there is little information about their sensitivity to small differences in behaviour in normal children. Behaviour ratings have also been criticized for their focus on negative behaviours, which may not differentiate the normal (that is, all behaviour within the normal range) from the super-normal (that is, better behaviour).

There are a number of subdivisions of behaviour which have proved useful in discriminating types of behaviour disorder. The Rutter scales distinguish neurotic and antisocial behaviours, and this distinction has proved useful in classifying the behaviour disturbance associated with organic disorders such as phenylketonuria, for example. Behaviours such as hyperactivity are known to be situation-specific; that is, they may occur in one situation such as at home, but not at school (Schachar *et al.*, 1981). If a behaviour disorder is pervasive then it is more likely to be organically determined (and evidence for this comes from the finding that the characteristics of children showing pervasive behaviour disorder are different from those showing situation-specific behaviours), so it is clearly an advantage to have ratings made in more than one situation. Behaviour, like intelligence, is subject to a wide range of environmental and social influences.

Design and sampling issues

Studies of the effects of low levels of lead have in the main been carried out on normal (usually urban) children selected from a total population. The first epidemiological studies were cross-sectional studies (e.g. Needleman *et al.*, 1979; Yule *et al.*, 1981; Harvey *et al.*, 1984), but more recently a number of longitudinal studies have been set up, and are in progress.

Some of the design and sampling issues, such as the sample size, and selection bias or representativeness, apply equally to both these types of design, but there are also potential biases or problems which attach to different designs.

Representativeness of the sample, and selection biases
The age group, and age range, of the population studied has to be decided, and issues of the evaluation of body lead burden, and the suitability and predictive validity of outcome measures (which will be discussed separately) are of relevance here. Since it is clearly impractical to study all children, a group has to be selected for study.

It is also important that the sample selected is of adequate size to achieve the statistical power necessary to detect (what are likely to be) small differences, amid other potential influences. If the sample is too small, then there are problems in controlling for potentially confounding variables, and quite sizeable differences on outcome measures may not be statistically significant, as in Winneke's first study (1979).

All this implies a selection procedure from a larger pool of individuals. In all studies of normal populations it is important, if the results are to be valid and generally applicable, that the sample investigated is representative of the whole identified population both in terms of the lead distribution, and in social and demographic indices. Flaws in the research design, sampling bias, and a high or biased drop-out rate can all result in a non-representative sample. There are three main points in the selection of a sample for study, where biases can be important.

1. *Selection bias.* In an epidemiological study bias may occur if some children are excluded from the sample, for reasons such as not providing a blood sample or a tooth, or if subjects cannot be traced, or do not respond to the request to take part in the study. It has been shown that there is a systematic bias relating to the variable of interest, which differentiates those who do not participate (Cox et al., 1977; Beck et al., 1984). In the study of Smith et al. (1983), where some information on the total population studied was available, it was demonstrated that there were very small, but consistent, differences between the group of children who provided teeth for the research study (and thus made themselves available for inclusion in the intensively investigated sample), and those who did not. A similar pattern, although the differences are mostly non-significant, can be seen in the test results of children who took part in the Dunedin lead study, which involved providing a blood sample, and those who did not (Silva et al., 1984).

   Methods of recruitment such as newspaper advertisements for volunteers are also known to increase the risk of biased selection (Rosenthal and Rosnow, 1969).

2. *Exclusion bias.* If some children who are selected for the sample are not tested, this can also cause bias. It has been demonstrated that those who drop out are likely to be systematically different from those who participate in a study (Labouvie et al., 1974).

3. *Inclusion bias.* Bias can equally well result from the inclusion in the sample of children who are untypical of the population studied, either in terms of their body lead burden, or their test performance. Children whose lead level is untypical for a known reason, for example because they have recently moved into the area, should be excluded, as should children who are disadvantaged in their performance on the outcome measures by language or physical handicaps, for example. The WHO/CEC meeting (WHO, 1984) resulted in a list of recommendations for exclusion criteria to avoid this bias. These include low birthweight, neonatal problems; evidence of alcoholism or drug abuse, or rubella infection, in the mother during pregnancy; motor or sensory deficits, chronic disease, any reported severe head injury or CNS abnormality in the child; recent divorce or

death of the child's parents; and children who have not lived in the (study) area all their lives.

Longitudinal versus cross-sectional studies

A cross-sectional study investigates one group of children, usually, but not necessarily, in a fairly narrow age range, at one point in time. A longitudinal (or prospective) study follows one group of children over time. This has one particular advantage in lead studies, as by making repeated measures of environmental sources, and by obtaining serial blood measures, it allows a more precise estimate of the exposure history, and of the body burden of the child. Equally, by collecting information on the child's social environment and circumstances over a period of several years it is hoped to obtain a more accurate measure of these. Although this approach will undoubtedly provide more information on the relationship of environmental sources, or behaviour related to uptake, and later measures of body burden, it is not without its drawbacks. One is the problem of repeated measures, and the model used, if it is to take advantage of the serial estimations of body lead available, needs to take this into account. For psychometric reasons also, it is undesirable to carry out many tests repeatedly, and most tests are not designed for this. Secondly the likelihood of chance correlations increases, as the number of measures increases.

Another major problem which can afflict longitudinal studies, is that of loss or attrition of part of the sample over time. This is likely to be for a number of reasons, but, as discussed earlier, it is likely to be non-random in some respects. The effects of attrition are relevant in lead studies where it is difficult to carry out a reliable neurological assessment of a young child, and these have little predictive significance. This means that ideally the sample will have to be followed for 6 or 7 years in order to obtain measures of intelligence, and other outcomes of known predictive significance. There is also the ethical and practical problem of intervention in cases where children are discovered to have an unduly high lead body burden, and the effect this will have on the study design and results.

Questions of critical periods for lead exposure, and the reversibility, or persistence, of detected lead effects are potentially answerable by means of longitudinal studies. However, longitudinal studies are in no way immune to the problems of design or methodology which might affect cross-sectional studies. For example if there is inadequate control of confounders, or important potentially confounding variables are not measured, then the effect in a longitudinal study will be the same as in a cross-sectional study, except that it will be perpetrated at each measurement stage of the study.

One potential advantage of some longitudinal studies is that of investigating the concept of reverse causality. That is, the less intelligent, or behaviourally more active children, take in more lead as a result of their intellect or behaviour, rather than as a cause of it. Since both lead measures and intellectual (or developmental) and behavioural measures are obtained sequentially, it is possible to examine the temporal relationships between these in both directions.

In a cross-sectional study the sample may be chosen to represent the full

16

range of lead levels (a continuous sample) or groups of children representing discrete points along the lead distribution can be studied. A continuous sample makes maximum use of the observed lead measurements, and it reduces the chance of having a biased sample, but at the same time it provides a less accurate estimate on the outcome measures throughout the distribution. Since the lead measures in a population are likely to follow a log-normal distribution, a continuous sample will mean that most of the subjects studied will have lead levels which are clustered near the lower end of the lead distribution. By studying discrete groups, children from the extreme ends of the distribution can be selected to maximize the lead difference, and by identifying relatively homogeneous groups it is possible to obtain good estimates on the outcome measures for these groups. Since neither extreme group, by definition, is typical of the population studied, it is clearly an advantage to include a third intermediate group, representing a typical lead burden. It is also necessary to have three groups in order to test for dose effects. Although many of the cross-sectional studies have followed one or other of these designs, there are variations. Winneke (1979) and Hansen et al. (1985) used a matched-pair design, where two lead groups were selected, and then pairs of children, differing in lead level, but matched on a number of other variables, were selected from within these groups. Smith et al. (1983) used a discrete group design where the groups were stratified by social grouping. The Edinburgh study (Fulton et al., 1987) have studied all high-lead children (the top quartile of the distribution within each school) and a random one-in-three sample from the rest of the distribution.

The research design has implications for the statistical techniques used in data analysis, but this will be discussed in a later section.

The association between social disadvantage and lead uptake

The clinic studies indicated that lead was not randomly distributed in normal populations, as children identified by screening clinics as having high lead levels were more likely to be disadvantaged. Studies of normal populations in several different countries have confirmed this relationship of lead measures with broad social indicators of disadvantage (Mahaffey et al., 1982; Yule et al., 1981; Ewers et al., 1982). Apart from explaining why it should be so, this finding poses the central problem for research studies. We know that disadvantaged children perform worse on psychometric tests (independently of any lead effect), so it may be that lead is merely acting as a marker of social disadvantage: that is, that lead and IQ (or behaviour) are linked only through their common association with socially disadvantageous factors.

The process by which the association of social factors and lead uptake operates is not wholly understood. At its extreme it is not difficult to see how dilapidated housing, providing access to flaking leaded paint, would contribute to a child's lead burden. On a more subtle level it is likely that a number of factors operate to result in somewhat higher lead burdens in more disadvantaged children. For example, the lack of a suitable play area resulting in children playing in the street, in conjunction with a low standard of family

17

hygiene, or thumb or finger-sucking, may contribute to increased lead burden. There is some empirical evidence which suggests that poorer physical caretaking and poorer housekeeping are factors which are partly responsible for the association. Dietrich *et al.* (1985) have shown that parental behaviour is associated with blood lead levels in infants, aged 6 months or more, independently of the apparent availability of sources of lead in the child's environment. There is also increasing evidence that the source of at least some of the additional lead is dust and dirt in or around the children's homes (Bornschein, 1985; Brunekreef *et al.*, 1983).

Broad demographic indicators, such as measures of income or social class classification, are only convenient indicators to a large number of intercorrelated and interacting factors. Factors such as poor parental supervision or poor housekeeping, or parental interest in the child, may be correlated with broad indicators such as social class, but within any social class classification there will be variability, which may be considerable, in these more specific measures. Since it appears that these broad indicators are associated both with lead burden and outcomes, it is important to try to break them down into component parts, some of which 'explain' body burden, and some different variables which are thought to be causally associated with the outcome measures. The point of this is to access the hidden variance within broad demographic indicators. For example in terms of lead uptake a child of low social class might be 'advantaged' if he lived in a modern house in good repair, and where the standard of hygiene was high. Equally a child of high social class might be 'disadvantaged' in intellectual terms, if his parents were depressed, or were not interested in him, and did not spend much time with him.

Since many measured variables will be at least partly collinear between lead and outcomes, it is important that this separation is done by prior hypothesis, and not as a result of empirical findings, as this will reduce the potential for bias. Thus in explaining why children from similar environments have different body burdens of lead, it is desirable to collect information on variables such as the degree of parental supervision, thumb-sucking and other mouthing behaviour, as well as on sources of lead, such as flaking paint in the children's environment. In explaining the different behavioural or intellectual performance of children, variables such as parental intelligence, parental interest in the child, and the parental mental state are relevant.

Defining confounding variables, and their control

A confounding variable by definition is a variable which influences outcome, and is associated with the factor of interest, thus producing a spurious association or masking a true association. Ideally, in order to study the effects of lead, groups of children should be selected, differing in lead burden, but matched in other ways. In practice this is unlikely to happen as the association of lead and social disadvantage suggests that if children are selected merely on the basis of lead level it is likely that the high-lead children will be more disadvantaged than low-lead children. This is particularly pertinent when the

18

design is one of extreme groups representing different lead levels, but is also relevant to continuous designs.

The social variables described above are likely to be confounding variables in the association between lead and outcome measures. If lead and IQ appear to be correlated in a normal population through their common link with social variables, then it is important to control for these influences, by removing the variance associated with the outcome. The problem is to remove variance (causally) associated with the outcome, without at the same time removing variance which might be attributable to the effects of lead.

If the confounders controlled are broad indicators to a number of important characteristics in the child's home environment, some of which may be relevant to the uptake of lead, and others to explain the child's performance, then controlling for these will remove the 'shared variance' which might in fact be due to lead. By controlling for more specific variables the problem of shared variance is reduced, as the collinearity is likely to be less, but since it is precisely because there is some collinearity in these variables that they are controlled, it does not disappear. This highlights the importance of a priori separation of variables into those thought to be causally related to lead burden, and those thought to be causally related to outcomes.

Failure to remove variance attributable to other influences (under-controlling) can result in an apparent lead effect, when in reality the cause is uncontrolled social differences, while removing variance which is in fact attributable to lead is over-controlling, and can result in the failure to find an effect which is really there. Different analytical techniques make different assumptions about shared and residual variance, and the order in which the variance attributable to different covariates is calculated can also influence the way shared variance is treated.

From a measurement point of view there is also an error in all the measures. The lead measure used, whether it is blood or teeth, is only an estimate of the parameter of interest, which is the amount of lead to which the brain has been exposed. The error between this and the lead measure will tend to underestimate any lead effect. The psychometric tests carried out provide an estimate of the true ability of the child, and although the standard error of measurement of these tests is often known, it is still only a measure of performance in one situation, so an estimate of the child's real ability. Equally the social and environmental measures will only provide estimates of the factors which have actually influenced the child's performance and behaviour. The error in these measures will act to underestimate the true effect of other (non-lead) variables on the outcome measures.

There is no easy formula to avoid the possibility of over- or under-controlling in the treatment of confounding variables. Generally, given the complex interacting pattern of influences on body burden and outcomes, control for a small number of variables is more likely to underestimate the effect of confounders, while control for a large number is more likely to over-control, because of the removal of shared variance. The control of only broad demographic indicators is more likely to remove shared variance erroneously (and at the same time probably not control for the real confounders), while control for more specific measures is less likely to. Some statistical techniques or approaches make over- or under-control less likely, while others increase the possibility. The relevance of the analytic method employed makes it important that details of the design and statistical processes used are clearly described in presenting the results of research.

INTER-STUDY COMPARISONS AND INTERNATIONAL DIFFERENCES

One of the best tests of the validity of a research result is its independent replication. However, it is important to remember that a similar result can also be due to a replication of methodological flaws, so the methodology of any study must be judged independently, before the replication is seen to strengthen the finding.

Research carried out in different countries offers the opportunity of providing information on the possible effects of lead over a wider range of exposures than would be possible in any one country. Where the information collected is comparable dose effects of lead at different exposure levels can be investigated. However, it is not always feasible, particularly with studies utilizing tooth lead, to know how the populations studied compare in terms of body burden.

Where contradictory or inconsistent results are obtained by different studies, and different measures have been used, it remains a possibility that differences in the instruments or measures used are responsible for differences found. It is also true that a finding can be strengthened if it is replicated with a different measure. Similarly, as has been described in earlier sections, methodological differences may limit extrapolation from one situation to another.

Recently there have been two initiatives to design common study protocols to increase the comparative power of studies carried out in different countries, or in different areas. One of these has been initiated by WHO and is coordinated by the Medical Institute of Environmental Hygiene, the WHO Collaborating Centre in Düsseldorf. As a result, the CEC and WHO lead studies carried out in Belgium, Bulgaria, Denmark, Greece, Hungary, Italy, Romania and Yugoslavia are to a large extent following a common protocol (WHO, 1984). The second initiative, coordinated by the Cincinnati group, means that there is considerable comparability in the methods and measures used by the prospective studies in the USA, and in Australia.

There is also a potential danger in a common protocol, which is that it is based on the assumption that the relationship between lead, outcomes, and confounders, is the same in different countries and cultures, and this is not necessarily so. Although the relationship between lead uptake and social class has been reported frequently, it is not found in all samples. There was no relationship between blood lead and social class measures in the epidemiological sample investigated in Dunedin in New Zealand. It may be that the concept of social disadvantage has different manifestations in its implications for lead burden in different countries. There may also be societal or cultural differences in the relationship of social variables with outcome measures. It

20

is known that there are differences in child-rearing practices in different cultures, and these, as well as other factors such as national differences in education standards, and the degree of employment of women, may affect the association of social variables and outcomes.

The results from different studies carried out independently, or in collaboration, can be combined statistically by meta-analysis. Meta-analysis is the quantitative cumulation and analysis of descriptive statistics across studies (Hunter et al., 1982). Although methods for combining probabilities across studies have been available for some years, the methods and techniques of meta-analysis are recent, and have been developed within the last decade, mostly for experimental or quasi-experimental studies. The basic statistic of meta-analysis is d, which is computed as the difference between group means, divided by the pooled within-group standard deviation.

Meta-analysis has certain limitations in all its uses. Just as in a narrative review such as this, the conclusions can be biased by the selection of studies included in, or excluded from, the analysis. The quality of the individual studies included in the analysis is important, although there are techniques which will allow for (some) non-chance variation in d. A more important limitation, in the current context, is that meta-analysis cannot deal systematically with confounding variables, and so cannot answer questions of causality. In an area such as that of sex differences, where there are inconsistencies or methodological weaknesses in study results which do not allow consistent conclusions to be reached, meta-analysis can overcome problems of design differences, small sample sizes, and age differences, with the creation of 'moderator variables' to explain variation in d, and so provide a synthesis which furthers understanding (Hyde, 1986). In the case of lead studies, meta-analysis would simply confirm the results of individual studies, which in the large majority of cases point in the same direction. It would not answer the question of whether the relationship is causal or not. This depends, as was discussed in an earlier section, on whether confounding variables have been adequately controlled for. Meta-analysis, even with moderator variables, does not, as yet, have the power to deal with complex multivariate designs, where the interpretation rests on whether over- or under-control for confounding variables has occurred.

WHAT WE 'KNOW' SO FAR

Intelligence

1. There is, in most studies of the effects of low levels of lead, an association between uncontrolled IQ scores, and lead measures, with higher-lead children performing worse on IQ measures. This has been found when the lead measure used was teeth (Needleman et al., 1979; Winneke et al., 1979; Smith et al., 1983; Hansen et al., this volume), blood (Yule et al., 1981; Harvey et al.,1984; Raab et al., this volume) or hair (Thatcher et al., 1983). This association has been noted with WISC-R (and its various translations), the British Ability Scales, and (in earlier studies) the Stanford Binet Scales. The association is not always of significant magnitude (Silva

21

et al., 1984) and is sometimes barely evident (Lansdown *et al.*, 1986). However, in no study is the performance of the high-lead group (numerically) better than that of the low-lead group.

2. Despite, or perhaps because of, the broad scope of intelligence tests, and the fact that almost all studies include an intelligence test in their test battery, it is in tests of IQ that associations with lead are most consistently noted.

3. The difference between high- and low-lead groups (or equivalent) in uncontrolled data, varies between one and seven IQ points, but is usually between four and six points.

4. The differences are generally noted in both verbal and performance components of the IQ test, but are almost always larger in the verbal subtests – an exception is the small non-significant difference found in the second London study (Lansdown *et al.*, 1986), where the WISC-R performance difference is bigger than the verbal difference.

5. The association, where it is quoted, of social indicators such as social class, with IQ measures, is always stronger than any lead/IQ association.

6. A number of other social or familial variables which explain a significant part of the variance in IQ measures can also be identified. The measure which is usually found to explain the largest part of the variance in an IQ measure is maternal IQ, which correlates with child IQ at about 0.5.

7. The effects of controlling for social variables which differ between lead groups, or which are associated with IQ scores, is, in most cases, to reduce the strength of the association between IQ and lead measures. The exceptions to this are the studies of Yule *et al.* (1981) and Bellinger *et al.* (this volume) where the effect of controlling for social variables was to increase the difference between lead groups.

8. In some cases controlling for social variables has reduced the lead/IQ association to non-significance (Winneke, 1983; Smith *et al.*, 1983; Harvey *et al.*, 1984) although it remains in the same direction.

9. Where maternal IQ has not been controlled, the IQ differences tend to remain significant (e.g. Yule *et al.*, 1981; Hansen *et al.*, this volume; Vivoli *et al*, this volume) after controlling for other social variables. However, in some studies where maternal IQ has been controlled the IQ differences remain significant (Needleman, 1979; Raab *et al.*, this volume).

10. In comparisons between studies where the WISC has been used, there is little indication of a dose effect of lead, in the size of the high/low IQ difference. In the Danish study (Hansen *et al.*, this volume) where the available blood lead data indicate that the exposure was very low, and the difference between high- and low-lead groups would be small, there was an eight-point verbal IQ difference between high- and low-lead groups. This is larger than differences reported by other studies, where lead levels are higher, and group differences greater. The two studies carried out by Winneke *et al.* (1982a, 1983a) also demonstrate the lack of dose effect. In the second study carried out in Stolberg the difference between the tooth lead means for the high- and low-lead groups was twice the size of the difference in means in the Duisburg study, but the IQ findings were similar, with, if anything, a larger difference in the

22

Duisburg sample.
11. There is little evidence of a threshold or no-effect lead level below which the lead/IQ association is not found. IQ deficits have been reported in studies where the mean lead level is 13 µg/dl (Yule *et al.*, 1981), and similar deficits in the Danish study where the primary measure was tooth lead, but blood levels are lower, at around 7 µg/dl.

Educational attainment

1. Seven of the epidemiological studies have included reading tests in their test batteries. Five of these found lead-related differences in the uncontrolled data. The exceptions to this are the studies of Needleman *et al.* (1979), and Lansdown *et al.* (1986).
2. Only a few studies (Yule, 1981; Thatcher *et al.*, 1983; Silva *et al.*, 1984; and Lansdown *et al.*, 1986) have incorporated spelling tests in their measures, and the results are less consistent. Significant associations (before controlling) were found by Yule, Silva, and Thatcher, but not by Lansdown.
3. Several studies have included tests of mathematics, but only two of these (one using a test of number skills, rather than a mathematics test) have shown significant lead-related differences in uncontrolled data. There were no significant differences in the studies of Needleman, Yule, Smith, and Lansdown and their colleagues.
4. In those studies where initially significant differences have been reported, when social class has been the only social variable controlled the effect has been much the same as in measures of intelligence, and the significant differences between groups have remained (Yule *et al.*, 1981; Silva *et al.*, 1984). However, this is not so of the initially significant differences found by Thatcher *et al.* (1983) in tests of reading, spelling and maths, which were no longer significant once age, sex, race and socioeconomic status had been controlled.
5. In one of the studies in which a larger number of more specific variables was controlled (Smith *et al.*, 1983) the initially significant differences were reduced to a level where they were no longer statistically significant, although they remained in the same direction. This was not the case in the Edinburgh study (Raab *et al.*, this volume) where differences remained significant after control for a number of specific variables.

Measures of behaviour

1. All but one (Thatcher *et al.*, 1983) of the cross-sectional studies have included a measure of behaviour in the outcomes.
2. No significant lead-related differences in behaviour have been found in studies where behaviour was measured by direct observation. This includes the simple observational adaptation of the Conners scale made by Winneke

23

(1979), and the highly sophisticated observational measures made by Harvey *et al.* (this volume).

3. Where standardized behaviour ratings such as the Conners and Rutter scales have been used some studies have found significant lead-related differences in both mothers' and teachers' scales (Silva *et al.*, 1984) some with teachers' scales only (mothers' scales were not administered) (Lansdown *et al.*, 1983). Other studies have not found significant differences on either mothers' or teachers' scales (Smith *et al.*, 1983; Lansdown *et al.*, 1986) or found none where only a mother's rating was obtained (McBride *et al.*, 1982) (partial scoring only).

4. The most consistent relationships between lead and behaviour have been found where teachers have completed short forced-choice scales. This applies with the Needleman 11-item scale (e.g. Needleman *et al.*, 1979) or modifications of it (e.g. Hatzakis *et al.*, 1985; Hansen *et al.*, this volume), and where the total score is of borderline significance, with individual items of the scale (Lansdown, *et al.*, 1983). Not all studies using this scale have found significant differences related to lead (Lansdown *et al.*, 1986).

5. It has been shown that teachers completing the short forced-choice scales are influenced by children's social backgrounds (Winneke, 1983) and in most studies no social factors have been controlled (Needleman *et al.*, 1979; Lansdown *et al.*, 1983) or where they have been, only broad indicators such as social class or socioeconomic status have been allowed for (Silva *et al.*,1984; Hatzakis *et al.*, 1985). This probably reflects the fact that it is more difficult to obtain social data from school teachers than from parents.

6. It has been demonstrated that individual items from the Needleman short forced-choice scale are very significantly related to intelligence measures (Lansdown *et al.*, 1983). This suggests that the apparently greater sensitivity of the short forced-choice scales may be due to their relationship with IQ, and that what is being detected are differences in intelligence, rather than behavioural differences. (There are also relationships between IQ and reading scores, and the total scores on the teachers' ratings for the longer standardized behaviour scales such as the Conners and Rutter scales, but these are usually very modest.)

7. Parents' behaviour ratings such as the Conners and Rutter scales are usually found to be independent of broad social indicators, such as social class, so controlling for these would not be expected to have an effect on results.

8. Despite the large amount of detailed information on social, environmental and familial factors available from lead studies, there has been little investigation of the relationship of these factors with behaviour measures. For example, factors such as the mother's mental health, and the quality of the parental marital relationship, have been shown to be highly associated with mothers' ratings on the Conners scale. Teachers' ratings have been shown to be sensitive to the family type (single-parent or not) (Smith, 1988). No studies have controlled for factors such as these.

9. Several studies have reported apparent dose–response relationships between items from the Needleman scale (or a modification of it) and children grouped on the basis of lead measures. This has been shown with

24

a large sample of children divided into six groups of increasing tooth lead (Needleman *et al.*, 1979), and with children divided into four groups of increasing blood lead (Lansdown *et al.*,1983; Hatzakis *et al.*, 1985). For most of the items from the scale the number of negative ratings increases in a step-like manner, with increasing lead level. However in only one of these analyses (Hatzakis *et al.*, 1985) was any social information controlled, and then it was the single datum of social class. A later study by Needleman (1981) replicated this finding (although it was less marked) with a smaller group of children, but showed that the initial step-like pattern disappeared when socioeconomic information was controlled. This appears to indicate that the apparent dose response was due to a step-wise increase in social variance, rather than to increases in lead.

Other psychometric measures

1. Most epidemiological cross-sectional studies have included, in their test batteries, some tests other than IQ and educational attainment measures. Exceptions are the test batteries of Yule *et al.* (1981) and Silva *et al.* (1984). Test batteries have included tests of visuospatial skills and visual attention and memory, auditory discrimination and auditory memory, gross and fine motor coordination, and attentional or vigilance performance.
2. Generally fewer than half of the tests in this category included in test batteries have shown significant lead-related differences.
3. Where differences in these measures have been reported it tends to be in uncontrolled (other than age and sex) data, or in data controlled only for broad social indicators.
4. Measures of other skills are not independent of IQ and behavioural measures nor, in most cases, of social influences, such as social class.
5. There is little information in the literature on more specific influences on performance in these areas.
6. Not all studies have published details of non-significant results on these tests. On the whole, where details of non-significant results are given, the results follow the same trend as IQ and reading results, with higher-lead children doing worse, even if not significantly so. There are only a few reported instances where this is not so, and only a few instances of significant results which do not favour low-lead children (i.e. in the direction opposite to that expected).
7. Tests of motor abilities, including gross and fine motor coordination, where these have been used, appear insensitive to any lead-related differences (Needleman *et al.*, 1979; Winneke, 1979; McBride *et al.*, 1982; Smith *et al.*, 1983; Harvey *et al.*, 1984). There are exceptions to this: in the data of Thatcher and colleagues (1983) there was a significant association between measures of hair lead, and pegboard, with the preferred hand only, and in Winneke *et al.*'s Stolberg study (1983a) where there is a near significant assocation with wrist tapping speed with the non-preferred hand.

8. There is not a great deal of consistency in the areas of functioning where deficits are reported. Needleman *et al.* (1979) reported deficits in verbal performance and auditory processing, but these have not been found by other workers who have assessed the same area, and in the case of the Seashore Rhythm test, used the same test (Smith *et al.*, 1983; Hansen *et al.*, 1985).

   Winneke and co-workers (1979, 1983a) and others (Hansen *et al.*, 1985; Harvey *et al.*, this volume) have reported differences in a test of visuospatial abilities, but other studies (Needleman *et al.*, 1979; Smith *et al.*, 1983) which have also included tests of visuospatial abilities, have not confirmed this. Some researchers (Winneke *et al.*, 1983a) have interpreted the differences found as due to attentional deficits, but others (Smith *et al.*, 1983; Hansen *et al.*, this volume; Harvey *et al.*, this volume) who have investigated this area of functioning, have not found these.

9. The most consistent results relate to the Bender Gestalt test which has been included in the test batteries of a number of studies (including all those which report deficits in visuospatial skills). Significant differences in the (error) scores for this test have been found in five of the seven studies where it has been used. Other similar tests of visual–motor integration or shape copying (e.g. Visual Motor Integration test; Frosting test, BAS Shape Copying test, ITPA Visual Sequential Memory test) have not shown lead-related differences.

10. Tests of so-called 'reaction time' used in lead studies, cover a number of different areas of functioning. Most studies (Needleman *et al.*, 1979; Smith *et al.*, 1983; Hunter *et al.*, 1985; and Vivoli *et al.*, and Harvey *et al.*, this volume) measuring reaction time after intervals of varying delay, have assessed attentional or vigilance performance. Within this group different paradigms have been used, but two studies, following essentially the same paradigm, have produced consistent results (Needleman *et al.*, 1979; Hunter *et al.*, 1985). In the Vivoli *et al.* study there was a significant association between vigilance performance on a delayed reaction time task and measures of ALAD, although not with blood or tooth lead measures. Other studies assessing reaction time with delay (Smith *et al.*, 1983; Winneke *et al.*, and Harvey *et al.*, this volume) have not found lead-related differences. Other measures of vigilance performance, such as symbol cancellation tasks and continuous performance tests, have not, on the whole, been shown to be associated with measures of lead.

   The German group have used a different measure of 'reaction time', measured with the Weiner reaction time device. The task is a complex choice reaction time task where children have to respond to a random sequence of visual and auditory signals, by pressing the appropriate buttons. There were no differences detected in the speed of response (measured by the number of late responses), and only small differences in the number of correct responses. The main difference detected was in the number of false responses, and this difference became more marked as the complexity of the task increased. Studies carrying out tests of reaction time after delay have not reported (and indeed have probably not recorded) the numbers of false responses.

EEG and other neurophysiological measures

Electroencephalogram measures have been shown to be sensitive to some forms of neurological insult, and they have been used in the diagnosis of a variety of neurological disorders. Other neurophysiological measures, such as brainstem auditory evoked potential (BAEP), and pattern-reversal visual evoked potential (PREP), are supposed to be stable, relatively age-independent, and free from social or cultural influences.

A number of groups have made direct neurophysiological measures of children, and related these to lead measures. Two of these studies (Otto et al., 1983; Otto, 1988; and Guerit et al., 1981) studied children who were exposed to a particular source of lead, and had rather high lead levels.

Guerit et al. (1981)

Guerit and colleagues studied a group of approximately 150 11-year-old children who were pupils in five different schools in Belgium. Three of these schools were in the vicinity of a lead smelter, and the other two were some distance away. The mean lead level of children in the schools near the smelter was shown to be much higher (28 μg/dl) than that of children in the more distant schools (12 μg/dl).

Four electroencephalogram (EEG) measures, including a BAEP, a PREP, and a flash-evoked potential, and an eye movement measure, were obtained for each child, and these were rated from 0 (normal) to 4 (clearly abnormal) and summed to provide a composite score. Results were analysed by school. In the two schools away from the smelter, and in one of the three schools near the smelter, there was no association between blood lead and the summated scores. In one of the schools near the smelter there was a significant negative association between EEG scores and blood lead, indicating that higher lead was associated with fewer abnormalities, and in the other school the association, while non-significant, was in the opposite direction.

Otto et al. (1983, 1985) and Otto (this volume)

Otto and colleagues have carried out a number of EEG studies on a group of high-risk children, who were predominantly black, from lower-income families, and half of whom had parents who worked in a battery factory. The mean blood lead at the initial evaluation, was 29 μg/dl, with a range of 6–55 μg/dl. The children were aged between 1 and 6 when first evaluated.

EEG measures were obtained from three sites during a passive sensory conditioning task of 35 trials. The data for more than a third of the subjects (particularly younger ones) were rejected for medical, technical and behavioural reasons, and a slow-wave analysis was carried out on the data obtained from 41 children. Two years later some of these children were followed up and valid data, based on 100 trials, were obtained for 28 children. A multivariate regression analysis was carried out to allow for possible effects of sex, age, SES and IQ, and to test for nonlinear effects of age and blood lead. These analyses showed that slow-wave voltage varied as a linear function of blood lead, but that the slope of this relationship varied with age. In children aged under 5, slow-wave voltage tended to be positive at lead levels below

27

30 μg/dl, and negative at blood lead levels above this, while in older children the opposite pattern was found. In the initial analysis, but not in follow-up, EEG spectrum gain (the relative amplitude of synchonized EEG between the left and right hemispheres), was also found to increase as a function of blood lead. The change in slow-wave voltage was evident 2 years later, despite mean blood lead levels being 11 μg/dl lower, and also (in the younger children) a ten-point drop in mean IQ.

More recently, a 5-year follow-up on 49 of the children (now aged 6–12 years), and on an independent sample of 75 children 3–7 years old, also with high lead levels, has produced somewhat inconsistent results. Slow-wave activity during passive sensory conditioning was not found to be associated with blood lead measures in either study, which Otto and colleagues' comment (1985) is not surprising, as blood lead levels at follow-up were all below 30 μg/dl. However, in the follow-up sample only, slow-wave voltage measures obtained during active conditioning were found to vary with blood lead.

A number of other neurophysiological measures, such as BAEP and PREP, were obtained on these two later samples, and in each sample some components of these were found to be systematically associated with blood lead measures, although there was little consistency between the two samples on which components were affected.

The BAEP measures which produced the most significant results in the 5-year follow-up were found to be associated with HOME scores (which were controlled in the data analysis), and sex differences were noted in BAEP latencies.

Otto *et al.* urge that their findings should be interpreted with caution, since the functional significance of slow-wave voltage changes (found at higher lead levels) is not known. However, they point out that the slowing of nerve conduction in the auditory pathway, which they reported at lower lead levels, has been related to pathological lesions, and non-specific demyelinating diseases such as multiple sclerosis.

Burchfiel et al., *1980*
This group investigated a small subsample of the children studied by Needleman *et al.* (1979). EEG measures were obtained from a group of 19 high-lead children and 22 low-lead children. The measures of brain activity were made in twenty electrode recording sites, under four different conditions and subsequently divided into four EEG frequency bands, producing a total of 320 measures (expressed as percentage spectral energy) for each subject. Computer-assisted spectral analysis was used to increase the sensitivity of the EEG analysis.

There were no significant differences in measures obtained in two of the four conditions (hyperventilation, and post-hyperventilation), and in two of the frequency bands (beta and theta). Most of the significant differences were recorded when the subject was relaxed with eyes closed. Out of the 320 measures obtained, twenty measures were identified which differed between high- and low-lead groups at the 5% level. The EEG measures which best discriminated high- and low-lead children were added to the previously obtained psychometric data, and it was shown that the combination of these measures resulted in greater separation power in direct and step-wise discriminant analysis procedures, than either EEG measures, or psychometric data alone. However, this is not surprising, as the measures were selected from a large number simply because they had the greatest potential to discriminate between high- and low-lead groups.

Winneke et al. (this volume)

As well as the psychometric measures obtained on the Nordenham sample of children, measures of nerve conduction velocity and visual and somatosensory evoked potentials were obtained in 1982, and again in 1985. The children in this sample have generally low blood leads, with a mean level of 7.7 μg/dl, and a range from 4 to 21 μg/dl. Nerve conduction velocity was measured in the N. radialis and N. medianus. On both occasions higher lead was associated with longer latencies in N1 and P2 components of the visual evoked potential. In 1982 an increase in nerve conduction velocity with increasing lead was found in N. radialis. This finding was not replicated in 1985, although the direction of change remained the same.

The contribution of EEG and other electrophysiological findings

1. The interpretation of these findings is difficult, as some of the authors point out themselves. There is little comparability in the methods of measurement, the measures obtained, and the statistical treatment of these measures, which makes comparisons between these studies difficult.
2. Even within studies there is not a great deal of consistency in the replication of results (Otto, this volume).
3. A more basic problem is raised by Otto and colleagues (1983). This is that the paradigms used in EEG studies are experimental, and normative data for young children do not exist. Since there are no concurrent behavioural measures the functional significance of any findings is unknown.
4. It is clear from the work of Otto and colleagues, where BAEP measures were found to be related to HOME scores, that the culture-free nature of EEG measures cannot be assumed. It is likely that there are a number of influences on EEG measures. It is known, for example, that diet can affect EEG measurements.
5. Until further information on EEG and other neurophysiological outcomes is available, in particular the influence of other (i.e. non-lead) social and environmental variables, the functional significance, or meaning of EEG and other electrophysiological findings cannot be assessed.

Animal studies

Experimental studies of animals dosed with controlled amounts of lead can help to answer some of the questions which are not answerable in epidemiological studies of children. There are three reasons for carrying out studies on animals: they can provide information on structural or biochemical changes in the central nervous system in lead-exposed animals; they can

29

provide information relating the degree or severity of abnormality found, to the dose of lead producing it; and thirdly, they can provide information on changes in behaviour of animals exposed to lead either *in utero*, or in early life. Although all three types of study are clearly relevant to an understanding of the neurotoxic effects of lead in children, it is not proposed to discuss the findings from studies carried out for the first two reasons. The results of behavioural studies will be discussed very briefly, in order to highlight the potential benefits, and problems, of extrapolation from animal studies to humans.

A number of different behavioural paradigms have been used with rats, mice, and monkeys, to demonstrate deficits in learning in animals dosed with lead, but showing no signs of overt toxicity, such as weight loss. Bushnell and Bowman (1979a) have observed differences in a discrimination reversal learning task in monkeys. There were no differences in the time taken to reach the original discimination learning criteria, but there were significant differences associated with the reverse learning, with the lead-dosed animals performing worse. Rice (this volume) has also shown that lead-dosed monkeys performed worse on reversal discrimination learning tasks. Lilienthal *et al.* (1983) obtained a similar result, also with monkeys, but in a different task. They found that there were no differences between lead-dosed animals and controls in their ability to learn simple discrimination problems, but the performance of lead-dosed animals was inferior when they were required to solve a series of similar problems successively. This indicates that lead-dosed animals were less able to generalize from one situation to another. Using two different visual discrimination tasks with rats, Winneke *et al.* (1983b) have shown that there were no differences in the error decrease to criterion between lead-dosed rats and controls when the discrimination task was easy, involving discrimination of a horizontal stripe pattern from a vertical stripe pattern. However, when the discrimination task was more difficult, requiring the rat to discriminate between two different-sized circles, lead-dosed rats performed worse, and took longer to reach criterion.

Other changes in performance associated with lead have been noted. Cory-Slechta and Thompson (1979) have shown that in a fixed-interval lever-press task, animals dosed with moderate levels of lead showed increased rates of responding compared with controls, although at high lead doses response rates were lower. This finding is similar to one by Gross-Selbeck and Gross-Selbeck (1981), who found that animals exposed to lead *in utero* had higher bar-pressing rates than control animals, in an operant procedure involving differential reinforcement of high rates. The requirements of the operant task determine whether this change in behaviour could be considered adaptive or not. For example, where the animal is required not to respond for a period of time, lead-dosed animals will do worse on the whole. Lead-dosed animals are also reported to respond in bursts (i.e. with a shorter latency between bar presses) (Cory-Slechta *et al.*, 1981) and some operant schedules will reward this behaviour, while in others it will disadvantage the animal. Rice (this volume) has shown, in an operant schedule, that lead-dosed monkeys made more responses, and their response rate was more variable than that of control monkeys. Cavanagh *et al.* (1984) interpreted these changes in operant performance as being due to changes in the animal's ability to organize the temporal patterning of responses.

Winneke et al. (1982b) carried out an interesting study which demonstrates how relevant the nature of the learning task is. In their study rats were dosed pre- and post-natally with lead. Animals were tested on a two-way active avoidance task, and later on a visual discrimination task. In the discrimination task the performance of lead-dosed animals was inferior to the controls. In the avoidance task the performance of animals improved significantly in a dose-related fashion, with increasing lead level.

The authors suggest that increased behavioural reactivity may be the explanation for these differential effects. An alternative explanation is that the improvement on the two-way active avoidance task is due to damage to the hippocampus, or related structures, as this is known to improve performance on this task. This is thought to be because of deficits in spatial ability, so that the animal loses the sense of place, and does not remember, and therefore does not fear, the previously dangerous place.

Another study has also reported an improvement in two-way active avoidance tasks in lead-dosed animals, but this must be balanced against two studies where the performance of lead-dosed animals was worse, and another three studies reviewed by Cavanagh et al. (1984) found no differences at all.

In order to examine whether the hippocampus is sensitive to damage by lead, a number of researchers have tested the performance of lead-dosed animals on spatial learning tasks. Most of these studies have investigated the ability of rats to learn mazes of varying degrees of complexity. Generally these tests, as well as operant tests requiring spatial discrimination, have not been found to be sensitive to lead. Winneke (1986) has investigated the possibility of hippocampal damage further, by comparing the performance of lead-dosed rats, with that of animals with hippocampal lesions. Although there were differences in learning and retention between lead-dosed animals and controls, the lead-dosed animals did not behave in the same way as the animals with hippocampal lesions. The latter group showed superior learning performance, but retention deficit. Winneke and colleagues conclude that hippocampal damage does not provide an adequate explanation of the findings with respect to lead.

Rice (this volume) has demonstrated that the performance of lead-dosed monkeys is inferior to that of controls on tests of short-term memory and attention. In one test of spatial memory the animal was required to alternate responses, and in another test the monkey had to memorize a stimulus, and then choose the previously seen stimulus from three presented.

Passive avoidance tasks, where the animal is required to refrain from doing something in order to avoid an aversive stimulus, do not usually show a lead effect (Cavanagh et al., 1984).

It has been shown that if dosing occurs during periods of active brain maturation the effects may be persistent, or irreversible (Bushnell and Bowman, 1979b). In monkeys that had been dosed with one of two doses of lead for the first year of life, there were differences in reversal learning discrimination tasks when the animals were tested at 4 years old, despite the fact that the animals had not been dosed with lead for 3 years, and that their blood lead levels were similar to those of control animals.

Recent work from the German group (Munoz *et al.*, 1986) has also addressed the question of the persistence of lead effects. In this study all the experimental rats were exposed pre-natally to a dose of lead, but for half the animals (the maternally exposed group) it was stopped when they were weaned at 16 days. For the remainder of the experimental animals dosing continued until the time they were tested. At this time the blood and brain lead levels, and degree of ALAD-inhibition, for the maternally exposed animals was indistinguishable from that of controls. The animals were tested on a visual discrimination learning task, as before, but they were also tested on a spatial learning task. In addition the animals were re-tested on these tests some weeks later, in order to see if there were differences in retention of the task.

The results are inconsistent with those of the previous study, to the extent that there was no significant difference in the visual discrimination learning between the groups. In the spatial learning task there were significant differences in the number of days required to reach criterion, with the performance of both maternally and permanently exposed groups inferior to that of controls.

When retested the performance of both lead-dosed groups was inferior to that of controls, on both the tests. The performance of the maternally dosed animals resembled that of the permanently dosed animals despite the fact that their blood and brain levels were comparable to those of the controls. This implies that early damage is irreversible, and that further exposure does not exacerbate this effect. The study also highlights the functional difference between learning and memory, as there was no difference in the learning of the visual discrimination task, but there were differences in the retention of this skill.

Cory-Slechta (this volume) has suggested that in rats, vulnerability may actually increase, rather than decreasing with age.

Most research workers who have assessed motor coordination in rats have not found it to be affected by lead, even at high doses. Tests of coordination usually measure the animal's ability to remain on a slowly rotating rod. Exceptions are the studies of Overmann (1977) and Overmann *et al.* (1981). It has also been demonstrated that there were differences in performance on this test between rats allowed free access to water, and those where access was restricted. The rats allowed free access to water were physically slightly larger, and this was thought to be the reason for the differences in performance.

Some research workers have studied lead-associated changes in social behaviours, and behaviours such as aggression, in animals. Since under-nourishment produces changes in these behaviours it is not possible to discount this as a cause in studies where animals have been dosed with high levels of lead. In the few studies where moderate doses of lead have been used, there is little indication of changes in behaviour, with the exception of changes in aggression. Several workers have reported that animals exposed to moderate doses of lead show reduced aggression, and this has been noted in a number of different situations. On the other hand, animals dosed with high levels of lead are reported to show increased aggression.

The contribution of animal studies

1. One of the major benefits of animal studies is that since experimental animals are dosed with lead, intake can be assumed to be independent of any of the social factors associated with intake in children, and which complicate epidemiological research. However, animal studies are not free of confounding factors, and in some cases the cause or effect question is unanswerable. For example, it is now clear that many of the effects, such as hyperactivity, and delay in development, which have previously been attributed to lead, were probably due to under-nutrition in lead-dosed rats, and not necessarily to lead.

2. While animal studies can indicate the sorts of functioning which might be affected by low levels of lead, there are some reservations. Behavioural changes, and particularly subtle changes, are difficult to measure in animals, and the repertoire of testable behaviours is limited in terms of its extrapolation to functioning in humans. Most of the research on lead effects has been carried out on rats, and this limitation is particularly relevant to these studies.

3. A more important reservation, in terms of the focus of this review, is that it is not possible to extrapolate from doses of lead in rats, to measures of body burden in humans. This has implications in behavioural studies, for questions of thresholds, and no-effect levels, which are not clearly answerable by animal studies. In biochemical studies, or studies investigating CNS structure or abnormalities, the permanence or reversibility of an effect is likely to depend largely on whether the damage is structural (and therefore probably irreversible) or biochemical or neurochemical (and more probably reversible). If structural changes are identified, for example reduced fibre outgrowth from nerve cells, and fewer synaptic junctions, or structural damage resulting in alterations in the functioning of the blood–brain barrier in animals, it is not possible to know with any certainty at what lead level these would occur in humans. All that can be said is that these changes occur in animals at levels lower than those causing symptoms of poisoning, such as under-nutrition, or other biologically observable signs such as brain blood vessel change.

   It is known that in terms of absorption rats do not provide an appropriate animal model in some ways. Adult rats are relatively insensitive to lead, and absorb from the gut about 1% of a given dose (this caused problems in early studies in trying to induce encephalopathy in rats). There is enormous variety of dosing methods and schedules, and dietary and nutritional factors influence uptake in both young and adult rats. In the most commonly used dosing procedure for experiments on young rats, the mothers are dosed with lead (either in food, or in drinking water), and the suckling rat is dosed through the mother's milk. It has been shown that milk increases absorption of lead, and this dosing schedule can, with sufficient quantities of lead, produce classic lead encephalopathy in rats. Where blood lead measures for animals are given these cannot be equated to blood lead levels in children, and calculations, such as equating the degree of δ-aminolaevulinic acid dehydratase inhibition, can only provide rough estimates of equivalence. In most studies animals have been dosed to body levels which, although not causing clinical signs of toxicity, are likely to be higher (in terms of rough equivalence), than those to which normal urban children are exposed.

4. Animal studies cannot address questions equivalent to those posed by studies of normal urban children, but they do provide some indications of what functions should be assessed, and information on persistence or reversibility of behavioural effects found at moderately raised lead levels.

5. There are some points of similarity between results from animal studies, and epidemiological studies of children, although on the whole they are rather few. Extrapolation is further limited by the fact that lead exposures are not equivalent, and tend to be an order of magnitude higher in animal studies.

6. In epidemiological studies of children, psychometric tests which bear some relation to those used in animal studies, such as visual discrimination tasks, or memory tests, have generally proved insensitive to lead. The exceptions are the Bender Gestalt test and the Wiener reaction task. These have both fairly consistently shown lead-related differences, and in a somewhat similar way to animal studies, in that it is error scores, rather than correct responses, which show the relationship. A further similarity in results from the Wiener reaction device is that the differences are more marked as the difficulty of the task increases.

7. If animal studies do not greatly aid the interpretation of existing epidemiological studies of children, they do indicate some directions which might be fruitful to pursue in the future.

8. Animal studies suggest that it is important to pay more attention to the nature of the task underlying test performance. That is, that test results in terms of an outcome score may be less important than knowing how the child does the task. Support for this comes from the observation that generally, in the more focused tests, false responses, trials to criterion, and error scores have proved more sensitive than scores based simply on the number of correct responses. Whether differences in the way children perform tests are important, and whether they explain differences in the results of psychometric test scores such as IQ tests, is another question.

9. Another implication from animal studies is that differences become apparent (or more apparent) when performance is stretched to the limit. Thus some simple tasks do not show lead-associated differences, while more taxing tasks do. The animal results from Winneke et al. (1983b) with simple and difficult visual discrimination learning, the reversal learning differences in monkeys (Bushnell and Bowman, 1979a) and the learning set formation differences in monkeys studied by Lilienthal et al. (1983) all show this pattern. The results from children with the Wiener reaction device again support this, and suggest that merely recording the status of the child on an open-ended test is not sufficient, but that performance must be pushed to the limit. Tests of learning set formation, to test children's ability to generalize from one learned concept to another, have not been used in lead studies, although there have been claims that

34

these tests can distinguish brain-damaged children and environmentally disadvantaged children.

10. Several investigators studying children have included tests of specific functions such as (short-term) memory or attention, but none has investigated retention over a longer time scale of several weeks, for example. Animal studies appear to indicate that learning is not (or is less) disrupted than long-term retention. Another interpretation could be that this is another example of a difficult task (retention) being sensitive to differences, while a less difficult one (learning) was not. A difference in long-term memory could easily explain differences in IQ and educational attainment tests, which reflect learning and retention over long periods.

11. Animal studies appear to indicate that a much more focused attention to behavioural change is necessary, since the behaviours affected are quite specific. Changes in behavioural reactivity, as reflected by apparently enhanced learning on an active avoidance task, the increased open-field activity in rats, particularly in novel situations, noted by some investigators, as well as increases in bar-pressing rates, all deserve some investigation in epidemiological studies. So far, only one study of children (Harvey *et al.*, 1984) has included any measures which could be considered equivalent to these. It is possible that a task sensitive to differences in behavioural reactivity would pick up a behavioural difference which the broad behavioural ratings would miss.

PROBLEMS IN INTERPRETING EXISTING DATA FROM EPIDEMIOLOGICAL STUDIES

There are a number of problems in interpreting the existing data – some of these apply to individual studies, and some to comparisons between different studies.

The picture which emerges from epidemiological studies of children is that children with higher levels of lead generally perform worse on psychometric tests. However, if lead at the low levels currently being investigated affects the intelligence or behaviour of children, then this effect should be detectable at the same (threshold) level, and should be apparent in the same skills in children in different environments and from different populations. Furthermore, the effect should be able to be related to the relative exposure, so that it should be greater where the exposure, and consequently body levels are higher. The evidence presented so far does not readily point to this conclusion, but there are many reasons why this might be so, even if the conclusion is valid.

As discussed earlier, in the section on methodological issues, studies differ in sampling and design, in the tests used to assess the 'same' skills, in the measures and levels of body lead, in the age and type of population studied, in the degree to which information on potential confounding variables is collected and controlled, and in the statistical methods employed in the analysis of data. The effects of these variations between studies have to be ascertained. If a pattern emerges which is consistent across studies, and explains the variety and apparent inconsistency in the results, then this is likely to provide insight into the true relationship between lead and outcome measures.

Sampling and design differences

Studies differ in the inclusion and exclusion criteria they have employed in selecting a sample, and in the attention to the avoidance of selection bias. The representativeness of the sample in terms of the total population studied is important if the results are to be accepted as valid, and applicable to other similar situations, but where biases are found (or suspected) it is generally not possible to estimate what effect these would have on results.

Where samples are obtained by means such as newspaper advertisements (Thatcher et al., 1983; Winneke et al., 1982d) a sample of unknown representativeness is obtained. If a large proportion of the identified population are excluded from the sample because they cannot be traced (e.g. McBride et al., 1982; Harvey et al., 1984) this can create a bias, and unless information on the excluded chidren is obtained, the direction or effect of this bias is impossible to quantify. Similarly if a substantial proportion of the children selected for the sample are not tested (e.g. Needleman et al., 1979) or their results are not included in the data analysis (e.g. McBride et al., 1982) this can also create biased results. In studies where information on the identified population is available (Smith et al., 1983; Silva et al., 1984; Hatzakis et al., 1985) there is evidence that there are small but consistent biases, in the direction which is consistent with previously reported data (Cox et al., 1977). In one study it was demonstrated that the characteristics of children who make themselves eligible to take part in the study, by providing a tooth, are similar to those of adult volunteer populations. Adults who volunteer to participate are more likely to be better educated, of higher social class status, more sociable, higher in need for social approval, and more likely to be female (Rosenthal and Rosnow, 1969). Smith et al. (1983) found small but consistent differences in sex, social grouping, family size, educational attainment and behaviour rating scores, which are consistent with this. Similar biases have been found in a study where the lead measure was blood. Silva et al. (1984) showed social class differences (although not strongly directional) between children who provided blood samples and those who did not. There was also a significant difference in the teacher's behavioural rating scores, with children who provided blood showing fewer problems on average.

In one study (Hatzakis et al., 1985) there were differences in some of the items from the behaviour rating, in the opposite direction to that expected, in favour of children who did not provide a blood sample. A possible explanation for this is that the study was seen as a public health exercise, and middle-class parents were more likely to feel that it was not of relevance to them, so the differences observed are postulated to reflect a social class bias in the sample (Hatzakis, 1986, personal communication).

Where information on a larger population is available it is possible to estimate the degree of bias in the sample, and if necessary to recreate a representative sample. The indications are, from studies where this information is available, that the non-participating children are likely to be slightly more disadvantaged as a group (and therefore, because of the known link between lead and social disadvantage, to have slightly higher body lead levels). It is likely that this bias also affects studies where this information is not available, although in these cases the size of the bias cannot be estimated. It is not possible to estimate the effect of this bias on the results. It suggests that if a truly representative sample were obtained there might be greater variation in the lead distribution, but equally greater variation in socially disadvantageous variables.

The effect of drop-out bias, or the failure to test children selected for the sample, is also difficult to estimate. There is evidence that children identified as having higher lead levels are more likely to drop out, for a number of reasons, than lower lead children. Lyngbye et al. (1988) have estimated that the low (7%) non-participation rate in their study, would create a bias, in the direction of the null hypothesis. However, this estimation ignores the corollary to the higher lead levels, which suggests that children who drop out will also be more disadvantaged on average.

Differences in the type of population studied, that is whether it is a generally advantaged or disadvantaged sector of society, have been postulated as a possible reason for disparate results (e.g. Yule and Rutter, 1985; Lansdown et al., 1986). Most of the early lead studies were of socially disadvantaged populations, either living in close proximity to industrial premises, or in inner-city slum areas. It was postulated that the effects of lead might be greater in more socially disadvantaged sectors of the population. Support for this argument came from data such as Harvey et al.'s (1984) where the association between blood lead and (uncontrolled) IQ scores was greater in working-class than in middle-class children. Winneke and Kraemer (1984) also found a somewhat stronger association between lead and outcome measures in more socially disadvantaged children, although this differential association is not found in all studies.

It was further suggested that studies which had failed to find lead effects had investigated a relatively advantaged population, and therefore had minimized the likelihood of identifying the effect. This is proposed as a possible explanation for the different results from studies carried out by Yule and Lansdown (Lansdown et al. (1986). The first study was carried out on a disadvantaged population, and a significant association between lead and IQ was found. In the second study the population studied was relatively more advantaged, and there was no significant association between lead and outcome measures.

However, several studies which have investigated mixed, or relatively advantaged, populations have found an association between (uncontrolled) outcome scores, and lead measures (Smith et al., 1983; Bellinger et al., 1986; Hansen et al., 1985), so this seems an unlikely explanation. Furthermore, in the Smith et al. study the strength of the lead/IQ association was the same for both social groups.

An alternative explanation of these findings might be that there is greater social homogeneity in middle classes than there is within the working class.

The implication of this, if lead is seen as a marker for different disadvantaging factors, is that there will be a greater range and variety of these factors in a working-class population, and so a stronger association with lead measures. In a middle-class population lead would be a less accurate marker since the disadvantageous factors would occur less often. This could also explain the Lansdown *et al.* (1986) result, as where there is little social variation, lead would not be an effective marker, and so for social reasons there would be no association between lead and outcomes. While not supporting this interpretation, the data of Bellinger *et al.* (1986), investigating a population of upper- and middle-class children, does suggest that the relationship of social variables, lead, and outcomes, may be different in more advantaged sectors of society. In this group controlling for social factors had the opposite effect to that usually found, in that it increased the difference between groups. This does not argue for social factors rather than lead as the causative influence, but it does indicate that the relationship of social factors and lead in an advantaged population may be different to that in a disadvantaged population (that is, that lead is not acting as a marker to the same disadvantageous factors which are associated with poorer performance on outcome measures). The further implication of this is that the relationship of environmental and familial variables to uptake should be studied separately in different groups of children, as the factors associated with uptake in socially disadvantaged children may not be the same as those associated with uptake in advantaged children.

Differences in psychometric measures

Apart from WISC-R, which has been used by most research groups as a measure of intelligence, the variety of tests used in lead test batteries is large. It is not possible to estimate how much the use of different tests has contributed to the disparate results obtained. It could also be said that the different and unstandardized translations of the WISC might explain the variation in the size of the high/low lead IQ difference found in different populations (although Winneke's disparate results, on two different samples of German children, would seem to argue against this). On the small number of occasions where the same tests have been used, disparate results have been obtained (with the Seashore rhythm test, for example), and relatively consistent results (with the Bender Gestalt test). This indicates that the use of different tests, while it may contribute to inter-study differences, is not a sufficient explanation for different results.

Statistical techniques and the control for confounding variables

Probably the most crucial difference between studies of lead effects, and now the most debated subject in epidemiological studies, is the statistical treatment of data, and the appropriate control of confounding variables.

Studies vary enormously in the extent to which they have collected information on potentially confounding variables. Generally there is a trend towards collecting more detailed information, and more specific information. Some studies have not controlled for any social variables (McBride et al., 1982). In other studies the only control (or matching) has been for social class or socioeconomic status (Yule et al., 1981; Winneke et al., 1982a; Thatcher et al., 1983). Studies such as those of Needleman et al. (1979) and Winneke et al. (1983a) have collected more detailed information which is largely of a descriptive nature; for example information on the age of the mother, the number of pregnancies, and details of parental education. Needleman et al. also obtained an estimate of the mother's verbal ability, with a Peabody Picture Vocabulary test. The studies of Smith et al. (1983), Harvey et al. (1984), Lansdown et al. (1986) and Fulton et al. (1987) have also collected this descriptive information, but in addition information on predictive variables has also been collected. These are variables which are hypothesized to be causally related to the outcomes, for example information on the mother/child relationship, the quality of the parents' marital relationship, and maternal mental health, and variables causally related to body lead burden, such as the state of the paintwork in the house.

There are other variations within this general pattern. Studies such as the one carried out in Århus in Denmark (Lyngbye et al., 1988) have collected information on a number of predominantly medical variables, in order to exclude children who were felt to be untypical in some way, but having adhered to these stringent exclusion criteria, socioeconomic status, school and neighbourhood were the only social variables matched between high- and low-lead groups. Vivoli et al. have similarly collected information in order to exclude atypical chidren, but the only social variable controlled was a combined measure of parental education and occupation (Vivoli et al., this volume). In Athens, Hatzakis and colleagues have collected information on area of residence, but they also have an estimate of maternal IQ.

Broad demographic indicators, while relevant to explain variance in the outcomes, will provide a rather gross indication of the actual influences on the outcome measures, so that studies which have controlled only for these are likely to under-control for social influences. In the studies which have collected more detailed information on potential confounders, the criteria for choosing which variables should be controlled also differs between studies, and this is partly reflected in the type of confounders investigated. Where information on descriptive variables has been obtained, the aim has been to show that the lead groups were similar in composition, and the variables controlled were those which were found to differ significantly between the lead groups or to be associated with lead measures (e.g. Needleman et al., 1979; Winneke, 1983). This approach has two disadvantages: since the variables are chosen precisely because they correlate with lead, variance which is attributable to lead may be removed; and secondly, variance which is relevant to explain differences in performance on the outcome is not controlled, since the relationship of 'confounders' with outcomes is not taken into account. A variable which correlated strongly with the outcome but non-significantly with the lead measure would not be controlled, while one that correlated strongly with the lead measure (and might be important in determining it) but weakly, or non-significantly with the outcomes, would.

Research studies which have collected more predictive information have tended to divide the information into that which is thought to predict lead burden, and that which is hypothesized to predict performance on the outcome measure. In these studies the variables controlled have been those found to be associated with performance on the outcome measures (Harvey *et al.*, 1984), those hypothesized and subsequently found to be associated with outcomes (Smith *et al.*, 1983) or those hypothesized to be associated with the outcomes (Fulton *et al.*, 1987). The effect of these procedures is that more of the variance in the outcome is explained, and (in the Smith and Fulton studies) the probability of removing variance which is actually attributable to lead is reduced, since the variables are selected on the basis of their hypothesized relationship with the outcomes.

In some ways the problem of interpretation hangs on the assessment of whether the control for confounders has been carried out correctly and adequately. Since we know that lead and outcomes are usually linked through their common association with social factors, the question of control is crucial to the interpretation of study results. Where significant (or indeed, non-significant) differences remain after controlling for covariates, these could be due to lead, or they could be due to social factors which have not been (or have been inadequately) controlled. Equally, where initially significant differences are reduced to non-significance after control, is a real effect of lead being masked by over-control?

Over- or under-controlling, and the problem of shared variance

As discussed earlier, studies which have controlled only for 'umbrella'-type variables, or variables which differ between lead groups, run the almost certain risk of under-control for social influences, and may attribute an effect to lead, when it is in fact due to other uncontrolled factors. Similarly, because of its high correlation with child IQ, studies which have not controlled for maternal IQ may under-correct for this influence.

It has been said that controlling for a large number of variables, and particularly interrelated variables, can result in over-control, that is removing variance due to lead, and masking a real effect. It is certainly true that controlling for a large number of variables adds noise, and by reducing the degrees of freedom, reduces the power to detect a real effect. The unnecessary inclusion of large numbers of control variables could reduce the power to detect what is a real effect. There are a number of statistical techniques, such as optimal regression, and the use of Mallow's C_p criterion which are designed to optimize the control for confounders, and to produce the 'least-noisy' adjustment. These techniques have been used in some analyses (e.g. Pocock and Ashby, 1985; Raab, 1986, personal communication). The results in one of these studies (the Institute of Child Health study) are very comparable whether the analysis is carried out by multivariate analyses of variance (MANOVA) techniques, step-wise regression, or optimal regression procedures.

40

The psychological and psychiatric literature provides ample evidence of the large number and variety of influences on intelligence, academic achievement, and behaviour, (and rather less information on influences on other skills). There is also evidence that many of these influences are highly correlated with each other. An example is the usually high correlations found between parental education, qualifications, and social class. Longstreth and colleagues (1981) in the USA have shown that, once maternal IQ was controlled, the addition of other variables relating to the home intellectual environment made no significant contribution to the total variance in child IQ explained. This shows that the influence of maternal IQ on children's intellectual development is not simply a genetic one, but is also evident in the environment provided in the home. Thus maternal IQ provides a good surrogate measure to a number of other dimensions in the home environment, which independently would be correlated to child IQ. Controlling for these highly interrelated variables will add noise, and as Longstreth demonstrates, does not contribute to the variance explained. However, there are other variables, less highly interrelated, which are also known to be relevant to intelligence or behaviour in children. Controlling for these may explain relevant variance. Smith et al. (1983) have shown that variables such as the quality of the parental marital relationship, and the mother's mental state, accounted for a significant proportion of the variance in outcome scores after maternal IQ was controlled, and this indicates that variables such as these should also be taken into account.

It is also relevant to mention that studies cannot control for variables not measured or identified. The total variance explained by multivariate techniques, in measures of intelligence or behaviour, is never huge. This is partly a reflection of the errors inherent in the measures, but also indicates that many of the causative factors in behaviour, and to a lesser extent intelligence, are still unknown. In addition, some factors known to be causative, for example fathers' IQ, have not been controlled in lead studies. It is probable that if these additional variables were controlled, more of the variance would be explained, and group differences would be reduced.

Traditionally statistics is a conservative science, and this has a number of implications for lead studies, where the effect looked for is small, and there are a number of other partly-related influences, which are likely to be larger. The cautious convention in multivariate statistics is to attribute any shared variance to the confounder, so if no association is found after control for covariates, there is assumed to be no effect of lead. If a confounder is to some extent a cause of the child's lead burden, as well as being related to the outcome, then variance attributable to lead will be removed along with the 'social' variance, relevant to the outcome. Similarly to control for variables which are consequences of the outcomes will result in over-control.

It is because there is a collinearity between lead and social variables that it is necessary to control the results for other variables. The effect and magnitude of collinearity is evident in regression procedures where the amount of variance apparently accounted for by lead will depend on whether the lead variable is entered first, last, or allowed to enter unforced, in a stepwise procedure.

The problem of over-control by the removal of shared variance is not easily resolved. The best guard against erroneously removing a lead effect in this way would seem to be to make the control variables as specific as possible, and base them firmly on their known predictive significance to the outcome measure. In studies where information on variables relating to lead uptake has also been obtained, one further possibility which could reduce the amount and problem of shared variance, presents itself. In these studies 'social' variables which were found to be collinear could be controlled for the 'lead' component. To use an example from some data I am familiar with: in the Institute of Child Health study, maternal IQ was used as a covariate because it was hypothesized (and found) to be associated with child IQ. The family cleanliness score was not controlled, because it was deemed to be a 'source' variable. However, it could also be said that through her housekeeping practices, reflected in the family cleanliness score, the mother's intelligence has implications for the child's lead level, so controlling for the mother's IQ could be removing lead variance. In order to avoid this if the mother's IQ was controlled for the family cleanliness scale, and the residual used as a covariate, this would potentially remove the lead variance from the covariate, and so provide a purer social variable.

CONCLUDING REMARKS

Studies of the effects of lead on children are, for necessary ethical reasons, non-experimental in design. Such studies, particularly when they involve multivariate social data, pose problems in drawing causative inferences, and lead studies are no exception. Despite the wealth of data, and including data from experimental studies with animals, it is still not possible to conclude with any certainty that lead at low levels is affecting the performance or behaviour of children. It is clear, however, that any differences in a measure such as IQ, which might be attributed to lead are likely to be small, accounting for about 1 or 2% of the variance. The educational significance of even a small difference when applied to a total population is substantial, so the implication is not that such differences are unimportant: merely that they are difficult to detect amid the much larger influences of a number of interacting variables.

It is nearly 10 years since the publication of the results of the first epidemiological studies of the effects of low levels of lead on urban children. In that time studies have been carried out in many different countries, and covering a wide range of 'normal' urban lead exposures. There have also been changes in study design, and improvements and refinements in the methodology and in the statistical techniques employed – and there has been much debate and discussion on the correct treatment of data, and the interpretation of study findings! This review has attempted to chart the progress made during the period, and to review some of the issues which are still the subject of debate, and which hinder the interpretation of existing data. It is not proposed to draw formal conclusions, since the whole of this review has aimed to provide an overview of the current state of the art. The papers contained in this volume describe in more detail the current research and most recent findings, and together they provide a much fuller, and an international, view of the current state of the art. At the end of the volume is a chapter based on the final sessions at the workshop, in which the implications of the existing data are discussed, and directions for future research initiatives are explored. It is clear that much progress has been made in the past 10 years, but also that there is still a lot to do.

REFERENCES

Alexander, F.W., Delves, H.T. and Clayton, B.E. (1973) 'The uptake and excretion by children of lead and other contaminants.' *Proceedings of the International Symposium, Environmental Health Aspects of Lead*, Amsterdam, 2-6 October 1972. (Luxembourg; Commission of European Communities)

Angle, C.R. and McIntire, M.S. (1979) Environmental lead and children: the Omaha study. *J. Toxicol. Environ. Health*, **5**, 855–870

Applebaum, A. and Tuma, J. (1977) Social class and test results: comparative validity of the Peabody with the WISC and WISC-R for two socioeconomic groups. *Psychol. Rep.*, **40**, 139–145

Baloh, R., Sturm, R., Green, B. and Gleser, G. (1975) Neuropsychological effects of chronic asymptomatic increased lead absorption. *Arch. Neurol.*, **32**, 326–330

Bayley, N. (1970) The development of mental abilities. In: Mussen, P.H. (ed.) *Carmichael's Manual of Child Psychology*, Vol. 1 (New York: John Wiley)

Beck, S., Collins, L., Overholser, J. and Terry, K. (1984) A comparison of children who receive and who do not receive permission to participate in research. *J. Abnorm. Child Psychol.*, **12**, 573-580

Bellinger, D., Leviton, A., Needleman, H.L., Waternaux, C. and Rabinowitz, M. (1986) Low-level lead exposure and infant development in the first year. *Neurobehav. Toxicol. Teratol.*, **8**, 151–161

Berlin, A. and Schaller, K.H. (1974) European standardized method for the determination of δ-aminolevulinic acid dehydratase activity in blood. *J. Clin. Chem. Clin. Biochem.*, **12**, 389–390

Bloom, A., Raskin, L. and Reese, A. (1976) A comparison of WISC-R and Stanford-Binet Intelligence Scale classifications of developmentally disabled children. *Psychol. Schools,* **13**, 288–290

Bornschien, R.L. (1985) Influence of social factors on lead exposure and child development. *Environ. Health Perspect.*, **62**, 343–351

Bornschein, R., Succop, P., Dietrick, K., Que Hee, S., Clark, S. and Hammond, P. (1985) Dust lead, hand lead and blood lead levels in young children. *Environ. Res.*, **38**, 108–118

Brunekreef, B., Noy, D., Biersteker, K. and Boleij, J. (1983) Blood lead levels of Dutch city children and their relationship to lead in the environment. *J. Air Pollut. Control Assoc.*, **33**, 872–876

Burchfiel, J., Duffy, F., Bartels, P.H. and Needleman, H.L. (1980). Combined discriminating power of quantitative electroencephalography and neuropsychologic measures in evaluating CNS effects of lead at low levels, in Needleman, H.L. (ed), *Low Level Lead Exposure: The Clinical Implications of Current Research* (New York: Raven Press)

Bushnell, P.J. and Bowman, R.E. (1979a) Reversal learning deficits in young monkeys exposed to lead. *Biochem. Behav.*, **10**, 733–742

Bushnell, P.J. and Bowman, R.E. (1979b) Persistence of impaired reversal learning in young monkeys exposed to low levels of dietary lead. *J. Toxicol. Environ. Health*, **5**, 1015–1023

Byers, R.K. and Lord, E.E. (1943) Late effects of lead poisoning on mental development. *Am. J. Dis. Child.*, **66**, 471–494

Cavanagh, J.B. Lewis, P.D., Reading, H.W. and O'Keefe, J. (1984) Review of laboratory studies on the possible effects of lead on brain development. (Unpublished manuscript, Institute of Neurology, London)

Conners, C.K. (1969) A teacher rating scale for use in drug studies with children. *Am. J.*

Psychiatry, **126**, 884–888

Conners, C.K. (1973) Rating scales for using in drug studies with children. *Psychopharmacol. Bull.* (Special issue–Pharmacotherapy of Children), pp. 24–29

Cory-Slechta, D.A. and Thompson, T., (1979) Behavioural toxicology of chronic post-weaning lead exposure in the rat. *Toxicol. Appl. Pharmacol.*, **47**, 151–159

Cory-Slechta, D.A., Bissen, S.T., Young, A.M. and Thompson, T. (1981) Chronic post-weaning lead exposure and response duration performance. *Toxicol. Appl. Pharmacol.*, **60**, 78–84

Cox, A., Rutter, M., Yule, B. and Quinton, D. (1977) Bias resulting from missing information: some epidemiological findings. *Br. J. Prev. Soc. Med.*, **31**, 131–136

David, O., Clark, J. and Voeller, K. (1972) Lead and hyperactivity. *Lancet*, **1**, 900–903

David, O., Hoffman, S.P., Sverd, J. and Clark, J. (1977) Lead and hyperactivity: lead levels among hyperactive children. *J. Abnorm. Child. Psychol.* **5**, 405–416

David, O, Hoffman, S., Clark, J., Grad, G. and Sverd, J. (1983) Penicillamine in the treatment of hyperactive children with moderately elevated lead levels, in Rutter, M. and Russell Jones, R. (eds), *Lead versus Health* (Chichester: John Wiley)

de la Burdé, B. and Choate, M.S. (1972) Does early asymptomatic lead exposure in children have latent sequelae? *J. Pediatrics*, **81**, 1088–1091

de la Burdé, B. and Choate, M. S. (1975) Early asymptomatic lead exposure and development at school age. *J. Pediatrics*, **87**, 638–642

de la Burdé, B. and Shapiro, I.M. (1975) Tooth lead, blood lead and pica in urban children. *Arch. Environ. Health*, **30**, 281–284

Delves, H.T., Clayton, B.E., Carmichael, A., Bubear, M. and Smith, M. (1982) An appraisal of the analytical significance of tooth-lead measurements as possible indices of environmental exposure of children to lead. *Ann. Clin. Biochem.*, **19**, 329–337

Delves, H.T., Sherlock, J. C. and Quinn, M.J. (1984). The temporal stability of blood lead concentrations in adults exposed only to environmental lead. *Hum. Toxicol.*, **3**, 279–288

Dietrich, K.N., Krafft, K.M., Pearson, D.T., Harris, L.C., Bornschein, R.L., Hammond, P. and Succop, P.A. (1985) Contribution of social and developmental factors to lead exposure during the first year of life. *Pediatrics*, **75**, 1114–1119

Dobbing, J. and Smart, J.L. (1974) Vulnerability of developing brain and behaviour. *Br. Med. Bull.*, **30**, 164–168

Edmonds, M.I., Al-Naimi, T. and Fremlin, J.H. (1978) The distribution of lead in human teeth, using charged particle activation analysis. Paper read at Fifth Symposium on Developments in Activation Analysis, Oxford, July

Ewers, U., Brockhaus, A., Winneke, G., Freier, I., Jermann, E. and Kramer, U. (1982) Lead in deciduous teeth of children living in a non-ferrous smelter area and a rural area of the FRG. *Int. Arch. Occup. Environ. Health*, **50**, 139–151

Fosse, G. and Justesen, N-P.B. (1978) Lead in deciduous teeth of Norweigan children. *Arch. Environ. Health*, **33**, 166–175

Fulton, M., Raab, G., Thomson, G., Laxen, D., Hunter, R. and Hepburn, W. (1987) Influence of blood lead on the ability and attainment of children in Edinburgh. *Lancet*, **1**, 1221–1226

Grandjean, P., Hansen, O.N. and Lyngbye, T. (1985) Lead concentration in deciduous teeth: variation related to tooth type and analytical method. Paper presented at the Nordic Symposium on Metabolism of Trace Elements Related to Human Diseases, Loen, Norway

Gross-Selbeck, E. and Gross-Selbeck, M. (1981) Changes in operant behaviour of rats exposed to lead at the accepted no-effect level. *Clin. Toxicol.*, **18**, 1247–1256

Guerit, J.M., Meulders, M., Amand G. *et al.* (1981) Lead neurotoxicity in clinically asymptomatic children living in the vicinity of an ore smelter. *Clin. Toxicol.*, **8**, 1257–1267

Hansen, O.N., Lyngbye, T., Trillingsgaard, A., Beese, I. and Grandjean, P. (1985) A neuropsychological and behavioral assessment of children with low level lead exposure, in Lekkas, T.D. (ed.), *Heavy Metals in the Environment*, (Edinburgh: CEP Consultants)

Harvey, P.G., Hamlin, M.W., Kumar, R. and Delves, H.T. (1984) Blood lead, behaviour and intelligence test performance in preschool children. *Sci. Total Environ.*, **40**, 45–60

Hatzakis, A., Salaminios, F., Kokevi, A., Katsouyanni, K., Maravelias, K., Kalandidi, A., Koutselinis, A., Stefanis, K. and Trichopoulos, D. (1985) Blood lead and classroom behaviour of children in two communities with different degree of lead exposure: evidence of a dose-related effect?, in Lekkas, T.D. (ed.), *Heavy Metals in the Environment*, (Edinburgh: CEP Consultants)

HMSO (1983) *Royal Commission on Environmental Pollution* (ninth report): *Lead in the*

Environment. (London: HMSO)

Hunter, J., Urbanowicz, M.A., Yule, W. and Lansdown, R. (1985) Automated testing of reaction time and its association with lead in children. *Int. Arch. Occup. Environ. Health,* **57,** 27–34

Hunter, J.H., Schmidt, F.L. and Jackson, G.B. (1982) *Meta-Analysis: Cumulating research findings across studies.* (Beverley Hills: Sage)

Hyde, J.S. (1986) Introduction: meta-analysis and the psychology of gender, in Hyde, J.S. and Linn, M.C. (eds), *The Psychology of Gender: advances through meta-analysis,* (Baltimore: Johns Hopkins University Press)

Kaplan, M., Peresie, H.J. and Jeffcoat, M. (1980) Lead content of blood and deciduous teeth in lead-exposed Beagle pups, in Needleman, H.L. (ed.), *Low Level Lead Exposure: the clinical implications of current research,* (New York: Raven Press)

Kotok, D., Kotok, R. and Heriot, J.T. (1977) Cognitive evaluation of children with elevated blood lead levels. *Am. J. Dis. Children,* **131,** 791–793

Labouvie, E.W., Bartsch, T.W., Nesselroade, J.R. and Baltes, P. (1974) On the internal and external validity of simple longitudinal designs. *Child Dev.,* **45,** 282–290

Laker, M. (1982) On determining trace element levels in man: the uses of blood and hair. *Lancet,* **2,** 260–262

Lansdown, R.G., Shepherd, J., Clayton, B.E., Delves, H.T., Graham, P.J. and Turner, W.C. (1974) Blood lead levels, behaviour, and intelligence: a population study. *Lancet,* **1,** 538–541

Lansdown, R.G., Yule, W., Urbanowicz, M.-A., and Miller, I.B., (1983) Blood lead, intelligence, attainment and behaviour in school children: overview of a pilot study, in Rutter, M. and Russell Jones, R. (eds.), *Lead versus Health,* (Chichester: John Wiley)

Lansdown, R., Yule, W., Urbanowicz, M.-A. and Hunter, J. (1986) The relationship between blood-lead concentrations, intelligence, attainment and behaviour in a school population: the second London study *Int. Arch. Occup. Environ. Health,* **57,** 225–235

Levin, H.S., Benton, A.L. and Grossman, R.G. (1982) *Neurobehavioural Consequences of Closed Head Injury* (Oxford: Oxford University Press)

Lilienthal, H., Winneke, G., Brockhaus, A., Molik, B. and Schlipkoeter, H.W. (1983) Learning set formation in rhesus monkeys pre- and postnatally exposed to lead, in Lekkas, T.D. (ed.), *Heavy Metals in the Environment* (Edinburgh: CEP Consultants)

Longstreth, L.E., Davis, B., Carter, L., Flint, D., Owen, J., Rickert, M. and Taylor, E. (1981) Separation of home intellectual environment and maternal IQ as determinants of child IQ. *Dev. Psychol.,* **17,** 532–541

Lyngbye, T., Nørby Hansen, O. and Grandjean, P. (1988) Bias resulting from non-participation in childhood epidemiological studies: a study of low-level lead exposure. (Unpublished manuscript, Institute of Psychiatric Demography in Århus, Risskov, Denmark)

McBride, W.G. (1984) Prospective study of health effects of lead in urban children. Paper presented at International Conference on Prospective Lead Studies, Cincinnati, Ohio, April

McBride, W.G., Black, B.P. and English, B.J. (1982) Blood lead levels and behaviour of 400 preschool children. *Med. J. Australia,* **2,** 26–29

Mackie, A.C., Stephens, R., Townsend, A. and Waldron, H.A. (1977) Tooth lead levels in Birmingham children. *Arch. Environ. Health,* **32,** 178–185

Mahaffey, K.R., Annest, J.L., Roberts, J. and Murphy, R.S. (1982) National estimates of blood lead levels: United States, 1976-1980: association with selected demographic and socioeconomic factors. *N. Engl. J. Med.,* **307,** 149–159

Moore, M.R., Campbell, B.C., Meredith, P.A., Beattie, A.D., Goldberg, A. and Campbell, D. (1978) The association between lead concentrations in teeth and domestic water lead concentrations. *Clin. Chim. Acta,* **87,** 77–83

Munoz, C., Garbe, K., Lilienthal, H. and Winneke, G. (1986) Persistence of retention deficit in rats after neonatal lead exposure. *Neurotoxicology* (in press)

Needleman, H.L., Gunnoe, C., Leviton, A., Reed, R., Peresie, H., Maher, C. and Barrett, P. (1979) Deficits in psychologic and classroom performance of children with elevated dentine lead levels. *N. Engl. J. Med.,* **300,** 689–695

Needleman, H.L. (1981) *Studies in Children Exposed to Low Levels of Lead.* EPA-600/1-81-066, North Carolina, 27711

Otto, D., Benignus, V., Muller, K. and Barton, C. (1983) Electrophysiological evidence of changes in CNS function at low to moderate blood lead levels in children, in Rutter, M. and Russell Jones, R. (eds), *Lead versus Health* (Chichester: John Wiley)

Otto, D., Robinson, G., Baumann, S., Schroeder, S.R., Mushak, P., Kleinbaum, D. and Boone, L. (1985) Five-year follow-up study of children with low-to-moderate lead absorption: electrophysiological evaluation. *Environ. Res.*, **38**, 168–186

Overmann, S.R. (1977) Behavioural effects of asymptomatic lead exposure during neonatal development in rats. *Toxicol. Appl. Pharmacol.*, **41**, 359–471

Overmann, S.R., Zimner, L. and Woolley, D.E. (1981) Motor development, tissue weights and seizure susceptibility in perinatally lead-exposed rats. *Neurotoxicology*, **2**, 725–742

Perino, J. and Ernhart, C.B. (1974) The relation of subclinical lead level to cognitive and sensorimotor impairment in black preschoolers. *J. Learn. Disorders*, **7**, 26–30

Piomelli, S., Seaman, C., Zullow, D., Curran, A. and Davidson, B. (1982) Threshold for lead damage to heme synthesis in urban children. *Proc. Natl. Acad. Sci., USA*, **79**, 3335–3339

Pocock, S.J. and Ashby, D. (1985) Environmental lead and children's intelligence: a review of recent epidemiological studies. *Statistician*, **34**, 31–44

Pueschel, S.M., Kopito, L. and Schwachman, H. (1972) Children with increased lead burden: a screening and follow-up study. *J. Am. Med. Assoc.*, **222**, 462-466

Rabinowitz, M., Leviton, A., Needleman, H., Bellinger, D. and Waternaux, C. (1985) Environmental correlates of infant blood lead levels in Boston. *Environ. Res.*, **38**, 96–107

Ratcliffe, J.M. (1977) Development and behavioural functions in young children with elevated blood lead levels. *B. J. Prev. Soc. Med.*, **31**, 258-262

Rodin, J. (1983) *Will this Hurt?* (London: Royal College of Nursing Research Monograph)

Rosenthal, R. and Rosnow, R.L. (1969) The volunteer subject, in Rosenthal, R. and Rosnow, R.L. (eds), *Artifact in Behavioural Research* (New York: Academic Press)

Rubin, R.A. and Barlow, B. (1979) Measures of infant development and socioeconomic status as predictors of later intelligence and school achievement. *Dev. Psychol.*, **15**, 225–227

Rutter, M. (1967) A children's behaviour questionnaire for completion by teachers: preliminary findings. *J. Child Psychol. Psychiatry*, **8**, 1-11

Rutter, M., Chadwick, O. and Shaffer, D. (1983) Head injury, in Rutter M. (ed.), *Developmental Neuropsychiatry* (New York: Guilford Press)

Schachar, R., Rutter, M. and Smith, A. (1981) The characteristics of situationally and pervasively hyperactive children: implications for syndrome definition. *J. Child Psychol. Psychiatry*, **22**, 375–392

Schooler, D., Beebe, M. and Koepke, T. (1978) Factor analysis of WISC-R scores for children identified as learning disabled, educable mentally impaired and emotionally impaired. *Psychol. Schools*, **15**, 478–485

Silva, P.A., Hughes, P., Crosado, B. and Faed, J. (1984) A pilot study of blood lead levels, cognitive development, and behaviour problems in 579 Dunedin eleven year old children. Paper presented at Workshop on Lead Research, University of Auckland.

Smith, M., (1985) Taking blood from children causes no more than minimal harm. *J. Med. Ethics*, **11**, 127–131

Smith, M., (1988) Maternal depression, marital disharmony and ratings of children's behaviour (In press)

Smith, M., Delves, T., Lansdown, R., Clayton, B. and Graham, P. (1983) The effects of lead exposure on urban children: the Institute of Child Health/Southampton study. *Dev. Med. Child Neurol., Suppl.* **47**

Stack, M.V. and Delves, H.T. (1982) Tooth-lead analysis–an interlaboratory survey, in Egan, H. and West, T.S. (eds), *IUPAC Collaborative Interlaboratory Studies in Chemical Analysis* (Oxford: Pergamon Press)

Stark, A.D., Quah, R.F., Meigs, J.W. and Delouise, E.R. (1982) The relationship of environmental lead to blood-lead levels in children. *Environ. Res.*, **27**, 372-383

Thatcher, R.W., Lester, M.L., McAlaster, R., Horst, R. and Ignasias, S.W. (1983) Intelligence and lead toxins in rural children. *J. Learning Disabil.*, **16**, 355–359

Thurston, D.L., Middlekamp, J.N. and Mason, E. (1955) The late effects of lead poisoning. *J. Pediatrics*, **47**, 413–423

Vimpani, G., McMichael, A., Robertson, E. and Wigg, N. (1985) The Port Pirie study: a prospective study of pregnancy outcome and early childhood growth and development in a lead-exposed community. *Environ. Res.*, **38**, 19–23

Waber, D.P., Carlson, D., Mann, M., Merola, J. and Moylan, P. (1985) SES-related aspects of neuropsychological performance in children. *Child Dev.*, **55**, 1878–1886

Wechsler, D. (1974) *Wechsler Intelligence Scale for Children*, revised edition. (New York:

Psychological Corporation). (English edition, Windsor: NFER/Nelson)

WHO/CIOMS (1982) *Proposed International Guidelines for Biomedical Research Involving Human Subjects.* (Geneva: WHO/CIOMS)

WHO (1984) *Studies in Epidemiology*, Part 1: *Health Aspects of Chemical Safety*, Interim Document 15, (Copenhagen: WHO Regional Office for Europe)

Winneke, G. (1979) Neuropsychological studies in children with elevated tooth lead levels. Paper presented at the Conservation Society Symposium on Toxic Effects of Environmental Lead, London, May

Winneke, G. (1983) Neurobehavioural and neuropsychological effects of lead, in Rutter, M. and Russell Jones, R. (eds), *Lead versus Health* (Chichester: John Wiley)

Winneke, G. (1985) Update on the Nordenham longitudinal study, in Goldwater, L.J., Wysocki, L.M. and Volpe, R.A. (eds), *Lead Environmental Health: the current issues* (Duke University, Durham, NC: Duke University Press)

Winneke, G. (1986) Persistence and age-dependency of lead-induced brain dsyfunction. (Unpublished manuscript, Medizinisches Institut für Umwelthygiene an der Universitat Düsseldorf)

Winneke, G. and Kraemer, U. (1984) Neuropsychological effects of lead in children: interactions with social background variables. *Neuropsychobiology*, **11**, 195-202

Winneke, G., Hrdina, K.G. and Brockhaus, A. (1982a) Neuropsychological studies in children with elevated tooth-lead concentrations. I: Pilot study. *Int. Arch. Occup. Environ. Health*, **51**, 169–183

Winneke, G., Lilienthal, H. and Werner, W. (1982b) Task dependent neurobehavioural effects of lead in rats. *Arch. Toxicol.* (Suppl.), **5**, 84-93

Winneke, G., Kraemer, U., Brockhaus, A., Ewers, U., Kujanek, G., Lechner, H. and Janke, W. (1983a) Neuropsychological studies in children with elevated tooth-lead concentrations. II. Extended study. *Int. Arch. Occup. Environ. Health*, **51**, 231–252

Winneke, G., Lilienthal, H. and Zimmermann, U. (1983b) Neurobehavioural effects of lead and cadmium, in Hayes, A.W., Schnell, R.C. and Miya, T.S. (eds), *Developments in the Science and Practice of Toxicology* (Amsterdam: Elsevier)

Yule, W. and Rutter, M. (1985) Effects of lead on children's behaviour and cognitive performance: a critical review, in Mahaffey, K.R. (ed), *Dietary and Environmental Lead: Human Health Effects* (Amsterdam: Elsevier)

Yule, W., Lansdown. R., Millar, I. and Urbanowicz, M-A. (1981) The relationship between blood lead concentrations, intelligence and attainment in a school population: a pilot study. *Dev. Med. Child Neurol.*, **23**, 567-576

Yule, W., Urbanowicz, M-A., Lansdown, R. and Millar, I.B. (1984) Teachers' ratings of children's behaviour in relation to blood lead levels. *Br. J. Den Psychology*, **2**, 295-305

Ziegler, E.E., Edwards, B.B., Jensen, R.L., Mahaffey, K.R. and Fomon, S.J. (1978) Absorption and retention of lead by infants. *Ped. Res.*, **12**, 29-34

1.2

Effects of Low-Level Lead Exposure on Paediatric Neurobehavioural Development: Current Findings and Future Directions

L. D. GRANT and J. M. DAVIS

INTRODUCTION

The topic addressed at this Edinburgh Workshop, i.e., relationships between lead (Pb) exposure and neurobehavioural development effects in children, has been one of widespread interest and debate for many years. It has been of especially keen interest and importance in nations where extensive exposure of the general population (including paediatric segments) occurs as the result of mining, smelting, manufacturing processes, and/or consumer uses of lead or lead products. Toxic effects arising from exposures to lead of either adult or paediatric populations, whether directly or indirectly (secondarily) associated with occupational/workplace contamination or via various environmental pathways (e.g., air, water, soil, dust, food, etc.) have been a public health matter of longstanding concern to governmental bodies at the Federal, State, and local levels in the United States and at analogous governmental levels in many other nations as well.

The development of sound regulatory policies aimed at providing adequate public health protection against the toxic effects of lead is highly dependent upon the extent and quality of the scientific knowledge concerning sources, routes, and levels of the lead exposure for various population segments and the biological relationships involved in the uptake, distribution, retention, and consequent health effects of the metal or its compounds. Studies concerning the effects of lead exposure early in development on the physical and neurobehavioural development of children form an extremely important part of the scientific data base currently being drawn upon in the development of

49

regulatory policies for the control of lead exposure in the United States and elsewhere, including the United Kingdom, Canada, Australia, and various European countries.

The effects of early lead exposure on neurobehavioural and physical development of children are among numerous types of health effects evaluated as part of recent assessments of scientific bases for policy decisions by the United States Environmental Protection Agency (US EPA) concerning regulatory actions aimed at control of human lead exposure via the ambient air or water and/or due to more specific sources, e.g., the combustion of leaded gasoline. The most thorough and comprehensive evaluation of these and other lead health effects is presented in the US EPA document *Air Quality Criteria for Lead* (US EPA, 1986a) and an associated Addendum (US EPA, 1986b).

This paper attempts: (1) to provide a concise overview of the evaluations contained in these two EPA source documents and selected other emerging findings pertinent to the subject of the present meeting; (2) to note some policy considerations arising out of such evaluations; and (3) to highlight certain issues useful in defining future research directions. One major issue focussed on throughout this review is the delineation of exposure–effect (or dose–response) relationships for various types of lead effects on paediatric development, starting with those associated with severe high-level lead intoxication and proceeding to those seen with lesser exposure. Particular emphasis is placed on newly emerging results from ongoing prospective studies conducted by many of the research teams represented at this meeting and on issues that might be profitably investigated as part of their future research efforts.

OVERT LEAD INTOXICATION IN CHILDREN

The most serious outcomes of severe lead intoxication, encephalopathy and the associated high risk of death, have long been of much concern and study. Symptoms of encephalopathy similar to those that occur in adults have been reported in infants and young children (Oliver, 1911; Blackfan, 1917; McKhann and Vogt, 1926; Cumings, 1959; Chisolm, 1968), with much higher incidence of severe encephalopathic symptoms and deaths among them than in adults. This may reflect the greater difficulty in recognizing early symptoms in young children, thereby allowing intoxication to proceed to a more severe level before treatment is initiated (Lin-Fu, 1972). In regard to the risk of death in children, the mortality rate for encephalopathy cases was approximately 65% prior to the introduction of chelation therapy as standard medical practice (Greengard et al., 1965; National Academy of Sciences, 1972). The following mortality rates have been reported for children experiencing lead encephalopathy since the inception of chelation therapy as the standard treatment approach: 39% (Ennis and Harrison, 1950); 20–30% (Agerty, 1952); 24% (Mellins and Jenkins, 1955); 18% (Tanis, 1955); and 5% (Lewis et al., 1955). These data, and those tabulated more recently (National Academy of Sciences, 1972), indicate that once lead poisoning has progressed to the point of encephalopathy, a life-treatening situation clearly exists and, even with medical intervention, is apt to result in a fatal outcome.

Determining precise values for lead exposures necessary to produce acute symptoms, such as lethargy, vomiting, irritability, loss of appetite, dizziness, etc., or later neurotoxic sequelae in humans, is difficult in view of the paucity of data on environmental lead exposure levels, period(s) of exposure, or body burdens of lead existing prior to manifestation of symptoms. Nevertheless, enough information is available to permit reasonable estimates to be made regarding the range of blood lead (PbB) levels associated with acute encephalopathic symptoms or death. Available data indicate that lower PbB levels among children than among adults are associated with acute encephalopathy symptoms. The most extensive compilation of information on a paediatric population is a summarization (National Academy of Sciences, 1972) of data from Chisolm (1962, 1965) and Chisolm and Harrison (1956). This data compilation relates occurrence of acute encephalopathy and death in children in Baltimore to PbB levels determined by the Baltimore City Health Department between 1930 and 1970. Blood lead levels formerly regarded as 'asymptomatic' and other signs of acute lead poisoning were also tabulated. Increased lead absorption in the absence of detected symptoms was observed at PbB levels ranging from 60 to 300 μg/dl (mean = 105 μg/dl). Acute lead poisoning symptoms other than signs of encephalopathy occurred from 60 to 450 μg/dl (mean = 178 μg/dl). Signs of encephalopathy (hyper-irritability, ataxia, convulsions, stupor, and coma) were associated with PbB levels of 90 to 800 μg/dl (mean = 330 μg/dl). The distribution of PbB levels associated with death (mean = 327 μg/dl) was essentially the same as for levels yielding encephalopathy. These data suggest that PbB levels capable of producing death in children are essentially identical to those associated with acute encephalopathy and that such effects are usually manifested in children starting at approximately 100 μg/dl. Certain other evidence from scattered medical reports (Gant, 1938; Smith et al., 1938; Bradley et al., 1956; Bradley and Baumgartner, 1958; Cumings, 1959; Rummo et al., 1979), however, suggests that acute encephalopathy in the most highly susceptible children may be associated with PbB levels of 80 to 100 μg/dl (see US EPA, 1977).

Central nervous system (CNS) pathology findings vary in cases of fatal lead encephalopathy among children (Blackman, 1937; Pentschew, 1965; Popoff et al., 1963) and often include cerebral oedema, altered capillaries (endothelial hypertrophy and hyperplasia), and perivascular glial proliferation. Neuronal damage is variable and may be caused by anoxia. However, in some cases gross and microscopic changes are minimal (Pentschew, 1965). More detailed information on encephalopathic brain changes has been gained by studying animal models. Studies of lead intoxication in the CNS of developing rats have shown vasculopathic changes (Pentschew and Garro, 1966), reduced cerebral cortical thickness and reduced number of synapses per neuron (Krigman et al., 1974a), and reduced cerebral axonal size (Krigman et al., 1974b). Biochemical changes in the CNS of lead-treated neonatal rats have also demonstrated reduced brain lipid content but no alterations of neural lipid composition (Krigman et al., 1974a) and a reduced cerebellar DNA

51

content (Michaelson, 1973). In cases of lower-level lead exposure, subjectively recognizable neuropathological features may not occur (Krigman, 1978). Instead there may be subtle changes at the level of the synapse (Silbergeld et al., 1980) or dendritic field, myelin–axon relations, and organization of synaptic patterns (Krigman, 1978). Since the nervous system is a dynamic structure rather than a static one, it undergoes compensatory changes (Norton and Culver, 1977), maturation and aging (Sotelo and Palay, 1971), and structural changes in response to environmental stimuli (Coss and Glohus, 1978). Thus, whereas massive structural damage in many cases of acute encephalopathy would be expected to cause lasting neurotoxic sequelae, some other CNS effects due to severe early lead insult might be reversible or compensated for, depending upon age and duration of toxic exposure. This raises the question of whether effects of early overt lead intoxication are reversible beyond the initial intoxication or continue to persist.

In cases of severe non-fatal episodes of lead encephalopathy, the neurological sequelae that occur are qualitatively similar to those often seen after traumatic or infectious cerebral injury, with permanent sequelae being more common in children than in adults. The most severe paediatric sequelae are cortical atrophy, hydrocephalus, convulsive seizures, and severe mental retardation (Mellins and Jenkins, 1955; Perlstein and Attala, 1966; Chisolm, 1968). Children who recover from acute lead encephalopathy but are re-exposed to lead almost invariably show evidence of permanent CNS damage (Chisolm and Harrison, 1956). Even if further lead exposure is minimized, 25 to 50% show severe permanent sequelae, such as seizure disorders, blindness, and hemiparesis (Chisolm and Barltrop, 1979).

Lasting neurotoxic sequelae of overt lead intoxication in children in the absence of acute encephalopathy have also been reported. Byers and Lord (1943) reported that children with previous lead poisoning later made unsatisfactory progress in school. Sensorimotor deficits, short attention span, and behavioural disorders have been confirmed in children with known high lead exposures but without a history of life-threatening forms of acute encephalopathy (Chisolm and Harrison, 1956; Cohen and Ahrens, 1959; Kline, 1960). Perlstein and Attala (1966) also reported neurological sequelae in 140 of 386 children (37%) following lead poisoning without encephalopathy. Such sequelae included mental retardation, seizures, cerebral palsy, optic atrophy, and visual–perceptual problems in some children with minimal intellectual impairment. Numerous studies (Cohen et al., 1976; Fejerman et al., 1973; Pueschel et al., 1972; Sachs et al., 1978, 1979, 1982) suggest that, in the absence of encephalopathy, chelation therapy may ameliorate the persistence of neurotoxic effects of overt lead poisoning (especially cognitive, perceptual, and behavioural deficits). On the other hand, another study found a residual effect on fine motor performance even after chelation (Kirkconnell and Hicks, 1980).

In summary, pertinent literature demonstrates that lead poisoning with encephalopathy results in a greatly increased incidence of permanent neurological and cognitive impairments. Also, several studies showed that children with overt, symptomatic lead intoxication in the absence of encephalopathy experience persisting neurological and behavioural impairments.

NON-OVERT LEAD INTOXICATION IN CHILDREN

Besides neurotoxic effects associated with overt lead intoxication in children, much evidence indicates that lead exposures not leading to overt paediatric lead intoxication can induce neurological dysfunctions. This issue has attracted much attention and controversy during the past 10 to 20 years. The evidence concerning occurrence of significant neurotoxic deficits at relatively low lead exposure levels is quite mixed and interpretable only after a thorough critical evaluation of methods employed in the various important studies (see chapter by Smith on methodological issues, this volume). Based on five criteria (adequate markers of exposure to lead, sensitive measures, appropriate subject selection, control of confounding covariates, and appropriate statistical analysis), the population studies summarized in Table 1 were conducted rigorously enough to warrant review in the EPA Criteria Document (US EPA, 1986a). Even so, no epidemiological study is completely flawless and, therefore, overall interpretation of such findings must be based on evaluation of the following: (1) the internal consistency and quality of each study; (2) the consistency of results obtained across independently conducted studies; and (3) the plausibility of results in view of other available information.

Rutter (1980) classified studies evaluating neurobehavioural effects of lead exposure in non-overtly lead intoxicated children according to several types, including four categories reviewed below: (1) clinic-type studies of children thought to be at risk because of high lead levels; (2) other studies of children drawn from general (typically urban or suburban) paediatric populations; (3) samples of children living more specifically in close proximity to lead-emitting smelters; and (4) studies of mentally retarded or behaviourally deviant children. Major attention is accorded here to studies falling under the second and third categories. A final section discusses some initial results beginning to emerge from long-term prospective studies, which relate effects on early neuropsychological development and later neuropsychological functioning to lead exposure histories for children documented back to birth or prenatally.

Clinic-type studies of children with high lead levels

Clinic-type studies are typified by evaluation of children with high lead body burdens as identified through lead screening programmes or other large-scale programmes focussing on mother–infant health relationships and early childhood development. The key features and most salient results emerging from such studies are summarized in Table 1. Comments on important points concerning such studies follow.

De la Burde and Choate (1972) found neurological dysfunctions, fine motor dysfunction, impaired concept formation, and altered behavioural profiles in 70 Richmond, VA preschool children exhibiting pica and elevated PbB levels (all $> 30 \mu g/dl$; mean $= 59 \mu g/dl$) compared to matched non-pica control subjects. All mothers were followed during pregnancy, and the children were postnatally evaluated by regular paediatric neurological examinations, psychological testing, and medical interviews. Children subject to prenatal,

Table 1 Summary of studies on neurobehavioural functions of lead-exposed children[a]

Reference	Population studied	N/group	Age at testing, year (range)	Mean blood lead, μg/dl (range or S.D.)	Psychometric tests employed	Summary of results	Levels of significance[b]
Clinic-type studies of children with high lead levels							
de la Burde and Choate (1972)	Inner city (Richmond, VA)	C = 72 Pb = 70	4.0 4.0	?[c] 58 (30–100)[d]	IQ (Stanford–Binet) Fine motor Gross motor Concept formation Behaviour profile	Score: C 94 Pb 89 % subnormal[e]: 10 25 26 45 7 16 10 15 10 30	<0.05 <0.05 N.S. N.S. <0.01
de la Burde and Choate (1975)	Follow-up same subjects	C = 67 Pb = 70	7–8 7–8	PbT: 112 μg/g 202 μg/g	WISC Full Scale IQ Verbal IQ Performance IQ Bender Gestalt Reading Spelling Arithmetic Goodenough–Harris draw test Auditory vocal assoc. Tactile recognition Behaviour profile	Score: C 90 Pb 87 % subnormal[e]: 6 24 9 18 13 24 27 49 7 12 11 16 7 12 1 13 13 31 3 15 3 25	0.01 N.S. N.S. 0.01 N.S. N.S. N.S. 0.02 0.01 0.05 0.001
Rummo (1974); Rummo *et al.* (1979)	Inner city (Providence, RI)	C = 45 Pb_1 = 15 Pb_2 = 20 Pb_3 = 10	5.8 5.6 (4–8) 5.6 5.3	23 (8) 61 (7) 68 (13) 88 (41)	McCarthy Scales: Gen. cognitive Verbal Perceptual Quantitative Memory Motor Parent ratings Neurological exam	C Pb_1 Pb_2 Pb_3 93 94 88 77 46 46 44 37 48 49 46 38 45 44 41 35 47 46 43 36 52 52 50 40 8 10 10 18 7/12 measures sig. different	<0.01 <0.05 <0.05 <0.01 <0.01 <0.01 <0.01

continued

Table 1 *continued*

Reference	Population studied	N/group	Age at testing, year (range)	Mean blood lead, μg/dl (range or S.D.)	Psychometric tests employed	Summary of results				Levels of significance[b]
						Norm	*C*	*Pb*		
Kotok (1972)	Inner city (New Haven, CT)	C = 25	2.7 (1.1–5.5)	38 (20–55)	Denver Developmental:	1.00	1.02	1.06		N.S.
		Pb = 24	2.8 (1.0–5.8)	81 (58–137)	Gross motor	1.00[f]	0.82	0.81[f]		<0.01[f]
					Fine motor	1.00[f]	0.82	0.73[f]		<0.01[f]
					Language					
						C		*Pb*		
Kotok et al. (1977)	Inner city (Rochester, NY)	C = 36	3.6 (1.9–5.6)	28 (11–40)	IQ Equivalent:	126		124		>0.10
		Pb = 31	3.6 (1.7–5.4)	80 (61–200)	Social	101		92		<0.10
					Spatial	93		92		>0.10
					Spoken vocal	96		94		>0.10
					Info–comprehension	93		90		>0.10
					Visual attention	100		93		>0.10
					Auditory memory					
						Low		*Mod.*		
Perino and Ernhart (1974)[f]	Inner city (New York, NY)	Low Pb = 50	3–6	(10–30)	McCarthy Scales:	90		80		<0.01
		Mod. Pb = 3C	3–6	(40–70)	Gen. cognitive	44		39		<0.05
					Verbal	44		37		<0.05
					Perceptual	48		44		N.S.
					Quantitative	45		42		N.S.
					Memory	46		42		N.S.
					Motor					
						Low		*Mod.*		
Ernhart et al. (1981)[f]	Follow-up same subjects	Low Pb = 31	8–13	21 (4)[g]	McCarthy Scales:	94		82		<0.05
		Mod. Pb = 32		32 (5)	Gen. cognitive	48		41		<0.05
					Verbal	43		40		N.S.
					Perceptual	43		38		N.S.
					Quantitative	44		39		N.S.
					Memory	49		46		<0.05
					Motor					
					Reading tests	Not reported				N.S.
					Conners teacher ratings	Not reported				N.S.
					Various experimental tests	Not reported				N.S.

continued

55

Table 1 *continued*

Reference	Population studied	N/group	Age at testing, year (range)	Mean blood lead, μg/dl (range or S.D.)	Psychometric tests employed	Summary of results C	Summary of results Pb	Levels of significance[b]
General population studies								
Needleman et al.	Urban (Boston, MA)	C = 100	7	PbT: <10ppm[i]	WISC Full Scale IQ	106.6	102.1	0.03
		Pb = 58	7	>20 ppm	Verbal IQ	103.9	99.3	0.06
					Performance IQ	108.7	104.9	0.12
					Seashore Rhythm Test	21.6	19.4	0.002
					Token Test	24.8	23.6	0.09
					Sentence Repetition Test	12.6	11.3	0.04
					Delayed Reaction Time	C > Pb on 3/4 blocks		<0.01
					Teacher Ratings	9.5	8.2	0.02
McBride et al. (1982)	Urban/suburban (Sydney, Australia)	Low Pb = >100	4/5	(2–9)		*Low* ~105	*Mod.* ~104	
		Mod. Pb = >100	4/5	(19–29)	Peabody Picture Vocab. Test	~105	~104	N.S.
					Fine Motor Tracking	C > Pb 1/4 comparisons		<0.05
					Pegboard	~20	~20	N.S.
					Tapping Test	~30	~31	N.S.
					Beam Walk	~5	~4	N.S.
					Standing Balance	C > Pb 1/4 comparisons		<0.05
					Rutter Activity Scale	~1.9	~2.1	N.S.
Yule et al. (1981)	Urban (London, England)	Group 1 = 34	9	8.8[j] (7–10)	WISC-R Full Scale IQ	103 103	96 96	0.027
		Group 2 = 48	9 (6–12)	11.6 (11–12)	Verbal IQ	101 101	95 94	0.043
		Group 3 = 49	8	14.5 (13–16)	Performance IQ	106 103	98 99	0.102
		Group 4 = 35	8	19.6 (17–32)	Vernon Spelling Test	104 98	92 89	0.001
					Vernon Math Test	97 97	95 95	N.S.
					Neale Reading Accuracy[k]	121 110	96 89	0.001
					Neale Reading Compre.[k]	117 110	95 88	0.001
Yule et al. (1984)	Same subjects in Yule et al. (1981)	Same	Same	Same	Needleman Teacher Ratings	1.53 1.54	2.45 2.63	0.096
					(4/11 items sig. different)			
					Conners Teacher Ratings	0.26	0.37	0.04
					(3/4 factors sig. at p < 0.05)			
					Rutter Teacher Ratings, including "Overactivity" factor			
					(2/26 items sig. at p ≦ 0.05)			
					(5/26 items differ at 0.05 < p < 0.10)			
					6% 4%	20% 17%		

Table 1 continued

Reference	Population studied	N/group	Age at testing, year (range)	Mean blood lead, µg/dl (range or S.D.)	Psychometric tests employed	Summary of results Low	Med	High	Levels of significance[b]
Lansdown et al. (1986)	Urban (London, England)	Low = 80 High = 82	9 9	7–12 13–24	WISC-R Full Scale	Low 107		High 105	N.S.
					Verbal IQ	104		103	N.S.
					Performance IQ	108		106	N.S.
					Neale Reading Accuracy	115		112	N.S.
					Neale Reading Comprehension	113		109	N.S.
					Vernon Spelling	101		99	N.S.
					Vernon Math	100		99	N.S.
Smith et al. (1983)	Urban (London, England)	High = 155 Med = 103 Low = 145	6,7 6,7 6,7	PbT ≥ 8.0 PbT = 5–5.5 PbT < 2.5 (All in µg/g) $\bar{X}$ PbB = 13.1 µg/dl	WISC-R Full Scale	Low 107	Med 105	High 105	N.S.
					Verbal IQ	105	103	103	N.S.
					Performance IQ	108	106	106	N.S.
					Word Reading Test	45	42	40	N.S.
					Seashore Rhythm Test	21	20	20	N.S.
					Visual Sequential Memory	20	19	20	N.S.
					Sentence Memory	9	9	9	N.S.
					Shape Copying	14	14	14	N.S.
					Mathematics	16	15	15	N.S.
					Mean Visual RT (seconds)	0.37	0.37	0.39	N.S.
					Conners Teacher Ratings	11	11	13	N.S.
Harvey et al. (1983, 1984)	Urban (Birmingham, England)	189	2.5	15.5 (6–30)		Regression F ratio[l]			
					British Ability Scales				
					Naming	<1			N.S.
					Recall	1.26			N.S.
					Comprehension	<1			N.S.
					Recognition	<1			N.S.
					IQ	<1			N.S.
					Standford–Binet Items				
					Shapes	<1			N.S.
					Blocks	2.34			N.S.
					Beads	2.46			N.S.
					Playroom Activity	?			N.S.

57

continued

Table 1 continued

Reference	Population studied	N/group	Age at testing, year (range)	Mean blood lead, µg/dl (range or S.D.)	Psychometric tests employed	Summary of results		Levels of significance[b]
Silva et al. (1986b)	Urban (Dunedin, New Zealand)	579	11	11.1 (4–50)	WISC-R Full Scale IQ	$r = -0.06$		N.S.
					Performance IQ	$= -0.03$		N.S.
					Verbal	$= -0.05$		N.S.
						R^2	Incrs. by Pb	
					Rutter Behavior Rating			
					Parent	0.21	1.38	0.003
					Teacher	0.10	1.23	0.008
					Inattention Rating			
					Parent	0.24	0.26	N.S.
					Teacher	0.25	1.51	0.001
					Hyperactivity Rating			
					Parent	0.12	1.01	0.015
					Teacher	0.12	0.82	0.028
					Burt Reading Test	0.43	0.28	N.S.
Schroeder et al. (1985)	Rural/urban (Wake County, North Carolina)	104	<2.5 or >2.5 (0.8–6.5)	6–59	Bayley MDI or Stanford–Binet	Regression analysis of sources for IQ effect:		
						Lead: $F = 7.689$		<0.01
						SES: $F = 20.159$		<0.001
	Follow-up same subjects	50	6–12	≦30	Stanford–Binet	Lead: $F < 1$		N.S.
Schroeder and Hawk (1987)	Rural/urban (Lenoir and Hanover Counties, North Carolina)	75	2	21 (6–47)	Stanford–Binet	Regression analysis of IQ against:		
						Current PbB: $F = 12.31$		<0.0008
						Max. PbB: $F = 10.55$		<0.0018
						Mean PbB: $F = 10.08$		<0.002
Smelter area studies						C	Pb	
Landrigan et al. (1975)	Smelter area (El Paso, TX)	C = 78	9.3 (3.8–15.9)	<40	WISC Full Scale IQ[m]	93	89	N.S.
		Pb = 46	8.3	40–68	WPPSI Full Scale IQ[n]	91	86	N.S.
					WISC + WPPSI Combined	93	88	N.S.
					WISC + WPPSI Subscales	C > Pb on 13/14 scales 7/14 scales sig. different		<0.05
					Neurological testing	C > Pb on 7/8 tests 1/8 tests sig. different		<0.01

58

Table 1 *continued*

Reference	Population studied	N/group	Age at testing, year (range)	Mean blood lead, μg/dl (range or S.D.)	Psychometric tests employed	Summary of results		Levels of significance[b]
McNeil and Ptasnik (1975)	Smelter area (El Paso, TX)	C = 37 Pb = 101	9 (1.8–18) 9	29 (14–39) 58 (40–93)	McCarthy General Cognitive	*C* 82	*Pb* 81	N.S.
					WISC-WAIS Full Scale IQ	89	87	N.S.
					Oseretsky Motor Level	101	97	N.S.
					California Personality	C > Pb, 6/10 items		<0.05
					Frostig Perceptual Quotient	100	103	N.S.
					Finger–Thumb Apposition	27	29	N.S.
Ratcliffe (1977)	Smelter area (Manchester, England)	Mod. Pb = 23 High Pb = 24	4.7 (4.1–5.6) 4.8 (4.2–5.4)	28 (18–35) 44 (36–64)	Griffiths Mental Dev.	*Mod.* 108	*High* 102	N.S.
					Frostig Visual Perception	14.3	11.8	N.S.
					Pegboard Test Dominant hand	17.5	17.3	N.S.
					Nondominant hand	19.5	19.8	N.S.
Winneke et al. (1982)	Smelter area (Duisberg, FRG)	C = 26 Pb = 26	8 8	PbT = 2.4 ppm[h] PbT = 9.2 ppm No PbB	German WISC Full Scale	*C* 122	*Pb* 117	N.S.
					Verbal IQ	130	124	N.S.
					Performance IQ	130	123	N.S.
					Bender Gestalt Test	17.2	19.6	<0.05
					Standard Neurological Tests	2.7	7.2	N.S.
					Conners Teacher Ratings	?	?	N.S.
Winneke et al. (1983)	Smelter area (Stolburg, FRG)	89	9.4	PbT: 6.16 ppm[h] PbB: 14.3 μg/dl	German WISC Full Scale IQ	% Variance due to PbT −0.0		N.S.
					Verbal IQ	−0.5		N.S.
					Performance IQ	+0.6		N.S.
					Bender Gestalt Test	+2.1		<0.05
					Standard Neurological Tests	+1.2		N.S.
					Conners Teacher Ratings	0.4–1.3		N.S.
					Wiener Reaction Performance	+2.0		N.S.

continued

59

Table 1 *continued*

Reference	Population studied	N/group	Age at testing, year (range)	Mean blood lead, μg/dl (range or S.D.)	Psychometric tests employed	Summary of results % Variance due to Pb	Levels of significance[b]
Winneke et al. (1984)	Smelter area (Nordenham, FRG)	122	6.5	8.2 (4.4–22.8)	German WISC		
					Short form	−0.3	N.S.
					Verbal IQ	+0.3	N.S.
					Performance	−2.4	N.S.
					Bender Gestalt Test	+0.5	N.S.
					Signalled Reaction Time		
					Short	+0.1	N.S.
					Long	−0.2	N.S.
					Wiener Reaction Time		
					Easy	+4.3	<0.05
					Difficult	+11.0	<0.01

[a]Abbreviations: C = control subjects; Pb = lead-exposed subjects; MDI = mental development index; N.S. = nonsignificant ($p > 0.05$); PbT = tooth lead; WISC = Wechsler Intelligence Scale for Children; WPPSI = Wechsler Preschool and Primary Scale of Intelligence; RT = reaction time

[b]Significance levels are those found after partialling out confounding covariates

[c]Urinary coproporphyrin levels were not elevated

[d]Some with positive radiological findings, suggesting earlier exposure in excess of 40–60 μg/dl

[e]Percentage of each group scoring 'borderline', 'suspect', 'defective', or 'abnormal'

[f]Reanalysis of data by Ernhart correcting for methodological problems in earlier published analyses described here mainly did not substantiate significant differences between control and lead-exposed children indicated in last two columns to the right (see chapter text)

[g]Dentine levels not reported for statistical reasons

[h]Reanalyses of Needleman data correcting for methodological problems in earlier published analyses confirmed significant differences between study groups indicated in last two right-hand columns for WISC IQ test result (see chapter text)

[i]Main measure was dentine lead (PbT)

[j]Blood lead levels taken 9–12 months prior to testing; none above 33 μg/dl

[k]Data not corrected for age

[l]This F ratio is result of testing the difference in sums of squares for two regression equations (one including and one excluding blood lead levels as an independent variable) against the residual mean square of the equation including blood lead

[m]Used for children over 5 years of age

[n]Used for children under 6 years of age

Source: US EPA (1986)

perinatal, and early postnatal insults were excluded from the study; and all included children had normal neurological examinations and Bayley tests at 8–9 mo of age. Follow-up studies of the same children at 7–8 y (de la Burde and Choate, 1975) revealed continuing CNS impairment in the lead-exposed group. Also, seven times as many lead-exposed children were repeating grades in school or being referred to the school psychologist, despite many of their PbB levels having dropped significantly from at the time of initial study.

In general, the de la Burde and Choate (1972, 1975) studies have many features that argue for the validity of their findings despite shortcomings avoided by many more recent studies. There were appreciable numbers of children (67 lead-exposed and 70 controls) whose PbB values were obtained in preschool years, the psychometric tests employed were well standardized and acceptable as sensitive indicators of neurobehavioural dysfunction, and testing was conducted blind. These studies, on the other hand, can be criticized on several points, although none are sufficient to reject their results. For example, PbB values were not determined for control subjects in the initial study; but the lack of pica history, as well as results of later tooth lead analyses in the follow-up study, render it improbable that lead-exposed subjects were wrongly assigned to the control group. A second problem was use of multiple chi-square statistical tests; but the fact that the control subjects did significantly better on nearly all measures makes it unlikely that all observed effects were due to chance alone. One last problem concerns ambiguities in subject selection which complicate interpretation of the results obtained. Because the lead-exposed group included children with PbB levels of 40 to 100 μg/dl, or of at least 30 μg/dl with "positive radiographic findings of Pb lines in the long bones, metallic deposits in the intestines, or both", observed deficits might best be attributed to PbB levels exceeding 40 μg/dl based on other evidence (Betts et al., 1973) indicating that lead lines are usually seen only if PbB levels exceed 40 to 60 μg/dl.

In another clinic-type study, Rummo (1974) and Rummo et al. (1979) found significant neurobehavioural deficits (hyperactivity, lower scores on McCarthy scales of cognitive function, etc.) among Providence, RI inner-city children who had previously experienced high lead exposure that had produced acute lead encephalopathy. Mean maximum PbB levels recorded at the time of encephalopathy were 88 $\pm$ 40 μg/dl. However, children with moderate PbB elevation but not manifesting symptoms of encephalopathy did not differ significantly (at $p < 0.05$) from controls on any measure of cognitive functioning, psychomotor performance, or hyperactivity. Still, when data from the Rummo et al. (1979) study for performance on the McCarthy General Cognitive Index or several McCarthy Subscales are compared (see Table 1), the scores for long-term moderate-exposure subjects consistently fall below those for control subjects and lie between the latter and the encephalopathy group scores. Thus, long-term moderate lead exposure, in fact, apparently exerted dose-related neurobehavioural effects. The overall dose–response trend may have been shown to be statistically significant by other types of analyses, if larger samples had been assessed, or if control subjects had PbB values <5–10 μg/dl. Note that (1) the maximum PbB levels for the short-term and long-term exposure subjects were all greater than $40 \, \mu g/dl$ (means = 61 ± 7 and $68 \pm 13 \, \mu g/dl$, respectively), whereas control subjects all had PbB levels below $40 \, \mu g/dl$ (mean = $23 \pm 8 \, \mu g/dl$), and (2) the control and lead-exposed subjects were inner-city children well matched for socioeconomic background, parental education levels, incidence of pica, and other pertinent factors except for parental IQ (not ascertained).

Kotok *et al.* (1977) found a similar pattern of results in a study in which 36 Rochester, NY, control-group children with PbB levels $< 40 \, \mu g/dl$ were compared with 31 children with distinctly elevated blood lead levels (61 to $200 \, \mu g/dl$) but no classical lead intoxication symptoms. Both groups were well matched on important background factors. Again, no clearly statistically significant differences between the two groups were found on numerous tests of cognitive and sensory functions. However, mean scores of control-group children were consistently higher than those of the lead-exposed group for all of the ability classes listed, although the control group children had notably elevated PbB values by current standards. Kotok (1972) had reported earlier that developmental deficiencies (using the Denver Development Screening Test) in a group of children with elevated PbB levels (58 to $137 \, \mu g/dl$) were identical to those in a control group similar in age, sex, race, environment, neonatal condition, and presence of pica, but with lower PbB levels (20 to $55 \, \mu g/dl$). The lead-exposed group, however, had PbB levels as high as $137 \, \mu g/dl$, whereas some control children had levels as high as $55 \, \mu g/dl$. Thus, the study essentially compared two groups with different degrees of markedly elevated lead exposure and had no true control group.

Perino and Ernhart (1974) reported relationships between neurobehavioural deficits and PbB levels ranging from 40 to $70 \, \mu g/dl$ in a group of 80 inner-city preschool black children, based on the results of a cross-sectional study of children with elevated PbB levels found through the New York City lead screening programme. They reported that the high-lead children had McCarthy Scale IQ scores markedly lower than those of the low-lead group (mean IQ = 80 versus 90, respectively). Also, the normal correlation of 0.52 between parents' intelligence and that of their offspring was found to be reduced to only 0.10 in the lead-exposed group, presumably because of the influence of another factor (lead) that interfered with normal intellectual development of the lead-exposed children. Another possible explanation, however, might be differences in educational backgrounds of parents of control subjects versus lead-exposed subjects, because parental education level was significantly negatively related to PbB levels of children in the study.

Ernhart *et al.* (1981) carried out follow-up evaluations on 63 of the 80 preschool children of the Perino and Ernhart (1974) study once they reached school age, using the McCarthy IQ scales, various reading achievement tests, the Bender–Gestalt test, the Draw-A-Child test, and the Conners Teacher's Questionnaire for hyperactivity. The children's PbB levels were significantly correlated with FEP ($r = 0.51$) and dentine lead levels ($r = 0.43$), but mean PbB levels of the moderately elevated group had decreased after five years. When control variables of sex and parental IQ were extracted by multivariate analyses, observed differences were greatly reduced (albeit still statistically significant) for three of seven tests on the McCarthy scales in relation to concurrently measured PbB levels but not in relation to earlier PbB levels or dentine lead levels for the same children. This led Ernhart et al. (1981) to reinterpret their 1974 (Perino and Ernhart, 1974) IQ results (in which they had not controlled for parental education) as either not likely being due to lead or, if due to lead, then representing only minimal effects on intelligence.

Reanalyses of the data set reported on by Perino and Ernhart (1974) and Ernhart et al. (1981) were carried out to correct certain methodological problems associated with the earlier published analyses, as reported by Ernhart (1983, 1984; Ernhart et al., 1985). Reanalysis of relationships between preschool-age children's PbB levels and concurrently obtained McCarthy Scales scores revealed no significant differences (at $p < 0.05$) due to lead; however, lower scores for the higher Pb exposure group on the General Cognitive Index (GCI) did approach significance at $p < 0.09$. Also, reanalysis of relationships between preschool PbB levels and 5-year later school-age outcome variables yielded no indication of persisting lead effects in terms of reading test results or scores on the McCarthy GCI or most of the McCarthy Subscales (except $p = 0.10$ for Verbal Index scores). The reanalysis of school-age PbB levels (newly corrected for haematocrit variation effects) and concurrent reading test and McCarthy Scales scores only found significant differences attributable to lead for lower McCarthy Verbal Index scores ($p < 0.036$ with a 'deviant case' included in the analysis, and $p < 0.07$ with the case excluded). Similar results were found with a different analysis using a 'lead construct index' as a measure of lead exposure that combined preschool- and school-age PbB levels and free erythrocyte protoporphyrin levels. Based on these results, Ernhart et al. (1985) concluded that "the reanalyses provide no reasonable support for an interpretation of lead effects in these data". However, they also noted that there was a certain level of unreliability in the measures used and that the sample size limited the power of the statistical analyses. Given such limitations and extensive attention accorded to statistical control of potentially confounding variables in the reanalyses, it is notable that an association between lead and lower Verbal Index scores was still found across several of the analyses (at p values <0.04 to 0.10) and that an association between preschool-age PbB levels and GCI scores approached significance at $p < 0.09$.

Other investigators (Shapiro and Marecek, 1984; Marecek et al., 1983) studied relationships between lead exposures and psychometric testing outcomes among black children from low socioeconomic status (SES) families in Philadelphia, PA. From among a large target sample of eligible children invited to participate, 199 families enrolled their children. Primary and/or circumpulpal dentine lead levels from shed deciduous teeth (mainly molars) were used to index lead exposure for 188 children (aged 10.6 to 14.7 y; $\bar{X} = 11.8$ y) who underwent neuropsychologic testing. Data on SES and several other potentially confounding variables were obtained for all children and IQ scores for parents of a subset of the children studied. Data analyses (heirarchical multiple regression analyses) first evaluated relationships between dentine lead exposure indices and test scores obtained several years earlier (at age 7 y) on the Bender–Gestalt, Wechsler Intelligence Scale for Children (WISC) subtests, and other tests; other analyses used dentine lead data and

63

results from concurrently administered psychometric tests. For tests at seven years of age, significant associations were found between dentine lead and performance IQ scores, but not for WISC verbal IQ scores. Similarly, significant relationships (at $p < 0.05$) were found between dentine lead values and concurrently obtained test results for performance abilities on the Bender–Gestalt, WISC, and other tests but not for verbal abilities. This study, while qualitatively suggesting that lead may affect cognitive performance, suffers from several methodological problems, including inadequate control for sampling bias, covarying social factors, and parental IQ, and retrospective estimation of lead exposure at age seven.

Odenbro et al. (1983) studied psychological development of children (aged 3 to 6 y) seen in Chicago Department oɪ Health Clinics (August 1976 to February 1977), evaluating scores on the Denver Developmental Screening Test (DDST) and two subtests of the Wechsler Preschool and Primary Scale of Intelligence (WPPSI) in relation to PbB levels obtained by repeated sampling during three previous years. A significant correlation ($r = -0.435, p < 0.001$) was found between perceptual visual–motor ability and mean PbB levels. Statistically significant ($p < 0.005$) deficits in verbal productivity and perceptual visual–performance (measured by the WPPSI) were found for groups of children with mean PbB levels of 30 to 40 μg/dl and 40 to 60 μg/dl versus control children with mean PbB levels < 25 μg/dl, using two-tailed Student's t-tests; however, significant associations ($p < 0.05$) between PbB levels and developmental retardations in language and fine-motor functions were found only for the 40 to 60 μg/dl group, using the DDST and chi-square analyses. These results suggest neuropsychological deficits associated with PbB levels of 40 to 60 μg/dl in preschool children. However, parental IQs were not measured, and the adequacy of the statistical analyses employed is questionable, especially in regard to lack of use of multivariate analyses that sufficiently control for confounding covariates.

In another study (Molina et al., 1983), high-risk children from families making lead-glazed pottery in a Mexican village were evaluated for lead-associated neuropsychological deficits, using an appropriately adapted Spanish language version of the revised WISC (WISC-R) test and the Bender–Gestalt test. Test results for 33 high-lead children ($\bar{X}$ age: 10 y, 7 mo $\pm$ 2 y, 7 mo) randomly selected from 64 school children with PbB levels > 40 μg/dl ($\bar{X}$: 63.4 $\pm$ 15.8 μg/dl) were compared with those for 30 lower lead children ($\bar{X}$ age: 10 y, 2 mo $\pm$ 2 y, 6 mo) with PbB levels below 40 μg/dl ($\bar{X}$: 26.3 $\pm$ 8.0 μg/dl), using two-tailed Student's t-test and the Mann–Whitney U test. The high-lead children had significantly lower WISC-R full-scale IQ ($p < 0.01$), verbal IQ ($p < 0.01$), and performance IQ ($p < 0.025$) than did the low-lead control children drawn from among the same low SES families as the high-lead children. A significant negative linear correlation was also observed for the same types of test scores among the high-lead children, but not for such scores among the low-lead children. These results, highly suggestive of lead-related neuropsychological deficits with PbB values > 40 μg/dl, must be viewed with caution in light of failure to include parental IQ levels and lack of adequate multivariate analyses controlling for age, sex, and other factors.

In summary, the above studies generally found that high-risk lead-exposure groups did more poorly on IQ or other types of psychometric tests than referent control groups with lower Pb exposures. Many of the studies did not control for important confounding variables or, when such were taken into account, found that the differences between lead-exposed and control subjects were reduced or were no longer statistically significant. Still, the consistency of finding the lower IQ values and other types of neuro-psychological deficits among at-risk higher lead exposure children across most of the studies lend credence to cognitive deficits occurring in apparently asymptomatic children with markedly elevated PbB levels (i.e., starting at 40 to 60 μg/dl and ranging upwards to 70 to 80 μg/dl or higher values).

The magnitude of lead's effects on IQ at the high exposure levels evaluated in these studies is difficult to estimate due to variations in measurement instruments used, variations in adequacy of control for confounding factors, and the fact that many of the referent control groups had what are now recognized to be elevated PbB levels (i.e., averaging in the 20 to 40 μg/dl range). Focussing on estimates of full-scale IQ deficits, Rummo (1974; Rummo et al., 1979) observed a decrement of about 16 IQ points on the McCarthy GCI for postencephalopathic children with PbB values exceeding 80 μg/dl. Asymptomatic children with long-term lead exposures yielding mean PbB values of 68 μg/dl experienced an average 5-point IQ (GCI) decrement, whereas short-term lead-exposed subjects with PbB levels around 60 μgdl showed no decrement compared to controls. The de la Burde subjects, with PbB levels averaging 58 μg/dl, had a mean Stanford–Binet IQ decrement of 5 points upon first testing (de la Burde and Choate, 1975). Ernhart originally reported an average 10-point IQ (GCI) decrement for children with PbB values in the 40 to 70 μg/dl range upon first testing (Perino and Ernhart, 1974) and 12 points upon follow-up 5 years later (Ernhart et al., 1981). However, these reported large decrements were likely due in part to confounding by uncontrolled covariates in the original analyses and, upon reanalysis of the data, are notably reduced. While it could be argued that the Rummo and de la Burde decrements would also be reduced in size if better control for confounding variables were employed, use of control subjects with lower lead exposure (e.g., < 10 μg/dl) would also logically be expected to result in offsetting influences on IQ. Thus, it seems warranted to conclude that the average decrements of about 5 IQ points observed in the de la Burde and Rummo studies represent a reasonable minimal estimate of the magnitude of full-scale IQ decrements associated with notably elevated PbB levels ($\bar{X} \approx$ 50 to 70 μg/dl) in asymptomatic children.

General population studies

These studies evaluated samples of non-overtly lead-intoxicated children selected to be representative of general paediatric populations. They focus mainly on asymptomatic children with lower lead body burdens than those of high-risk children in clinic-type studies.

A pioneering general population study by Needleman et al. (1979) used shed deciduous teeth to index lead exposure. Teeth were donated from 70% of 3329 first and second grade children from two towns near Boston. Almost all children who donated teeth (2146) were rated by their teachers on an 11-item classroom behaviour scale used by the authors to assess attention disorders. An apparent dose–response function was reported for ratings on the behaviour scale, not taking potentially confounding variables into account. After excluding various subjects for control reasons, two groups (< 10th and > 90th percentiles of non-circumpulpal dentine lead levels) were provisionally selected for further in-depth neuropsychological testing. Later, some provisionally eligible children were also excluded for various reasons, leaving 100 low-lead (< 10 ppm dentine lead) children for comparison with 58 high-lead (> 20 ppm dentine lead) children. A preliminary analysis on 39 non-lead variables showed significant differences between the low- and high-lead groups for age, maternal IQ and education, maternal age at time of birth, paternal SES, and paternal education. Some of these variables were entered as covariates along with lead into an analysis of covariance. Significant effects ($p < 0.05$) were reported for full-scale WISC-R IQ scores, for WISC-R verbal IQ scores, for 9 of 11 classroom behaviour scale items, and for several experimental measures of perceptual–motor behaviour.

Additional papers published by Needleman and coworkers report on results of the same or further analyses of the data discussed by Needleman et al. (1979). For example, a paper by Needleman (1982) provided a summary of findings from the Needleman et al. (1979) study, and Burchfiel et al. (1980) reported findings concerning EEG patterns for a subset of children from the 1979 study. Needleman (1982) also summarized results of an additional analysis of the 1979 data set, showing a downward shift across the entire cumulative frequency distribution of verbal IQ scores for high-lead subjects. Another paper, by Bellinger and Needleman (1983), provided still further follow-up analyses of the 1979 data set, focussing mainly on comparison of the low- and high-lead children's observed versus expected IQs based on their mother's IQ; regression analyses showed that IQs of children with elevated dentine lead levels (> 20 ppm) fell below those expected based on their mothers' IQs and the amount by which a child's IQ fell below the expected value increased with increasing dentine lead levels in a nonlinear fashion. Scatter plots of IQ residuals by dentine lead levels and regression analyses for the control children with dentine below 10 ppm and for high-lead children with 20 to 29.9 ppm dentine lead did not reveal significant associations between increasing Pb levels in that range and IQ residuals, in contrast to statistically significant correlations between IQ residuals and dentine lead for high-lead group children with 30 to 39.9 ppm dentine lead levels.

Reanalyses of Needleman et al. (1979) study data have been done to correct certain methodological problems with some earlier published analyses. Needleman (1984), Needleman et al. (1985), and US EPA's Office of Policy and Analysis (1984) reported that the reanalyses confirm the published findings on significant associations between elevated dentine lead levels and decrements in IQ, after correcting data calculation errors detected in earlier published analysis and using alternative model specifications incorporating better control for potentially confounding factors. The average magnitude of the full-scale IQ decrement attributable to lead was estimated in the 1979 analyses to be ~ 4 points after control for confounding factors. Based on the later reanalyses, the size of the full-scale lead effect remained about the same (i.e., around 4 points) after controlling for confounding variables. It is, however, very difficult to define quantitative dose–response relationships based on these data, beyond the statement that an average IQ decrement of about 4 points appears to be associated with lead exposure levels experienced by the high-lead group. Among that group, statistically significant IQ decrements appear to remain (after controlling for confounding variables) for children with 30 to 39.9 ppm dentine lead levels, but not for children with 20 to 29.9 ppm or lower dentine lead levels, as reported by Bellinger and Needleman (1983). Only limited data exist by which to estimate lead values likely associated with the observed IQ effects; that information points broadly toward an average PbB concentration in the 30 to 50 μg/dl range.

Bellinger et al. (1984b) later studied the academic performance of some children initially evaluated by Needleman et al. (1979). Of the 118 first and second grade children originally classified into low (< 10 ppm) and elevated ($\geq$ 20 ppm) dentine lead groups, 70 were evaluated 4 years later. Also, 71 children with midrange dentine lead levels (10.0 to 19.9 ppm) were included in the follow-up investigation. Contemporary PbB levels could not be obtained. Four types of outcome measures were assessed: (1) standardized IQ measures, e.g., most recently available scores for the Otis–Lennon Mental Ability Test, as routinely administered by the school system; (2) teacher ratings, comprising a 24-item pupil-rating scale and the same 11-item scale used by Needleman et al. (1979); (3) indices of school failure, i.e., remedial instruction or grade retention; and (4) direct observation of classroom behaviour patterns reflecting inattention, distractibility, etc. Various statistical analyses suggested that grade retention was clearly associated with past dentine lead levels; and other outcomes showed the predicted direction of effect, but mostly at p values between 0.05 and 0.15. The teacher rating scale revealed no lead effect, a finding in contrast to earlier results of Needleman et al. (1979) and a more recent replication by Yule et al. (1984).

A study of urban children in Sydney, Australia (McBride et al., 1982) involved 454 preschoolers (aged 4 to 5 y) with PbB levels of 2 to 29 μg/dl. PbB levels were evaluated at the time of neurobehavioural testing, but earlier exposure history was apparently not assessed. Using a multiple statistical comparison and Bonferroni correction to protect against study-wise error, no statistically significant differences were found between two groups with PbB levels more than one standard deviation above or below the mean (> 20 μg/dl versus < 9 μg/dl) on the Peabody Picture Vocabulary IQ Test, on Rutter's parent rating scale of hyperactivity, or on three tests of motor ability (pegboard, standing balance, and finger tapping). In one test of fine motor coordination (tracking), five-year-old boys in the higher lead group performed worse than boys in the lower lead group. In a test of gross motor skill (walking balance), results for the two age groups were conflicting. This study suffers from many methodological weaknesses and cannot be taken as providing evidence for or against an effect of low-level lead exposures in non-overtly lead intoxicated children. For example, a comparison of socioeconomic status (father's occupation and mother's education) of the study sample with the general population showed that it was higher than Bureau of Census statistics for the Australian work force as a whole. Also, there was apparently some self-selection bias due to a high proportion of professionals living near the hospital where the children were born, and certain other important demographic variables (e.g., mother's IQ) were not evaluated.

Another large-scale study (Smith et al., 1983) of tooth lead, behaviour, intelligence, and cognitive skills evaluated a general population sample of over 4000 children aged 6 to 7 years in three London boroughs. Of the 2663 children who donated shed teeth for analysis, 403 children were selected to form six groups, one each of high ($8 \mu g/g$ or more), intermediate (5 to 5.5 $\mu g/g$), and low (2.5 $\mu g/g$ or less) tooth lead levels for two socioeconomic groups (manual versus non-manual workers). Parents were intensively interviewed at home regarding parental interest and attitudes toward education and family characteristics and relationships. The early history of the child was then studied in school using tests of intelligence (WISC-R), educational attainment, attention, and other cognitive tasks. Teachers and parents completed the Conners behaviour questionnaires. Results showed that intelligence and other psychological measures were strongly related to social factors, especially social grouping. Lead level was linked to a variety of factors in the home, especially the level of cleanliness and, to a lesser extent, maternal smoking. Before correcting for confounding factors, there were significant associations between lead and full-scale IQ scores; however, upon correcting for confounding factors, there were no statistically significant associations between lead level and IQ or academic performance. Also, when rated by teachers (but not by parents), there were small, reasonably consistent (but not statistically significant) tendencies for high-lead children to show more behavioural problems after the different social covariables were taken into account statistically.

The Smith et al. (1983) study has much to recommend it: (1) a well-drawn sample of adequate size; (2) three tooth lead groupings based on well-defined classifications minimizing overlaps of exposure groupings based on whole-tooth lead values, including quality-controlled replicate analyses for the same tooth and duplicate analyses across multiple teeth from the same child; (3) PbB levels on a subset of 92 children which correlated reasonably well with tooth lead levels ($r = 0.45$); (4) cross-stratified design of social groups; (5) extensive information on social covariates and exposure sources; and (6) statistical control for potentially confounding covariates in the analyses of study results. It should also be noted that further statistical analyses of the Smith data, using tooth lead as a continuous variable or finer-grain categorization of subjects into eight tooth lead exposure groups, have recently been reported (Pocock and Ashby, 1985) to confirm no statistically significant associations between tooth lead and IQ across the entire spectrum of lead exposure levels present among the study population. Interestingly, the average full-scale IQ values for the medium- and high-lead groups in the Smith study were 2 points below the average value for the control group. Also, PbB values for subsets of the children in the medium and high groups averaged 12 to 15 μg/dl (with all but one < 30 μg/dl) upon sampling within a few months of neuropsychological testing around age six. Somewhat higher PbB values might have been obtained if sampled at earlier ages for these children (given typical peaking of blood leads seen in preschool children), but they probably would have still fallen mainly in the 15 to 30 μg/dl range.

Harvey et al. (1983, 1984) reported a study involving 189 children, average age 2.5 years and 15.5 μg/dl PbB, from the inner city of Birmingham, England. A wide range of psychometric tests, behavioural measures of activity level, and psychomotor performance were used. Blood lead made no significant contribution to IQ decrements after appropriate allowance had been made for social factors, although, consistent with findings from the Lansdown et al. (1986) study discussed below, a stronger correlation between IQ and PbB levels was found in children of manual workers ($r = -0.32$) than in children of non-manual workers ($r = +0.06$). Strengths of this study are the following: (1) a well-drawn sample; (2) extensive evaluation of 15 confounding social factors; (3) a wide range of abilities evaluated; and (4) blind evaluations. The finding of no significant associations between lead and IQ decrements at the relatively low PbB levels evaluated are consistent with the results of Smith et al. (1983), discussed above, for children in the same exposure range.

Yule et al. (1981) conducted a pilot study of effects of low-level lead exposure on 85% of a cohort of 195 children aged 6 to 12 years, whose PbB concentrations were determined nine months earlier as part of a European Economic Community survey. The PbB concentrations ranged from 7 to 32 μg/dl; 11 to 12 μg/dl; 13 to 16 μg/dl; and 17 to 32 μg/dl. The tests of achievement and intelligence were similar to those used in studies by Lansdown et al. (1974) and Needleman et al. (1979). Significant associations were found between PbB levels and decrements in IQ (full-scale IQ scores averaged ~ 7 points lower for the highest lead group), as well as lower scores on tests of reading and spelling, but not mathematics (Yule et al., 1981). These differences in performance (although reduced in magnitude) largely remained statistically significant at $p < 0.05$ after age, sex, and father's occupation were taken into account. However, other potentially confounding social factors such as parental IQ were not controlled in this study, and the investigators cautioned against interpretation of their results as evidence of relationships between lead and IQ or functioning at school without further confirmatory results after better control for social factors.

Lansdown et al. (1986) replicated their earlier pilot study (Yule et al., 1981) with 194 children ($\bar{X}$ age = 8.8 y) living in a mainly working-class area of London near a busy roadway. In this second, better designed study, a lengthy structured interview yielded data on sources of exposure, medical history, and many potentially confounding variables, including parental IQ and social factors. Analyses of covariance were used to evaluate the effects of lead and other factors on WISC-R verbal, performance, and full-scale IQ scores, as well as reading accuracy and comprehension scores, for children with low (7 to 12 μg/dl) versus elevated (13 to 24 μg/dl) PbB levels. No significant lead effect was evident even before considering social class. However, there was some suggestion of a trend in effects on IQ in the children of manual workers when compared with children of non-manual workers.

In another study, Yule and Lansdown (1983) evaluated 302 chldren ($\bar{X}$ age = 9 y) living in Leeds, England. Tests and procedures similar to those employed in the previous two studies were used and, in addition, a reaction time test was employed (Hunter et al., 1985). The Leeds children were divided, for statistical analyses of the data, by (1) social class (manual versus non-manual) and (2) blood lead level (low = 5 to 11 μg/dl; high = 12 to 26 μg/dl). As in the London replication study, no statistically significant relationships for any of the IQ or reading performance scores were found even before social class was controlled for in the statistical analyses. The high-lead children averaged nearly identical or slightly better than control subjects on several outcomes. However, small but statistically significant ($p < 0.05$) changes in reaction time (shorter for 3-s delays; longer for 12-s delays) were found and paralleled similar reaction time effects of larger magnitude found by Needleman et al. (1979) for American children with higher lead exposures. Analysis of covariance, controlling for age, revealed that the reaction-time differences between low- and high-lead children in Leeds were only significant for the younger children (aged 6 to 10 y) but not for the older children (aged 11 to 14 y). Yule et al. (this volume) have extended these findings and developed other assessments of neurobehavioural function in lead-exposed children with some interesting preliminary resutls.

Yule et al. (1984) also used three different teacher questionnaires (Needleman, Rutter, and Conners) to assess attention deficits in the same children evaluated in their earlier report (Yule et al., 1981). While there were few differences between groups on the Rutter scale, the summed scores on the Needleman questionnaire across the PbB groupings approached significance ($p = 0.096$). Three of the questionnaire items showed a significant dose–response function ("Day Dreamer", "Does not Follow Sequence of Direction", "Low Overall Functioning"). Nine of 11 items were highly correlated with children's IQ. Therefore, the Needleman questionnaire may be tapping IQ-related attention deficits as opposed to measures of conduct disorder and socially maladaptive behaviour (Yule et al., 1984). The hyperactivity factors of the Conners and Rutter scales were reported to be related to PbB levels (7 to 12 versus 13 to 32 μg/dl), but the authors noted that caution is necessary in interpreting their findings in view of the crude measures of social factors available and the differences between countries in diagnosing attention deficit disorders. Also, since the PbB values reported were determined only once (nine months before psychological testing), earlier lead exposure may not have been fully reflected in the reported PbB levels; however, even if higher earlier, the PbB values would likely have still fallen mainly in the 15 to 30 μg/dl range for the higher two quartile groups.

Two reports by Schroeder and colleagues (Schroeder et al., 1985; Schroeder and Hawk, 1987) are of particular importance for the issue of lead's effects on children's cognitive functioning. Although these studies dealt with children identified through lead-screening programmes or who were potentially at risk for elevated lead exposure, actual PbB levels in these children were close to or not much higher than levels in the above general population studies. Schroeder et al. (1985) evaluated 104 lower SES children in North Carolina, ages 10 months to 6.5 years. About half of the children (aged < 30 months) were tested on the Bayley Scales of Mental Development; the rest of the subjects (age > 30 months) were tested on the Stanford–Binet Intelligence Scale. Several other variables were also assessed, including Caldwell and Bradley (1979) HOME scores and parental IQ, SES, education, and employment. Venous blood samples obtained on the day of testing ranged from 6 to 59 μg/dl ($\bar{X} \approx 30\ \mu$g/dl). Statistical analysis of the data involved a form of hierarchical backward stepwise regression. Lead was found to be a significant ($p < 0.01$) source of effect on IQ scores in these children after controlling for SES, HOME score, maternal IQ, and other social factors. SES was the only other variable to reach statistical significance ($p < 0.001$); other variables apparently failed to reach significance because of collinearity with SES. A corollary study of the same children by Milar et al. (1981) found no association between lead exposure and hyperactivity. Fifty of the children were re-examined 5 years later, at which time all PbB levels were < 30 μg/dl. In addition to re-evaluating the children with the Stanford–Binet IQ test, the investigators repeated SES and maternal IQ (but not HOME) measurements. Although the 5-year follow-up IQ scores were negatively correlated with both contemporary and initial PbB levels, the lead effect was not significant after covariates (especially SES) were included in the regression model. It is interesting to note also that the correlation between maternal and child IQ was only ~0.06 for children with initial PbB levels of 31 to 56 μg/dl, but returned to a nearly normal value of 0.45 after 5 years, when PbB levels had dropped. Similar findings were reported by Perino and Ernhart (1974) and Bellinger and Needleman (1983), and have been used to argue that an environmental factor (i.e., lead) disrupts the normal mother–child IQ correlation of ~0.50. Thus, this Schroeder et al. (1985) finding provides further, indirect evidence of lead's disruptive effect on children's cognitive functioning at PbB levels in the range of ~30 to 60 μg/dl.

Schroeder and Hawk (1987) replicated the above study with 75 black children from North Carolina, all of low SES and aged 3 to 7 years. Blood lead levels averaged 21 μg/dl (range: 6 to 47 μg/dl). Backward stepwise multivariate regression analysis revealed a highly significant relationship between contemporary PbB level and IQ ($p < 0.0008$); the effect was nearly as striking ($p < 0.002$) whether maximum or mean PbB values (from health department records) were used. No other covariate achieved significance at $p = 0.05$ in this analysis, although maternal IQ was closest. SES was not a significant covariate in this study because SES was uniformly low. (Further analyses showed HOME scores to be significantly correlated with PbB levels and to be collinear with maternal IQ and SES.) The effect of PbB level on IQ appeared to extend linearly across the entire range of PbB concentrations. In fact, 78% of the subjects had PbB levels below 30 μg/dl. More details on the Schroeder studies are provided elsewhere in these proceedings.

In another study discussed elsewhere in this volume, Fulton et al. (1987) evaluated cognitive abilities and educational attainment in a population of school-age children from central Edinburgh, Scotland. The geometric mean average PbB level for the 501 children in the study sample was 11.5 μg/dl (range 3.3–34.0 μg/dl). Multiple regression analyses indicated significant relationships between log-transformed PbB levels and composite scores on the British Ability Scales and between PbB levels and attainment test scores for quantitative and reading skills, with allowance for 33 possible confounding variables. Grouping the subjects by PbB levels showed a clear dose–response relationship without any evident threshold down to the lowest subgroup mean PbB level of 5.6 μg/dl.

Silva *et al.* (1988) investigated cognitive development and behaviour problems in 579 11-year-old children in Dunedin, New Zealand. Higher SES groups were significantly over-represented in this sample, but the correlation between PbB levels and SES was near zero. The mean PbB level at age 11 was 11.1 μg/dl (SD = 4.91). No significant effects on IQ were evident from an analysis of WISC-R scores. Regression analyses and multiple correlations were performed on scores from a reading ability test, the Rutter parent and teacher questionnaires, and other assessments of children's inattention and hyperactivity derived from parent and teacher reports. The contribution of PbB levels to the explained variance for the reading ability scores was non-significant. However, five of the six remaining assessments of children's behaviour showed significant increases in the amount of explained variance when the PbB variable was added. Although PbB accounted for only 0.8 to 1.2% of the additional variance, the results nonetheless indicate some association between lead exposure and small but significant adverse effects on behaviour in older children, even after allowance for certain background factors (e.g., maternal verbal ability, maternal depression, a composite index of social disadvantage). Another report by Silva *et al.* (1986) noted that some of the children in the Dunedin pilot study had had significant exposure to lead through paint-stripping activities in the home. Although only two subjects had PbB levels above 30 μg/dl at the time of testing, this information highlights the need for earlier and more precise histories of long-term lead exposure for accurate interpretation of the Dunedin findings.

The general population studies reviewed here do not individually provide definitive evidence for or against neuropsychological deficits being associated with low body lead burdens in non-overtly lead-intoxicated children representative of general paediatric populations. However, the overall pattern of results certainly substantiates such an association, with two recent studies (Schroeder and Hawk, 1987; Fulton *et al.*, 1987) especially indicating a highly significant linear relationship between measures of IQ and PbB levels over a broad range (6–47 μg/dl and 3–34 μg/dl, respectively). In the Schroeder and Hawk study this effect was almost equally as strong regardless of whether contemporary, past maximum, or mean PbB levels were used in the analysis. Because the subjects were all black children of uniformly low socioeconomic status, SES was not a significant covariate in the analysis. It is possible that SES and lead exposure interact such that IQ is affected by PbB at lower SES levels but not at higher SES levels (*cf.* Schroeder *et al.*, 1985). Findings of stronger correlations between IQ and PbB levels in children of manual working class fathers (Harvey *et al.*, 1983, 1984; Yule and Lansdown, 1983; Lansdown *et al.*, 1986) are consistent with this hypothesis (*cf.* Winneke and Kraemer, 1984). If true, this interactive relationship would suggest that lower SES places children at greater risk for deleterious effects of low-level lead exposure on cognitive ability. However, as results from Schroeder *et al.* (1985) and Schroeder and Hawk (1987) indicate, other variables such as HOME scores and maternal IQ may covary with SES. Other work (e.g., Milar *et al.*, 1980; Dietrich *et al.*, 1985) points to the home environment as a significant predictor of lead exposure. This close relationship between SES, quality of home environment, and lead exposure suggests that low SES may not be the sole determiner of increased risk for cognitive impairment. (See also the discussion by Bellinger *et al.*, 1986b, and elsewhere in this volume.) Further research is needed to disentangle the relative contributions of these variables to the neurotoxic effects of lead.

In regard to the magnitude of lead effects on IQ, the Needleman analyses point toward full-scale IQ deficits of about 4 points and other neurobehavioural deficits in American children being associated with lead exposures resulting in dentine lead values above 20 to 30 ppm and likely average PbB values in the 30 to 50 μg/dl range. The report of recent analyses by Schroeder *et al.* (1985) further supports this conclusion, even after the major influence of SES was allowed for in the analyses. However, their findings indicate that the effect of PbB on IQ could not be detected five years after the original assessment. A follow-up by Bellinger *et al.* (1984b) of the children studied by Needleman *et al.* (1979) suggests that other measures of classroom performance may show long-term effects of early lead exposure more effectively than IQ measures (see also Silva *et al.*, 1988). Shaheen (1984) has also questioned the sensitivity of IQ scores and has suggested that the variability of outcomes of studies of lead's effects on neuropsychological functioning in children may relate to differences in the ages at which children are subjected to toxic lead exposures.

For the most part, the remaining general population studies reviewed in this section report a lack of statistically significant effects on IQ or other neuropsychological measures. Most of those studies found slightly lower IQ scores for higher-lead exposure groups than for low-lead control groups before correcting for confounding variables, but the differences were typically reduced to 1 to 2 IQ points and were non-significant (usually even at $p < 0.10$) upon correction for confounding factors. The following conclusions may be stated about these latter results: (1) they tend to suggest relatively minimal effects of lead on IQ in general populations, especially in comparison to much larger effects of other factors (e.g., social variables), at the exposure levels evaluated in the studies (PbB values mainly in the 15 to 30 μg/dl range); and (2) they are not incompatible with other findings of significant lead effects on IQ at higher average PbB levels (≥ 30 μg/dl).

Exceptions to the general pattern noted above are beginning to emerge and warrant comment here. Specifically, Schroeder and Hawk's findings for a population of low-SES US children complement those of Fulton *et al.* for a relatively more affluent population in Edinburgh. The average and range of PbB levels in the Edinburgh study were somewhat lower than those in the Schroeder and Hawk study: 11.5 μg/dl (3.3–34.0 μg/dl) in Edinburgh versus 21 μg/dl (6–47 μg/dl) in North Carolina. Even so, Fulton *et al.* reported significant lead-related effects on covariate-adjusted scores of cognitive ability and educational attainment. Since only 2% of the Edinburgh study sample

73

had PbB levels above 25 µg/dl and since a dose–response analysis showed no evident threshold (down to an average PbB level of 5.6 µg/dl) for either ability or attainment scores, these findings, in conjunction with the results of Schroeder and Hawk, point to notable deficits in cognitive performance at PbB levels well below 30 µg/dl and possibly extending to levels below 10 µg/dl. However, as with other cross-sectional studies, a complete history of past blood lead levels was not obtained, and so the possibility remains that a higher degree of lead exposure at some earlier period of development (and not reflected by contemporary PbB levels) was responsible for the outcomes measured in these studies. Also, the findings of altered reaction time patterns by Hunter et al. (1985), which parallel those reported by Needleman at higher exposure levels, are notable and appear to argue for probable effects of lead on attention or vigilance functions at levels extending below 30 µg/dl and, possibly, down to as low as 15 to 20 µg/dl.

Other recent cross-sectional studies of neurobehavioural performance in general populations of children are described elsewhere in this volume by Cludyts, Hansen et al., and Vivoli et al. These studies also point to deficits in neurobehavioural function at relatively low levels of lead exposure, primarily reflected by tooth lead concentration as an indicator of cumulative lead exposure.

Smelter area studies

Smelter studies evaluated children with elevated lead exposures associated with residence in cities or elsewhere in close proximity to lead-emitting smelters. Most of the early studies, conducted in the 1970s, found mixed results even though evaluating children with PbB levels typically in excess of 30 µg/dl. Because of methodological weaknesses, however, most of the early studies must be viewed as inconclusive. For example, in an early study of this type, Lansdown et al. (1974) reported a relationship between PbB level in children and the distance they lived from lead-processing facilities, but no relationship between PbB level and mental functioning. However, only a minority of the lead-exposed cohort had PbB levels markedly differing from control subjects with elevated PbB levels (< 40 µg/dl), and the study did not adequately control for important confounding factors.

In another study, Landrigan et al. (1975) found the lead-exposed children living near an El Paso, Texas, smelter scored significantly lower than matched controls on measures of performance IQ and finger–wrist tapping. The control children in this study were, however, not well matched by age or sex to the lead-exposed group, although the results remained statistically significant after adjustments were made for age differences. In contrast, NcNeil and Ptasnik (1975) found little evidence of lead-associated decrements in cognitive abilities in another sample of children living near the same El Paso smelter. These children were generally comparable medically and psychologically to matched controls living elsewhere in the same city, but for direct effects of lead (PbB level, free erythrocyte protoporphyrin levels, and X-ray findings). An extensive critique of these two El Paso studies was performed by an

74

expert committee (see Muir, 1975), which concluded that no reliable conclusions could be drawn from either of the published studies in view of various methodological and other problems affecting their conduct and statistical analyses.

A study by Ratcliffe (1977) of children living near a battery factory in Manchester, England found no significant associations between PbB levels sampled at two years of age ($28 \mu g/dl$ versus $44 \mu g/dl$ in low- versus high-lead groups) and testing done at age five on the Griffiths Mental Development Scales, the Frostig Developmental Test of Visual Perception, a pegboard test, or a behavioural questionnaire. The scores, although not very different in magnitude, were somewhat better for the low-lead exposure children than for the higher exposure group. The small sample size (23 low-lead and 24 high-lead children), inadequate control for parental IQ, and the failure to repeat PbB assays at age five weaken this study. Variations in PbB levels occurring after age two among control children may have lessened exposure differences between the low- and high-lead groups, and larger sample sizes would have better allowed for detection of any lead effects present.

More recent smelter studies provide assessments that accord greater attention to control for potentially confounding factors, and many also assessed larger samples of children, allowing for more power to detect lead effects. Two studies by Winneke and colleagues, the first a pilot study (Winneke et al., 1982) and the second an extended study (Winneke et al., 1983), used tooth lead analyses analogous to some studies described above. In the pilot study, incisor teeth were donated by 458 children aged 7 to 10 years in Duisburg, Germany, an industrial city with airborne lead concentrations of 1.5 to $2.0 \mu g/m^3$. Two extreme exposure groups were formed, a low-lead group with $2.4 \mu g/g$ mean tooth lead level ($n = 26$) and a high-lead group with $7 \mu g/g$ mean tooth lead level ($n = 16$). These groups were matched for age, sex, and father's occupational status. The two groups did not differ significantly on confounding covariates, except that the high-lead group showed more perinatal risk factors. Parental IQ and quality of the home environment were not among the 52 covariables examined. The authors found a marginally significant decrease ($p < 0.10$) of 5 to 7 IQ points and a significant decrease in perceptual–motor integration ($p < 0.05$), but no significant differences in hyperactivity as measured by the Conners Teachers' Questionnaire. As with the Yule et al. (1981) study, the inadequacy of statistical or other control for background social variables and parental IQ (as well as group differences in perinatal factors) weaken this study; the investigators cautioned against interpretation of their results as evidence for low-level lead effects in the absence of further, confirmatory results from larger, better controlled studies.

In their second study, Winneke et al. (1983) evaluated 115 children ($\bar{X}$ age: 9.4 y) living in the lead smelter town of Stolberg, Germany. Tooth lead ($\bar{X}$: 6.16 ppm, range: 2.0 to 38.5 ppm) and PbB levels ($\bar{X}$: $13.4 \mu g/dl$; range: 6.8 to $33.8 \mu g/dl$) were significantly correlated ($r = 0.47$; $p < 0.001$) for the children studied. Using stepwise multiple regression analysis, the authors found significant ($p < 0.05$) or marginally significant ($p < 0.10$) associations between tooth lead and measures of perceptual–motor integration, reaction-time performance, and four behavioural rating dimensions, including distractibility, even after controlling for age, sex, duration of labour at birth, and socio-hereditary background. However, the proportion of explained variance due to lead never exceeded 6% for any of these outcomes, and no significant association was found between tooth lead and WISC verbal IQ after the effects of socio-hereditary background were eliminated.

A third study by Winneke et al. (1984) evaluated neuropsychological functioning and neurophysiological parameters for 122 children (aged 6 to 7 y) living in the Nordenham, FRG area. Performance on various neuropsychological tests (shortened form of the Hamburg–Wechsler IQ test; reaction-behaviour and reaction-time tests, etc.) was evaluated in relation to both concurrently sampled PbB values ($\bar{X} = 8 \, \mu g/dl$; max. $= 23 \, \mu g/dl$) and umbilical cord PbB levels (max. $= 31 \, \mu g/dl$). A variety of potentially confounding factors (such as socio-hereditary variables, pre- and postnatal risk factors, etc.) were also assessed and taken into account in a series of stepwise multiple regression analyses in which the effects of confounding factors were successively eliminated and the lead effects then checked for significance. No significant associations (at $p < 0.05$) were found between either umbilical cord or current PbB levels and verbal, performance, or total IQ scores estimated from the Hamburg–Wechsler subtests (only the correlation for performance IQ with current PbB level reached $p < 0.10$). On the other hand, much larger and highly significant correlations were found between socio-hereditary factors and all three types of IQ scores. The investigators remarked on the heavy dependence of the IQ measurements on the social environment and noted that, as in their prior large-scale study (Winneke et al., 1983), it was not possible to convincingly show a lead-dependent decrease in intelligence. Nor were any lead effects found on the Goettinger shape reproduction test of psychomotor performance or for various reaction-time measures. Only in the case of reaction behaviour, as indexed by increased errors on the Wiener (Vienna) serial stimulus reaction test, were significant deficits in neuropsychological functioning detected at the low exposure levels (PbB < 25 to $30 \, \mu g/dl$) evaluated in this study. Certain statistically significant effects on electrophysiological measures of neurophysiological functioning were also observed. Retesting of 76 of the Nordenham children at age 9, with PbB levels approximately equal to those measured 3 years earlier, indicated persisting lead-related deficits in performance on the Wiener reaction test (see Winneke et al., this volume).

Hatzakis et al. (this volume) also conducted neuropsychological testing on more than 500 children living near a lead smelter in Lavrion, Greece, and found impairments in WISC-R IQ scores and reaction performance scores, including performance on the Wiener reaction device. These effects were significantly associated with PbB levels after controlling for 17 covariates, including parental IQ, in a multiple regression model. Blood lead concentrations ranged from 7.4 to $63.9 \, \mu g/dl$ and averaged 23.7. Grouping of subjects by PbB levels showed dose–response relationships for IQ as well as reaction performance scores, with no evident threshold for reaction performance effects.

The above smelter area studies, particularly the more recent, better conducted studies of populations with average PbB levels well below 30 μg/dl, supplement findings from general population studies of neurobehavioural function in children. Although the Hatzakis study provides additional evidence of IQ deficits in children with PbB levels < 30 μg/dl, the strongest effects to emerge from these studies appear to be in the area of reaction performance. As such, these findings are consistent with the results of Hunter *et al.* (1985) and Needleman *et al.* (1979) and point to lead-induced neurobehavioural effects in children at PbB levels below 30 μg/dl, possibly extending to as low as 15 μg/dl.

Studies of neuropsychiatrically disordered children

Rather than starting with a known lead-exposed population and attempting to discover evidence of neurobehavioural dysfunction, a number of studies have first identified a population with some recognized disorder and then looked for evidence of elevated lead exposure. For example, a series of studies by David *et al.* (1974; 1976a,b; 1977; 1979a,b; 1982a,b; 1983; 1985) measured lead levels in diagnosed hyperkinetic children and showed an association between hyperactivity and elevated lead levels. However, whether a disorder such as hyperactivity is the effect or the cause of elevated lead exposure is difficult to resolve. It is possible, for example, that hyperactive children might ingest more lead than normal children because of a greater incidence of pica or because they stir up more dust-borne lead by their activity. David *et al.* (1977) reported that PbB levels of hyperactive children with a probable aetiology of an organic nature were lower than those of children with no apparent cause (other than lead). This finding suggests that hyperactivity does not necessarily result in elevated lead exposure, but it does not rule out the possibility of a third factor causing both hyperactivity and elevated PbB levels (see discussion of Gittelman and Eskenazi, 1983, below). Also, a problem common to the studies in question is the lack of adequate information on the children's past lead exposure, particularly during preschool years when children tend to be at greatest risk for higher exposure levels. As David *et al.* (1976a) have acknowledged, it is difficult to establish an aetiological relationship between lead and behavioural disorders on the basis of retrospective estimations of lead exposure.

Another study by David *et al.* (1983) appeared to obviate some correlational approach problems by experimentally manipulating body lead levels, i.e., by reducing PbB concentrations through the administration of a chelating agent, penicillamine. The objective was to determine if decreases in body lead burden would be accompanied by improvements in children's hyperactive behaviour, and in short, this was essentially the conclusion drawn by David and his colleagues. In addition, the study compared the effect of the chelating agent with a therapeutic drug of known efficacy, methylphenidate, and found the two treatments to be roughly equivalent in reducing symptoms of hyperactivity. Although this study was in many respects well designed and executed, certain problems nevertheless cloud its interpretation. As noted by Needleman and Bellinger (1984), the number of subjects per treatment group was rather

77

limited (maximum of 31) and quite unbalanced due in part to a high and disproportionate subject attrition rate. Subjects were particularly prone to drop out of the placebo group, and this imbalance was exacerbated by a 'chance preponderance' of subjects assigned to the penicillamine treatment and by later reassignment of some placebo and methylphenidate subjects to the penicillamine group. Questions also arise concerning the appropriateness of the statistical treatment of data by David et al. (1983). For example, multivariate analysis of variance (MANOVA) would seem to be more appropriate than separate ANOVAs and multiple t-tests applied to the various outcome measures used to assess the children's behaviour. Use of MANOVA would also have helped alleviate the problem of regression toward the mean, which in this case may have created the false impression that 'improvements' in behaviour, i.e., changes toward more normal behaviour, were due to an effect of the treatment. Rutter (1983, p. 313) has also noted that David's multiple group comparisons are not as convincing as an analysis that would utilize individual PbB values and behaviour scores (presumably, multivariate regression analysis). Finally, as David et al. (1983) themselves point out, it is clear that lead could be only one of several aetiological factors in the causation of hyperkinesis or attention deficit disorders in children and that, at best, their findings pertain only to recognized hyperactive children, not to the general population.

An attempt by Gittelman and Eskenazi (1983) to replicate earlier work by David et al. (1974, 1977) was only partly supportive of the latter's findings. A large group of hyperactive children ($n = 103$) showed a trend ($p = 0.06$) toward higher chelated lead levels in their urine, but a clear-cut ($p = 0.02$) elevation in lead levels was evident only in paired comparisons with 33 non-hyperkinetic siblings. As Gittelman and Eskenazi (1983) noted, this finding raises the question of why the hyperactive children had higher lead levels than their siblings, given that they shared the same water, air, and home environment. The possibility of a third factor, e.g., a metabolic difference that might affect the ability to excrete lead as well as the occurrence of hyperactivity, cannot be dismissed.

A study of 98 Swedish children with various minor neuropsychiatric disorders (e.g., perceptual–motor dysfunctions, speech disorders, attention-deficit problems) found no correlation between the children's disorders and their tooth lead levels (Gillberg et al., 1982). However, comparing the 10 highest and 10 lowest lead-burdened children did reveal a significant difference in a clinical measure of their mean reaction times.

Youroukos et al. (1978) compared PbB as well as ALA-D values of 60 Greek children with mental retardation of unknown aetiology against 30 mentally retarded children with a known aetiology and 30 normal children. The average values of the mentally retarded children with unknown aetiology were significantly different from both the other groups in two regards: their mean PbB level was higher (30 μg/dl versus 21 μg/dl in both control groups) and, in 24 patients with elevated ($\geq 40\,\mu$g/dl) PbB levels, ALA-D activity was significantly lower. Although pica was noted to be common in both groups of mentally retarded children, no child in the study was known to have ever been lead-poisoned.

78

Work in Scotland has provided information tending to link prenatal lead exposures to the later development of mental retardation. Beattie *et al.* (1975) identified 77 retarded children and 77 normal children matched on age, sex, and geography. The residence during the gestation of the subject was determined, and a first-flush morning sample of tap water was obtained from the residence. Of 64 matched pairs, no normal children were found to come from homes served with water containing high lead levels ($> 800 \mu$g/L), whereas 11 of the 64 retarded children came from homes served with such high-lead water. The authors concluded that pregnancy in a home with high lead in the water supply increases by a factor of 1.7 the risk of bearing a retarded child. In follow-up work, Moore *et al.* (1977) obtained lead values from blood samples drawn during the second week of life from children studied by Beattie *et al.* The samples were obtained as part of routine screening for phenylketonuria and kept stored on filter paper. Blood samples were available for 41 of the retarded and 36 of the normal children in the original study by Beattie *et al.* (1975). PbB concentrations in the retarded children were significantly higher than values measured in normal children: the mean for retardates was $1.23 \pm 0.43 \mu$mol/L ($25.5 \pm 8.9 \mu$g/dl) and for normals was $1.0 \pm 0.38 \mu$mol/L ($20.9 \pm 7.9 \mu$g/dl). The difference in PbB levels was significant ($p = 0.02$) by the Mann–Whitney test.

These latter two studies suggest that fetal lead exposure during the critical period of brain development may cause perturbations in brain organization that are expressed later in mental retardation syndromes, and they raise for careful scrutiny the issue of postnatal risks associated with intrauterine exposure to lead. Long-term prospective studies of the type described later are beginning to produce results which address that issue.

Studies of association of neuropsychological effects and hair lead levels

Several studies have reported significant associations between hair lead levels and behavioural or cognitive testing endpoints (Pihl and Parkes, 1977; Hole *et al.*, 1979; Hansen *et al.*, 1980; Capel *et al.*, 1981; Ely *et al.*, 1981; Thatcher *et al.*, 1982; Marlowe *et al.*, 1982, 1983, 1985; Marlowe and Errera, 1982). Measures of hair lead are easily contaminated by external exposure and are generally questionable in terms of accurately reflecting internal body burdens (see Chapter 9 of US EPA, 1986a). Such data, therefore, cannot be credibly used to evaluate relationships between absorbed lead and nervous system effects, and they are not discussed further here.

ELECTROPHYSIOLOGICAL STUDIES OF LEAD EFFECTS IN CHILDREN

In addition to psychometric and behavioural approaches, electrophysiological studies of lead neurotoxicity in non-overtly lead-intoxicated children have been conducted. One such study (Thatcher *et al.*, 1984) reported significant effects on various measures of auditory and visual evoked potentials in lead-exposed children, but the only measure of lead exposure was hair lead, which, as previously noted, is not a suitable index of lead exposure.

Burchfiel et al. (1980) used computer-assisted spectral analysis of a standard EEG examination on 41 children from the Needleman et al. (1979) study and reported significant EEG spectrum differences in percentages of alpha and low-frequency delta activity in spontaneous EEGs of the high-lead children. Percentages of alpha and delta frequency EEG activity and results for several psychometric and behavioural testing variables (e.g., WISC-R full-scale IQ and verbal IQ, reaction time under varying delay, etc.) for the same children were then employed as input variables (or 'features') in direct and stepwise discriminant analyses. The separation determined by these analyses for combined psychological and EEG variables ($p < 0.005$) was reported to be strikingly better than the separation of low-lead from high-lead children using either psychological ($p < 0.041$) or EEG ($p < 0.079$) variables alone. Unfortunately, no dentine lead or PbB values were reported for the specific children from the Needleman et al. (1979) study who underwent the EEG evaluations reported by Burchfiel et al. (1980). Lead-exposure levels associated with the observed EEG effects would appear likely to fall within the same broad 30 to 50 µg/dl PbB range estimated earlier for the Needleman IQ deficit observations.

Guerit et al. (1981) examined 79 11-year-old children attending three different schools near a lead smelter and presenting PbB levels up to 44 µg/dl (averaging less than 30 µg/dl). Children from two distant urban and rural schools served as controls. A neurophysiological function score for each child was based on measures of EEGs, visual evoked potentials, brainstem auditory evoked potentials, and eye movements. Neurophysiological scores were negatively correlated ($p < 0.05$ by Spearman rank correlation coefficient) with PbB and FEP levels for the children from one of the smelter area schools, but the authors attributed this finding to the inclusion of four children who were left-handed or suffering from external ear pathology. Chi-square tests of neurophysiological scores as a function of PbB or FEP groupings based on the total study population were all non-significant. Note that comparatively low-power non-parametric statistical tests were employed in this study because of the qualitative or ordinal nature of the data. However, the use of more detailed quantitative measures of neurophysiological function would have enabled the investigators to employ more powerful parametric statistics, with possibly different outcomes from their analyses.

The relationship between low-level lead exposure and neurobehavioural function (including electrophysiological responses) in children aged 13 to 75 months was extensively explored in another study, conducted by the University of North Carolina and the US Environmental Protection Agency. Psychometric evaluation revealed a significant lead-related IQ decrement at the time of initial evaluation (Schroeder et al., 1985), as noted previously. No relationship between PbB and hyperactive behaviour (as indexed by standardized playroom measures and parent–teacher rating scales) was observed in these children (Milar et al., 1981). On the other hand, electro-physiological assessments, including analyses of low cortical potentials during sensory conditioning (Otto et al., 1981) and EEG spectra (Benignus et al., 1981), did provide evidence of lead CNS effects in the same children. A significant linear relationship between PbB (ranging from 6 to 59 μg/dl) and slow wave voltage during conditioning trials was observed (Otto et al., 1981). Analyses of quadratic and cubic trends, moreover, did not reveal any evidence of a threshold for this effect. The slope of the PbB × slow wave voltage function, however, varied systematically with age. No effect of PbB on EEG power spectra or coherence measures was observed, but the relative amplitude of synchronized EEG between left and right hemispheres (gain spectra) increased relative to PbB levels (Benignus et al., 1981). A significant cubic trend for gain between the left and right parietal lobes was found with a major inflection point at 15 μg/dl. This finding suggests that EEG gain is altered at PbB levels as low as 15 μg/dl, although the clinical and functional significance of this measure has not been established.

A follow-up study of slow cortical potentials and EEG spectra in a subset (28 children aged 35 to 93 months) of the original sample was carried out two years later (Otto et al., 1982). Slow wave voltage during sensory conditioning again varied as a linear function of blood lead, even though the mean lead level had declined by 11 μg/dl (from 32.5 μg/dl to 21.2 μg/dl). Although the EEG gain effect did not persist, the similarity of slow wave voltage results obtained at initial and follow-up assessments suggests that the observed alterations in this parameter of CNS function were persistent, despite a significant decrease in the mean PbB level during the two-year interval.

In a five-year follow-up study on a subset of the same children, Otto et al. (1985) found that slow wave voltage varied as a function of current PbB level during active conditioning, but not during the passive conditioning test used in earlier studies. In the passive test, a tone was paired with a short blackout of a silent cartoon. The active test was similar except that children pressed a button to terminate the blackout and resume the cartoon. Although the brain response elicited by the active test is greater than that produced by the passive test, the active test cannot be performed reliably by children under five years of age.

In addition to the experimental conditioning tests, Otto et al. (1985) used two clinically validated measures of sensory function, the pattern-reversal visual evoked potential (PREP) and the brainstem auditory evoked potential (BAEP). Exploratory analysis of PREPs revealed increased amplitude and decreased latency of certain components as a linear function of original PbB levels. Although these results were contrary to predictions, the findings are consistent with the results of Winneke et al. (1984), who found an association between increased PbB levels and decreased latency in the primary positive component of PREPs in children. BAEP results of the five-year follow-up study also indicated significant associations between original PbB levels and increased latencies of two components (waves III and V), indicative of auditory nerve conduction slowing.

Otto and his coworkers (Otto, 1985; Robinson et al., 1985) also reported results of a replication study with an independent group of children 4 to 7 years old; PbB levels ranged from 6 to 47 μg/dl at the time of testing.

Psychometric data from this study (Schroeder and Hawk, 1987) have been reviewed above. Sensory conditioning was limited to the passive test due to the age range of the children. Contrary to earlier findings (Otto *et al.*, 1981, 1982), slow wave voltage did not vary with PbB levels. Differences between the two groups studied, however, may have contributed to the discordant results. Children in the earlier studies were somewhat younger (1 to 6 versus 3 to 7 years) and were exposed by different routes (secondary occupational exposure versus lead paint and contaminated soil) than children in the replication study (see review by Otto, 1985). More recent analyses of these slow wave data and their implications, as well as other results, are discussed by Otto elsewhere in this volume.

Results from Otto's replication study also indicated that hearing threshold, a reflection of peripheral auditory system function, increased directly with lead levels. Although hearing threshold did not vary with blood lead level in the five-year follow-up study (Otto *et al.*, 1985), this finding bears further investigation in view of other reports suggesting impaired auditory processing in lead-exposed children (de la Burde and Choate, 1975; Needleman *et al.*, 1979); and in fact, additional new analyses reported elsewhere in this volume by Otto and by Schwartz and Otto (1987) provide further evidence for lead-induced auditory system effects.

In summary, these electrophysiological studies provide emerging evidence for lead-related effects on CNS function in children at PbB levels considerably below 30 μg/dl, but inconsistent findings across studies require clarification. Linear dose–response relations have been observed in slow wave voltage during conditioning (Otto *et al.*, 1981, 1982, 1985), BAEP latency (Otto *et al.*, 1985), PREP latency (Otto *et al.*, 1985; Winneke *et al.*, 1984), and PREP amplitude and direction of effect varied across studies. Sensory evoked potentials, in particular, hold considerable promise as sensitive, clinically valid nervous system measures unaffected by social factors that tend to confound traditional psychometric measures (Halliday and McDonald, 1981; Prasher *et al.*, 1981). BAEPs, for instance, are not altered by changes in attention or level of consciousness. Reliable BAEPs can be recorded in (sedated) children between the ages of one and five, the most vulnerable period for lead poisoning as well as the most difficult period for most types of neurobehavioural testing. The current electrophysiological evidence concerning lead exposure and brain function in children, however, is too fragmentary to draw any firm conclusions. The use of evoked potential measures in prospective paediatric lead studies would provide a useful adjunct to other neurobehavioural tests and would help to better establish any neurobehavioural threshold for lead toxicity.

The adverse effects of lead on peripheral nerve function in children remain to be considered. Lead-induced peripheral neuropathies, although often seen in adults after prolonged exposures, are rarely noted in children. Several articles (Anku and Harris, 1974; Erenberg *et al.*, 1974; Seto and Freeman, 1964), however, describe case histories of children with lead-induced peripheral neuropathies, as indexed by electromyography, assessment of nerve conduction velocity, and observation of other overt neurological signs, such as tremor and wrist or foot drop. Frank neuropathic effects have been observed at PbB levels of 60 to 80 μg/dl (Erenberg *et al.*, 1974). In one case study

(Seto and Freeman, 1964), signs indicative of peripheral neuropathy were reported to be associated with PbB values of 30 µg/dl; however, lead lines in long bones suggested probable past exposures leading to peak PbB levels at least as high as 40 to 60 µg/dl and probably in excess of 60 µg/dl (based on the data of Betts et al., 1973). In all these case studies, some, if not complete, recovery of affected motor functions was reported after treatment for lead poisoning. A tentative association has also been hypothesized between sickle cell disease and increased risk of peripheral neuropathy as a consequence of childhood lead exposure. Half of the cases reported (10 out of 20) involved inner-city black children, several with sickle cell anaemia (Anku and Harris, 1974; Lampert and Schochet, 1968; Seto and Freeman, 1964; Imbus et al., 1978). In summary, evidence exists for frank peripheral neuropathy in children, and such neuropathy can be associated with PbB levels at least as low as 60 µg/dl and, possibly, as low as 40 to 60 µg/dl.

Further evidence for lead-induced peripheral nerve dysfunction in children is provided by two studies by Feldman et al. (1973a,b, 1977) of inner city children and from a study by Landrigan et al. (1976) of children living close to a smelter in Idaho. No clearly abnormal conduction velocities were observed, although a statistically significant negative correlation was found between peroneal NCV and PbB levels ($r = -0.38$, $p < 0.02$ by one-tailed t-test). These results, therefore, provide evidence for significant slowing of nerve conduction velocity (and, presumably, for advancing peripheral neuropathy as a function of increased PbB levels), but do not allow clear statements regarding a threshold for pathological slowing of NCV.

In a recent study mentioned earlier, Winneke et al. (1984) evaluated neurophysiological functions as well as neuropsychological performance in children from Nordenham, FRG. Results from a standard neurological examination and sensory nerve conduction velocities of the radial and median nerves were analysed in relation to concurrent PbB values and umbilical cord PbB levels sampled approximately six years earlier. Contrary to expectations, increasing conduction velocities for radial and median nerves were found to be significantly associated with current PbB levels (at $p < 0.01$ and <0.10, respectively). As noted above, visual evoked potentials showed a significantly decreased latency in one component, which suggested more rapid conduction in the visual pathway, consistent with the peripheral nerve conduction findings. Somatosensory evoked potentials showed no significant effect; nor were associations found between any of the electrophysiological measures and cord PbB levels or any of a number of socio-hereditary background variables (the latter of which were strongly related to neuropsychologic outcome results).

The lead-associated increases in nerve conduction observed by Winneke et al. (1984) for children with PbB levels below 25 to 30 µg/dl differ from previously noted findings of slowed NCVs being associated with increasing PbB values above 30 µg/dl. However, the apparently paradoxical findings were noted by the investigators as being consistent with those of Englert (1978), who similarly found an increase in the motor NCV of the median nerve among lead-exposed children in Nordenham. Davis and Svendsgaard (1987a) have discussed these and other examples of 'U-shaped' dose–response

83

relationships for lead as well as other toxic agents. However, as Winneke *et al.* (1984) have noted, these findings still require experimental confirmation before a bi-phasic effect of lead on peripheral nervous functions can be assumed. See additional discussion of these results and related findings by Winneke and colleagues elsewhere in these proceedings.

EFFECTS OF LOW-LEVEL LEAD EXPOSURE ON EARLY DEVELOPMENT

Prospective studies of human populations

That lead can affect the survival and development of the fetus and infant has been known since at least the 1800s (Paul, 1860). Indeed, around the turn of the century, lead was routinely sold as an abortifacient (Hall and Cantab, 1905). Studies of experimental animals have also amply demonstrated lead's gametotoxic, embryotoxic, and teratogenic properties (US EPA, 1986a). Most of this evidence, however, has involved relatively high levels of exposure, at least by today's standards, and may have been confounded by factors such as nutritional deficits. Also, the relevance of findings from animal studies, e.g., malformations in chicks (Gilani, 1973a,b), is not always clear. Some studies have pointed to a number of effects in humans at ambient exposure levels, including decreased birth weight, shortened gestation, and stillbirths (Fahim *et al.*, 1976; Nordstrom *et al.*, 1979; Khera *et al.*, 1980). But other investigations have not supported these findings (Clark, 1977; Alexander and Delves, 1981; Roels *et al.*, 1978).

One of the difficulties in drawing conclusions from many of the past studies of the reproductive and developmental effects of lead derived from problems in accurately measuring PbB levels (see Chapter 9, US EPA, 1986a). In addition, the statistical power of earlier studies was often limited by the small number of subjects employed. In recent years there have been notable improvements in the design and methodology of studies of lead effects. These improvements owe a great deal to the exchange of information among investigators in this area of research and the careful examination of their results by one another and by other 'interested parties', such as scientists for government agencies or other organizations with a direct interest in the implications of this work. Meetings such as the present international workshop and past conferences (e.g., Bornschein and Rabinowitz, 1985) have contributed to these beneficial interactions among scientists.

Although cross-sectional epidemiological studies, particularly those discussed earlier in this paper and elsewhere in this volume, provide important information on the health effects of environmental lead exposure, the emergence of prospective studies of lead's developmental effects has offered a notable advantage over the cross-sectional approach, namely a more precise characterization of the history of lead exposure during the period of development. The primary focus here is therefore on emerging prospective investigations of the relationship between lead and early development.

Although it may go without saying that early human development is influenced by many variables, early studies of lead's effects did not always succeed in dealing with these 'extraneous' factors. The studies to be discussed here have taken into consideration an impressive number of such variables as potential covariates or confounders of a relationship between lead and developmental outcomes. In general, current studies demonstrate a high degree of sophistication in design, methodology, and data analysis.

Of the several prospective studies currently under way in various parts of the world, three in the United States – in Boston, Cincinnati, and Cleveland – and one in Port Pirie, South Australia have progressed far enough to provide published findings for the purposes of this review. Since these studies are already quite well represented by other papers in this volume and have been discussed in greater detail in US EPA (1986b) and by Davis and Svendsgaard (1987b), only the major features of these studies are summarized here. Attention is devoted primarily to the convergences in these studies and to their collective implications for public health. Additional information on other prospective studies not yet fully underway or complete in data collection and analysis is also provided elsewhere in this volume (see Graziano *et al.*, McBride *et al.*, Moore *et al.*, and Rothenberg *et al.*).

Table 2 summarizes some of the main features of the study populations for each of the four prospective studies to be examined here. Note that the study populations are generally adequate in size, with *n*'s numbering in the hundreds. However, the actual number of subjects used in specific analyses may be somewhat less than the enrolled population. For the most part, prenatal lead exposure was indicated by the maternal PbB level prior to or at delivery, or cord PbB level at delivery. Note that these average PbB levels were all below 15 μg/dl and are probably representative of past and/or still prevalent levels in various parts of the world.

The studies to be reviewed here have independently assessed many of the same endpoints of physical and/or neurobehavioural development. For example, gestational age, birth weight, and postnatal neurobehavioural development were commonly evaluated. One of the strengths of these studies

Table 2 Summary of population characteristics of prospective lead studies

Location	*n* *	Exposure indicator**	Mean blood lead (range), μg/dl	Reference
Boston	249	Cord	6.5 (0–25)	Bellinger *et al.* (1984a, 1986a, 1987)
Cincinnati	305	Maternal-pre Neonatal	8.0 (1–27) 4.5 (1–28)	Dietrich *et al.* (1986, 1987b)
Cleveland	359	Maternal-del Cord	6.5 (2.7–11.8) 5.8 (2.6–14.7)	Ernhart *et al.* (1986, 1987)
Port Pirie	831	Maternal-del Cord 6-mo	11 (?) 10 (?) ~ 14 (?)	McMichael *et al.* (1986); Vimpani *et al.* (1985)

*Actual number of subjects used for specific analyses may be somewhat less than number enrolled in study.
**Maternal blood lead measured at delivery (del) or at prenatal clinic visit (pre).

is their use of comparable or even the same assessment techniques. In particular, all four prospective studies used the Bayley Scales of Infant Development, particularly the Mental Development Index, to measure postnatal neurobehavioural development. The Bayley Scales comprise three indices of mental, motor, and emotional development. Of the three, the Mental Development Index (MDI) has the greatest reliability and validity, and was designed to assess: "senory-perceptual acuities, discriminations, and the ability to respond to these; the early acquisition of 'object constancy' and memory, learning, and problem-solving ability; vocalizations and the beginnings of verbal communication; and early evidence of the ability to form generalizations and classifications, which is the basis of abstract thinking" (Bayley, 1969).

Table 3 summarizes the neurobehavioural results from the prospective studies. Note that the magnitude of the deficit in Bayley MDI scores is fairly consistent across studies: about 2 to 8 points per 10-μg/dl increase in blood lead level. Also to be noted are the lowest-observed-effect levels (LOELs) for these effects. Since each study deals with data in a slightly different way, the studies will be discussed individually to explain how the information in Table 3 was derived.

In the case of the Boston study (Bellinger et al., 1987), a difference of 4 to 8 points, after control for potential confounders, between low (mean = 1.8 μg/dl) and high (mean = 14.6) cord PbB groups has been found at 6-month intervals over the first two years of life. Since the deficit in the high-exposure group was evenly distributed throughout that group (that is, the decrease in MDI scores was not associated primarily with the subjects having the highest PbB levels), it appears that the effect occurred at PbB levels as low as 10 μg/dl (range for the high-exposure group was 10 to 25 μg/dl).

Somewhat different approaches were used in analysing and reporting the neurobehavioural results from the other prospective studies. Instead of grouping subjects into different levels of exposure, regression analyses were applied to data across the entire range of PbB levels. This approach does not identify a 'threshold' at which effects occur, but it does provide a useful estimate of the quantitative relationship between PbB levels and changes (in this case, decrements) in Bayley MDI scores. Recent results from the Cincinnati study indicate, for example, that 6-month-old male infants show an 8-point decrease in the MDI for every 10-μg/dl increase in PbB level (Dietrich et al.,

Table 3 Summary of neurobehavioural findings from prospective lead studies

Study	MDI deficit pts.	Average PbB (range), μg/dl
Boston	4 to 8*	14.6 (10−25)
Cincinnati	8	~12.5 (7−18)
Cleveland	?	? (3−15)
Port Pirie	2	~14 (?)

*Differences between high- and low-exposure groups in Boston at 6-month intervals during first 2 years; other studies report deficit per 10-μg/dl increment in blood lead level.

1987b). Separate analyses of the Cincinnati data led Bornschein *et al.* (this volume) to conclude that a threshold for reductions in birth weight related to prenatal lead exposure existed at about 12 to 13 μg/dl. Since structural equation models indicated that birth weight mediated, at least in part, the effect of prenatal lead exposure on MDI, by inference one could conclude that the MDI effect had the same threshold. As a rough estimate, then, 12 to 13 μg/dl PbB can be taken as the LOEL for MDI effects in the Cincinnati study.

Reported analyses of the Cleveland data have not provided information on either the magnitude of the lead effect or the level at which it occurs. Indeed, Ernhart *et al.* (1986, 1987) have repeatedly concluded that their data show no clear indication of an effect of low-level lead exposure on fetal or child development. Nevertheless, results from the Cleveland study show some consistency with findings from the other prospective studies. Assessment of neonatal neurobehavioural function indicated that scores on the Graham–Rosenblith Neurological Soft Signs Scale were significantly related to cord PbB levels, even after reducing the data set to only 132 cases. While this single result in itself does "not provide a reasonable level of support for the hypothesis of adverse effects due to intrauterine low-level lead exposure", as Ernhart *et al.* (1986) said, it does provide an intriguing link to another finding from the Cleveland study. Wolf *et al.* (1985) reported that the 12-month MDI scores of subjects from this study were significantly related to Neurological Soft Signs scores shortly after birth. Thus, one could infer that prenatal lead exposure (as reflected in cord PbB level) is associated, indirectly, with performance on the Bayley MDI at 12 months of age. The Cleveland investigators are properly cautious about interpreting these specific results from their study, but in the larger context provided by the other prospective studies these findings are entirely consistent with and supportive of the conclusion that intrauterine lead exposure results in impaired postnatal neurobehavioural development. Moreover, the comparatively low levels of exposure (mean PbB ~ 6 μg/dl) and reduced number of subjects actually used in the analyses ($n = 132$), suggest that the effect would have had to be fairly robust to be detected at all in the Cleveland study. The fact that the highest individual PbB level in this study was only 14.7 μg/dl necessarily implies that the LOEL had to be below 15 μg/dl, and could have even been below 10 μg/dl.

The Port Pirie study also demonstrates an effect of lead exposure on the Bayley MDI. In this case, the MDI was administered only at 2 years of age, but PbB measurements were taken at various points starting with the mother during pregnancy and from birth onward in the infants. The only PbB measurement to show a significant relationship to 24-month MDI performance, after correcting for covariates such as maternal intelligence and HOME scores, was the 6-month postnatal PbB level. The first report of this finding indicated that for an increase of 10 μg/dl in mean blood lead level, there was a 4-point decline in MDI performance (Vimpani *et al.*, 1985). More recent analyses (Vimpani *et al.*, this volume) suggest that the decrease in MDI scores may be closer to two points. While the magnitude of deficit is consistent with other findings, the contrast between prenatal and postnatal exposure indicators in the Port Pirie study does seem at odds with the other studies. However, it should be noted that a clearcut relationship between prenatal lead exposure and pregnancy outcome (in particular, risk of pre-term delivery) was in fact found in this same cohort (McMichael *et al.*, 1986). These findings will be discussed in greater detail below. For now, it is enough to point out that prenatal exposure did have a significant effect on fetal development at mean PbB levels above 14 μg/dl (and possibly starting at somewhat lower levels). By the time of testing on the Bayley MDI at 24 months of age, however, PbB levels had risen to approximately 21 μg/dl. It seems plausible that earlier testing on the Bayley MDI, i.e., before the rather precipitous increase in PbB levels between birth and 24 months, might have revealed a relationship between prenatal exposure indicators and MDI performance that was no longer detectable at 24 months.

Some of the other developmental effects that have been revealed in the prospective studies are summarized in Table 4. The duration of gestation is reduced as a function of lead exposure in two of these studies. In the Port Pirie study (McMichael *et al.*, 1986), this effect was reflected in a categorical measure, pre-term delivery (i.e., before the 37th week of pregnancy). The relative risk of pre-term delivery was noted to increase 2.8-fold for every 10-μg/dl increase in maternal PbB levels. Alternatively, at PbB levels above 14 μg/dl, the risk of pre-term delivery was 4.4 times that at 8 μg/dl or below. When late fetal deaths were excluded, the risk was even greater: an 8.7-fold increase in relative risk. These findings indicate that the effect occurred at PbB levels at least as low as 15 μg/dl.

The Cincinnati study also has found an effect of prenatal lead exposure on gestational age, measured in weeks as a continuous variable. One analysis (Dietrich *et al.*, 1986) indicated that gestational age was reduced by approximately 0.6 week for each natural log unit of prenatal maternal blood lead (PbB measurements were transformed to natural logarithms for these analyses to better approximate a normal distribution). Also related to these findings is the cross-sectional study by Moore *et al.* (1982), which has shown a significant relationship between pre-term delivery and either maternal or cord PbB levels in Glasgow, Scotland. This relationship held even after adjustment for a number of possible confounders.

Fetal growth also appears to be affected. Head circumference was reduced approximately 0.3 cm for every 10 μg/dl of blood lead in Port Pirie mothers

Table 4 Summary of other developmental findings related to lead exposure

Study	Effects	Magnitude of effects*
Port Pirie	Pre-term delivery	2.8 × Rel. Risk
	Head circumference	−0.3 cm
Cincinnati	Gestational age	−0.6 wk
	Birth weight	−225 g
	Birth length	−2.5 cm

*Per 10-μg/dl increment in PbB in Port Pirie; per natural log unit PbB in Cincinnati.

(McMichael *et al.*, 1986). Birth weight and length were also significantly reduced in Cincinnati infants (Dietrich *et al.*, 1986; Bornschein *et al.*, this volume), although the effect on length was evident only in white infants.

A variety of other findings related to fetal development and growth have been provided by the prospective studies, but are perhaps less clearcut. These findings have been discussed in greater detail by US EPA (1986b) and Davis and Svendsgaard (1987b).

The evidence summarized in this section is remarkably consistent in indicating that exposure to lead during early development is linked to disturbances in fetal and postnatal development. Specifically, these studies indicate statistically significant deficits of 2 to 8 points on the Bayley Mental Development Index for every 10-μg/dl increase in PbB level. In addition, gestational age, birth weight, and possibly other aspects of fetal growth and development appear to be reduced by prenatal lead exposure. Taken collectively, the evidence suggests that PbB concentrations of 10 to 15 μg/dl, and possibly even lower, constitute a level of concern for developmental deficits arising from early lead exposure. Note that this level of concern has heretofore been considered well within the safe or even 'normal' range of PbB values.

Given these conclusions, the obvious question is, "What are the implications for the public health?" First, what portion of the population is at risk? Based on data from the National Center for Health Statistics (1982), approximately 3.6 million live births occurred in the United States in 1980. Data from the US National Health and Nutrition Examination Survey for about the same period (February 1979 to February 1980) indicate that about 27% of the women of child-bearing age had PbB concentrations of 10 μg/dl or more (*cf.* Schwartz *et al.*, 1985). Thus, nearly 1 million infants may have been born in the United States around 1980 to mothers with maternal PbB levels high enough to put the infants at risk for developmental impairments. Blood lead levels in the United States have probably declined somewhat since then due to reduced ambient levels (Schwartz *et al.*, 1985), but the scope of potential concern is still significant, particularly in parts of the world where ambient levels may be greater. .

In assessing the public health significance of the above findings, one may also ask what is the significance of a 2- to 8-point decline on the Bayley Mental Development Index? The Bayley MDI has been the most reliable and valid indicator available for assessing the current state of an infant's development (Honzik, 1977). Although its ability to predict later cognitive or intellectual function has been debated (Wilson, 1973; Lewis and McGurk, 1973), the MDI generally shows moderate, positive, and statistically significant correlations with later childhood IQ test scores (e.g., Wilson and Harpring, 1972). At this time, however, it is impossible to say to what extent later academic, cognitive, or other neurobehavioural performance might be affected by early lead exposure, based on deficits in 6- to 12-month Bayley MDI scores. Clearly, though, such deficits in themselves cannot be assumed to be inconsequential. It is also important to note that these changes represent *average* decrements. Thus, for a population of children, a 4-point downward shift in a normal distribution of MDI scores would result in 50% more children scoring below 80 (*cf.* Needleman, 1983). Although a 4-point change in an individual child would not generally be considered clinically important, such an effect on a population basis should not be ignored.

Similar considerations apply to the findings on gestational age and fetal growth. In general, reductions in fetal growth are a major risk factor in perinatal morbidity (Yerushalmy, 1970; Usher and McLean, 1974). Moreover, as the work of Dietrich *et al.* (1986, 1987a) has shown, even slight reductions in duration of gestation and birth weight are related to declines in MDI performance. Some recent work also finds a positive relationship between children's height and intelligence (Wilson *et al.*, 1986), which would also suggest that lead-induced effects on growth may have broader health implications.

Lead effects on physical growth/development and their interrelationships with delayed neurobehavioural development have only recently begun to be recognized as being of likely concern at low levels of lead exposure. Among the earliest indications of lead effects on stature in children are observations reported by Nye (1929) regarding 'runting', along with squint and foot drop, as physical signs characteristic of overtly lead-poisoned Australian children seen in the 1920s. Remarkably, since then relatively few systematic evaluations of possible stunting of physical growth have been included among the health endpoints examined in the numerous epidemiological studies of lead effects on early human development. With regard to such studies, some have provided suggestive evidence of associations between relative decreases in height and PbB levels in the range of 30 to 80 μg/dl in comparison to 'low-lead' groups (PbB range = 10–30 μg/dl) from among children aged 1–6 y (Mooty *et al.*, 1975; Johnson and Tenuta, 1979; Routh *et al.*, 1979). However, given certain differences in racial composition and mean age of the control and comparison groups in these studies they do not allow clear determination of the relative contribution of lead to the observed smaller stature of the high-lead subjects.

Much stronger evidence for lead exposure producing retardation of growth and decreased stature has more recently emerged in the 1980s from both animal toxicology studies and evaluation of larger scale epidemiological data sets. In regard to the latter, work by Lauwers *et al.* (1986) in Belgium points to associations between lead exposure and disturbed physical growth in young children. Biometric measurements made on 312 children (aged 2.5 to 16 years) included stature, weight, total arm length, biacromial and bicristal diameter, upper arm circumference, thigh circumference, head length and breadth, and bizygomatic diameter; PbB levels were measured an average of 9.5 months earlier and SES was ranked by parental occupation. Univariate and multivariate analyses indicated that low-PbB (0 to 30 μg/dl) and high-PbB (40 to 60 μg/dl) children were significantly different in their biometric profiles. These differences were greatest in children below 8 years of age. Although few specific measures differed significantly between high- and low-PbB groups, the overall differences in profiles are consistent with findings from other studies described above. Also, Schwartz *et al.* (1986) have reported results of analyses of data from the large scale National Health and Nutrition Evaluation Survey (NHANES II) conducted in the United States during 1976–

1980. More specifically, results for anthropometric measurements, as well as numerous other factors (age, race, sex, dietary, etc.) likely to affect rates of growth and development, among the NHANES II children were analysed. Linear regressions of adjusted data from 2695 children (aged 7 y or younger) indicated that 9% of the variance in height, 72% of the variance in weight, and 58% of the variance in chest circumference were explained by the following six variables: age, race, sex, blood lead, total calories or protein, and haematocrit or transferrin saturation. The step-wise multiple regression analyses further indicated that PbB levels were a statistically significant predictor of children's height ($p < 0.0001$), weight ($p < 0.001$), and chest circumference ($p < 0.026$), after controlling for age (in months), race, sex, and nutritional covariates. The strongest relationship was found between PbB and height, with threshold regressions indicating no evident threshold for the relationship down to the lowest observed blood lead level of 4 μg/dl. At their average age (59 mo.), the mean PbB level of the children appears to be associated with a reduction of about 1.5% below the height expected if their PbB level had been zero, and the relative impacts on weight and chest circumference were of the same magnitude. Overall, these findings appear to be highly credible, being based on well-conducted statistical analyses of a large-scale national survey data set that was subjected to rigorous quality assurance procedures and took into account numerous potentially confounding variables.

Although the full ramifications of early developmental impairments due to lead cannot be stated at present, the *prima facie* indications are that such effects should be avoided. One factor to be considered in evaluating the public health implications of these findings is their relative permanence or irreversibility. Broadly speaking, ontogeny is characterized both by plasticity and by sequential dependency. Developing organisms are often able to compensate for deficiencies, even major neurological impairments, if they occur early enough in the maturation of the individual. Catch-up growth spurts in children are a well-known example of such compensatory phenomena (Ashworth and Millward, 1986). Thus, one might suppose that early developmental lags, particularly those that are fairly subtle (as suggested by the findings reviewed here), could 'disappear' at later ages.

On the other hand, even if a lead-induced lag in cognitive or physical development were no longer *detectable* at a later age, this would not necessarily imply that the earlier impairment was without consequence. Decades of research in developmental psychology have affirmed and extended the early work of Carmichael (1926, 1927), who showed that the actualization of behavioural capabilities as basic as a tadpole's swimming movements requires appropriate periods of functional neural activity for proper development. Of more immediate relevance, perhaps, is recent work on the subtle impairments of language acquisition in children whose hearing has been affected by intermittent otitis media (e.g., Needleman, 1977). Although much remains to be learned about this particular issue, it illustrates the potential for serious and long-lasting sequelae of deficits that may be only transient and, in themselves, reversible during early development. Moreover, secondary effects of early developmental perturbations need not be strictly sequential. Given the complex interactions that figure in the cognitive, emotional, and social development of children, it could well be that attempts to compensate for lead-induced deficits in one area of a child's development may exact a cost in another area of development. Thus, even if lead-induced deficits on the Bayley scales do not eventually predict other specific deficits, such as reduced IQ test performance in later childhood, one needs to be careful in assessing the full and ultimate cost to the developing child, and hence the public health.

Continued research is obviously needed to determine the ultimate impact of early developmental lead exposure. Such work needs to follow current cohorts of subjects with appropriate assessments of cognitive, emotional, social, and physical development. In addition, interactive effects involving variables such as socioeconomic status (Bellinger et al., this volume), gender (Dietrich et al., 1986), and race (Dietrich et al., this volume) need to be investigated. Much remains to be learned about the critical periods during development for the induction of lead's effects and the levels of exposure responsible for these effects. Estimating fetal lead exposure from maternal or cord PbB levels, for example, is far from precise. More accurate indicators of fetal exposure are needed if early developmental effects are to be detected reliably. In addition, the possible contribution of paternal lead exposure to these effects needs to be investigated (cf. Uzych, 1985; Cohen, 1986). The findings reviewed here provide more than adequate impetus for pursuing these questions.

INTERPRETIVE SUMMARY AND EVALUATION

Assessment of the impact of lead on human physical and neurobehavioural development raises a number of issues. Among the key points addressed here are the following: (1) the internal lead exposure levels, as indexed by PbB levels, at which various effects on physical and neurobehavioural development occur; (2) the reversibility of such deleterious effects; and (3) the populations that appear to be most susceptible to neural damage. In addition, note is made that animal toxicology studies provide parallels to the human study results.

Internal exposure levels associated with effects on neurobehavioural development

Markedly elevated PbB levels are associated with readily detectable neurotoxic effects (including severe, irreversible brain damage as indexed by the occurrence of acute and/or chronic encephalopathic symptoms) in both humans and animals. For most adult humans, such damage typically does not occur until PbB levels exceed 100 to 120 μg/dl. In children, effective PbB levels for producing encephalopathy or death are somewhat lower, encephalopathy signs and symptoms having been reported for some children at PbB levels as low as 80 to 100 μg/dl. In addition, numerous studies show that children with high blood lead levels (over 80 to 100 mg/dl), but not observed to manifest acute encephalopathic symptoms, are permanently cognitively impaired, as are most children who survive acute episodes of frank lead encephalopathy.

Other evidence reviewed here confirms that various types of neural dysfunction also exist in apparently asymptomatic children across a broad range of PbB levels. The body of studies on low- or moderate-level lead effects on neurobehavioural functions, as summarized in Table 1, presents a rather impressive array of data pointing to that conclusion. It is true that numerous types of methodological problems or weaknesses are associated with many of the studies in Table 1. Such problems, at times, limit acceptance of their resulting published findings or conclusions and make overall interpretation of their results difficult. However, careful examination of the studies both individually, weighing specific limitations against other (sometimes offsetting) considerations, and collectively nevertheless yields useful information on the effects of lead on neurobehavioural functions in non-overtly lead-intoxicated children.

Figure 1, for example, illustrates the general pattern that seems to emerge from most of the available studies in terms of the magnitude of lead effects on one commonly employed measure of children's mental abilities, i.e., full-scale IQ. Clearly, many caveats are in order in regard to the interpretation presented in Figure 1. First, 'IQ' was measured by many different specific test instruments across the various studies reviewed earlier and those upon which the figure is based. The tests, especially their subscales, may be tapping different specific abilities and, thus, it could be argued that no quantitative comparison across studies can be made. On the other hand, full-scale IQ scores derived from various test instruments, overall, generally tend to reflect roughly similar constellations of mental capabilities and some reasonable, albeit crude, comparisons should be warranted across various studies. Secondly, the magnitudes of the IQ decrements shown in Figure 1 at different PbB levels are based on the study results reflecting varying degrees of corrections for potentially confounding variables. Some, for example, do not reflect correction for parental IQ whereas others do. Still, the overall pattern of results is revealing.

For comparison's sake, the magnitude of IQ decrements observed by Rummo for postencephalic children is also included, that being about 16 points at mean PbB levels in the range of 80 to 100 μg/dl. At somewhat lower exposure levels, several studies (e.g., Rummo; de la Burde) point to average 5-point IQ decrements in asymptomatic children at average PbB levels in the range of 50 to 70 μg/dl. Other evidence from Needleman's studies is indicative of average IQ decrements of up to 4 points being associated with PbB levels in a 30 to 50 μg/dl range. Below 30 μg/dl, the evidence for IQ decrements has been relatively mixed, with most of the recent British and Winneke's studies showing no statistically significant associations with lead once other confounding factors are controlled. Still, the 1 to 2 point differences in IQ often reported for PbB levels in the 15 to 30 μg/dl range are suggestive of small lead effects that are dwarfed or, quite possibly, masked by other social factors. The complex interrelationships between lead exposure and confounding variables (e.g., lower parental IQ,

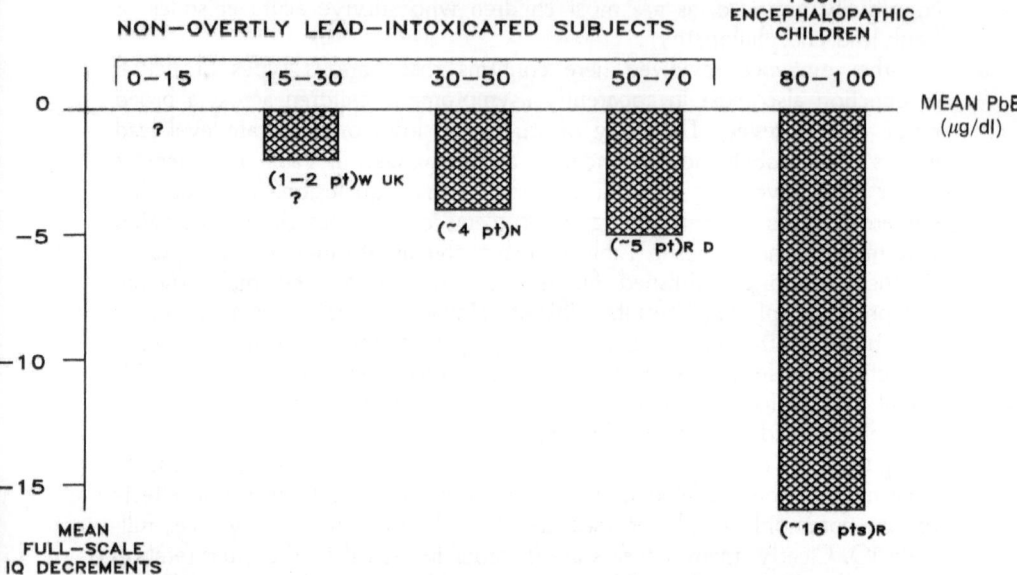

Figure 1 General pattern of results from clinic, smelter, and general population studies of lead exposure effects on cognitive function, as reflected by deficits in IQ scores on various standardized tests. The magnitude of IQ decrements associated with a broad range of blood lead levels is estimated here based on evaluation of studies noted in figure key and discussed in text. Note that latest results from certain newer studies point toward lead effects on IQ across a broad range of PbB levels, down to as low as 10–15 μg/dl or perhaps lower (as illustrated in Figure 2). *Key*: R = Rummo studies; D = de la Burde studies; N = Needleman studies; W = Winneke studies; UK = Recent British studies by Smith, Lansdown, Yule, Harvey, etc.

poorer HOME situations and/or socioeconomic status) complicates conceptual modelling and statistical evaluation of lead effects.

Some investigators, in fact, argue that 'overcorrection' for many confounding factors, which may themselves reflect the impact of lead, tends to lead to underestimation of the magnitude of lead effects. Of interest in that regard are the findings of Schroeder and Hawk (1987) and Fulton *et al.* (1987) plotted in Figure 2*. The Schroeder and Hawk (1987) finding of a highly statistically significant linear relationship between IQ and PbB over the range of 6 to 47 μg/dl found in uniformly low-SES black children indicates that notable IQ effects may be detected without evident threshold even at these low levels, at least in this population of children where variation in SES levels does not confound the lead effects. Results from the Fulton et al. (1987) study described elsewhere in this volume are also plotted in Figure 2. Their results indicate a 5–6 point decrement in British Ability Scale composite and reading attainment scores as average PbB levels increased from 5.6 to 22.1 μg/dl. In addition, other behavioural (e.g., reaction time, psychomotor performance) and electrophysiological (altered EEG patterns, evoked potential measures, and peripheral nerve conduction velocities) effects are consistent with a dose–response function relating neurotoxic effects to lead exposure levels as low as 15 to 30 μg/dl and possibly lower. Also, although the comparability of PbB concentrations across species is uncertain, animal studies (such as those of Rice and Cory-Schlecta reported elsewhere in these proceedings) show neurobehavioural effects in rats and monkeys at maximal PbB levels below 20 to 30 μg/dl.

The medical or health significance of neuropsychological and electro-physiological effects associated with low-level lead exposure as reported in the above studies remains a matter of debate. Observed IQ deficits and other behavioural changes, although statistically significant in some studies, tend to be relatively small as reported by the investigators, but nevertheless may still affect the intellectual development, school performance, and social development of the affected children sufficiently to be regarded as adverse. This would be especially true if such impaired intellectual development or school performance and disrupted social development were reflective of persisting, long-term effects of low-level lead exposure in early childhood.

The question of irreversibility

Relatively little research on children is available on persistence of effects. However, although the issue of persistence of such lead effects remains to be

---

*Figure 2 presents regression lines relating PbB levels and covariate-adjusted scores from the studies of Schroeder and Hawk (1987) and Fulton et al. (1987). The lines were derived from information provided in the original reports as follows. The β coefficient (-0.396) for the sixth model in Table 7 from Schroeder and Hawk (1987) was used to generate a line that passes through the mean average PbB (20.65 μg/dl) and the average Stanford–Binet IQ score (estimated as 87) for that study. Fulton et al. (1987) reported a regression coefficient of -3.70 for the relationship between log-transformed PbB levels and adjusted British Ability Scale Composite (BASC) scores in the 'optimum model' in Table III of their report. A curve was therefore constructed to represent this relationship for arithmetic blood lead values to provide comparability to the results of Schroeder and Hawk. The curve was constructed by passing a line through the geometric mean blood lead level (11.5 μg/dl) and the overall mean BASC score (112) in the Fulton et al. study. A straight line fitted to that curve over the observed range of blood lead levels, with an average slope of -0.247, is shown in Figure 2. Although these lines are not based on the raw data, they are reasonable derivations and are consistent in showing a negative relationship between PbB and cognitive performance extending to PbB levels well below 10 μg/dl, even in different populations of children whose performance was assessed by different tests.

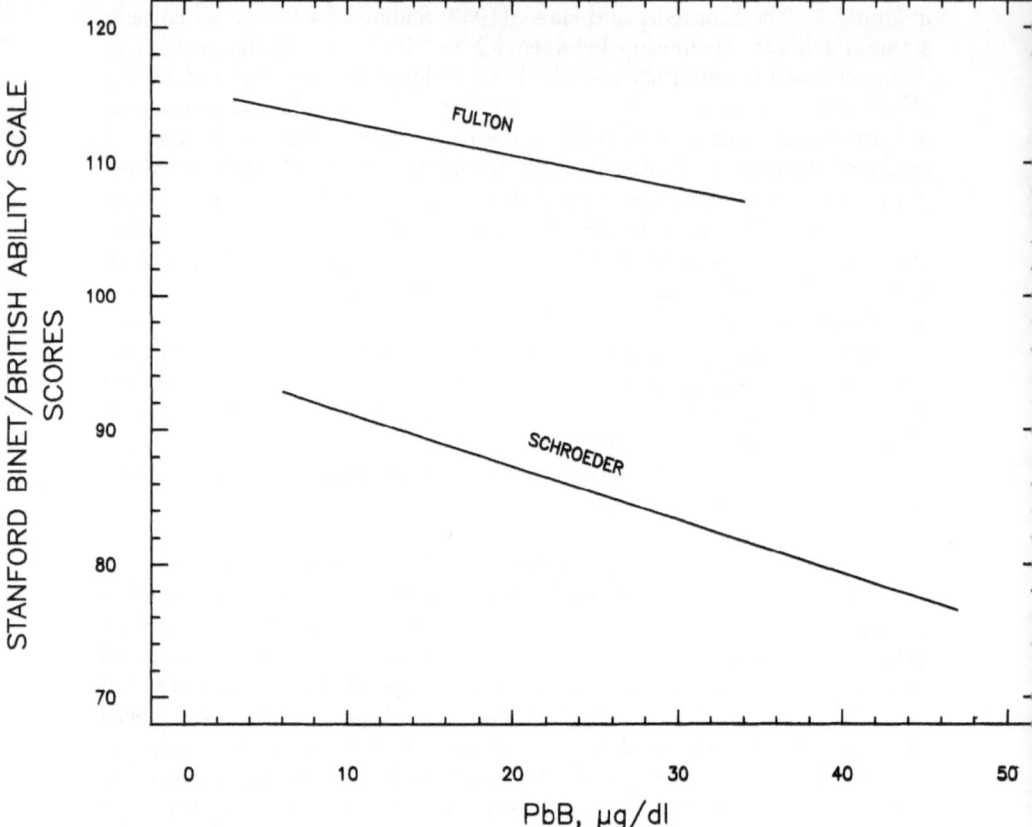

Figure 2 Regression lines relating PbB levels and covariate-adjusted scores for the Stanford-Binet IQ (Schroeder and Hawk, 1987) and the composite British Ability Scale (Fulton *et al.*, 1987). Lines are estimated from the original sources (see discussion in footnote to text)

more clearly resolved, some study results reviewed above suggest that significant low-level lead-induced neurobehavioural and electrophysiological effects may, in fact, persist at least into later childhood. Results from the longitudinal study in Boston indicate a persistent effect of prenatal lead exposure (cord PbB) on postnatal neurobehavioural development (Bayley MDI scores) up to at least 24 months of age. Similarly, the Cincinnati study has thus far observed comparable effects up to 12 months of age. It remains to be seen how long the effects of prenatal lead exposure can be detected in these cohorts at later ages.

The series of studies by Otto and colleagues on a group of lead-exposed children also indicate persistent relationships between PbB and altered electrophysiological responses, e.g., slow wave cortical potentials at two- and five-year follow-ups. However, IQ deficits in the same group of subjects were no longer evident at the five-year follow-up. Some work suggests that other measures of classroom performance may be more sensitive indicators of lead-induced effects in other children. Evaluation of school age IQ, classroom behaviour, and academic performance in prospective longitudinal studies on lead's developmental effects of the type presented at this meeting will likely be needed to answer questions on the persistence or reversibility of neurotoxic effects of early lead exposure.

Various animal studies provide evidence that alterations in neurobehavioural function may be long-lived, with such alterations being evident long after PbB levels have returned to control levels. These persistent effects have been demonstrated in monkeys as well as rats under a variety of learning performance test paradigms.

Early development and susceptibility to prenatal or early postnatal lead exposure effects

On the question of early childhood vulnerability, the neurobehavioural data are consistent with morphological and biochemical studies of the susceptibility of the haeme biosynthetic pathway to perturbation by lead. Various lines of evidence suggest that the order of susceptibility to neurotoxic effects of lead is: young > adult, and female > male. Animal studies also have pointed to the perinatal period of ontogeny as a particularly critical time for a variety of reasons: (1) it is a period of rapid development of the nervous system; (2) it is a period where good nutrition is particularly critical; and (3) it is a period where the caregiver environment is vital to normal development. However, the precise boundaries of a critical period for lead exposure are not yet clear and may vary depending on the species and function or endpoint that is being assessed. One analysis of lead-exposed children suggests that differing effects on cognitive performance may be a function of the different ages at which children are subjected to neurotoxic exposures. Nevertheless, there is general agreement that human infants and toddlers below the age of three years are at special risk because of *in utero* exposure, increased opportunity for exposure because of normal mouthing behaviour of lead-containing objects, and increased rates of lead absorption due to various factors, e.g., iron and calcium deficiencies. The results emerging from long-term prospective studies reviewed earlier in this paper and presented in more detail by the investigators at this meeting also highlight the vulnerability of the human fetus to lead and reinforce the importance of viewing women of childbearing age as being a population group at special risk as well as young children.

Figure 3 provides a schematic depiction of relationships that have been demonstrated or can be hypothesized to exist between prenatal lead exposure, other factors, and the developmental status of infants, based on results emerging from the long-term prospective studies reviewed here. Significant effects of prenatal lead exposure at maternal and neonatal PbB levels in the range of 10 to 20 μg/dl have been reported for several studies in relation to pregnancy outcomes, with increased spontaneous abortions and stillbirths among the effects observed in some and obstetric complications and/or pre-term deliveries in the same or other studies. As for the offspring, reduced birth weight has been reported by several investigators and lower neurological development scores, e.g., on the Bayley MDI and PDI scales, in relation to maternal or cord PbB levels. These types of effects may be directly due to prenatal lead or, as hypothesized by some investigators, may be mediated indirectly by lead-induced shortening of the gestation period and, hence, gestational age. Whether prenatal lead exposure induces minor physical malformation at the low exposure levels evaluated by the current studies, as suggested by at least one of them, remains to be more clearly established. The other relationships noted generally appear to have been detectable even when taking into account many other potentially confounding variables, e.g., alcohol and tobacco usage, but may also be related to certain other factors, e.g., parental size, not fully accounted for in some studies.

Proper control for various confounding variables remains an issue of much debate among researchers conducting the prospective studies. One viewpoint is to accept lead effects as being demonstrated only if lead measures are

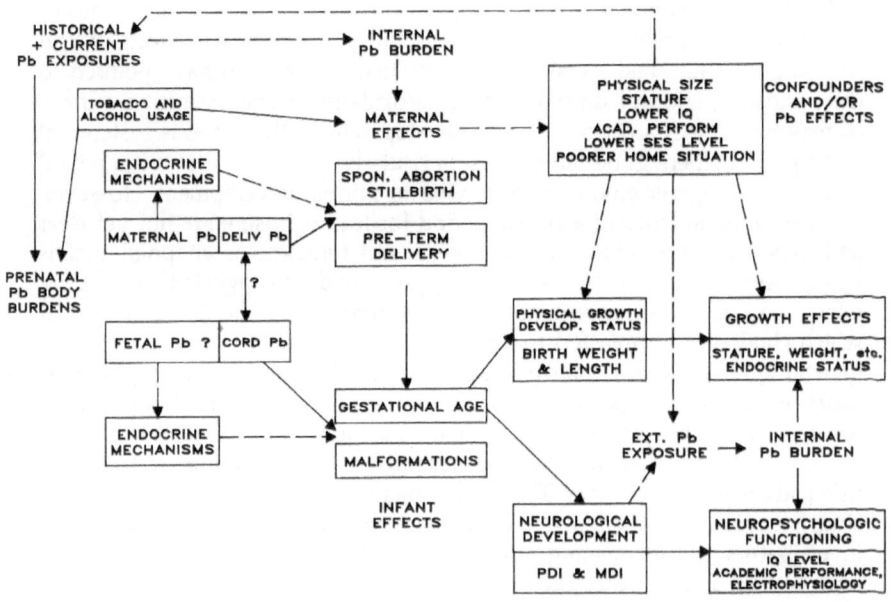

Figure 3 Hypothesized relationships among lead (Pb) and other factors affecting fetal and postnatal development. As discussed in more detail in text, historical and current maternal lead exposures contribute to prenatal lead body burdens, indexed typically by maternal blood lead (PbB) levels during pregnancy or umbilical PbB levels at delivery. Resulting impacts of prenatal exposures include both maternal and infant effects at birth, as well as postnatal effects persisting into later childhood that may be due to the prenatal exposures and/or early postnatal exposures. Potential confounding variables (upper right) make it difficult to quantify precisely effects of lead on dependent variables indicated. An alternative view holds that control for certain confounders may lead to underestimation of lead effects on currently studied subjects, due to 'transgenerational' impacts of lead exposure on the parents of such subjects contributing to negative impacts of the 'confounders' on the lead exposure measures and health effect endpoints

shown to be significantly associated (at $p < 0.05$) with dependent variable outcomes after all possible confounding variables have been accounted for, including variables of the type shown in the upper right of Figure 3. Another viewpoint is that many of the same variables may themselves be determined in part by virtue of past or present lead exposures and, therefore, correction for them may partly obscure otherwise significant lead effects. Also, some of the 'confounders' contribute to increased lead levels in the environment, thus increasing exposure to both parents and children, further complicating separation of the relative contribution of various factors to observed effects.

In addition to highlighting such issues as the above, note should be made of interconnections that may become apparent from diverse areas of investigation reviewed in the present paper. For example, gestational-age-mediated effects on physical size at birth may be related to reduced-stature effects documented for children at later ages and paralleled by observations from animal studies. The earlier discussion of reduced stature effects raises the possibility that neuroendocrine mechanisms underlie effects on postnatal growth or stature; also, attention should be drawn to the possible involvement of prenatal lead effects on endocrine mechanisms in producing both pregnancy outcome effects and/or the observed 'gestational-age' mediated effects on the fetus. Lastly, one might note the possibility of effects of altered neurological development during the early postnatal period resulting in behavioural patterns that may increase lead exposure of the developing child and thereby exacerbate further the effects of earlier prenatal lead exposure.

One other implication of the conceptual scheme in Figure 3 is that early lead exposure of parents may contribute to neurobehavioural and other effects that result in poorer school performance and social behaviour, consequent lower financial or economic success, or other behaviours that place their offspring in more heavily lead-contaminated environments. Their offspring, in turn, may be placed at greater risk for increased lead exposure and continue the experience of their parents, thus manifesting increasingly negative 'transgenerational' effects of lead unless the cycle is broken.

Utility of animal studies in drawing parallels to the human condition

Animal models are used to shed light on questions where it would be impractical or ethically unacceptable to use human subjects. This is particularly true in the case of exposure to environmental toxins such as lead.

Studies using rodents and monkeys have provided a variety of evidence of neurobehavioural alteration induced by lead exposure. In most cases these effects suggest impairment in 'learning', i.e., the process of appropriately modifying one's behaviour in response to information from the environment. Such behaviour involves the ability to receive, process, and remember information in various forms. Some studies indicate behavioural alterations of a more basic type, such as delayed development of certain reflexes. Other evidence suggests changes affecting rather complex behaviour in the form of social interactions. See papers by Rice and by Cory-Schlecta (this volume) for more detailed discussions of such types of effects found in animal toxicology studies.

Many of the above types of effects are evident in rodents and monkeys with PbB levels exceeding 30 μg/dl, but some effects on learning ability are apparent even at maximum PbB exposure levels below 20 μg/dl. The problem of extrapolating exposures, and therefore the results of animal research to human populations are discussed in another review by Smith (this volume). Until the function describing the relationship of exposure indices in different species is available, the utility of animal models for deriving dose–response functions relevant to humans may be limited. However, consistent observations of altered behaviour across several species and humans at PbB levels below 30 μg/dl tend to converge to indicate lead effects on CNS function at lead levels previously considered 'safe'.

Another neurobehavioural endpoint of interest in comparing human and animal neurotoxicity of lead is electrophysiological function. Alterations of electroencephalographic patterns and cortical slow wave voltage have been reported for lead-exposed children, and various electrophysiological alterations both *in vivo* (e.g., in rat visual evoked response) and *in vitro* (e.g., in frog miniature endplate potentials) have also been noted in laboratory animals. Thus far, however, these lines of work have not converged sufficiently to allow for much in the way of definitive conclusions regarding electrophysiological aspects of lead neurotoxicity.

In addition, lead has been shown to have subcellular effects in the CNS at the level of mitochondrial function and protein synthesis. In particular, some work has indicated that delays seen in cortical synaptogenesis and metabolic maturation following prenatal lead exposure may well underlie the delayed development of exploratory and locomotor function seen in other studies of lead's neurobehavioural effects. Further studies on the correlation between human PbB values and lead-induced disruptions of tetrahydrobiopterin metabolism indicate that subsequent interference with neurotransmitter formation may be linked to small reductions in IQ scores.

Given the difficulties in formulating a comparative basis for internal exposure levels among different species, the primary value of many animal studies, particularly *in vitro* studies, may be in the information they can provide on basic mechanisms involved in lead neurotoxicity. A number of key *in vitro* studies are summarized in US EPA (1986a). These studies show that significant, potentially deleterious, effects on nervous system function occur at *in situ* lead concentrations of 5 μmol/L and possibly lower. This suggests that, at least on an intracellular or molecular level, there may exist essentially no threshold for certain neurochemical effects of lead. The relationship between PbB levels and lead concentrations at extra- or intracellular sites of action, however, remains to be determined.

Despite the problems in generalizing from animals to humans, both the animal and the human studies show considerable internal consistency in that they both support a continuous dose–response functional relationship between lead and neurotoxic biochemical, morphological, electrophysiological, and behavioural effects.

IMPLICATIONS FOR PUBLIC HEALTH PROTECTION

The results of studies reviewed here are very important with regard to their implications for effective actions to protect against health effects associated with lead exposure. These findings should not be viewed in isolation but rather within a context of a wide array of effects associated with exposure of children to lead. It is clear from a wealth of available literature reviewed in Chapter 12 of US EPA (1986a) that there exists a continuum of biological effects associated with lead across a broad range of exposure. At rather low levels of lead exposure, biochemical changes, e.g., disruption of certain enzymatic activities involved in haeme biosynthesis and erythropoietic pyrimidine metabolism, are detectable. Haeme biosynthesis is a generalized process in mammalian species, including humans, with importance for normal physiological functioning of virtually all organ systems. With increasing lead exposure, there are sequentially more intense effects on haeme synthesis as well as a broadening of effects to additional biochemical and physiological mechanisms in various tissues. In addition to haeme biosynthesis impairment at relatively low levels of lead exposure, disruption of normal functioning of the erythropoietic and nervous systems occurs, and additional organ systems are affected, resulting, for example, in manifestation of renal effects, disruption of reproductive functions, and impairment of immunological functions. At sufficiently high levels of exposure, the damage to the nervous system and other effects can be severe enough to result in death or, in some cases of nonfatal lead poisoning, long-lasting sequelae such as permanent mental retardation.

Of particular importance for deriving criteria and developing government policies to protect human health are findings which have bearing on the establishment of quantitative dose–effect or dose–response relationships that can be potentially viewed as adverse health effects likely to occur among the general population at or near existing ambient air exposure levels. Dose–response information for the wide variety of observed lead health effects and their implications for children are discussed in detail elsewhere (US EPA, 1986a). Emphasis is placed on the delineation of internal lead exposure levels, as defined mainly by PbB levels likely associated with the occurrence of such effects. Also discussed are characteristics of these effects that are of crucial importance in determining 'adverse health effects' in human populations.

Over the years, there have been superimposed on the continuum of lead-induced biological effects various judgments as to which specific effects observed in humans constitute 'adverse health effects'. Such judgments involve not only medical consensus regarding the health significance of particular effects and their clinical management, but also incorporate societal value judgments. Such societal value judgments often vary depending upon the specific overall contexts in which they are applied, e.g., in judging permissible exposure levels for occupational versus general population lead exposures. For some lead exposure effects, e.g., severe nervous system damage resulting in death or serious medical sequelae consequent to intense lead exposure, there exists little or no disagreement as to these being significant 'adverse health effects'. For many other effects detectable at sequentially lower levels

101

of lead exposure, however, the demarcation lines as to what constitutes being 'adverse' and the lead exposure levels at which they reliably occur are neither sharp nor fixed, having changed markedly during the past several decades. That is, from an historical perspective, levels of lead exposure deemed to be acceptable for either occupationally exposed persons or the general population have been steadily revised downward as more sophisticated biomedical techniques have revealed formerly unrecognized biological effects and concern has increased in regard to the medical and societal significance of such effects.

As for dose–response relationships, lowest-observed-effect levels for a variety of important health effects observed in children are discussed in US EPA (1986a). It can be seen there that lead impacts many different organ systems and biochemical/physiological processes across a wide range of exposure levels. These include severe, irreversible CNS damage (manifested in terms of encephalopathic signs and symptoms), permanent severe mental retardation, and other marked neurological deficits among lasting neurological sequelae typically seen in cases of non-fatal childhood lead encephalopathy. Other overt neurological signs and symptoms of subencephalopathic lead intoxication are evident in children at lower PbB levels. Chronic nephropathy, indexed by animoaciduria, is most evident at high exposure levels over 100 μg/dl, but may also exist at lower levels (e.g., 70 or 80 μg/dl). In addition, colic and other overt gastrointestinal symptoms clearly occur at similar or still lower PbB levels in children, at least down to 60 μg/dl. Frank anaemia is also evident by 70 μg/dl, representing an extreme manifestation of the reduced haemoglobin synthesis observed at PbB levels as low as 40 μg/dl, along with other signs of marked inhibition of haeme synthesis at that exposure level. All of these effects are reflective of the widespread marked impact of lead on the normal physiological functioning of many different organ systems, and some are evident in children at PbB levels as low as 40 μg/dl; all of them are widely accepted as being clearly adverse health effects.

Additional studies demonstrate evidence for further, important health effects occurring in non-overtly lead-intoxicated children at similar or lower PbB levels than those indicated above for overt intoxication effects. Among the most important of these are neuropsychological and electrophysiological effects. While the precise medical or health significance of some neuropsychological and electrophysiological effects remain to be more fully defined, IQ deficits and other behavioural changes likely impact the intellectual development, school performance, and social development of the affected children sufficiently to be regarded as adverse. This is especially true if such impaired intellectual development or school performance and disrupted social development are reflective of persisting, long-term effects of low-level lead exposure in early childhood. The issue of persistence of such lead effects still remains to be more clearly resolved, with some study results reviewed above suggesting relatively short-lived or markedly decreasing lead effects on neuropsychological functions from early to later childhood and other studies suggesting that significant low-level lead-induced neurobehavioural and EEG effects may, in fact, persist into later childhood.

Research concerning lead-induced effects on haeme synthesis also provides

102

information of importance in evaluating what PbB levels are associated with significant health effects in children. As discussed in US EPA (1986a) lead affects haeme synthesis at several points in its metabolic pathway with consequent impact on the normal functioning of many body tissues. Of special interest at low PbB levels are lead effects on haeme synthesis beyond metabolic steps involving ALA. The level of erythrocyte protoporphyrin (EP) in the blood is one commonly employed index of lead exposure used for medical screening purposes. The threshold for elevation of erythrocyte protoporphyrin (EP) levels is well-established as being 25 to 30 μg/dl in adults and approximately 15 μg/dl for young children, with significant EP elevations (> 1 to 2 standard deviations above reference normal EP mean levels) occurring in 50% of all children studied as PbB approaches or moderately exceeds 30 μg/dl.

Recently, it has also been shown in children that lead interferes with vitamin D metabolism, with the negative association existing down to 12 μg/dl PbB. This lead effect is of considerable significance on two counts: (1) altered vitamin D metabolism not only impacts calcium homeostasis (affecting mineral metabolism important in bone formation and growth) but also likely impacts calcium's known roles in immunoregulation and tumorigenesis processes; and (2) the effect of lead on vitamin D is a particularly robust one, with PbB levels of 30 to 50 μg/dl resulting in effects that overlap comparable degrees of impairment seen with severe kidney injury or certain genetic diseases.

Also adding to the concern about low level lead exposures are results of an expanding array of animal toxicology studies which demonstrate the following: (1) persistence of lead-induced neurobehavioural alterations well into adulthood long after termination of perinatal lead exposure early in development of several mammalian species; (2) evidence for uptake and retention of lead in neural and non-neuronal elements of the CNS, including long-term persistence in brain tissues after termination of external lead exposure and return to 'normal' PbB levels; and (3) evidence from various *in vivo* and *in vitro* studies indicating that, at least on a subcellular–molecular level, no threshold may exist for certain neurochemical effects of lead.

Given the above new evidence that is now available, indicative of significant lead effects on nervous system functioning and other important physiological processes as PbB levels increase above 10 to 20 μg/dl, the rationale for considering 30 μg/dl as a 'maximum safe' blood lead level, as was the case in setting the 1978 EPA lead National Ambient Air Quality Standards (Federal Register, 1978), is called into question and substantial impetus is provided for revising the criteria level downward. At this time, it is difficult to identify specifically what PbB criteria level would be appropriate in view of the existing medical information. Clearly, however, 30 μg/dl does not afford any margin of safety before reaching PbB levels associated with unacceptable risk of notable adverse health effects in some children. This is based on at least two grounds: (1) blood lead levels in the 30 to 40 μg/dl range are now known to 'mask', for some children, markedly elevated chelatable body lead burdens that are comparable to lead burdens seen in other children displaying overt signs and symptoms of lead intoxication, and (2) PbB levels in the 30

103

to 40 μg/dl range are also associated with the onset of deleterious effects in several organ systems which are either individually or collectively seen as being adverse. These and other considerations have led the medical community (US Centers for Disease Control, 1985) to define 25 μg/dl PbB as a level associated with unacceptable risk for paediatric lead toxicity and to note that even lower PbB levels should not be taken as 'safe'.

At levels below 25 to 30 μg/dl, many of the different smaller effects reported as being associated with lead exposure might be argued as separately not being of clear medical significance, although each is indicative of interference by lead with normal physiological processes. On the other hand, the collective impact of all of the observed effects (representing potentially impaired functioning and depleted reserve capacities of many different tissues and organs) can, at some point distinctly below 25 to 30 μg/dl, be seen as representing an adverse pattern of effects worthy of avoidance. The onset of signs of detectable haeme synthesis impairment in many different organ systems at PbB levels starting around 10 to 15 μg/dl, along with increasing indications of altered nervous system activity, might be viewed as such a point. The demonstration of significant prenatal or early postnatal lead exposure effects of the type being found by prospective studies of the type reviewed here is increasingly discussed as providing the bases for viewing even lower PbB levels (e.g., 10 to 15 μg/dl or, perhaps, lower) as being associated with unacceptable risk.

FUTURE RESEARCH DIRECTIONS

The extensive and widely varying studies reviewed in the present paper have provided extremely valuable information regarding low level lead effects on the neuropsychological development of children. Still, many issues remain to be resolved and it is useful to highlight some considerations here which may assist in shaping future research in the field.

Findings of recent prospective studies from Boston, Cincinnati, Port Pirie, and Cleveland show consistent declines in Bayley Scales performance and in other aspects of growth and development (gestational age, birth weight, and possibly other outcomes) as a function of low-level lead exposure early in development. Despite the notable methodological advances and convergent results these studies exemplify, further questions arise from this work. Although PbB concentrations appear to be measured reliably and accurately in recent prospective studies, the assessment of 'prenatal lead exposure' requires further elucidation. The fact that different indices of prenatal exposures were used by different research groups is the first sign that matters may be a bit more complex than they appear at first glance. The Boston study obtained only cord blood lead. The Cincinnati study collected cord blood, but used only maternal blood leads obtained at the first prenatal visit (generally first or second trimester) for the initial reported analyses. The Port Pirie study collected maternal blood leads at various points during pregnancy and at delivery, as well as cord blood lead. The Cleveland study used both cord and maternal blood lead at delivery.

104

All of these studies continued to monitor postnatal exposure through periodic PbB levels of the children. In every study some effect of prenatal exposure was demonstrated, although the effect on Bayley Scales performance in the Port Pirie study was more clearly associated with postnatal rather than prenatal exposure. While the Port Pirie study would appear to be the anomaly in this respect, that study also had the largest study population and the most frequent PbB measurement protocol, facts which make it difficult to disregard its finding in this regard. Of course, there are noteworthy differences among the study populations and their sources of exposure that could underlie this apparent discrepancy. Further study might resolve this matter.

More importantly, even though the preponderance of work shows an effect of prenatal exposure, it is not clear which index of prenatal exposure is the most valid or useful. The basic problem in accurately gauging prenatal lead exposure is that the dynamics of the situation make single determinations of PbB levels a questionable basis for judging the overall level of prenatal exposure. First of all, there may be changes in exposure during the course of gestation that are not adequately reflected in a PbB measurement at delivery (or any other single point in time). In addition, the dynamics of the mother–fetus transfer of lead make it difficult to determine the fetal portion of the shared lead burden. Some evidence from the Port Pirie study as well as other work suggests the possibility that the fetus may serve as a sink for the mother's body burden, at least in some cases. What is needed is a more frequent assessment of mothers during the course of pregnancy and delivery. Such research would be particularly useful to those concerned with the formulation of regulatory standards for lead, as it would help show whether maternal PbB concentrations are an adequate index of fetal lead exposure at the population level.

Another aspect of these prospective studies that bears further investigation is the long-term consequences of demonstrated early developmental effects. Previous basic research has shown that the Bayley Scales, although reliable and valid (particularly for below-average children), are only moderately good at predicting later intelligence measures or academic performance. Thus, the implications of small decreases (approximately 0.4 point on the Bayley MDI for every μg/dl of blood lead) in early development for later cognitive and academic performance are not clear at present. Continued assessment of cognitive, social, and emotional development, along with academic performance, seems advisable as long as any effects are detectable.

Physical growth and stature ought to be included here as well, not only because of findings relating reduced gestational age and birth weight to prenatal lead exposure, but in view of recent analyses (Schwartz et al., 1986; Lauwers et al., 1986) indicating effects on growth associated with PbB levels in children up to 7 or 8 years of age and parallel animal study findings (e.g., Grant et al., 1980) demonstrating effects of prenatal lead exposure on birth weight and length in neonatal rats. Results from the Grant study indicate persisting slower growth rates with continuing postnatal lead exposures. Thus, prospective study researchers may have an unusual opportunity to tease out analogous physical development sequelae that heretofore have largely escaped detection.

Investigators in this field might also wish to consider assessing other endpoints as well. Recent analyses of NHANES data by Schwartz and Otto (1987) suggest that various developmental milestones (age at which a child first sat up, walked, spoke) were related to lead exposure. In addition, hearing thresholds of children were significantly higher as lead exposure increased. The latter finding is particularly noteworthy in view of previous work relating brainstem auditory evoked potentials to low-level lead exposure in children. Investigators might consider assessing these and other electrophysiological endpoints having demonstrated clinical utility. Electrophysiological measures may yet prove to be a useful neurotoxicological assay for detecting lead effects at very low exposure levels.

Not to be forgotten is the question of the mechanisms underlying the developmental deficits thus far demonstrated by prospective epidemiological studies. The interaction of physiological, genetic, socio-cultural, and nutritional factors involved in development and growth makes it very difficult to elucidate lead's role in such effects. This may explain why so little experimental work has been devoted to examining how lead might affect endocrine and other mechanisms related to growth and development. Elucidation of neuroendocrine mechanisms potentially involved in the mediation of perinatal and later lead effects on development would seem to be a particularly promising research direction.

The call to pursue underlying mechanisms raises a more general point related to research needs. As environmental exposure levels of lead continue to decline, there is sometimes a tendency to view lead studies as passé. Having identified a problem and taken major steps to eliminate it (if one may speak so simplistically about lead), we may not see any need to further understand it. Certainly this is an understandable point of view from a regulatory perspective. But from the standpoint of the science of environmental toxicology, it seems shortsighted to fail to follow through on unresolved questions about an environmental pollutant that has probably been investigated more than any other.

ACKNOWLEDGEMENTS

We thank the numerous colleagues who have commented on earlier versions or portions of this manuscript. We especially thank Dr Marjorie Smith for her extensive helpful comments and, also, Dr David J. Svendsgaard for his helpful discussions and advice on statistical matters and, in particular, for the analyses that were used to generate Figure 2 for this paper. We also appreciate the excellent assistance provided by Douglas Fennell, Miriam Gattis, Lorrie Godley, Lynette Davis, Allen Hoyt, Deborah Staves and Emily Lee in producing this paper and in other tasks related to the editing of this volume. This paper was reviewed by the US Environmental Protection Agency and approved for publication. Approval does not signify that the contents necessarily reflect the views or policies of the Agency.

REFERENCES

Agerty, H.A. (1952). Lead poisoning in children. *Med. Clin. North Am.*, **36**, 1587–1597

Alexander, F.W. and Delves, H.T. (1981). Blood lead levels during pregnancy. *Int. Arch. Occup. Environ. Health*, **48**, 35–39

Anku, V.D. and Harris, J.W. (1974). Peripheral neuropathy and lead poisoning in a child with sickle-cell anemia. *J. Pediatr. (St. Louis)*, **85**, 337–340

Ashworth, A. and Millward, D.J. (1986). Catch-up growth in children. *Nutr. Rev.*, **44**, 157–163

Bayley, N. (1969). *Bayley Scales of Infant Development.* (New York, NY: Psychological Corp.)

Beattie, A.D., Moore, M.R., Goldberg, A., Finlayson, M.J.W., Graham, J.F., Mackie, E.M., Main, J.C., McLaren, D.A., Murdoch, K.M. and Stewart, G.T. (1975). Role of chronic low-level lead exposure in the aetiology of mental retardation. *Lancet* (7907), 589–592

Bellinger, D.C. and Needleman, H.L. (1983). Lead and the relationship between maternal and child intelligence. *J. Pediatr. (St. Louis)*, **102**, 523–527

Bellinger, D.C., Needleman, H.L., Leviton, A., Waternaux, C., Rabinowitz, M.B. and Nichols, M.L. (1984a). Early sensory-motor development and prenatal exposure to lead. *Neurobehav. Toxicol. Teratol.*, **6**, 387–402

Bellinger, D., Needleman, H.L., Bromfield, R. and Mintz, M. (1984b). A follow-up study of the academic attainment and classroom behavior of children with elevated dentine lead levels. *Biol. Trace Elem. Res.*, **6**, 207–223

Bellinger, D., Leviton, A., Needleman, H.L., Waternaux, C. and Rabinowitz, M. (1986a). Low-level lead exposure and infant development in the first year. *Neurobehav. Toxicol. Teratol.*, **8**, 151–161

Bellinger, D., Leviton, A., Rabinowitz, M., Needleman, H. and Waternaux, C. (1986b). Correlates of low-level lead exposure in urban children at 2 years of age. *Pediatrics*, **77**, 826–833

Bellinger, D., Leviton, A., Waternaux, C., Needleman, H. and Rabinowitz, M. (1987). Longitudinal analyses of prenatal and postnatal lead exposure and early cognitive development. *N. Engl. J. Med.*, **316**, 1037–1043

Benignus, V.A., Otto, D.A., Muller, K.E. and Seiple, K.J. (1981). Effects of age and body lead burden on CNS function in young children: II. EEG spectra. *Electroencephalogr. Clin. Neurophysiol.*, **52**, 240–248

Betts, P.R., Astley, R. and Raine, D.N. (1973). Lead intoxication in children in Birmingham. *Br. Med. J.*, **1**(5850), 402–406

Blackfan, K.D. (1917). Lead poisoning in children with especial reference to lead as a cause of convulsions. *Am J Med. Sci.*, **153**, 877–887

Blackman, S.S., Jr. (1937). The lesions of lead encephalitis in children. *Bull. Johns Hopkins Hosp.*, **61**, 1–43

Bornschein, R.L. and Rabinowitz, M.B. (eds.) (1985). The second international conference on prospective studies of lead; April 1984; Cincinnati, OH. *Environ. Res.*, **38**(1).

Bradley, J.E. and Baumgartner, R.J. (1958). Subsequent mental development of children with lead encephalopathy, as related to type of treatment. *J. Pediatr. (St. Louis)*, **53**, 311–315

Bradley, J.E., Powell, A.E., Niermann, W., McGrady, K.R. and Kaplan, E. (1956). The incidence of abnormal blood levels of lead in a metropolitan pediatric clinic with observation on the value of coproporphyrinuria as a screening test. *J. Pediatr. (St. Louis)*, **49**, 1–6

Burchfiel, J.L., Duffy, F.H., Bartels, P.H. and Needleman, H.L. (1980). The combined discriminating power of quantitative electroencephalography and neuropsychologic measures in evaluating central nervous system effects of lead at low levels. In: Needleman, H.L. (ed.) *Low Lead Exposure: The Clinical Implications of Current Research*, pp. 75–89. (New York, NY: Raven Press)

Byers, R.K. and Lord, E.E. (1943). Late effects of lead poisoning on mental development. *Am. J. Dis. Child.*, **66**, 471–494

Caldwell, B.M. and Bradley, R.H. (1979). *Home Observation for Measurement of the Environment.* (Little Rock, AR: University of Arkansas at Little Rock)

Capel, I.D., Pinnock, M.H., Dorrell, H.M., Williams, D.C. and Grant, E.C.G. (1981). Comparison on concentrations of some trace, bulk, and toxic metals in the hair of normal and dyslexic children. *Clin. Chem. (Winston-Salem, NC)*, **27**, 879–881

Carmichael, L. (1926). The development of behavior in vertebrates experimentally removed from the influence of external stimulation. *Psychol. Rev.*, **33**, 51–58

Carmichael, L. (1927). A further study of the development of behavior in vertebrates experimentally removed from the influence of external stimulation. *Psychol. Rev.*, **34**, 34–47

Chisolm, J.J., Jr. (1962). Aminoaciduria as a manifestation of renal tubular injury in lead intoxication and a comparison with patterns of aminoaciduria seen in other diseases. *J. Pediatr.* (St. Louis), **60**, 1–17

Chisolm, J.J., Jr. (1965). Chronic lead intoxication in children. *Dev. Med. Child Neurol.*, **7**, 529–536

Chisolm, J.J., Jr. (1968). The use of chelating agents in the treatment of acute and chronic lead intoxication in childhood. *J. Pediatr.* (St. Louis), **73**, 1–38

Chisolm, J.J., Jr. and Barltrop, D. (1979). Recognition and management of children with increased absorption. *Arch. Dis. Child.*, **54**, 249–262

Chisolm, J.J., Jr. and Harrison, H.E. (1956). The exposure of children to lead. *Pediatrics*, **18**, 943–958

Clark, A.R.L. (1977). Placental transfer of lead and its effects on the newborn. *Postgrad. Med. J.*, **53**, 674–678

Cohen, F.L. (1986). Paternal contributions to birth defects. *Nurs. Clin. North Am.*, **21**, 49–64

Cohen, G.J. and Ahrens, W.E. (1959). Chronic lead poisoning. A review of seven years' experience at the Children's Hospital, District of Columbia. *J. Pediatr.* (St. Louis), **54**, 271–284

Cohen, D.J., Johnson, W.T. and Caparulo, B.K. (1976). Pica and elevated blood lead level in autistic and atypical children. *Am. J. Dis. Child.*, **130**, 47–48

Coss, R.G. and Glohus, A. (1978). Spine stems on tectal interneurons in jewel fish are shortened by social stimulation. *Science* (Washington, DC), **200**, 787–790

Cumings, J.N. (1959). *Heavy Metals and the Brain*. Part 3: Lead, pp. 93–155. (Springfield, IL: Thomas)

David, O.J. (1974). Association between lower lead concentrations and hyperactivity in children. *EHP Environ. Health Perspect.*, **7**, 17–26.

David, O.J., Hoffman, S.P., Sverd, J., Clark, J. and Voeller, K. (1976a). Lead and hyperactivity: behavioral response to chelation: a pilot study. *Am. J. Psychiatry*, **133**, 1155–1158

David, O., Hoffman, S., McGann, B., Sverd, J. and Clark, J. (1976b). Low lead levels and mental retardation. *Lancet*, **2**, 1376–1379

David, O.J., Hoffman, S.P., Sverd, J. and Clark, J. (1977). Lead and hyperactivity: lead levels among hyperactive children. *J. Abnorm. Child Psychol.*, **5**, 405–416

David, O.J., Clark, J. and Hoffman, S. (1979a). Childhood lead poisoning: a re-evaluation. *Arch. Environ. Health*, **34**, 106–111

David, O.J., Hoffman, S. and Kagey, B. (1979b). Sub-clinical lead levels and behavior in children. In: Hemphill, D.D. (ed.) *Trace Substances in Environmental Health – XIII*: [proceedings of University of Missouri's 13th annual conference on trace substances in environmental health]; June; Columbia, MO, pp. 52–58. (Columbia, MO: University of Missouri-Columbia)

David, O.J., Wintrob, H.L. and Arcoleo, C.G. (1982a). Blood lead stability. *Arch. Environ. Health*, **37**, 147–150

David, O.J., Grad, G., McGann, B. and Koltun, A. (1982b). Mental retardation and "nontoxic" lead levels. *Am. J. Psychiatry*, **139**, 806–809

David, O.J., Hoffman, S., Clark, J., Grad, G. and Sverd, J. (1983). Penicillamine in the treatment of hyperactive children with moderately elevated lead levels. In: Rutter, M. and Russell Jones, R. (eds.) *Lead versus Health: Sources and Effects of Low level Lead Exposure*, pp. 297–317. (New York, NY: John Wiley & Sons)

David, O.J., Katz, S., Arcoleo, C.G. and Clark, J. (1985). Chelation therapy in children as treatment of sequelae in severe lead toxicity. *Arch. Environ. Health*, **40**, 109–113

Davis, J.M. and Svendsgaard, D.J. (1987a). U-shaped dose-response functions. Presented at: 26th annual meeting of the Society of Toxicology; February; Washington, DC. *Toxicologist*, **27**, 184

Davis, J.M. and Svendsgaard, D.J. (1987b). Lead and child development. *Nature* (London), **329**, 297–300

de la Burde, B. and Choate, M.S., Jr. (1972). Does asymptomatic lead exposure in children have latent sequelae? *J. Pediatr.* (St. Louis), **81**, 1088–1091

de la Burde, B. and Choate, M.S., Jr. (1975). Early asymptomatic lead exposure and development at school age. *J. Pediatr.* (St. Louis), **87**, 638–642

Dietrich, K.N., Krafft, K.M., Pearson, D.T., Harris, L.C., Bornschein, R.L., Hammond, P.B. and Succop, P.A. (1985). Contribution of social and developmental factors to lead exposure during the first year of life. *Pediatrics*, **75**, 1114–1119

Dietrich, K.N., Krafft, K.M., Bier, M., Succop, P.A., Berger, O. and Bornschein, R.L. (1986). Early effects of fetal lead exposure: neurobehavioral findings at 6 months. *Int. J. Biosoc. Res.*, **8**, 151–168

Dietrich, K.N., Krafft, K.M., Bornschein, R.L., Hammond, P.B., Berger, O., Succop, P.A. and Bier, M. (1987a). Effects of low-level fetal lead exposure on neurobehavioral development in early infancy. *Pediatrics*, **89**, 721–730

Dietrich, K.N., Krafft, K.M., Shukla, R., Bornschein, R.L. and Succop, P.A. (1987b). The neurobehavioral effects of early lead exposure. In: Schroeder, S.R. (ed.) *Toxic Substances and Mental Retardation: Neurobehavioral Toxicology and Teratology*, pp. 71–95. (Washington, DC: American Association on Mental Deficiency) (Begab, M.J. (ed) Monographs of the American Association on Mental Deficiency: no. 8).

Ely, D.L., Mostardi, R.A., Woebkenberg, N. and Worstell, D. (1981). Aerometric and hair trace metal content in learning-disabled children. *Environ. Res.*, **25**, 325–339

Englert, N. (1978). Messung der peripheren motorischen Nervenleitgeschwindigkeit an Erwachsenen und Kindern mit erhoehtem Blutbleispiegel [Measurement of peripheral motor nerve conduction velocity in adults and children with elevated blood lead levels]. *BGA Ber.*, **(1)**, 108–117

Ennis, J.M. and Harrison, H.E. (1950). Treatment of lead encephalopathy via BAL (2,3-dimercaptopropanol). *Pediatrics*, **5**, 853–868

Erenberg, G., Rinsler, S.S. and Fish, B.G. (1974). Lead neuropathy and sickle cell disease. *Pediatrics*, **54**, 438–441

Ernhart, C.B. (1983). Lead versus intelligence. *J. Pediatr.* (St. Louis), **103**, 830–833

Ernhart, C.B. (1984). Comments on chapter 12, air quality criteria for lead. Available for inspection at: US Environmental Protection Agency, Central Docket Section, Washington, DC; docket no. ECAO-CD-81-2IIA.E.C.1.30.

Ernhart, C.B., Landa, B. and Schell, N.B. (1981). Subclinical levels of lead and developmental deficit – a multivariate follow-up reassessment. *Pediatrics*, **67**, 911–919

Ernhart, C.B., Landa, B. and Wolf, A.W. (1985). Subclinical lead level and developmental deficit; reanalyses of data. *J. Learn. Disabil.*, **18**, 475–479

Ernhart, C.B., Wolf, A.W., Kennard, M.J., Erhard, P., Filipovich, H.F. and Sokol, R.J. (1986). Intrauterine exposure to low levels of lead: the status of the neonate. *Arch. Environ. Health*, **41**, 287–291

Ernhart, C.B., Morrow-Tlucak, M., Marler, M.R. and Wolf, A.W. (1987). Low level lead exposure in the prenatal and early preschool periods: early preschool development. *Neurotoxicol. Teratol.*, **9**, 259–270

Fahim, M.S., Fahim, Z. and Hall, D.G. (1976). Effects of subtoxic lead levels on pregnant women in the state of Missouri. *Res. Commun. Chem. Pathol. Pharmacol.*, **13**, 309–331

Federal Register (1978). National ambient air quality standard for lead: final rules and proposed rulemaking. *Fed. Reg.*, **43** (October 5), 46246–46263

Fejerman, N., Gimenez, E.R., Vallejo, N.E. and Medina, C.S. (1973). Lennox's syndrome and lead intoxication. *Pediatrics*, **52**, 227–234

Feldman, R.G., Haddow, J. and Chisolm, J.J. (1973a). Chronic lead intoxication in urban children: motor nerve conduction velocity studies. In: Desmedt, J. and Karger, S. (eds.) *New Developments in Electromyography and Clinical Neurophysiology*, vol. 2, pp. 313–317. (Basel, Switzerland: S. Karger)

Feldman, R.G., Haddow, J., Kopito, L. and Schwachman, H. (1973b). Altered peripheral nerve conduction velocity. *Am. J. Dis. Child.*, **125**, 39–41

Feldman, R.G., Hayes, M.K., Younes, R. and Aldrich, F.D. (1977). Lead neuropathy in adults and children. *Arch. Neurol.*, **34**, 481–488

Fulton, M., Rabb, G., Thomson, G., Laxen, D., Hunter, R. and Hepburn, W. (1987). Influence of blood lead on the ability and attainment of children in Edinburgh. *Lancet*, (8544), 1221–1226

Gant, V.A. (1938). Lead poisoning. *Ind. Med.*, **7**, 679–699

Gilani, S.H. (1973a). Congenital anomalies in lead poisoning. *Obstet. Gynecol.*, **41**, 265–269

Gilani, S.H. (1973b). Congenital cardiac anomalies in lead poisoning. *Pathol. Microbiol.* (Basel), **39**, 85–90

Gillberg, C., Noren, J.G., Wahlstrom, J. and Rasmussen, P. (1982). Heavy metals and neuropsychiatric disorders in six-year-old children: aspects of dental lead and cadmium. *Acta Paedopsychiatr.*, **48**, 253–263

Gittelman, R. and Eskenazi, B. (1983). Lead and hyperactivity revisited: an investigation of nondisadvantaged children. *Arch. Gen. Psychiatry*, **40**, 827–833

Grant, L.D., Kimmel, C.A., West, G.L., Martinez-Vargas, C.M. and Howard, J.L. (1980). Chronic low-level lead toxicity in the rat. II. Effects on postnatal physical and behavioral development. *Toxicol. Appl. Pharmacol.*, **56**, 42–58

Greengard, J., Adams, B. and Berman, E. (1965). Acute lead encephalopathy in young children. Evaluation of therapy with a corticosteroid and moderate hypothermia. *J. Pediatr.* (St. Louis), **66**, 707–711

Guerit, J.M., Meulders, M., Amand, G., Roels, H.A., Buchet, J.P., Lauwerys, R., Bruaux, P., Claeys-Thoreau, F., Ducofre, G. and Lafontaine, A. (1981). Lead neurotoxicity in clinically asymptomatic children living in the vicinity of an ore smelter. *Clin. Toxicol.*, **18**, 1257–1267

Hall, A. and Cantab, M.D. (1905). The increasing use of lead as an abortifacient: a series of thirty cases of plumbism. *Br. Med. J.*, **1**, 584–587

Halliday, A.M. and McDonald, W.I. (1981). Visual evoked potentials. In: Stalberg, E. and Young, R.R. (eds.) *Clinical Neurophysiology*, pp. 228–258. (Boston, MA: Butterworths) (Butterworths International Medical Reviews: Neurology 1).

Hansen, J.C., Christensen, L.B. and Tarp, U. (1980). Hair lead concentration in children with minimal cerebral dysfunction. *Dan. Med. Bull.*, **27**, 259–262

Harvey, P., Hamlin, M. and Kumar, R. (1983). The Birmingham blood lead study. Presented at: annual conference of the British Psychological Society, symposium on lead and health: some psychological data; April; University of York, United Kingdom.

Harvey, P.G., Hamlin, M.W. and Kumar, R. (1984). Blood lead, behavior and intelligence test performance in preschool children. *Sci. Total Environ.*, **40**, 45–60

Hole, K., Dahle, H. and Klove, H. (1979). Lead intoxication as an etiologic factor in hyperkinetic behavior in children: a negative report. *Acta Paediatr. Scand.*, **68**, 759–760

Honzik, M.P. (1977). Value and limitations of infant tests: an overview. In: Lewis, M. (ed.) *Origins of Intelligence: Infancy and Early Childhood*, pp. 59–95. (New York, NY: Plenum Press)

Hunter, J., Urbanowicz, M.A., Yule, W. and Lansdown, R. (1985). Automated testing of reaction time and its association with lead in children. *Int. Arch. Occup. Environ. Health*, **57**, 27–34

Imbus, C.E., Warner, J., Smith, E., Pegelow, C.H., Allen, J.P. and Powars, D.R. (1978). Peripheral neuropathy in lead-intoxicated sickle cell patients. *Muscle Nerve*, **1**, 168–171

Johnson, N.E. and Tenuta, K. (1979). Diets and lead blood levels of children who practice pica. *Environ. Res.*, **18**, 369–376

Khera, A.K., Wibberley, D.G. and Dathan, J.G. (1980). Placental and stillbirth tissue lead concentrations in occupationally exposed women. *Br. J. Ind. Med.*, **37**, 394–396

Kirkconnell, S.C. and Hicks, L.E. (1980). Residual effects of lead poisoning on Denver developmental screening test scores. *J. Abnorm. Child Psychol.*, **8**, 257–267

Kline, T.S. (1960). Myocardial changes in lead poisoning. *Am. J. Dis. Child.*, **99**, 48–54

Kotok, D. (1972). Development of children with elevated blood lead levels: a controlled study. *J. Pediatr.* (St. Louis), **80**, 56–71

Kotok, D., Kotok, R. and Heriot, T. (1977). Cognitive evaluation of children with elevated blood lead levels. *Am. J. Dis. Child.*, **131**, 791–793

Krigman, M.R. (1978). Neuropathology of heavy metal intoxication. *EHP Environ. Health Perspect.*, **26**, 117–120

Krigman, M.R., Druse, M.J., Traylor, T.D., Wilson, M.H., Newell, L.R. and Hogan, E.L. (1974a). Lead encephalopathy in the developing rat: effect upon myelineation. *J. Neuropathol. Exp. Neurol.*, **33**, 58–73

Krigman, M.R., Druse, M.J., Traylor, T.D., Wilson, M.N., Newell, L.R. and Hogan, E.L. (1974b). Lead encephalopathy in the developing rat: effect on cortical ontogenesis. *J. Neuropathol. Exp. Neurol.*, **33**, 671–686

Lampert, P.W. and Schochet, S.S., Jr. (1968). Demyelineation and remyelination in lead neuropathy: electron microscopic studies. *J. Neuropathol. Exp. Neurol.*, **27**, 527–545

Landrigan, P.J., Whitworth, R.H., Baloh, R.W., Staehling, N.W., Barthel, W.F. and Rosenblum, B.T. (1975). Neuropsychological dysfunction in children with chronic low-level lead absorption. Lancet (7909), 708–712

Landrigan, P.J., Baker, E.L., Jr., Feldman, R.G., Cox, D.H., Eden, K.V., Orenstein, W.A., Mather, J.A., Yankel, A.J. and von Lindern, I.H. (1976). Increased lead absorption with anemia and slowed nerve conduction in children near a lead smelter. J. Pediatr. (St. Louis), 89, 904–910

Lansdown, R.G., Shepherd, J., Clayton, B.E., Delves, H.T., Graham, P.J. and Turner, W.C. (1974). Blood-lead levels, behavior, and intelligence – a population study. Lancet, 1(7857), 538–541

Lansdown, R., Yule, W., Urbanowicz, M.-A. and Hunter, J. (1986). The relationship between blood-lead concentrations, intelligence, attainment and behavior in a school population: the second London study. Int. Arch. Occup. Environ. Health, 57, 225–235

Lauwers, M.C., Hauspie, R.C., Susanne, C. and Verheyden, J. (1986). Comparison of biometric data of children with high and low levels of lead in the blood. Am. J. Phys. Anthropol., 69, 107–116

Lewis, B.W., Collins, R.J. and Wilson, H.S. (1955). Seasonal incidence of lead poisoning in children in St. Louis. South. Med. J., 48, 298–301

Lewis, M. and McGurk, H. (1973). [Response to letter by R.S. Wilson]. Science (Washington, DC), 182, 737

Lin-fu, J.S. (1972). Undue absorption of lead among children – a new look at an old problem. N. Engl. J. Med., 286, 702–710

Maracek, J., Shapiro, I.M., Burke, A., Katz, S.H. and Hediger, M.L. (1983). Low-level lead exposure in childhood influences neuropsychological performance. Arch. Environ. Health, 38, 355–359

Marlowe, M. and Errera, J. (1982). Low lead levels and behavior problems in children. Behav. Disord., 7, 163–172

Marlowe, M., Folio, R., Hall, D. and Errera, J. (1982). Increased lead burdens and trace-mineral status in mentally retarded children. J. Spec. Educ., 16, 87–99

Marlowe, M., Errera, J. and Jacobs, J. (1983). Increased lead and cadmium burdens among mentally retarded children and children with borderline intelligence. Am. J. Ment. Defic., 87, 477–483

Marlowe, M., Stellern, J., Moon, C. and Errera, J. (1985). Main and interaction effects of metallic toxins on aggressive classroom behavior. Aggressive Behav., 11, 41–48

McBride, W.G., Black, B.P. and English, B.J. (1982). Blood lead levels and behavior of 400 preschool children. Med. J. Aust., 2, 26–29

McKhann, C.F. and Vogt, E.C. (1926). Lead poisoning in children: with notes on therapy. Am. J. Dis. Child., 32, 386–392

McMichael, A.J., Vimpani, G.V., Robertson, E.F., Baghurst, P.A. and Clark, P.D. (1986). The Port Pirie cohort study: maternal blood lead and pregnancy outcome. J. Epidemiol. Commun. Health, 40, 18–25

McNeil, J.L. and Ptasnik, J.A. (1975). Evaluation of long-term effects of elevated blood lead concentrations in asymptomatic children. In: Recent Advances in the Assessment of the Health Effects of Environmental Pollution, Vol. 2, pp. 571–590. Proceedings, international symposium; June 1974; Paris, France. (Luxembourg: Commission of the European Communities)

Mellins, R.B. and Jenkins, C.D. (1955). Epidemiological and psychological study of lead poisoning in children. J. Am. Med. Assoc., 158, 15–20

Michaelson, I.A. (1973). Effects of inorganic lead on RNA, DNA and protein content in the development neonatal rat brain. Toxicol. Appl. Pharmacol., 26, 539–548

Milar, C.R., Schroeder, S.R., Mushak, P., Dolcourt, J.L. and Grant, L.D. (1980). Contributions of the caregiving environment to increased lead burden of children. Am. J. Ment. Defic., 84, 339–344

Milar, C.R., Schroeder, S.R., Mushak, P. and Boone, L. (1981). Failure to find hyperactivity in preschool children with moderately elevated lead burden. J. Pediatr. Psychol., 6, 85–95

Molina, G., Zuniga, M.A., Cardenas, A., Alvarez, R.M., Solis-Camara, P., Jr. and Solis-Camara, P. (1983). Psychological alterations in children exposed to a lead-rich home environment. Bull. Pan Am. Health Org., 27, 186–192

Moore, M.R., Meredith, P.A. and Goldberg, A. (1977). A retrospective analysis of blood-lead in mentally retarded children. Lancet, 1(8014), 717–719

Moore, M.R., Goldberg, A., Pocock, S.J., Meredith, A., Stewart, I.M., Macanespie, H., Lees,

R. and Low, A. (1982). Some studies of maternal and infant lead exposure in Glasgow. *Scot. Med. J.*, **27**, 113–122

Mooty, J., Ferrand, C.F. and Harris, P. (1975). Relationship of diet to lead poisoning in children. *Pediatrics*, **55**, 636–639

Muir, W.R. (1975). A review of studies on the effects of lead smelter emissions in El Paso, Texas. In: *International Conference on Heavy Metals in the Environment*: symposium proceedings, Vol. 3, pp. 297–304. October; Toronto, Ontario, Canada. (Toronto, Ontario, Canada: University of Toronto, Institute for Environmental Studies)

National Academy of Sciences. (1972). *Lead: Airborne Lead in Perspective*. (Washington, DC: National Academy of Sciencies) (Biologic effects of atmospheric pollutants).

National Center for Health Statistics. (1982). Births, marriages, divorces, and deaths for 1981. Hyattsville, MD: US Department of Health and Human Services; DHHS publication no. (PHS) 82-1120. (NCHS monthly vital statistics report vol. 30 no. 12).

Needleman, H. (1977). Effects of hearing loss from early recurrent otitis media on speech and language development. In: Jaffe, B.J. (ed.) *Hearing Loss in Children: a Comprehensive Text*, pp. 640–649. (Baltimore, MD: University Park Press)

Needleman, H.L. (1982). The neurobehavioral consequences of low lead exposure in childhood. *Neurobehav. Toxicol. Teratol.*, **4**, 729–732

Needleman, H.L. (1983). Low level lead exposure and neuropsychological performance. In: Rutter, M. and Russell Jones, R. (eds.) *Lead versus Health*, pp. 229–248. (New York, NY: John Wiley & Sons)

Needleman, H.L. (1984). Comments on chapter 12 and appendix 12c, air quality criteria for lead (external review draft # 1). (Pittsburgh, PA: Children's Hospital of Pittsburgh) Available for inspection at: US Environmental Protection Agency, Central Docket Section, Washington, DC; docket no. ECAO-CD-81-2 IIA.E.C.1.20.

Needleman, H.L. and Bellinger, D. (1984). The developmental consequences of childhood exposure to lead: recent studies and methodological issues. In: Lahey, B.B. and Kazdin, A.E. (eds.) *Advances in Clinical Psychology*, Vol. 7, pp. 195–220. (New York, NY: Plenum Press)

Needleman, H.L., Gunnoe, C., Leviton, A., Reed, R., Peresie, H., Maher, C. and Barrett, P. (1979). Deficits in psychologic and classroom performance of children with elevated dentine lead levels. *N. Engl. J. Med.*, **300**, 689–695

Needleman, H.L., Geiger, S.K. and Frank, R. (1985). Lead and IQ scores: a reanalysis [letter]. *Science* (Washington, DC), **227**, 701–704

Nordstrom, S., Beckman, L. and Nordenstrom, I. (1979). Occupational and environmental risks in and around a smelter in northern Sweden: V. spontaneous abortion among female employees and decreased birth weight in their offspring. *Hereditas*, **90**, 291–296

Norton, S. and Culver, B. (1977). A Golgi analysis of caudate neurons in rats exposed to carbon monoxide. *Brain Res.*, **132**, 455–465

Nye, L.J.J. (1929). An investigation of the extraordinary incidence of chronic nephritis in young people in Queensland. *Med. J. Aust.*, **2**, 145–159

Odenbro, A., Greenberg, N., Vroegh, K., Bederka, J. and Kihlstrom, J.-E. (1983). Functional disturbances in lead-exposed children. *Ambio*, **12**, 40–44

Oliver, T. (1911). Lead poisoning and the race. *Br. Med. J.*, **1**(2628), 1096–1098

Otto, D.A. (1985). The relationship of event-related brain potentials and lead absorption: a review of current evidence. In: Goldwater, L., Wysocki, L.M. and Volpe, R.A. (eds.) *Edited Proceedings: Lead Environmental Health – the Current Issues*; May; Durham, NC, pp. 151–164. (Durham, NC: Duke University)

Otto, D.A., Benignus, V.A., Muller, K.E. and Barton, C.N. (1981). Effects of age and body lead burden on CNS function in young children. I. Slow cortical potentials. *Electroencephalogr. Clin. Neurophysiol.*, **52**, 229–239

Otto, D., Benignus, V., Muller, K., Barton, C., Seiple, K., Prah, J. and Schroeder, S. (1982). Effects of low to moderate lead exposure on slow cortical potentials in young children: two year follow-up study. *Neurobehav. Toxicol. Teratol.*, **4**, 733–737

Otto, D.A., Baumann, S.B., Robinson, G.S., Schroeder, S.R., Kleinbaum, D.G., Barton, C.N. and Mushak, P. (1985). Auditory and visual evoked potentials in children with undue lead absorption [abstract]. *Toxicologist*, **5**, 81

Paul, C. (1860). Etude sur l'intoxication lente par les preparations de plomb, de son influence par le produit de la conception [Study of the effect of slow lead intoxication on the product of conception]. *Arch. Gen. Med.*, **15**, 513–533

Pentschew, A. (1965). Morphology and morphogenesis of lead encephalopathy. *Acta Neuropathol.*, **5**, 133–160

Pentschew, A. and Garro, F. (1966). Lead encephalo-myelopathy of the suckling rat and its implications on the porphyrinopathic nervous diseases, with special reference to the permeability disorders of the nervous system's capillaries. *Acta Neuropathol.*, **6**, 266–278

Perino, J. and Ernhart, C.B. (1974). The relation of subclinical lead level to cognitive and sensorimotor impairment in black preschoolers. *J. Learn. Dis.*, **7**, 616–620

Perlstein, M.A. and Attala, R. (1966). Neurologic sequelae of plumbism in children. *Clin. Pediatr.* (Philadelphia), **5**, 292–298

Pihl, R.O. and Parkes, M. (1977). Hair element content in learning disabled children. *Science* (Washington, DC), **198**, 204–206

Pocock, S.J. and Ashby, D. (1985). Environmental lead and children's intelligence: a review of recent epidemiological studies. *Statistician*, **34**, 31–44

Popoff, N., Weinberg, S. and Feigin, I. (1963). Pathologic observations in lead encephalopathy with special reference to the vascular changes. *Neurology*, **13**, 101–112

Prasher, D.K., Sainz, M. and Gibson, W.P.R. (1981). Binaural voltage summation of brainstorm auditory evoked potentials: an adjunct to the diagnostic criteria for multiple sclerosis. *Ann. Neurol.*, **11**, 86–95

Pueschel, S.M., Kopito, L. and Schwachman, H. (1972). Children with an increased lead burden. A screening and follow-up study. *J. Am. Med. Assoc.*, **222**, 462–466

Ratcliffe, J.M. (1977). Developmental and behavioral functions in young children with elevated blood lead levels. *Br. J. Prev. Soc. Med.*, **31**, 258–264

Robinson, G., Baumann, S., Kleinbaum, D., Barton, C., Schroeder, S., Mushak, P. and Otto, D. (1985). Effects of low to moderate lead exposure on brainstem auditory evoked potentials in children. In: *Environmental Health*, doc. 3: extended abstracts from the second international symposium on neurobehavioral methods in occupational and environmental health; August; Copenhagen, Denmark, pp. 177–182. (Copenhagen, Denmark: World Health Organization)

Roels, H., Hubermont, G., Buchet, J.-P. and Lauwerys, R. (1978). Placental transfer of lead, mercury, cadmium, and carbon monoxide in women: III. factors influencing the accumulation of heavy metals in the placenta and the relationship between metal concentration in the placenta and in maternal and cord blood. *Environ. Res.*, **16**, 236–247

Routh, D.K., Mushak, P. and Boone, L. (1979). A new syndrome of elevated blood lead and microcephaly. *J. Pediatr. Psychol.*, **4**, 67–76

Rummo, J.H. (1974). Intellectual and behavioral effects of lead poisoning in children [dissertation]. Chapel Hill, NC: University of North Carolina. Available from: University Microfilms, Ann Arbor, MI: publication no. 74–26, 930

Rummo, J.H., Routh, D.K., Rummo, N.J. and Brown, J.F. (1979). Behavioral and neurological effects of symptomatic and asymptomatic lead exposure in children. *Arch. Environ. Health*, **34**, 120–124

Rutter, M. (1980). Raised lead levels and impaired cognitive/behavioral functioning. *Dev. Med. Child Neurol.* (Suppl.), **42**, 1–26

Rutter, M. (1983). Scientific issues and state of the art in 1980. In: Rutter, M. and Russell Jones, R. (eds.) Lead versus health: sources and effects of low level lead exposure, pp. 1–15. (New York, NY: John Wiley & Sons)

Sachs, H.K., Krall, V., McCaughran, D.A., Rozenfeld, I.H., Youngsmith, N., Growe, G., Lazar, B.S., Novar, L., O'Connell, L. and Rayson, B. (1978). IQ following treatment of lead poisoning: a patient–sibling comparison. *J. Pediatr.* (St. Louis), **93**, 428–431

Sachs, H.K., McCaughran, D.A., Krall, V., Rozenfeld, I.H. and Youngsmith, N. (1979). Lead poisoning without encephalopathy: effect of early diagnosis on neurologic and psychologic salvage. *Am. J. Dis. Child.*, **133**, 786–790

Sachs, H.K., Krall, V. and Drayton, M.A. (1982). Neuropsychological assessment after lead poisoning without encephalopathy. *Percept. Motor Skills*, **54**, 1283–1288

Schroeder, S.R. and Hawk, B. (1987). Psycho-social factors, lead exposure, and IQ. In: Schroeder, S.R. (ed.) *Toxic Substances and Mental Retardation: Neurobehavioral Toxicology and Teratology*, pp. 97–137. (Washington, DC: American Association of Mental Deficiency) (Begab, M.J., ed. Monographs of the American Association on Mental Deficiency: no. 8).

Schroeder, S.R., Hawk, B., Otto, D.A., Mushak, P. and Hicks, R.E. (1985). Separating the effects of lead and social factors on IQ. In: Bornschein, R.L. and Rabinowitz, M.B. (eds.) *The Second International Conference on Prospective Studies of Lead*; April 1984; Cincinnati, OH. *Environ.*

Res., **38**, 144–154

Schwartz, J. and Otto, D. (1987). Blood lead, hearing thresholds, and neurobehavioral development in children and youth. *Arch. Environ. Health*, **42**, 153–160

Schwartz, J., Pitcher, H., Levin, R., Ostro, B. and Nichols, A.L. (1985). Costs and benefits of reducing lead in gasoline: final regulatory impact analysis. Washington, DC: US Environmental Protection Agency, Office of Policy, Planning and Evaluation; EPA report no. EPA-230/05-85-006.

Schwartz, J., Angle, C. and Pitcher, H. (1986). Relationship between childhood blood lead and stature. *Pediatrics*, **77**, 281–288

Seto, D.S.Y. and Freeman, J.M. (1964). Lead neuropathy in childhood. *Am. J. Dis. Child*, **107**, 337–342

Shaheen, S.J. (1984). Neuromaturation and behavior development: the case of childhood lead poisoning. *Dev. Psychol.*, **20**, 542–550

Shapiro, I.M. and Maracek, J. (1984). Dentine lead concentration as a predictor of neuropsychological functioning in inner-city children. *Biol. Trace Elem. Res.*, **6**, 69–78

Silbergeld, E.K., Hruska, R.E., Miller, L.P. and Eng, N. (1980). Effects of lead in vivo and in vitro on GABAergic neurochemistry. *J. Neurochem.*, **34**, 1712–1718

Silva, P.A., Hughes, P. and Faed, J.M. (1986). Blood lead levels in 579 Dunedin eleven year old children. *N.Z. Med. J.*, **99**, 179–183

Silva, P.A., Hughes, P., Williams, S. and Faed, J.M. (1988). Blood lead, intelligence, reading attainment, and behavior in eleven year old children in Dunedin, New Zealand. *J. Child Psychol. Psychiatry*, **29**, 43–52

Smith, F.L., 2nd, Rathmell, T.K. and Marcell, G.E. (1938). The early diagnosis of acute and latent plumbism. *Am. J. Clin. Pathol.*, **8**, 471–508

Smith, M., Delves, T., Lansdown, R., Clayton, B. and Graham, P. (1983). The effects of lead exposure on urban children: the Institute of Child Health/Southampton study. *Dev. Med. Child Neurol.*, **25(5)**, suppl. 47

Sotelo, C. and Palay, S.L. (1971). Altered axons and axon terminals in the lateral vestibular nucleus of the rat: possible example of axonal remodeling. *Lab. Invest.*, **25**, 653–671

Tanis, A.L. (1955). Lead poisoning in children. *Am. J. Dis. Child.*, **89**, 325–331

Thatcher, R.W., Lester, M.L., McAlaster, R. and Horst, R. (1982). Effects of low levels of cadmium and lead on cognitive functioning in children. *Arch. Environ. Health*, **37**, 159–166

Thatcher, R.W., McAlaster, R. and Lester, M.L. (1984). Evoked potentials related to hair cadmium and lead in children. *Ann. N.Y. Acad. Sci.*, **425**, 384–390

US Centers for Disease Control. (1985). Preventing lead poisoning in young children. Atlanta, GA: US Department of Health and Human Services, Centers for Disease Control; no. 99-2230.

US Environmental Protection Agency, Office of Policy and Analysis. (1984). Comments on issues raised in the analysis of the neuropsychological effects of low level lead exposure. Presented at: Clean Air Scientific Advisory Committee (CASAC) meeting; April; Research Triangle Park, NC. Available for inspection at: US Environmental Protection Agency, Central Docket Station, Washington, DC: docket no. ECAO-CD-81-2 IIA.F.19.

US Environmental Protection Agency. (1986a). Air quality criteria for lead. Research Triangle Park, NC: Office of Health and Environmental Assessment, Environmental Criteria and Assessment Office; EPA report no. EPA-600/8-83/028aF-dF. 4v. Available from: NTIS, Springfield, VA; PB87-142378.

US Environmental Protection Agency. (1986b). Lead effects on cardiovascular function, early development, and stature: an addendum to US EPA *Air Quality Criteria for Lead* (1986). In: Air quality criteria for lead. Research Triangle Park, NC: Office of Health and Environmental Assessment, Environmental Criteria and Assessment Office; pp. A1–A67.

Usher, R.H. and McLean, F.H. (1974). Normal fetal growth and the significance of fetal growth retardation. In: Davis, J.A. and Dobbing, J. (eds.) *Scientific Foundations of Paediatrics*, pp. 69–80. (London: Heinemann Medical Books)

Uzych, L. (1985). Teratogenesis and mutagenesis associated with the exposure of human males to lead: a review. *Yale J. Biol. Med.*, **58**, 9–17

Vimpani, G.V., Wigg, N.R., Robertson, E.F., McMichael, A.J., Baghurst, P.A. and Roberts, R.J. (1985). The Port Pirie cohort study: blood lead concentration and childhood developmental assessment. In: Goldwater, L.J., Wysocki, L.M. and Volpe, R.A. (eds.) *Edited Proceedings: Lead Environmental Health – the Current Issues*; May; Durham, NC, pp. 139–146. (Durham, NC:

Duke University)

Wilson, D.M., Hammer, L.D., Duncan, P.M., Dornbusch, S.M., Ritter, P.L., Hintz, R.L., Gross, R.T. and Rosenfeld, R.G. (1986). Growth and intellectual development. *Pediatrics*, **78**, 646–650

Wilson, R.S. (1973). Testing infant intelligence [letter]. *Science* (Washington, DC), **182**, 734–736

Wilson, R.S. and Harpring, E.B. (1972). Mental and motor development in infant twins. *Dev. Psychol.*, **7**, 227–287

Winneke, G. and Kraemer, U. (1984). Neuropsychological effects of lead in children: interactions with social background variables. *Neuropsychobiology*, **11**, 195–202

Winneke, G., Hrdina, K.-G. and Brockhaus, A. (1982). Neuropsychological studies in children with elevated tooth lead concentrations. Part I: Pilot study. *Int. Arch. Occup. Environ. Health*, **51**, 169–183

Winneke, G., Kramer, U., Brockhaus, A., Ewers, U., Kujanek, G., Lechner, H. and Janke, W. (1983). Neuropsychological studies in children with elevated tooth-lead concentrations. Part II: extended study. *Int. Arch. Occup. Environ. Health*, **51**, 231–252

Winneke, G., Beginn, U., Ewert, T., Havestadt, C., Kramer, U., Krause, C., Thron, H.L. and Wagner, H.M. (1984). Studies zur Erfassusng subklinischer Bleiwirkungen auf das Nervensystem bei Kindern mit bekannter praenataler Exposition in Nordenham [Study on the determination of subclinical lead effects on the nervous system of Nordenham children with known prenatal exposure] *Schriftenr. Ver. Wasser. Boden. Lufthyg.*, **(59)**, 215–229

Wolf, A.W., Ernhart, C.B. and White, C.S. (1985). Intrauterine lead exposure and early development. In: Lekkas, T.D. (ed.) *International Conference: Heavy Metals in the Environment*; September; Athens, Greece, Vol. 2, pp. 153–155. (Edinburgh: CEP Consultants)

Yerushalmy, J. (1970). Relation of birth weight, gestational age, and the rate of intrauterine growth to perinatal mortality. *Clin. Obstetr. Gynecol.*, **13**, 107–129

Youroukos, S., Lyberatos, C., Philippidou, A., Gardikas, C. and Tsomi, A. (1978). Increased blood lead levels in mentally retarded children in Greece. *Arch. Environ. Health*, **33**, 297–300

Yule, W. and Lansdown, R. (1983). Lead and children's development: recent findings. In: *International Conference Heavy Metals in the Environment*; September; Heidelberg, West Germany, Vol. 2, pp. 912–916. (Edinburgh: CEP Consultants)

Yule, W., Lansdown, R., Millar, I.B. and Urbanowicz, M.-A. (1981). The relationship between blood lead concentrations, intelligence and attainment in a school population: a pilot study. *Dev. Med. Child Neurol.*, **23**, 567–576

Yule, W., Urbanowicz, M.-A., Lansdown, R. and Millar, I.B. (1984). Teachers' ratings of children's behavior in relation to blood lead levels. *Br. J. Dev. Psychol.*, **2**, 295–305

Section 2

INTRODUCTORY PAPERS

2.1
Lead: Ancient Metal – Modern Menace?

G. KAZANTZIS

SUMMARY

The use of lead since prehistoric times, and its mobilization into the global environment has resulted in increased exposure to, and uptake of, this inessential trace metal. Acute lead poisoning following both occupational and general environmental exposure has been recognized since classical times and has become increasingly common following industrialization. While the control of the working environment has now resulted in a marked decline in the frequency of acute lead poisoning in industrialized societies, the development of indicators of absorption and effect has facilitated investigation of the more subtle effects of lead. Neurobehavioural deficits have been documented in children as sequelae of acute lead poisoning. The greater intake and absorption of lead by children, together with the sensitivity of the developing nervous system to the effects of lead, has stimulated extensive research on a possible causal relationship between low-level lead exposure and neurobehavioural effects in children. These studies have been beset with methodological difficulties requiring coordinated activity between investigators and careful consideration of the objectives of future research programmes.

This workshop has been convened to consider the effects of low-level lead absorption on the health of children, in particular on whether such absorption can give rise to subtle neuropsychiatric effects. In recent years an enormous amount of work has been carried out in this field, giving rise to over 3000 publications of varied worth. I will attempt to trace the stages in our understanding of the adverse health effects of lead, and will try to show how we have arrived at the stage in which we find ourselves at the present time.

Lead is, as far as we know, an inessential trace metal which is widely distributed in the global environment. The release of lead from human activities over millennia has been such that it is now difficult to estimate its natural concentration. Studies indicate that natural air-lead concentrations were some two to four orders of magnitude lower than present day values (Patterson, 1965). Current worldwide atmospheric lead emissions from human activities have been estimated at 450,000 tons/year compared with about 25,000 tons/year from natural sources. Indeed, the *International Register for Potentially Toxic Chemicals*, of the United Nations Environment Programme, lists lead as one of ten environmentally dangerous chemical substances and processes of global significance – cadmium and mercury being the other metals in this listing (UNEP, 1984).

THE USE OF LEAD THROUGH THE AGES

A historical account of the uses of lead has been given by Smith (1986) and in more detail, interestingly illustrated, to include the role of lead in art through the ages, by Krysko (1979). These sources have been drawn on here.

Lead may have been the first metal to have been smelted, probably from its sulphide ore, galena. Lead beads have been found, together with gold and copper ornaments, in Anatolia dating from 7000 to 6500 BC. There are several references to lead in the Old Testament of the Bible, lead was used in the construction of the Hanging Gardens of Babylon, and the Phoenicians mined lead in Spain from about 2000 BC. Lead ores were mined in ancient times, in large part for their silver content. In the process of cupellation the ore was heated to a higher temperature for the extraction of silver, producing lead oxide, used as a glaze in ceramics from about 5000 BC. Lead carbonate, known as cerussa, was used as a pottery glaze, and Xenophon referred to its use as a cosmetic to whiten the face. Lead was used since ancient times to improve the quality of glass.

The Romans used lead throughout their empire for the construction of aqueducts and cisterns. We can see an example of this in the city of Bath today. Cooking utensils were made of copper, lead or pewter, in Roman times a 50% lead–tin alloy. Lead was mined in Britain by the Romans for about three centuries, and the need for lead may have been one motive for the conquest of Britain.

Following the decline of the Roman Empire the use of lead diminished considerably, although lead was used for roofing and piping in the stately homes of England and France at the time of the Renaissance, and extensively in warfare. It was, however, the Industrial Revolution which saw a great upsurge in the use of lead. The manufacture of white lead by the stack process has been graphically described by Charles Dickens in *The Uncommercial Traveller* (1867). Women and children were employed indiscriminately in the manufacture of lead paints, in the smelting of lead ores and in pottery glazing. Good respirators were provided, Dickens wrote, 'made of flannel and muslin, gauntlet gloves and loose gowns and a female attendant to help them, and to watch that they do not neglect the cleansing of their hands before touching their food'. The transfer of lead from the work to the nearby home environment in the nineteenth century would have been considerable.

Between 1850 and 1855 the Analytical Sanitary Commission – set up by Thomas Wakley, editor of the *Lancet* – instituted a searching investigation into food adulteration. Their reports included analysis of 100 samples of children's sweets, 59 of which were coloured with chromate of lead and 12 with red lead (Hassall, 1855).

In our time, over the past decade, over 2.5 million metric tonnes of lead have been mined annually. The lead acid battery accounts for over half of this total. Other major uses of lead are in the manufacture of the petrol additive tetraethyl lead, in cable sheathing, lead sheet and pipe, pigments, bearings, solders, printing, shielding for ionizing radiation and for a variety of other purposes.

LEAD IN THE ENVIRONMENT

This extensive usage of lead has given rise to widespread environmental contamination. In rural areas ambient lead levels are usually below 0.2 $\mu g/m^3$; in remote areas of the world one or two orders of magnitude below this, and in urban areas one order of magnitude above, with values up to 10 $\mu g/m^3$ not infrequently recorded in dense traffic. Over one-half and up to 90% of the airborne lead is derived from vehicle exhausts, the remainder from refuse incineration, fossil fuel combustion and from industrial sources such as smelters, iron and steel works and lead processing plants.

Lead levels in drinking water are generally below 10 $\mu g/l$, but in soft-water areas with lead piping, concentrations have exceeded 1 mg/l, with higher values in first-draw samples (Moore, 1983). The lead content of soil is determined from natural and anthropogenic sources. The principal contributions to the latter come from mining activities, industrial sources and motor vehicle emissions. However, only a small fraction of the lead in soil is biologically available. Street dust can contain a considerable amount of lead derived from industrial sources, mines, old flaking paint and motor vehicle emissions, ranging from 500 to 5000 $\mu g/g$, and even higher values have been recorded in highly polluted areas (Duggan and Williams, 1977)

The lead content of different foodstuffs varies widely, plant-based foods being the major source. Total diet studies in industrialized countries indicate a lead intake of the order of 200–300 μg per day, although values ranging from less than 100 to more than 400 μg/day have been quoted (MAFF, 1982). Lead solder in cans, and the ingestion of dust by young children, make significant contributions to the daily lead intake, as does lead plumbing in areas with soft-water supplies.

Chamberlain (1983) estimated that about 10% of dietary lead is contributed by atmospheric fallout, but this was considered to be an underestimate by the Royal Commission on Environmental Pollution (1983). The factors influencing absorption of ingested and inhaled lead are complex and beyond the scope of this review. Current evidence suggests that some 75% of the total uptake of lead by the body is derived from dietary sources.

THE ADVERSE HEALTH EFFECTS OF LEAD

The earliest description of acute lead poisoning has been attributed to Hippocrates, who in 370 BC reported a severe attack of colic and constipation

121

in a worker who extracted metals, although lead was not identified. The Greek physician Nikander, in the second century BC, gave in the *Alexipharmac* a description of lead poisoning following exposure to lead oxide (cerussa) with pallor, colic, paralysis of limbs and ocular disturbance resulting in death (Major, 1945). Pliny, in the first century AD, described lead workers tying up their faces in loose bags to 'avoid inhaling the pernicious dust'. However, lead poisoning was more than an occupational disease in Roman times. Indeed Gilfillan (1965) suggested that lead poisoning resulting in a low birth rate, and high child mortality among the aristocracy, was responsible for the decline of the Roman empire. This theory was developed by Nriagu (1983), but the role of lead is here likely to have been overstated (Simms, 1984). Nevertheless, even as far back as classical times we have evidence of lead poisoning being both an occupational and an environmentally determined disorder.

Outbreaks of lead poisoning reaching epidemic proportions have been described occurring in medieval times. One such outbreak in seventeenth-century France became known as the Poitiers colic. In England the Devonshire colic was attributed by Sir George Baker in 1767 to contamination through the use of lead presses to crush cider apples. Baker was able to confirm the presence of lead in cider, but was roundly condemned by Devonshire folk for bringing their much-prized local product into disrepute.

In Britain in the mid-nineteenth century occupational lead poisoning was a not uncommon disorder. The Factories (Prevention of Lead Poisoning) Act 1883, which required white lead factories to conform to certain standards, was the first Act of Parliament to be directed against a specific occupational disease. The appointment of Thomas Legge as the first medical inspector of factories resulted in lead poisoning being made a notifiable disease in 1899. In the first 5 years of this century almost 4000 cases were notified, with over 100 deaths. The effect of notification in controlling acute lead poisoning can be seen in the steady decline of cases during the present century despite a marked increase in the consumption of lead.

Acute lead poisoning most commonly presents with severe abdominal colic accompanied by constipation. It has been mistaken for the acute surgical abdomen, the finding of anaemia with basophilic stippling of erythrocytes on a routine blood film making the correct diagnosis. The most dramatic presentation of acute lead poisoning is encephalopathy, which may present with convulsions resembling grand mal epilepsy, or with coma, delirium, a toxic Korsakow-type psychosis, transient pareses which may also involve one or more cranial nerves, aphasia or aphonia. A more chronic form of encephalopathy also occurs, characterized by headaches, mental dullness, transitory aphasia, hemianopia, and tremor (Hunter, 1978). Papilloedema and both primary and secondary optic atrophy may occur, particularly in children, who may present with headache, vomiting, occasional convulsions, gross papilloedema and paralysis of the external rectus of the eye. Among 200 cases of lead poisoning admitted to the Brisbane Children's Hospital, 54 showed marked papilloedema (Gibson, 1922, quoted by Hunter, 1978).

An account of cases of lead poisoning in girls in an institution caused by drinking water kept in a leaden cistern describes 'head and belly ache; loss of appetite; sickness; rapid pulse; hot, dry skin; flushed dusky countenance; confined bowels . . . several had fits described as being hysterical; some had faintings; the majority had a relapse, some even three times' (Robertson, 1851).

Another classic feature of acute lead poisoning is a motor neuropathy giving rise to weakness or paralysis, most commonly of the external muscles of the dominant hand, to produce the classical wrist-drop. Lead palsy less frequently affects the lower limbs giving rise to foot-drop, a condition seen more often in children than in adults.

Until the nineteenth century acute adverse health effects were attributed to lead exposure by associating the development of symptoms with such exposure. In 1839, Tanquerel des Planches published his classic description of acute lead poisoning based on 1213 admissions to La Charité Hospital in Paris. These cases occurred in workers engaged in the manufacture of lead compounds, painters, potters, copper and bronze founders and others in industries involving exposure to lead. He, and in 1840, Burton in London, described the leaden blue line seen on the gum in lead-poisoned patients, about a millimetre from the gingival margin. This then became an indicator of absorption and a rough guide to duration and intensity of exposure, but not to lead intoxication. About the same time Laennec described pallor of the tissues and thinness of the blood as a further feature of lead poisoning.

A mild to moderate anaemia is responsible for the pallor seen in classical cases of lead poisoning. The lowered haemoglobin is accompanied by basophilic stippling of erythrocytes, not specific to lead poisoning but most frequently seen in this condition. So consistent is the anaemia produced by over-exposure to lead that for a long time haemoglobin estimation has been used as a screening test for evidence of excessive lead absorption by workers. Until recently a 3-monthly haemoglobin estimation was the only investigation required by law for certain categories of lead worker in Britain.

So far only acute adverse effects which could be readily associated with excessive lead exposure have been considered. However, studies on lead workers have elicited symptoms of lassitude, anorexia, abdominal discomfort, constipation, insomnia, irritability, pallor and anaemia – complaints which are common in the general population. The recent development of environmental and biological monitoring procedures, and of epidemiological methodology, now enables us to investigate non-specific and subclinical effects in relation to lead exposure with greater precision.

ANALYTICAL CONSIDERATIONS

The development of analytical methods for the determination of lead concentration in environmental and biological samples has been a turning point in our understanding of the more subtle adverse health effects of lead. Early attempts to measure lead in body fluids were crude. An early study on lead poisoning in welders engaged on dismantling naval vessels estimated lead in urine by precipitation of lead as the chromate and determination of chromate content.

The presence of lead in bone was identified as early as 1861 by Gusserow in Germany. In an elegant series of experiments in the cat, Minot and Aub (1924) showed the quantitative deposition and storage of lead in the skeleton following respiratory absorption.

The development of colorimetric, polarographic and atomic absorption spectrophotometric techniques has enabled lead to be estimated in biological samples in increasingly low concentrations. Currently used measures of absorption and effect are reviewed in the next chapter, by Mushak.

In Britain, the estimation of blood lead is now common practice. Blood lead (PbB) estimations were performed on exposed workers by the Employment Medical Advisory Service from around 1974, in conjunction with the legally required haemoglobin estimation. PbB estimation at regular intervals for certain categories of lead worker became mandatory in 1980 (Control of Lead at Work Regulations, 1980).

For the periodic monitoring of workers exposed to lead, the Commission of the European Communities now recommends PbB level as a measure of internal dose and erythrocyte protoporphyrin (see Mushak, this volume) as an indicator of effect. It is further recommended that in male workers PbB levels should not exceed 60 µg/dl, and in women workers of childbearing age PbB should be no higher than 40 µg/dl because of a potential adverse effect on the fetus (Alessio and Foa, 1983).

While adherence to these levels ensures that the majority of lead-exposed adults would not experience clinical adverse effects, they cannot be taken as 'no-effect' levels. Over the years, with increasing understanding of the effects of lead, permissible PbB levels for workers have been systematically reduced. Some sensitive individuals have experienced adverse clinical effects at PbB levels below 60 µg/dl, a decrease in nerve conduction velocity has been demonstrated at levels between 30 and 60 µg/dl, and erythrocyte protoporphyrin has been shown to be raised in females at PbB levels of 15–20 µg/dl.

Children are more sensitive to the effects of lead than adults. Encephalopathy usually occurs in adults with PbB levels above 120 µg/dl, but in children at PbB levels of 80–100 µg/dl. Lead colic and peripheral neuropathy has occurred in children at PbB levels down to 60 µg/dl. Reduced haemoglobin synthesis may be seen in adults above 50 µg/dl but in children at levels as low as 40 µg/dl, and ZPP elevation at PbB levels of 15–20 µg/dl.

THE MORE SUBTLE ADVERSE EFFECTS OF LEAD

An adverse pregnancy outcome was recognized in the previous century in women occupationally exposed to lead, and reported in more recent studies of women with heavy lead exposure. In the earlier studies, first-trimester abortions and stillbirths were reported, with macrocephaly and seizures in livebirths. A lowered fertility rate has also been claimed. However at current UK levels of occupational lead exposure in females an adverse effect on pregnancy outcome or on fertility has not been documented. The evidence for a possible association between lead exposure and chromosomal aberration is contradictory.

Lead-induced nephropathy was first reported more than a century ago. However, the condition remains to be clearly defined. A study from Queensland, Australia, described 34 patients with a chronic nephropathy who had suffered from lead palsy in childhood following exposure to lead paints (Nye, 1933). Interstitial fibrosis, tubular atrophy and dilation have been observed in workers with heavy long-term exposure to lead. Renal tubular dysfunction characterized by glycosuria and aminoaciduria has been observed in lead-exposed children (Chisholm and Leahy, 1962). Lead exposure should be considered in the differential diagnosis of glycosuria occurring in childhood.

An increased mortality from cerebrovascular disease has been observed in a study on lead battery workers (Dingwall-Fordyce and Lane, 1963). An association between lead absorption and the development of hypertension has been claimed, initially in lead-exposed workers. In a US population-based study on adult males, lead was found to be significantly related to both systolic and diastolic blood pressure after controlling for a number of confounding variables (Schwartz, 1985). However, a British population-based study on men aged 40–59 found only a very weak association between PbB and either systolic or diastolic blood pressure. The investigators commented on the problem of adjusting adequately for all relevant confounders, and concluded that it is premature to consider that an elevated lead body burden has a causal influence on blood pressure (Pocock et al., 1985).

Lead acetate, subacetate and lead phosphate administered in high doses can induce adenocarcinoma of the kidney in rats and mice. With sufficient animal data, IARC (1987) assigned lead and inorganic lead compounds to Group 2B, the group of chemicals with insufficient evidence regarding their carcinogenicity in humans. In a recent cohort study of over 7000 workers in lead battery and lead production plants in the USA, a significant excess mortality has been found for both lung and stomach cancer (Cooper et al., 1985). In this study account could not be taken of important confounding factors, and data were inadequate to seek evidence of a dose–effect relationship. It would be premature to postulate at this stage a causal relationship between lead exposure and cancer in humans.

Consideration must now be given to the neurotoxic effects of lead. Mention has already been made of encephalopathy as a cardinal feature of acute lead poisoning. The nature of the pathological changes – which include perivascular haemorrhage, increased intracranial pressure as evidenced by papilloedema, and neuronal degeneration as evidenced by optic atrophy – indicate the occurrence of neuronal damage and destruction, and it is likely that such effects will have been initiated before the onset of symptoms. As cellular regeneration within the central nervous system does not occur, permanent functional deficits must result. This in fact is the case, postencephalic sequelae in children ranging from clinical convulsions and idiocy in severe cases to a lack of motor coordination and sensory perception in milder cases. Encephalopathy occurs most frequently in children between the ages of 1 and 3 years with a history of pica, with access to flakes of lead-containing paint, lead sulphide-containing eye cosmetics or lead dust brought from the workplace on clothing.

It occurs more often during the summer, and may possibly be related to vitamin D activation of lead from skeletal stores.

Classic lead palsy results from axonal degeneration or segmental demyelination of peripheral nerve. Interference with central neurotransmitter function may also be involved (Fullerton, 1966; Silbergeld, 1983). Impaired nerve conduction velocity has been observed in lead workers who were without evidence of any clinical adverse effect (Seppäläinen and Hernberg, 1972) and in children with clinical lead poisoning but without evidence of neuropathy (Feldman et al., 1973). An improvement in nerve-conduction velocity following chelation therapy with calcium EDTA has also been reported (Araki et al., 1980). Good correlations of nerve conduction velocity with PbB have not been reported, but PbB estimated at the time of nerve conduction measurement may not have been indicative of past exposure. Nevertheless, here we have evidence for functional involvement of the nervous system with moderately raised PbB levels, not associated with clinical symptoms or signs.

In 1943, Byers and Lord followed up 20 children who had been hospitalized for lead poisoning, only two of whom had evidence of encephalopathy characterized by convulsions. While all had made a complete recovery from the known effects of lead poisoning, all but one subsequently developed deficits in perceptual motor function, experienced difficulties at school and suffered from emotional problems. Such studies, together with the recognition that body burdens of lead in present-day populations greatly exceed those in what might be termed the 'natural state', and the observation in children of a higher intake and absorption per unit weight, stimulated research into possible neurobehavioural effects of lead in young children without any preceding history of lead poisoning.

Studies in the 1970s indicated that, in children, PbB levels persistently raised above 60 μg/dl tended to be associated with a three- to four-point reduction in intelligence quotient, even if the children were asymptomatic. However, below this level, research has been beset with a number of major epidemiological problems related to the inadequacy of the available indicators of exposure and effect; to study design and statistical interpretation, and to the lack of understanding of underlying biological mechanisms.

With regard to the first of these, while tooth lead levels provide information on lead body burden, teeth have not been sampled in a standardized manner, and neither blood nor tooth lead values give information on the biologically active fraction of lead or on lead uptake by the nervous system. With regard to effect indicators, measures of neurobehavioural function have been in general insensitive and in some instances inappropriate. Many studies showed serious defects in their design – selection bias, small sample size, multiple significance testing, inadequate control of confounding variables. Furthermore, in the absence of a sound theoretical model on which to base observations, studies have tended to become increasingly data-driven rather than model-driven. Not knowing what to measure, the tendency has been to measure as much as possible, and to search for a pattern in the data collected, thus introducing the risk of inferring causation from statistical association.

The major studies will be reviewed later in this volume. At the present time a no-effect level for lead on the nervous system cannot be given, in

126

particular with regard to intelligence and behaviour of children. It is sincerely hoped that the result of this Workshop will be to stimulate increasing coordination of research activities between investigators in the relevant scientific disciplines, and that the most careful consideration will be given to the objectives and design of future research programmes.

REFERENCES

Alessio, L. and Foa, V. (1983) Lead, in Alessio, L., Berlin, A., Roi, R. and Boni, M. (eds), *Human Biological Monitoring of Industrial Chemicals* series (Luxembourg: Commission of the European Communities)

Araki, S., Honma, T., Yanagihara, S. and Ushio, K. (1980) Recovery of slowed nerve conduction velocity in lead exposed workers. *Int. Arch. Occup. Environ. Health*, **46**, 151–157

Byers, R.K. and Lord, E.E. (1983) Late effects of lead poisoning on mental development. *Am. J. Dis. Child.*, **66**, 471–494

Chamberlain, A.C. (1943) Fallout of lead and uptake by crops. *Atmos. Environ.*, **17**, 693–706

Chisholm, J.J. and Leahy, N.B. (1962) Aminoaciduria as a manifestation of renal tubular injury in lead intoxication and a comparison with patterns of aminoaciduria seen in other diseases. *J. Pediat.*, **60**, 1–17

Cooper, W.C., Wong, O. and Kheifets, L. (1985) Mortality among employees of lead battery plants and lead producing plants, 1947–1980. *Scand. J. Work Environ. Health*, **11**, 331–345

Dingwall-Fordyce, I. and Lane, R.E. (1963) A follow-up study of lead workers. *Br. J. Ind. Med.*, **20**, 313–315

Duggan, M.J. and Williams, S. (1977) Lead in dust in city streets. *Sci. Total Environ.*, **7**, 91–97

Feldman, R.G., Haddow, J., Kopito, L. and Schwachman, H. (1973) Altered peripheral nerve conduction velocity. *Am. J. Dis. Child.*, **125**, 39–41

Fullerton, P.M. (1966) Chronic peripheral neuropathy produced by lead poisoning in guinea pigs. *J. Neuropathol. Exp. Neurol.*, **25**, 214–236

Gilfillan, S.C. (1965) Lead poisoning and the fall of Rome. *J. Occup. Med.*, **7**, 53–60

Hassall, A.H. (1855) *Food and its Adulterations; comprising the reports of the Analytical Sanitary Commission of* The Lancet (London: Longman, Brown, Green and Longmans)

Hunter, D. (1978) Lead, in *The Diseases of Occupations* (London: Hodder & Stoughton)

IARC (1987) Monographs on the Evaluation of the Carcinogenic Risk of Chemicals to Humans, IARC Monographs supplement 7 (Lyon: International Agency for Research on Cancer)

Krysko, W.W. (1979) *Lead in History and Art* (Stuttgart: Dr Riederer)

MAFF (1982) *Survey of Lead in Food: Second Supplementary Report*. Food Surveillance Paper No. 10, Ministry of Agriculture, Fisheries and Food (London: HMSO)

Major, R.H. (1945) *Classic Descriptions of Disease*, 3rd edn (Illinois: Thomas)

Minot, A. and Aub, J.C. (1924) Lead studies: the distribution of lead in the human organism. *J. Ind. Hygiene*, **6**, 149

Moore, M.R. (1983) Lead exposure and water plumbosolvency, in Rutter, M. and Jones, R. (eds), *Lead Versus Health: Sources and Effects of Low-level Lead Exposure*, pp. 79–106 (Chichester: Wiley)

Nriagu, J.O. (1983) *Lead and Lead Poisoning in Antiquity* (New York: Wiley)

Nye, L.J.J. (1933) *Chronic Nephritis and Lead Poisoning* (Sydney: Angus & Robertson)

Patterson, C.C. (1965) Contaminated and natural environments of man. *Arch. Environ. Health*, **11**, 322–360

Pocock, S.J., Shaper, A.G., Ashby, D. and Delves, T. (1985) Blood lead and blood pressure in middle-aged men. *International Conference: Heavy metals in the Environment* (Athens: CEP Consultants), vol. 1, pp. 303–305

Robertson, J. (1851) An account of cases of chronic lead poisoning caused by drinking water kept in a leaden cistern. *Lancet*, **1**, 202

Royal Commission on Environmental Pollution (1983) *Lead in the Environment*, Ninth Report, Cmd 8852 (London: HMSO)

Schwartz, J.J. (1985) The relationship between blood lead and blood pressure. *International*

Conference Heavy Metals in the Environment (Athens: CEP Consultants), vol. 1, pp. 300–302

Seppäläinen, A.M. and Hernberg, S. (1972) Sensitive technique for detecting subclinical lead neuropathy. *Br. J. Ind. Med.*, **29**, 443–449

Silbergeld, E. (1983) Experimental studies of lead neurotoxicity: implication for mechanisms, dose–response and reversibility, in Rutter, M. and Russell Jones, R. (eds), *Lead Versus Health: Sources and Effects of Low-level Lead Exposure* (Chichester: Wiley)

Simms, D.L. (1984) Lead in history, leaden history, lead or history? *Sci. Total Environ.*, **37**, 259–266

Smith, M. (1986) Lead in history, in Lansdown, R. and Yule, W. (eds), *The Lead Debate: The Environment, Toxicology and Child Health*, (London: Croom Helm)

UNEP (1984) List of environmentally dangerous chemical substances and processes of global significance. *International Register for Potentially Toxic Chemicals* (Geneva: United Nations Environment Programme)

2.2
Biological Monitoring of Lead Exposure in Children: Overview of Selected Biokinetic and Toxicological Issues

P. MUSHAK

SUMMARY

The biological monitoring of lead exposure in paediatric and adult human populations has usually involved one of two approaches: (1) measurement of the internal or systemic dose of lead itself in some indicator medium, or (2) quantification of some 'subcritical' effect of lead. The extent to which biological monitoring in humans accurately states both exposure risk and relative health risk remains the subject of much research. Of particular interest are (1) the biokinetic characteristics of the common indicators of exposure, (2) the development and use of kinetic models of lead metabolism, and (3) the relative merits of the use of biological effect indicators versus measurement of the toxicant in some medium.

Any successful study of the adverse effects of lead exposure in children rests heavily on the quality of the methods used to monitor the type and extent of lead exposure in these subjects, and how well such exposures can be quantitatively related to adverse health risk and population response.

In general, there are several ways to monitor the exposure of human populations to lead or other environmental pollutants. The traditional approach has been that of environmental monitoring, in which the level of toxicant is measured in those environmental media which also serve as routes of human exposure (e.g., ambient or workplace air, food, drinking water, soil). Currently, however, increasing preference is being given to biological monitoring, in which measurements are taken of the level of a pollutant, one or more of the pollutant's metabolites, or some metabolic change relatively specific for the substance, in some biological medium obtained from an exposed subject (e.g., blood, mineralizing or keratinizing tissues, excreta). Although the use of certain biological effect indicators as exposure indices in the case of lead has been frequently recorded, this type of monitoring is more appropriately placed under the heading of health surveillance monitoring.

There are a number of recognized advantages to biological versus environmental monitoring, although the two approaches should not be viewed as being mutually exclusive. One virtue of biological monitoring is that it represents the systemic or internal level of exposure of the subject, being the result of the integration of all exposure routes and toxicokinetic parameters relating to intake and uptake of the substance.

With the increasing popularity of biological monitoring of lead exposure in children and other human populations, there is also recognition of some problems of both utility and interpretation, and these centre around the following issues: (1) the relative ease and reliability of the quantitative analysis of the toxicant; (2) the strength of the relationship between internal and external (environmental) exposure as well as interrelationships among various biological indicators of lead exposure, e.g., lead in whole blood (PbB) versus lead in teeth (PbT) or lead in hair (Pb-Hair); and (3) the relationship of the particular internal exposure measure to any quantitative health risk assessment.

Since biological monitoring is now commonly employed to assess both lead exposure and health risk relationships in young children and adult populations, and this includes the various prospective studies currently under way, it is of interest to consider some issues specific to biological monitoring of this particular toxicant. These areas of discussion include: (1) the quantitative relationship between some environmental medium and the amount present in some biological medium, e.g., the relationship of lead in air to lead in blood; (2) the state of development of various biokinetic models to provide theoretical underpinnings for lead's biokinetic behaviour in organisms; (3) the characteristics of the various methods of biological monitoring as determined by both experiment and modelling exercises, including the interrelationships among various biological indicators; (4) the quantitative relationship of exposure indices such as lead in blood to target or critical organs for lead's effects and associated dose–effect and dose–population response relationships; and (5) the relative value of lead levels in some biological medium compared to the use of certain early biological effect indicators of lead exposure. Although the quantitative relationship of lead in biological, versus lead in environmental, media is an important topic and comprises an extensive literature, this area is somewhat outside the interests of this report.

BIOKINETIC MODELLING OF THE BEHAVIOUR OF LEAD *IN VIVO*

In the broadest sense, modelling exercises use abstract and mathematical frameworks to reduce complex biological relationships into manageable and categorical descriptions. The use of models has as its purpose the rationalization of experimental information and the prediction of lead kinetics *in vivo*. Such models may be qualitative, i.e., purely descriptive in nature, or they may provide quantitative information about the discrete steps involved in the

130

biological handling of lead, such as the size of the transfer coefficients that govern the movement of lead among body compartments.

From the perspective of biological monitoring and the interests of the toicologist or the clinician, the relative merits of biokinetic models for lead increase with the ability of such exercises to (1) describe the actual exposure of humans and that level of apparent exposure signalled by some biological indicator; (2) provide guidance as to the best biological indicator to reflect toxicologically significant internal exposure; (3) connect biological indicator levels with amounts of toxicant in the actual target or critical organs; and finally (4) assist in the evolution of dose–effect and dose–response relationships.

In the specific case of lead metabolism, a number of models have been proposed and published over the years to rationalize the biological behaviour of lead in human subjects and experimental animals. The development and predictive utility of these models rest in large part on the considerable amount of empirical information available in the literature, relating to lead absorption, distribution, excretion, and retention in humans and test species.

The earliest models of lead toxicokinetics are typified by that of Rabinowitz *et al.* (1976, 1977), using stable lead isotope in human volunteers, and which indicate that there are at least three kinetically distinct body compartments for lead disposition *in vivo*. These compartments consist of a central blood compartment, a second lead depository in peripheral soft tissues, and, finally, the large bone compartment for lead. Lead in blood is the most kinetically labile, whereas lead in soft tissues has a somewhat larger biological half-life. The bone compartment retains lead for the longest time. Blood and soft tissues contain relatively small burdens of lead, *ca.* 1.9 and 0.6 mg respectively, while the vast majority of the body burden of lead is sequestered in a kinetically slow compartment of bone, with levels that can exceed 200 mg of the toxicant.

Kneip *et al.* (1983) developed a multi-organ compartment model based on single and chronic oral exposures of juvenile and infant baboons that allowed the estimation of different transfer coefficients for lead among body compartments in both developing and adult organisms. Using the same modelling approach and estimates for human subjects up to 20 years of age, Harley and Kneip (1984) have attempted to develop an integrated model of lead kinetics in humans of various ages. They provide estimates of organ lead levels and selected tissue lead half-lives for ages 1 through 20 in 1-year increments. Some of these estimates for selected ages are given in Tables 1 and 2.

The above modelling approaches assume well-mixed, interconnected pools under essentially steady-state conditions, and they employ first-order kinetics using coupled differential equations and linear exponential solutions. As such, the models collectively provide a reasonable description of biological disposition under rather well-defined circumstances, e.g. a low level of exposure over an extended time. In addition, the modelling approach of Harley and Kneip (1984) provides some estimation of age differences for the tissue burdens of lead in humans.

Linear models of lead biokinetics in humans and test species encounter

131

Table 1 Estimated biological half-life values for age-dependent tissue lead burdens[a]

	Tissue Half-Life, (days)		
Age (years)	Bone	Kidney	Liver
1	1135	10	23
3	1135	10	23
6	1135	10	23
8	2560	10	23
13	3421	10	23
15	3421	10	23
20	3421	10	23

[a] Adapted from Harley and Kneip, 1984

Table 2 Estimated tissue lead burdens as a function of age[a,b]

Age (years)	Blood ($\mu g/dl$)	Bone ($\mu g/g$ ash)	Kidney ($\mu g/g$ wet)
1	11.9	35.5	0.7
2	16.2	38.1	1.0
3	14.6	42.6	0.9
5	14.5	51.0	0.9
7	13.0	57.9	0.8
10	10.4	57.6	0.9
15	11.3	41.7	0.7

[a] Adapted from Harley and Kneip, 1984
[b] Based on 40% uptake/100 μg intake in males

difficulty when one must consider such phenomena as dose-dependent uptake and tissue distribution of lead and the very labile biokinetics of lead in young children. Related to the issue of dose-related biokinetics, of course, is the fact that there is a curvilinear relationship between plasma and blood lead that indicates a higher fraction of blood lead present in plasma with increasing blood lead (DeSilva, 1981; Manton and Cook, 1984).

In a series of reports, Marcus (1985a, b, c) has discussed linear and nonlinear multicompartment models of lead kinetics in mammalian systems with particular emphasis on the relationship of plasma lead to whole blood lead, a relationship which is nonlinear in nature, and the nonlinear relationship of lead in exposure media to lead in blood. Marcus (1985c) proposed four discrete pools for lead within the blood compartment: shallow and deep erythrocyte pools, diffusable lead in plasma, and protein-bound lead in plasma. In this model, Marcus employed data for a volunteer subject who ingested lead under tightly controlled conditions for a period of time (DeSilva, 1981). Different versions of the model, differing as to the mechanisms underlying the nonlinear plasma lead/whole blood lead relationship, were tested, and the one based on site-limited absorption provided the best fit for the 103 subjects studied by DeSilva (1981). The tightness of fit is particularly good at higher blood lead values, while plasma lead is underestimated at or below 30 μg Pb/dl.

Chamberlain (1985) employed a nonlinear modelling approach to focus upon the nonlinear relationships of lead in ambient air, drinking water or diet, and blood lead. In Chamberlain's approach the nonlinearity to the uptake–

blood lead relationship is ascribed to a dose-dependent renal excretion rate for body lead. Nonlinear renal clearance of lead over a broad exposure range is not inconsistent with the plasma lead results of Manon and Cook (1984), DeSilva (1981), and Marcus (1985c), in that an increased renal excretion rate occurs with a proportionately increased lead fraction in plasma at higher exposure levels; i.e., all transfer coefficients are increased with elevated blood lead, as suggested by Chamberlain (1985).

In summary, both linear and nonlinear models have been applied to lead biokinetics under mainly steady-state conditions and mainly employing information from limited numbers of subjects. In many cases, depending upon the demands on the particular model, there may not be any added virtue of nonlinear over linear models, e.g., study of subjects in steady state at relatively low level of exposure. On the other hand, the various nonlinear relationships that are known to exist for external media/biological media relationships and further refined body compartments, e.g., plasma and erythrocyte pools for blood lead, require more complex approaches. The approaches of Marcus (1985c) and Chamberlain (1985) are particularly helpful in extending the use of modelling in rationalizing the various observed nonlinear relationships.

With the exception of the somewhat tenuous estimates of Harley and Kneip (1984) for biological half-times and tissue lead burdens of individuals from the ages of 1 to 20 years (Tables 1 and 2), few biokinetic models have focused on the developing organism, which is a major limitation, since young children are recognized as the key risk population for the adverse health effects of lead. Any attempt to produce precise models, however, is severely impeded by the highly labile nature of lead toxicokinetics in young children.

BIOLOGICAL MONITORING AND THE BIOKINETIC CHARACTERISTICS OF BIOLOGICAL INDICATORS FOR LEAD

Lead in blood

Blood lead (PbB) is the most commonly used biological indicator of both lead exposure and health risks in humans and experimental animals. It is also the indicator for which most data are available in terms of external versus internal exposure relationships, dose–effect and dose–population response relationships, etc.

Based on experimental data (Griffin et al., 1975; Rabinowitz et al., 1976; Chamberlain et al., 1978) and epidemiological studies (O'Flaherty et al., 1982; Kang et al., 1983; Hryhorczuk et al., 1985), PbB has been found to be a relatively dynamic and labile measure, and this biokinetic characteristic governs this indicator's merits and drawbacks in any exposure picture.

Blood lead reflects, biokinetically, both relatively recent lead exposure and the toxicologically active fraction of lead body burden in various soft tissues, at least under steady-state conditions or near steady state.

The degree to which PbB reflects the large body burden of lead sequestered in bone, and which has the potential to become toxicologically active, appears to depend on the subject's exposure status, age, and/or mineral metabolism. In one study of retired lead workers, for example, the level of lead in bone,

133

as determined *in vivo* by X-ray fluorescence spectrometry (Christoffersson *et al.*, 1984), was found to be strongly positively correlated with the PbB of the subjects, indicating that the primary determinant of PbB in these older individuals was the resorption of lead sequestered in bone. By contrast, workers still employed showed no correlation between PbB and the lead level in bone, indicating that current exposure was probably the main determinant of PbB in this group.

Manton (1985) demonstrated that lead isotope ratio data for the blood lead of two subjects followed for *ca.* 9 years was in accord with a contribution of *ca.* 70% of lead from bone to PbB. Also, the PbB elimination rate studies of O'Flaherty *et al.* (1982) and Hryhorczuk *et al.* (1985) show a dependence of elimination half-life on length of exposure time, a parameter directly related to bone lead burden.

The relative contribution of current uptake versus bone content of lead to PbB in young children, unlike the case for adults, is not well understood. The probability exists that lead resorption from bone to blood in children would be a more dynamic process than in adults, given the biological half-life of lead in bone of young children as estimated by Harley and Kneip (1984) and shown in Table 1 as being *ca.* 30% that of teenagers.

It is generally understood that PbB reflects a shorter exposure time than, say, lead in teeth, but it is not widely known just what this means in quantitative terms. Hence, it is of interest to examine the response of PbB with changes in exposure, particularly reduction in lead uptake as occurs when children grow older, and the relative stability of PbB as a function of time and/or development.

Available information on elimination rates for lead from blood to tissues and excreta consists of both experimental exposures under controlled conditions and surveys of PbB behaviour in human subjects with changes in exposure.

Using various experimental exposure methods, including isotopic tracer (Rabinowitz *et al.*, 1976; Chamberlain *et al.*, 1978) and chamber techniques (Griffin *et al.*, 1975), the biological half-life of PbB has been estimated as being on the order of 16–28 days, as depicted in Table 3.

The experimental results noted above mainly reflect the relatively fast component of what would appear to be a two-component PbB decay curve (O'Flaherty *et al.*, 1982; Kang *et al.*, 1983; Hryhorczuk *et al.*, 1985), since these studies were short in duration. It is therefore expected that an increase in the survey period and the number of sampling points (as well as biological differences) would be associated with considerable variability and increases

Table 3 Experimental studies of blood lead elimination rates in humans[a]

Conditions	Half-life (days)	Reference
1. Oral Pb-204, five adults	25	Rabinowitz *et al.*, 1976
2. Pb-203, all routes, 10 adults	16	Chamberlain *et al.*, 1978
3. Inhaled Pb aerosol,	28 (10.9 $\mu g/m^3$)	Griffin *et al.*, 1975
18 adults, two doses	26 (3.2 $\mu g/m^3$)	
3.2 or 10.1 $\mu g/m^3$		

in estimated half-lives for PbB. This appears to be the case in epidemiological surveys of PbB changes in human subjects having reduced exposure, as seen in Table 4.

Lead workers who were removed from active exposure for various reasons showed PbB decay half-lives that varied considerably: 20–130 days (O'Flaherty et al., 1982); 79–133 days (estimated by the author from the elimination rate constants reported in the paper of Kang et al., 1983); and a median of 619 days (Hryhorczuk et al., 1985). Non-occupational subjects, who have also been studied in terms of alterations in lead exposure, had PbB half-life values on the order of 180–210 days (Thomas et al., 1979; Delves et al., 1984).

Data pertaining to the opposite process, the rate of PbB increase with increase in exposure, have been less well studied in human subjects since most of the available data have been derived from animal studies. However, from studies of newly employed lead workers (Tola et al., 1973) and non-occupational volunteers (Griffin et al., 1975) who inhaled metred lead aerosols in exposure chambers, it appears that an upward change in lead uptake leads to a plateau in higher PbB at ca. 60 days.

In summary, the PbB decay rates reported under experimental and epidemiological survey conditions indicate relatively short biological half-lives. The values of the half-lives vary with the type of study, e.g., length of survey and number of measurement points. For example, the lead-poisoned workers of Hryhorczuk et al. (1985) showed a median PbB decay half-life of 619 days when followed for more than 5 years. The PbB curves for these subjects probably included more of the slow decay component than in any of the other reports. With an increase in lead exposure, adults appear to require ca. 60 days to return to exposure steady state, i.e., a rise in the PbB curve followed by a plateau.

Turning to a related issue, the temporal stability of PbB over various intervals and differing exposure settings appears to differ in infants, children, and adults.

In infants, PbB is very unstable in the first year of life but increases in

Table 4 Epidemiological studies of blood lead elimination rates in humans

Study population	Exposure conditions	$T_{1/2}$ (days)	Reference
Lead workers, $n = 68$	Removed from exposure by work stoppage	20–130 (exposure-dependent)	O'Flahety et al., 1982
Lead workers, $n = 77$, four smelters	Medical removal for elevated PbB	79–133[a]	Kang et al., 1983
Workers with Pb poisoning $n = 65$	Medical removal with Pb intoxication	619 (median)	Hryhorczak et al., 1985
Adult women	Pb in tapwater; Pb plumbing removed	180	Thomas et al., 1979
Adult men	Oral exposure, reduced intake	180–120	Delves et al., 1984

[a] Calculated from rate constants in report

stability during the second year (Rabinowitz *et al.*, 1984). As seen in Table 5, correlation among PbB levels at 6-month intervals is poor the first year, but the Spearman coefficients increase significantly in the second year, particularly from 18 to 24 months ($r = 0.61$). Furthermore, concordance as to the PbB category, in 6-month increments, showed that only 38% of the infants remained in their original exposure class (low, medium, or high) from birth to 24 months. The report of Winneke *et al.* (1985) supports the previous discussion in that children examined as to cord blood versus PbB 6–7 years later showed only modest correlation in the two measures ($r = 0.27, p < 0.05$).

Among older subjects, PbB stability over time is considerably greater, at least in terms of rank order. Figure 1 depicts a plot of 5-year follow-up PbB values for a group of children ($n = 50$) compared to their original concentrations, recorded when they were 10 months to 6.5 years of age (Schroeder *et al.*, 1985). A good correlation was obtained between the two measures ($r = 0.72$). Similarly, Lansdown *et al.* (1986) reported that the PbB values for 162 school-aged children drawn *ca.* 20 months apart showed a correlation of 0.52 between the two measures. In adults the temporal stability

Table 5 Spearman correlation coefficients for PbB at different ages (r)[a]

Age	Birth	6 months	12 months	18 months	24 months
Birth	—	0.10	0.20	0.09	0.19
6 mo	0.10	—	0.19	0.28	0.25
12 mo	0.20	0.19	—	0.41	0.36
18 mo	0.09	0.28	0.41	—	0.61
24 mo	0.19	0.25	0.36	0.61	—

[a] From Rabinowitz *et al.*, 1984, with permission

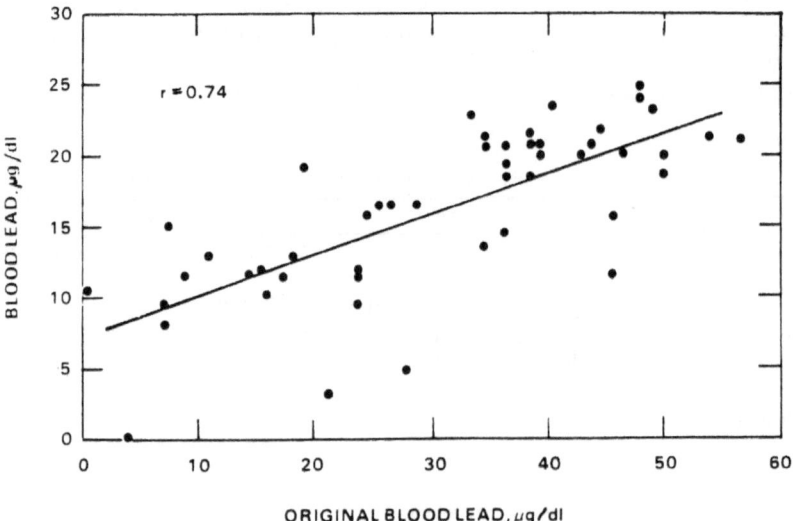

Figure 1 Five-year follow-up PbB levels plotted against original values in a group of lead-exposed children ($n = 50$). Adapted from Schroeder *et al.*, 1985

136

of PbB in 21 adults having relatively low environmental exposure was examined for periods of up to 11 months by Delves *et al.* (1984), and the variance of serial measurement was found to be less than 0.5 μg Pb/dl, where the male mean PbB was 12.2 and that of females was 8.5 μg Pb/dl. Hence, in the absence of major exposure changes, PbB values appear to be quite stable in adults.

In summary, the temporal stability of PbB is a function of age and stage of development. PbB values are most labile in infancy and tend to become more stable with age. In older children this stability is mainly in the form of preservation of rank order, whereas in adults there is also rather good preservation of absolute PbB values. These data suggest that single PbB measurements are least reliable in infancy but become more reliable with increasing age of the subject. The stability of the rank order in children as they get older may represent the relative level of body lead burden in bone. This would parallel what is seen in retired lead workers, where the main determinant of PbB is the bone lead burden (Hryhorczuk *et al.*, 1985).

Lead in teeth

The use of lead in mineralizing tissue, especially in teeth, as a biological indicator of lead exposure is based on the accumulation of the toxicant in these matrices as a function of both age and level of exposure. Hence, lead in teeth or bone provides a cumulative index of exposure over very extended time frames. Lead levels in shed teeth as an exposure indicator have been employed in a number of studies of the effects of lead on paediatric populations (e.g., Needleman *et al.*, 1979; Delves *et al.*, 1982; Ewers *et al.*, 1982; Grandjean *et al.*, 1984). Elevated levels of the element have been reported in whole teeth or their constituents as a function of poisoning history, point source proximity, or geographical location (Shapiro *et al.*, 1973; Needleman *et al.*, 1979; Steenhout and Pourtois, 1981; Ewers *et al.*, 1982; Delves *et al.*, 1982; Grandjean *et al.*, 1984).

The biokinetic aspects of lead deposition and relative distribution in dentition appear to be relatively complicated, and a number of factors governing the behaviour of lead in mineralizing tissue need to be recognized. The level of lead in whole teeth varies with the type of dentition, highest in incisors and decreasing to the premolars (e.g., Mackie *et al.*, 1977). In addition, the distribution of lead in tooth regions is heterogeneous and is variable in concentration stability over time, reflecting in part the developmental anatomy and physiology of dentition. The highest concentrations of lead are present in the inner and outer surfaces, i.e., the outer layer of enamel, and the circumpulpal dentine (Shapiro *et al.*, 1972, 1973; Brudevold *et al.*, 1977). Circumpulpal dentine is directly interfaced with the blood supply and provides the best index of lead accumulation as a function of systemic exposure. Enamel seems to remain relatively invariant in lead content, although one Finnish study of children with modest cumulative lead exposure suggests that enamel may adsorb lead from saliva in proportion to environmental exposure (Haavikko *et al.*, 1984).

The deposition of lead in primary dentine, the major component of dentine

137

on a mass basis (Al-Naimi *et al.*, 1980), remains unclear in terms of lead deposition rate, the time frame for lead deposition, and the mechanisms of deposition. Although lead in primary dentine is only *ca.* 10–30% that of circumpulpal dentine, this region accumulates lead with increased exposure (Shapiro *et al.*, 1973) and with postnatal age (Al-Naimi *et al.*, 1980). In the latter report, for example, primary dentine lead levels in young subjects up to 16 years of age, who lived in different areas of the United Kingdom, were significantly below corresponding values for individuals 40–72 years of age. In one subset of subjects the mean difference was *ca.* sevenfold. The mechanisms by which lead is postnatally deposited within the matrix of primary dentine is not clear. Carroll *et al.* (1972) have demonstrated, by electron microprobe techniques, that lead in mineralized dentine is not uniformly distributed but is laid down in interconnected pockets or channels with lead enrichment. These areas also correspond to regions of low mineralization. Hence, small amounts of lead may possibly move from circumpulpal to primary dentine along these lead-enriched channels.

Any detailed assessment of lead in dentition as a useful indicator is confounded by the fact that the various relevant studies have not employed a standard sampling protocol. Some researchers have employed whole tooth or crowns (Pinchin *et al.*, 1978; Steenhout and Pourtois, 1981; Delves *et al.*, 1982; Ewers *et al.*, 1982; Smith *et al.*, 1983), while others have employed lead levels in regions of teeth, generally secondary (circumpulpal) dentine (Shapiro *et al.*, 1973, 1975; Needleman *et al.*, 1979; Grandjean *et al.*, 1984). In most cases, lead levels in whole or dissected teeth have been used as such, but reporting of lead burden as a function of age has also been done.

Although marked differences in lead content across types of dentition have been recognized, there is also the question of how much variance exists in the measure within dentition type for tooth exfoliation in children, e.g., the two upper central incisors. Using central and lateral incisor crowns, Delves *et al.* (1982) noted that the extent to which lead values in central–central, lateral–lateral, or central–lateral pairs of shed incisors from a group of children exceeded relative analytical variance was 23, 35, and 54%, respectively. Subsequently, the same group found that the differences are maximized with differing jaw position, i.e., upper versus lower (Smith *et al.*, 1983). Variance within the jaw was considerably less. By contrast, variation within-tooth-type lead level appeared to be rather modest in the studies of Pinchin *et al.* (1978) and Ewers *et al.* (1982). However, a close comparison of these three studies is not readily made.

The relevance of the results of Delves *et al.* (1982) for some of the major surveys of the effects of lead exposure in children, employing tooth lead analysis, remains unclear. For example, in the study of Needleman *et al.* (1979), dentine zone analysis was carried out using concordance criteria for acceptability of replicate measurements. The relative impact of variation in lead level within tooth type may be increased at very low levels of concentration and decreased with higher concentration. There is no evidence to indicate that the relative biological variance of the type seen by Delves *et al.* persists with increasing concentration. As Delves *et al.* have acknowledged, their mean and median lead levels are lower than those noted elsewhere in

138

the United Kingdom, in Europe, and in the United States.

One key question is the degree to which lead levels in shed dentition correlate with the more common biological indicator, lead in blood. Since lead accumulates in teeth over a period of years (from formation through eruption until shedding), one might expect a moderate correlation with an indicator of more recent exposure such as PbB. Ewers *et al.* (1982) reported a correlation coefficient of 0.47 between PbB and incisor crowns in a group of 83 children. Similarly, in the report of Smith *et al.* (1983), a correlation coefficient of 0.50 was obtained for 92 children across all teeth analysed. Further analysis as a function of jaw position (lower or upper incisors) or exposure category produced a value of 0.58 for lower teeth. Correlations by exposure group produced more widely ranging values, from -0.09 for medium lead exposure to a value of 0.43 for the high-lead group.

In summary, the use of shed dentition as a biological indicator of cumulative exposure to lead in children would appear to be appropriate under certain conditions. These conditions include rigorous steps to minimize variance in the measure: multiple tooth sampling restricted to the same type (and location if possible), or use of concordance criteria for acceptance or rejection of lead levels in replicate sampling. By its nature, measurement of lead in teeth is a retrospective index of exposure to lead, and this measure is not as inherently useful for regulatory policy or clinical intervention/management of lead exposure and intoxication as is PbB. The various prospective studies currently under way in different countries for lead exposure/effects in children include some that utilize serial measurement of PbB in the paediatric subjects as they develop. Comparison of these multiple measurements with lead in shed dentition in the future would be valuable in establishing blood lead–tooth lead relationships.

Chelatable lead

Chelatable lead refers to that fraction of the body lead burden that is mobilized into urine by a single dose of the chelating agent Ca-Na$_2$ EDTA, with the dose standardized as to body surface or weight of the subject. It is an exposure monitoring term operationally distinct from chelation therapy, a clinical procedure employed to reduce the toxicological capacity of a given lead exposure. Since the EDTA challenge test is an invasive procedure and one having other constraints (Piomelli *et al.*, 1984), it is only employed when elevated body lead burden has been established by other means (PbB and erythrocyte zinc protoporphyrin).

Evidence of lead intoxication is taken as the ratio of urinary lead excreted over 8 h to milligrams of chelant in excess of 0.60. With a ratio of 0.60–0.69, either further monitoring or treatment is carried out, depending on the child's age. A ratio of 0.70 or higher dictates a course of chelation therapy in all cases (Piomelli *et al.*, 1984).

Chelatable lead is widely viewed as the most useful index of toxicologically active lead burden in adults and children (US Centers for Disease Control, 1985; World Health Organization, 1977), and it is of interest to consider this

139

exposure indicator compared to PbB in childhood lead toxicity.

Chelatable lead is widely accepted as representing removal from soft tissue (e.g., Chisolm and Barltrop, 1979), but some mobilizable compartment for lead storage in bone must also be providing a sizeable contribution. Evidence for the bone source includes (1) the age dependency of chelatable lead in non-occupationally exposed subjects, whereas lead in soft tissue is rather invariant with age (Araki, 1973; Araki and Ushio, 1982); (2) experimental animal (Hammond, 1971, 1973) and *in vitro* bone culture data (Rosen and Markowitz, 1980) showing removal of lead from bone; and (3) the tracer modelling data of Rabinowitz *et al.* (1977), which define a bone compartment for lead which is kinetically well mixed with those for blood and soft tissue.

Given the above indications that a sizeable fraction of mobilizable lead exists in bone, and that this portion of body burden is indexed by chelatable lead testing, the question arises as to exactly how chelatable lead is related to PbB in assessment of overall systemic exposure risk. In the detailed report of Piomelli and co-workers (1984) describing the management of childhood lead intoxication, a survey of 210 children from four lead poisoning centres in the United States in terms of chelatable lead versus PbB, suggests that PbB may indeed understate toxicity risk level. Table 6 notes the percentages of these children whose chelatable lead ratios exceed 0.60, a ratio showing lead intoxication, as a function of different PbB values. As can be seen, PbB levels below 30 μg/dl are not associated with worrisome mobilizable lead levels, while at somewhat higher PbB values the percentage of such children is significant and increases considerably with PbB. These data also provide an additional argument for viewing PbB values below 30 μg/dl as the upper limit of permissible exposure (US Centers for Disease Control, 1985).

Table 6 Percentage of children exceeding EDTA challenge ratio as a function of PbB ($n = 210$)[a]

PbB (μg/dl)	Percentage exceeding
< 30	0
30–39	11.5
40–49	37.9
50–59	49.2

[a] From Piomelli *et al.*, 1984

Lead in hair

In theory, lead in hair would appear to be an ideal biological indicator. The sampling is noninvasive, the medium is indefinitely stable in storage, and a temporal profile of exposure along the hair length is available. Hair has been used in a number of surveys of lead exposure in children (e.g., Marlow and Errera, 1982; Thatcher *et al.*, 1982).

In practical terms, however, there are some severe limits on the use of hair lead as a systemic or internal indicator of exposure, one of which is methodological and the other metabolic. With hair, it is virtually impossible to avoid external contamination by ubiquitous lead, and there are no accurate validation techniques for assessing hair cleaning techniques. This is not to say that hair cannot be used as an external indicator, where it would still be expected to show some correlation with various health end-points. For example, fallout of particulate lead onto hair surface or uptake of lead from bathing water would reflect air lead and water lead. The question here, however, is usefulness as an internal indicator. In addition to methodological hazards, the biokinetics of lead in hair is not understood to the extent required for its reliable use as a biological indicator. This is especially true at low levels of exposure associated with subtle effects in children.

Lead in bone

Lead accumulates in the trabecular and cortical bone as a function of both age and exposure. It represents the major repository of lead in the human body, accounting for at least 95% of total body burden. While the overall biokinetics of lead in bone suggest a compartment with a long biological half-life, of the order of a decade or so, some fraction of this amount can be remobilized via various bone resorption processes as noted earlier in this report.

The direct use of bone lead levels as a biological indicator was not possible in the past, and much of our information on lead in this matrix has involved autopsy sampling. More recently, however, a number of laboratories have been occupied with the development and use of *in vivo* methods for measurement of lead in bone. For example, Christoffersson *et al.* (1984) have developed an X-ray fluorescence technique for the measurement of lead in long bones, and have applied the method to lead exposure status of both active and retired lead workers. Similarly, *in vivo* X-ray fluorescence techniques are being developed for assessment of lead in the long bones of children (Wielpolski *et al.*, 1983).

Until the newly developed *in vivo* methods described above can be applied in relatively large-scale survey schemes, it is not possible to say what the practical merits of such an approach would be in the biological montoring of lead exposure. Certainly, the tandem use of *in vivo* bone lead measurement with serial PbB sampling would provide a potent measure of both circulating, biologically active lead and simultaneously, potentially toxic, mobilizable toxicant.

USE OF BIOLOGICAL EFFECT INDICATORS IN THE MONITORING OF LEAD EXPOSURE

When referring to the early or 'subcritical' effects of lead in humans as biological indicators of exposure, the primary concern is the alterations in those levels of intermediates in the haem biosynthesis pathway that are known to be affected by the presence of lead. Three processes that have lent themselves to examination in the context of biological monitoring include: (1) the inhibition of delta-aminolaevulinic acid dehydratase (δ-ALA-D);

(2) the accumulation of delta-aminolaevulinate in urine (δ-ALA-U) due to inhibition of the δ-ALA dehydratase enzyme and the feedback-mediated derepression of delta-aminolaevulinate synthetase enzyme; and (3) the accumulation of zinc protoporphyrin (ZPP) in erythrocytes owing to inhibited action of ferrochelatase or iron transport to the iron-insertion site. Detailed discussions of these effects can be found in the documents of the US Environmental Protection Agency (1977) and the World Health Organization (1977).

Early effect indicators, whatever their limitations in a preventive context of lead exposure, have the virtue of indicating that fraction of measurable lead that is actually biologically active. Also, given the widespread use of measurement of erythrocyte protoporphyrin prior to actual PbB determinations in the large-scale screening of children, these effect indicators will remain on the scene.

Employed as an index of lead exposure, the inhibition of δ-ALA-D in erythrocytes would appear to offer little advantage over direct measurement of PbB. In erythrocytes the enzyme is vestigial, and its inhibition requires the presence of lead ion interacting with the sulphydryl group in the proximity of the active site (Mitchell et al., 1977). In addition, a number of methodological problems abound that would further serve to minimize this measure's attraction as a substitute for PbB.

On a group basis, the elevation of ALA level in the urine of children and adults is taken as an effect indicator of lead exposure. The effect becomes most pronounced above a 'threshold' of ca. 40 μg/dl PbB, and the relationship of the measure to PbB below this value is clouded in some disagreement (USEPA, 1977). Since much of the current interest in lead exposure of children involves PbB values below 40 μg/dl, δ-ALA-U may not be sensitive enough to be of much use. There are also some methodological limitations, including the desirability of obtaining 24-h urine samples.

At present, the most popular biological effect indicator of lead exposure is erythrocyte ZPP. Elevation of ZPP is a sensitive indicator, showing a threshold of response in children of ca. 15 μg/dl PbB (Piomelli et al., 1982; Hammond et al., 1985) and shows a tight correlation with PbB (log-transformed ZPP data). ZPP elevation occurs also in the presence of iron deficiency, a common occurrence in young children, and any use of this measure for exposure monitoring would require correction for, and determination of, the level of iron deficiency. In older children, ZPP levels are a cleaner measure.

Elevation of erythrocyte ZPP lags any increases in PbB due to increased exposure. ZPP levels, furthermore, remain elevated when exposure has ceased. The former arises from ZPP insertion into cells occurring only during active intoxication of bone marrow, whereas ZPP decay, when exposure ceases, is governed to some degree by the rate of erythrocyte turnover.

Various studies have been directed to the relative merits of ZPP versus other indicators in studies of effect outcomes. These have produced something of a mixed picture (Fischbein et al., 1980; Hammond et al., 1980; Saenger et al., 1982). For example, Fischbein and co-workers (1980) reported that ZPP was elevated in those workers showing central nervous system or gastrointestinal symptoms. By contrast, only 5% of these workers had PbB levels in excess of 40 μg/dl. Hammond *et al.* (1980) used ZPP, δ-ALA-U, and PbB as exposure indicators, and found that PbB was not particularly advantageous in predicting subjective neurological symptoms compared to the haematological effect indicators.

REFERENCES

Al-Naimi, T., Edmonds, M.I. and Fremlin, J.H. (1980) The distribution of lead in human teeth, using charged particle activation analysis. *Phys. Med. Biol.*, **25**, 719–726

Araki, S. (1973) On the behaviour of 'active deposit of lead (Teisinger)' in the Japanese free from occupational exposure to lead. *Ind Health*, **11**, 203–224

Araki, S. and Ushio, K. (1982) Assessment of the body burden of chelatable lead: a model for application to workers. *Br. J. Ind. Med.*, **39**, 157–160

Brudevold, F., Aasenden, R., Srinivasien, B.N. and Bakhos, Y. (1977) Lead in enamel and saliva, dental caries and the use of enamel biopsis for measuring past exposure to lead. *J. Dental Res.*, **56**, 1165–1171

Carroll, K.G., Needleman, H.L., Tuncay, O.C. and Shapiro, I.M. (1972) The distribution of lead in human deciduous teeth. *Experientia*, **28**, 434–445

Chamberlain, A.C. (1985) Prediction of response of blood lead to airborne and dietary lead from volunteer experiments with lead isotopes. *Proc. R. Soc. Lond.*, *B*, **224**, 149–182

Chamberlain, A.C., Heard, M.J., Newton, D., Wells, A.C. and Wiffen, R.D. (1978) *Investigations into Lead from Motor Vehicles*. AERE Report 9198 (London: HMSO)

Chisolm, J.J., Jr and Barltrop, D. (1979) Recognition and management of children with increased lead absorption. *Arch. Dis. Childh.*, **54**, 249–262

Christoffersson, J.O., Schutz, A., Ahlgren, L., Haeger-Aronsen, B., Mattsson, S. and Skerfving, S. (1984) Lead in finger-bone analyzed *in-vivo* in active and retired lead workers. *Am. J. Ind. Med.*, **6**, 447–457

Delves, H.T., Clayton, B.E., Carmichael, A., Bubear, M. and Smith, M. (1982) An appraisal of the analytical significance of tooth-lead measurements as possible indices of environmental exposure of children to lead. *Ann. Clin. Biochem.*, **19**, 329–337

Delves, H.T., Sherlock, J.C. and Quinn, M.J. (1984) Temporal stability of blood lead concentrations in adults exposed only to environmental lead. *Human Toxicol.*, **3**, 279–288

DeSilva, P.E. (1981) Determination of lead in plasma and studies on its relationship to lead in erythrocytes. *Br. J. Ind. Med.*, **38**, 209–217

Ewers, U., Brockhaus, A., Winneke, G., Freier, I., Jermann, E. and Krämer, U. (1982) Lead in deciduous teeth of children living in a non-ferrous smelter area and a rural area of the FRG. *Int. Arch. Occup. Environ. Health*, **50**, 139–151

Fischbein, A., Thornton, J., Blumberg, W.E., Bernstein, J., Valciukas, J.A., Moses, M., Davidow, B., Kaul, B., Sirstas, M. and Selikoff, I.J. (1980) Health status of cable splicers with low-level exposure to lead: results of a clinical survey. *Am. J. Public Health*, **70**, 697–700

Grandjean, P., Hansen, O.N. and Lyngbye, G. (1984) Analysis of lead in circumpulpal dentine of deciduous teeth. *Ann. Clin. Lab. Sci.*, **14**, 270–275

Griffin, T.B., Coulston, F., Wills, H., Russell, J.C. and Knelson, J.H. (1975) Clinical studies on men continuously exposed to airborne particulate lead, in Griffin, T.B. and Knelson, J.H. (eds), *Lead* (New York: Academic Press)

Haavikko, K., Antilla, A., Helle, A. and Vuori, E. (1984) Lead concentrations of enamel and dentine of deciduous teeth of children from two Finnish towns. *Arch. Environ. Health*, **39**, 78–84

Hammond, P.B. (1971) The effects of chelating agents on the tissue distribution and excretion of lead. *Toxicol. Appl. Pharmacol.*, **18**, 296–310

Hammond, P.B. (1973) The effects of D-penicillamine on the tissue distribution and excretion of lead. *Toxicol. Appl. Pharmacol.*, **26**, 241–246

Hammond, P.B., Lerner, S.I., Gartside, P.S., Hanenson, I.B., Roda, S.B., Foulkes, E.C., Johnson, D.R. and Pesce, A.J. (1980) The relationship of biological indices of lead exposure to the health status of workers in a secondary lead smelter. *J. Occup. Med.*, **22**, 475–484

Hammond, P.B., Bornschein, R.L. and Succop, P. (1985) Dose–effect and dose–response relationships of blood lead to erythrocytic protoporphyrin in young children. *Environ. Res.,* **38**, 187–196

Harley, N.H. and Kneip, T.H. (1984) *An Integrated Metabolic Model for Lead in Humans of All Ages.* Final Report to the US Environmental Protection Agency: Contract No. B44899 with New York University School of Medicine, 30 December, 1984

Hryhorczuk, D.O., Rabinowitz, M.B., Hessl, S.M., Hoffman, D., Hogan, M.M., Mallin, K., French, H., Arris, P. and Berman, E. (1985) Elimination kinetics of blood lead in workers with chronic lead intoxication. *Am. J. Ind. Med.,* **8**, 33–42

Kang, H.K., Infante, P.F. and Carra, J.S. (1983) Determination of blood-lead elimination patterns of primary lead smelter workers. *J. Toxicol. Environ. Health,* **11**, 199–210

Kneip, T.J., Mallon, R.P. and Harley, N.H. (1983) Biokinetic modelling for mammalian lead metabolism. *Neurotoxicology,* **4**, 189–192

Lansdown, R., Yule, W., Urbanowicz, M.-A. and Hunter, J. (1986). The relationship between blood-lead concentrations, intelligence, attainment and behaviour in a school population. The second London study. *Int. Arch. Occup. Environ. Health,* **57**, 225–235

Mackie, A.C., Stephens, R., Townsend, A. and Waldron, H.A. (1977) Tooth lead levels in Birmingham children. *Arch. Environ. Health,* **32**, 178–185

Manton, W.I. (1985) Total contribution of airborne lead to blood lead. *Br. J. Ind. Med.,* **42**, 168–172

Manton, W.I. and Cook, J.D. (1984) High accuracy (stable isotope dilution) measurements of lead in serum and cerebrospinal fluid. *Br. J. Ind. Med.,* **41**, 313–319

Marcus, A.H. (1985a) Multicompartment kinetic models for lead. I. Bone diffusion models for long term retention. *Environ. Res.,* **36**, 441–458

Marcus, A.H. (1985b) Multicompartment kinetic models for lead. II. Linear kinetics and variable absorption in humans without excessive lead exposures. *Environ. Res.,* **36**, 459–472

Marcus, A.H. (1985c) Multicompartment kinetic models for lead. III. Lead in blood plasma and erythrocytes. *Environ. Res.,* **36**, 473–489

Marlowe, M. and Errrera, J. (1982) Low lead levels and behaviour problems in children. *Behav. Disorders,* **7**, 163–172

Mitchell, R.A., Drake, J.E., Wittlin, C.A. and Rejent, T.A. (1977) Erythrocyte porphobilinogen synthase (delta-aminolevulinate dehydratase) activity: a reliable and quantitative indicator of lead exposure in humans. *Clin. Chem.,* **23**, 105–111

Needleman, H.L., Gunnoe, C., Leviton, A., Reed, R., Peresie, H., Maher, C. and Barrett, P. (1979) Deficits in psychologic and classroom performance of children with elevated dentine lead levels. *N. Engl. J. Med.,* **300**, 689–695

O'Flaherty, E.J., Hammond, P.B. and Lerner, S.I. (1982) Dependence of apparent blood lead half-life on the length of previous lead exposure in humans. *Fund. Appl. Toxicol.,* **2**, 49–54

Pinchin, M.J., Newham, J. and Thompson, R.P.J. (1978) Lead, copper and cadmium in teeth of normal and mentally retarded children. *Clin. Chim. Acta,* **85**, 89–94

Piomelli, S., Seaman, C., Zullon, D., Currin, A. and Davidow, B. (1982) Threshold for lead damage to heme synthesis in urban children. *Proc. Natl. Acad. Sci. USA,* **79**, 3335–3339

Piomelli, S., Rosen, J.F., Chisolm, J.J., Jr and Graef, J.W. (1984) Management of childhood lead poisoning. *J. Pediat.,* **105**, 523–532

Rabinowitz, M.B., Wetherill, G.W. and Kopple, J.D. (1976) Kinetic analysis of lead metabolism in healthy humans. *J. Clin. Invest.,* **58**, 260–270

Rabinowitz, M.B., Wetherill, G.W. and Kopple, J.D. (1977) Magnitude of lead intake from respiration by normal man. *J. Lab. Clin. Med.,* **90**, 238–248

Rabinowitz, M.B., Leviton, A. and Needleman, H. (1984) Variability of blood lead concentrations during infancy. *Arch. Environ. Health,* **39**, 74–77

Rosen, J.F. and Markowitz, M.E. (1980) D-penicillamine: its actions on lead transport in bone organ culture. *Pediat. Res.,* **14**, 330–335

Saenger, P., Rosen, J.F. and Markowitz, M.E. (1982) Diagnostic significance of edetate disodium calcium testing in children with increased lead absorption. *Am. J. Dis. Child.,* **136**, 312–315

Schroeder, S.R., Hawk, B., Otto, D.A., Mushak, P. and Hicks, R.E. (1985) Separating the effects of lead and social factors on IQ. *Environ. Res.,* **38**, 144–154

Shapiro, I.M., Needleman, H.L. and Tuncay, O.C. (1972) The lead content of human deciduous and permanent teeth. *Environ. Res.,* **5**, 467–470

Shapiro, I.M., Dobkin, B., Tuncay, O.C. and Needleman, H.L. (1973) Lead levels in dentine and circumpulpal dentine of deciduous teeth of normal and lead poisoned children. *Clin.*

144

Chim. Acta, **46**, 119–123

Shapiro, I.M., Mitchell, G., Davidson, I. and Katz, S.H. (1975) The lead content of teeth. Evidence establishing new minimal levels of exposure in a living preindustrialized human population. *Arch. Environ. Health*, **30**, 483–486

Smith, M., Delves, T., Lansdown, R., Clayton, B. and Graham, P. (1983) The effects of lead exposure on urban children: The Institute of Child Health/Southampton study. *Dev. Med. Child Neurol.*, **25** (Suppl. 47), 1–54

Steenhout, A. and Pourtois, M. (1981) Lead accumulation in teeth as a function of age with different exposures. *Br. J. Ind. Med.*, **38**, 297–303

Thatcher, R.W., Lester, M.L., McAlaster, R. and Horst, R. (1982) Effects of low levels of cadmium and lead and cognitive functions in children. *Arch. Environ. Health*, **37**, 159–166

Thomas, H.F., Elwood, P.C., Welsby, A. and St Leger, A.S. (1979) Relationship of blood lead in women and children to domestic water lead. *Nature*, **282**, 712–713

Tola, S., Hernberg, S., Asp, S. and Nikkänen, J. (1973) Parameters indicative of absorption and biological effect in new lead exposure: a prospective study. *Br. J. Ind. Med.*, **30**, 134–141

US Centers for Disease Control (1985) Preventing Lead Poisoning in Young Children: A statement by the Centers for Disease Control – January 1985. US Department of Health and Human Services, Public Health Service, Atlanta, Ga.

US Environmental Protection Agency (1977) Air Quality Criteria for Lead. Criteria and Special Studies Office, Research Triangle Park, N.C. EPA Report No. EPA-600/8-77-017, December

Wielpolski, L., Rosen, J.F., Slatkin, D.N., Vartsky, D., Ellis, K.J. and Cohn, S.H. (1983) Feasibility of noninvasive analysis of lead in the human tibia by soft X-ray fluorescence. *Med. Phys.*, **10**, 248–251

Winneke, E., Beginn, U., Ewers, T., Havestadt, C., Kraemer, U., Krause, C., Thron, H.L. and Wagner, H.M. (1985) Comparing the effects of perinatal and later childhood lead exposure on neuropsychological outcome. *Environ. Res.*, **38**, 155–167

World Health Organization (1977) *Environmental Health Criteria*, 3 (Geneva, Switzerland)

Section 3
CROSS-SECTIONAL EPIDEMIOLOGICAL STUDIES OF CHILDREN

Introduction

The first research studies of the effects of low levels of lead were cross-sectional in design, investigating a group or groups of children at one point in time. These studies established the association between lead at low levels and outcomes such as intelligence. The studies reported in this section are mainly 'second-generation' cross-sectional studies, that is, exploring further the nature and extent of the relationship. There are investigations of the relation between body lead burden and outcomes in a number of different countries, in diverse situations, over a range of body lead levels, assessed by different measures of lead, and on a variety of outcome measures.

The research reported here has been carried out in Belgium, Denmark, Germany, Greece, Italy, the UK, and USA. It represents a wide range of different situations, reflected in the range of body lead levels found. In urban Denmark (Hansen *et al.*) the overall mean blood lead level was 5 μg/dl, while the mean blood lead of children living near a lead smelter in Greece, studied by Hatzakis, was 24 μg/dl. Vivoli *et al.* have investigated in Italy the relationship of different measures of body lead burden to outcomes. Different types of outcome measure have been explored by Yule *et al.*, with the automated assessment of attention, vigilance and learning. Otto has reviewed the evidence relating to electrophysiological outcome measures. The paper by Schroeder examines the relationship of child caregiving practices to body lead burden and outcomes, and the papers by Pocock *et al.* and Raab *et al.* explore the role of a range of social variables in the association between lead levels and outcome measures.

Although strictly longitudinal, the study by Winneke *et al.* has been included in this section. This was a three-year follow-up of children originally seen at six years of age. It was not a prospective study, and the age group investigated and measures used make it in some ways more comparable with the cross-sectional studies.

3.1

Lead Exposure and Children's Intellectual Performance: the Institute of Child Health/Southampton Study

S. J. POCOCK, D. ASHBY and M. A. SMITH

SUMMARY

The Institute of Child Health/Southampton Study is one of the largest cross-sectional surveys of lead exposure and children's intelligence. 402 6-year-olds in London, with tooth lead concentration in three predefined ranges, were selected for neuropsychological testing. This paper presents new findings on the relationship between child IQ and tooth lead levels which build on previous findings (Smith *et al.*, 1983) in four respects: (1) Rather than simply classifying children into high, medium and low lead groups the actual concentrations of lead in each child's tooth have been used to provide a more powerful assessment of the association between IQ and body lead burden. (2) The influence of parental and social factors on child IQ is explored in detail in order to see if any residual lead–IQ association exists after allowance for such confounders. (3) The methods of multiple regression, including an 'optimal' statistical policy, are more fully described. (4) The possibility of interactions between lead and confounders is explored.

Findings are that parental IQ is the most important influence on child IQ, though several other factors (e.g. family size, social class and quality of marital relationships) were also significantly related. There was no overall evidence that tooth lead concentrations were related to child IQ once these other factors were taken into account. However, a significant interaction between tooth lead and sex of child indicates that the lead–IQ association appears much more pronounced in boys. This unexpected finding needs cautious interpretation and further exploration in other studies.

This paper is a modified version of a paper first published in the *International Journal of Epidemiology* (1987, **16**, 57–67), and included here by permission of the editor.

INTRODUCTION

The potential influence of low-level lead exposure on child IQ has been investigated in many epidemiological studies and several reviews are available (Medical Research Council, 1984; Environmental Protection Agency, 1985; Pocock and Ashby, 1985). The evidence has been conflicting, as might be anticipated by differences in sample selection, small size of studies, different extents of allowance for confounding factors and various methods of statistical analysis. A further problem is that publications have usually reported on several other neuropsychological measures as well, so that detailed insight into the lead–IQ association has not been possible.

The objective of this paper is to explore fully the associations of lead and confounding factors on child IQ, using data from the Institute of Child Health/Southampton Study, one of the largest cross-sectional surveys of this kind.

METHODS

The design of the Institute of Child Health/Southampton Study has been described in detail elsewhere (Smith et al., 1983). Briefly, 6875 6-year-old children in the top infant classes at 168 schools in three areas of London were recruited into the study. In order to be eligible for neuropsychological testing a child had to be without major disability, should have attended a school in the area since age 5, and both child and parents needed to be UK-born. 4293 children satisfied these criteria. All children were asked to donate milk teeth as they were shed. 2663 (62%) eligible children gave at least one tooth, and 890 of them had at least one incisor tooth analysed for lead concentration. Tooth lead estimations were made using atomic absorption spectroscopy on whole tooth crowns, such analysis being on duplicate portions.

Children were selected for neuropsychological testing if their tooth lead concentration was low ($< 2.5\,\mu g/g$), medium ($5.0-5.5\,\mu g/g$) or high ($\geqslant 8.0\,\mu g/g$). Criteria were slightly different for the first area sampled: in particular there was no medium lead group. One important aim of this paper is to make fuller use of the lead data by using the actual tooth lead concentration as a continuous variable rather than simply classifying children into three lead groups. This should increase statistical power since the high lead group had concentrations ranging from 8 to $34\,\mu g/g$.

Since tooth lead has a skew distribution, a log transform is used in statistical analysis. Also, upper incisor teeth have a higher geometric mean for lead concentration ($5.01\,\mu g/g$, $n = 829$) compared with lower incisors ($3.86\,\mu g/g$, $n = 1061$) so that in statistical analysis concentrations for upper teeth have been divided by 1.30. Altogether 431 children were selected. With eight children moving out of the area, six refusals, six non-responders and nine subsequently found to be ineligible, the final sample comprised 402 children. The child's primary caretaker (usually the mother) was given a structured interview by a psychologist to provide information on potential confounding factors. A different psychologist tested the child for several neuropsychological

150

items, including the child's IQ using the revised Wechsler Intelligence Scale for Children (Wechsler, 1974).

Confounding factors

Many facets of the family and social environment are potentially related to a child's IQ. Some are simple factual items, e.g. family size, sex of child. Others, e.g. mother's IQ, can be quantified using standard procedures. However, information about the family's circumstances can be obtained only by a structured interview of the mother. Hence several measures (e.g. parental interest in the child, quality of marital relationships, mother's mental health) have been defined by combining the mother's responses to specific questions at interview into a quantifiable score. It is impossible to summarize perfectly such complex issues. Nevertheless, it is important to characterize such influences on child IQ as best as one can. The principal confounding factors used in this study are now described. All confounders were chosen because of their potential relationship with child IQ, rather than any direct association with lead exposure *per se*:

Sex of child has proved relevant, but age is not considered because of the narrow age range and the age-standardization of IQ scores.

Social group of the child is determined by whether the father's occupation was manual or non-manual, and *social class* is a more detailed breakdown of father's occupation, using the Registrar General's classification of occupations (Great Britain Office of Population Censuses and Surveys, 1970). If the father was absent, the mother's occupation determined the child's social group. If the father was not currently employed, the father's last occupation (manual or non-manual) was noted.

Family size is the number of children in the family and *birth order* indicates the child's position in the family. A measure of overcrowding in the child's household was given by the *occupation ratio*, the number of habitable rooms per person.

The mother's recall of neonatal problems has been summarized by three indicators: *length of gestation* < 38 weeks, *birth weight* < 6 lb (2.7 kg) or length of *hospital stay* after birth > 11 days.

Mother's IQ was assessed using two subtests of the Weschler Adult Intelligence Scale: the vocabulary test and the block design test. These are the two subtests that correlate most highly with the verbal and performance scores respectively of the WAIS.

The quality of *marital relationships* was assessed from questions about father's help with the children, quarrels, separations, and from the interviewer's assessment of the quality of marriage. The score had values ranging from 1 to 14, with higher scores indicating marital problems.

The *family characteristics* score measures how far the family structure departs from that of a nuclear family. This incorporates questions about marital status of the child's natural parents and present parents/step-parents, whether other people live with the family, including step-children, and whether any children live away from home.

151

Mother's mental health was assessed by a questionnaire on neurotic and depressive symptoms, and by interview questions on depression, suicidal thoughts, psychiatric treatment, anxiety, and personality disorders. High scores are indicative of mental ill-health.

Social background of the child is a composite score describing the child's home: whether it is rented or owned, whether a house or flat, how old and what amenities are available (e.g. inside lavatory, cooker, television, telephone). Higher scores indicate a poorer social background.

Parental education was measured in terms of type of school attended, examinations taken, the age of leaving school and any further education. This information was collected for each parent, and the scores combined. High scores indicate a more extensive education.

Parental interest was assessed by whether the child went to a childminder, nursery or playgroup and why, the parents' contact with the school, the number of outings the children went on, their toys, storage space, books and use of public library. Higher scores indicate a lack of contact and facilities.

Parental attitude is a score intended to reflect the degree of responsibility parents show towards a child's care, incorporating questions on the child's diet, dental visits, immunizations and parental restraint on child behaviour.

Use of multiple regression

Multiple regression techniques are commonly used to explore how allowance for confounding factors affects the association between tooth lead and child IQ. For such complex data there are many possible regression methods and it is important to define an objective *analysis strategy*. We have adopted an 'optimal' regression method which proceeds in two stages. First one determines for each possible number of variables p ($p = 1$ up to 18 in this case) the linear combination of variables that minimizes the residual sum of squares. Since tooth lead is of fundamental interest, such optimality is made conditional on log (tooth lead) being included in every model. Calculations were done using the RSQUARE procedure in the SAS statistical package. The second stage is to decide how many variables to include in the final model. The following rule defined by Mallows (1973) has been adopted. For each optimal regression for $p = 1, \ldots, 18$ covariates one defines

$$C_p = \frac{\text{residual sum of squares}}{\hat{\sigma}^2} - n + 2p$$

where n = the total no. of subjects = 377 (25 subjects excluded because of missing values or one or more confounders), and $\hat{\sigma}^2$ = the residual sum of squares obtained from the regression fitting all covariates. The final model is that optimal regression for the number of variables p which minimizes C_p. The principle here is to allow variables of borderline significance to enter the model, but to exclude variables whose contributions are well within chance variation.

Forwards or backwards stepwise procedures are simpler alternatives to the above approach, but can lead to conflicting results. With the increased

152

sophistication of computing packages, we feel that the above 'optimal' regression procedure is a better proposition for obtaining an informative and parsimonious model.

Nine confounding factors were used as continuous measurements in multiple regression. Two measures, social background and parental interest, have skew distributions requiring log transformations. Also eight dummy variables were defined for sex, the three neonatal factors, non-manual social class, social classes IV and V, family size 3, and married relationships not reported (i.e. not married or separated).

RESULTS

Tooth lead and child IQ (unadjusted for confounders)

Figure 1 shows the association between tooth lead concentration and full-scale IQ for the 402 children. The wide scatter in IQ at any level of tooth lead concentration reveals no obvious visual association between tooth lead and IQ. However, there is a highly significant negative correlation between log (tooth lead concentration) and IQ, with $r = -0.16$, $p < 0.01$. This is more clearly seen in Figure 2 where mean IQ is shown for children categorized into eight roughly equal groups (ordered by their tooth lead concentrations).

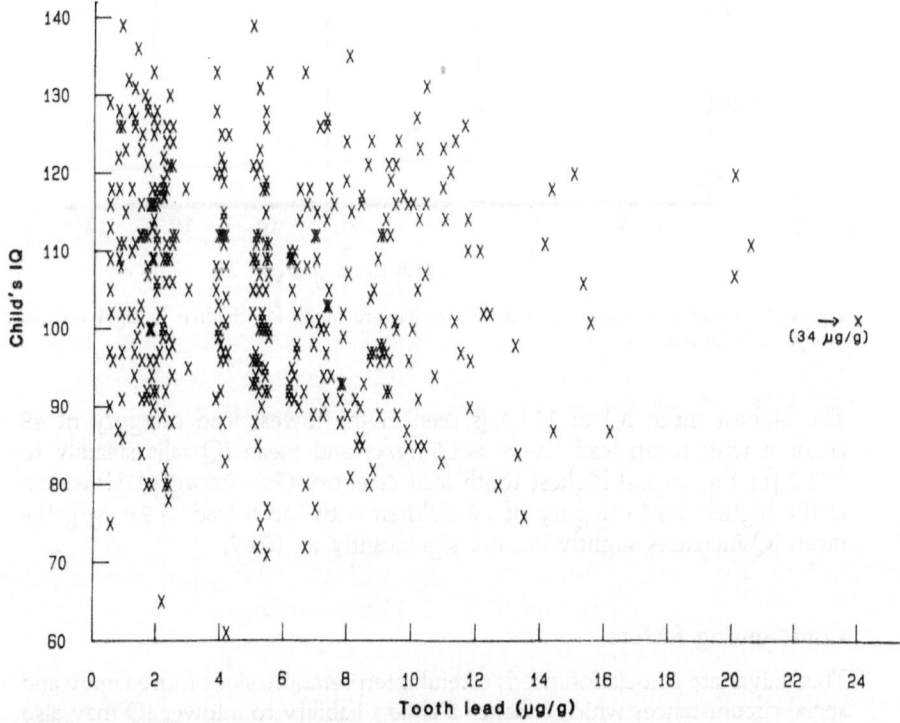

Figure 1 Full-scale IQ and tooth lead concentration (adjusted for tooth type) in 402 London schoolchildren

153

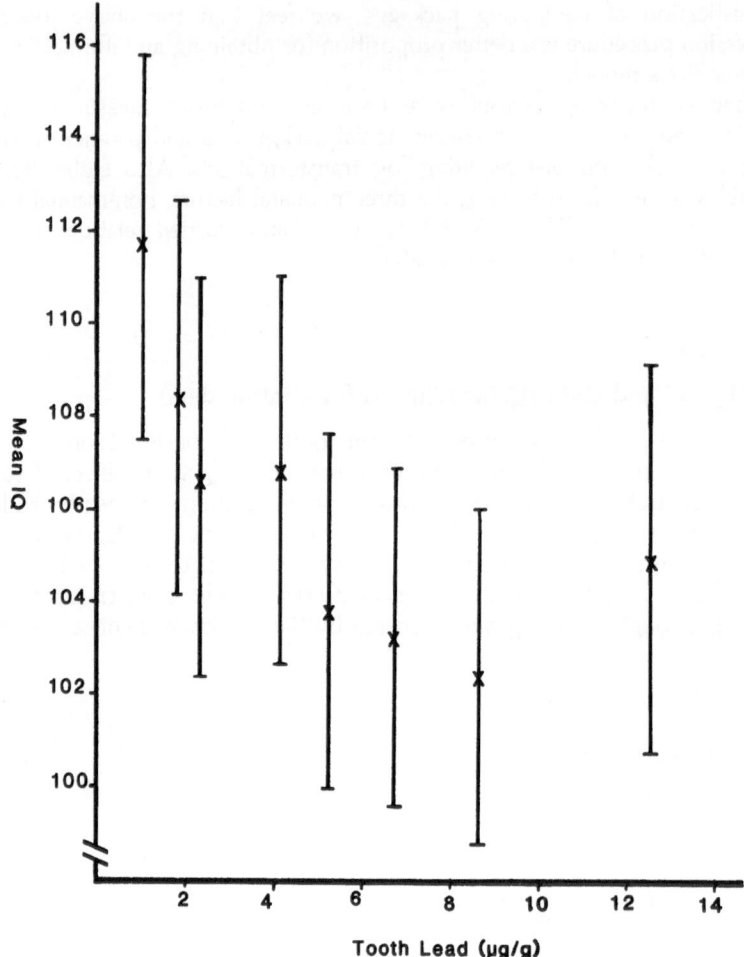

Figure 2 Unadjusted mean IQ and 95% confidence limits for children in eight ordered groups of tooth lead

The highest mean IQ of 111.4 is seen in the lowest lead category of 49 children with tooth lead levels ⩽1.5 μg/g, and mean IQ falls steadily to 102.2 for the second highest tooth lead category (7.8–9.6 μg/g). However, in the highest lead category of 49 children with tooth lead >9.6 μg/g the mean IQ increases slightly but not significantly to 104.7.

Confounding factors

This univariate association needs careful interpretation, since those family and social circumstances which enhance a child's liability to a lower IQ may also be associated with increased body lead burden. Thus, one needs to identify quantifiable confounding factors which reflect these non-lead influences on

IQ, and then use multiple regression techniques to see if there remains any residual lead effect on IQ after allowance for these confounders.

Table 1 shows 17 factors which were associated with child IQ. IQ scores tended to be higher in boys; in children whose fathers were in non-manual occupations; in children from smaller families, and in children whose families

Table 1 The associations of child IQ and tooth lead concentrations with various confounding factors

Confounding factor	No. of children	Mean IQ	Standard error	Geometric mean (μg/g) of tooth lead
Sex				
Female	220	103.6	0.9	4.02
Male	182	108.2	1.1	3.98
Social group				
Non-manual	154	111.1	1.0	3.48
Manual	248	102.3	0.9	4.36
Social class				
I professional	30	112.3	2.4	2.50
II managerial	78	112.7	1.2	3.61
III non-manual (clerical)	28	108.9	2.6	3.54
III manual (skilled)	152	104.4	1.2	4.29
IV semi-skilled manual	37	97.0	1.7	3.95
V unskilled manual	20	98.8	3.1	5.79
Other or unknown	57	102.6	1.9	4.60
Family size				
1	50	107.6	1.9	4.41
2	223	107.7	0.9	3.70
3	92	100.7	1.5	4.18
4 or more	37	103.1	2.2	4 97
Birth Order				
1	172	106.5	1.1	4.18
2	155	107.0	1.1	3.64
3	49	100.3	2.1	4.10
4 or more	26	102.3	2.2	5.02
Occupation ratio				
0–0.99	37	97.2	1.9	5.92
1–1.19	101	103.1	1.3	4.46
1.2–1.29	100	104.9	1.5	3.85
1.3–1.59	95	109.4	1.4	3.47
1.60–3.0	59	109.5	1.8	3.31
Length of gestation				
<38 weeks	45	102.6	2.0	3.66
≥38 weeks	350	106.2	0.8	4.07
Birth weight				
<6 lb (2.7 kg)	46	101.3	2.2	4.25
≥6 lb (2.7 kg)	351	106.3	0.7	3.97

continued

Table 1 *continued*

Confounding factor	No. of children	Mean IQ	Standard error	Geometric mean (µg/g) of tooth lead
Length of hospital stay				
0–11 days	360	106.5	0.7	4.02
>11 days	36	98.4	2.5	4.11
Mother's IQ				
7–15	82	98.2	1.4	4.90
16–18	72	102.3	1.6	4.11
19–21	93	106.5	1.4	3.41
22–24	79	107.3	1.5	3.77
25–35	68	116.6	1.2	3.92
Marital relationships quality				
Not reported	59	103.2	1.9	5.09
1–3	74	110.9	1.5	3.30
4–5	119	107.4	1.3	3.96
6–7	94	103.9	1.4	3.79
8–14	56	100.8	1.8	4.49
Family characteristics				
0	282	106.9	0.8	3.78
1–2	88	104.5	1.5	4.14
3–6	29	98.9	2.0	6.28
Mother's mental health				
0	107	107.9	1.3	3.82
1	82	106.29	1.52	3.658
2–3	109	106.44	1.30	3.938
4–6	52	104.48	1.93	4.452
7–14	49	99.08	2.23	4.747
Social background				
4–6	71	100.9	1.6	4.43
7–9	109	99.5	1.6	4.66
10–12	68	105.2	1.5	4.32
13–15	68	109.6	1.3	3.57
16–18	83	111.9	1.4	3.35
Parental education				
0–1	101	99.6	1.3	4.04
2–3	74	103.4	1.7	4.30
4–7	91	103.6	1.5	4.62
8–14	74	111.8	1.6	3.66
15–24	62	114.0	1.3	3.26
Parental interest				
7–10	73	95.1	1.7	6.41
11–14	130	102.0	1.7	4.49
15–18	92	105.1	1.4	3.87
19–22	60	107.7	1.2	3.49
23–38	41	112.4	1.6	3.67
Parental attitude				
2–10	49	97.5	1.7	5.15
11–13	79	103.1	1.6	4.58
14–15	89	103.2	1.5	3.87
16–17	91	109.1	1.4	3.57
18–21	90	111.6	1.3	3.56

had more spacious housing. Also, child IQ was positively associated with mother's IQ, the extent of parental education, the degree of parental interest in the child, a favourable parental attitude towards child care, the quality of marital relationships and the extent of social amenities. The child's IQ tended to be lower if there were neonatal problems (i.e. low birth weight, a long hospital stay after birth, a short gestation), a mother whose mental health was poor, or the family circumstances deviated from the nuclear family. Also, first or second births tended to have higher mean IQs but this was attributable to family size rather than birth order *per se* (see Table 2). Mother's IQ was the factor most strongly associated with child IQ ($r = +0.44$) and five other factors (social group, social background, parental education, parental interest and parental attitude) had substantial correlations with child IQ, i.e.: $0.3 < |r| < 0.4$.

It can be seen from Table 1 that most confounding variables were not strongly related to tooth lead levels. The most marked associations, statistically significant at the 1% level, were for family characteristics, parental interest and parental attitude, which suggests that these family measures may be the most relevant confounders. In order to explore the interrelationships between the confounding variables, Figure 3 shows a minimum spanning tree (Gower and Ross, 1969) whereby each variable is linked by a continuous line to the variable with which it is most highly correlated. The groups of variables so formed are linked by dotted lines reflecting the strongest pairwise connection between groups. The largest group of confounding variables comprised mother's IQ, parental education, social class, social background, family characteristics and occupation ratio. Four smaller groups were as follows: the neonatal variables; parental interest and attitude; marital relationships, mother's mental health and sex of child; family size and birth order. In general these interrelationships fit in with our logical understanding of the social and family aspects each variable is intended to reflect. No pairwise correlation between variables exceeds $r = 0.6$, except that between family size and birth order. This indicates that each variable has the potential to act as an independent contributor to the determination of child's IQ.

Tooth lead and child IQ adjusting for confounding factors

In this section the simultaneous influence of tooth lead and confounding factors on child IQ is assessed using the sequence of 'optimal' regression

Table 2 Mean IQ for 402 children by family size and birth order

Family size	Birth order		
	1	*2*	*3*
1	107.6		
	(50)		
2	106.9	108.5	
	(103)	(120)	
3	101.7	102.0	101.0
	(19)	(35)	(75)

n in parentheses

157

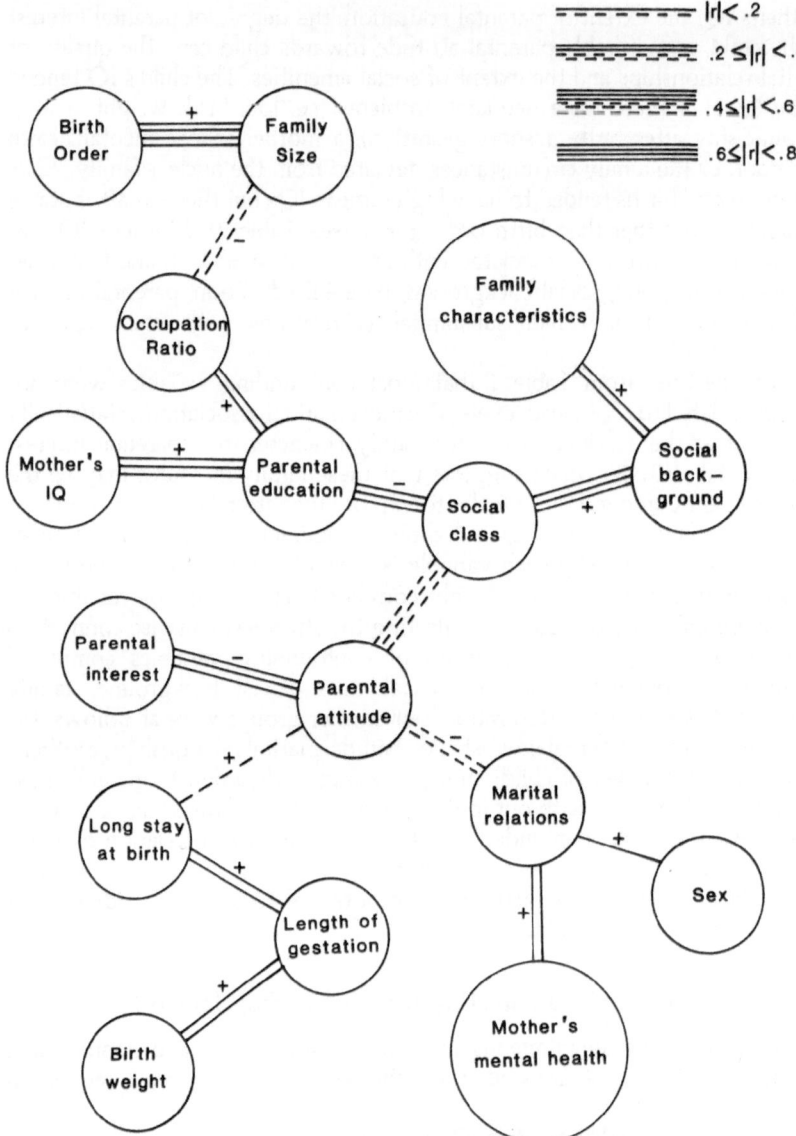

Figure 3 Minimum spanning tree for confounding variables

models presented in Table 3. Log (tooth lead) was forced to be the first variable included. Mother's IQ was the first confounder to enter the model, as would be anticipated from Table 1. Thereafter, variables enter the model in decreasing order of importance, such that only the first eight variables achieve at conventional levels of statistical significance. The regression coefficient for log (tooth lead) steadily decreases as one progresses through the sequence of optimal models so that it is no longer significant at the 5%

Table 3 The sequence of 'optimal' regression models

No. of variables	Optimal combination*	C_p	p value for added variable	p value for log Pb	Regression coefficient for log Pb
1	log(tooth lead)	135.8	0.002	0.002	−2.66
2	+mother's IQ	48.0	0.0001	0.01	−2.02
3	+marital relationships	35.1	0.0002	0.03	−1.72
4	+family size ⩾ 3	26.4	0.002	0.04	−1.58
5	+social class IV, V	19.8	0.004	0.05	−1.49
6	+low birth weight	15.5	0.01	0.06	−1.43
7	+non-manual social class	13.1	0.04	0.09	−1.27
8	+long hospital stay after birth	10.4	0.03	0.09	−1.27
9	+family characteristics	9.3	0.08	0.16	−1.06
10	+sex	8.8	0.11	0.16	−1.07
11	+parental interest	8.5	0.13	0.22	−0.94
12	+parental education	9.4	0.29	0.21	−0.95
13	+not married	10.7	0.41	0.21	−0.96
14	+gestation <38 weeks	12.1	0.43	0.20	−0.98
15	+mother's mental health	13.7	0.61	0.19	−1.00
16	−mother's mental health +social background +occupation ratio	15.4	0.53 0.49	0.18	−1.03
17	+mother's mental health	17.0	0.55	0.17	−1.05
18	+parental attitude	19.0	0.96	0.17	−1.05

*Conditional on log(tooth lead) being included

level after five confounders have entered the model. For all models with eight or more confounders the regression coefficient for log (tooth lead) remains around − 1.0 with a p value around 0.2.

The optimality criterion C_p reached its minimum when $p = 11$ variables, and this optimal model is presented in Table 4. Mother's IQ is by far the most important determinant of child IQ, even after allowance for all other factors. The increase in child IQ for a one standard deviation increase in mother's IQ is + 3.74 points. The other quantitative interview scores (marital relationships, family characteristics and parental interest) are all of borderline significance.

Children from large families, i.e. ⩾ 3 children, have a mean IQ 3.77 points lower than the rest, even after allowing for other factors. The adjusted mean IQ for children with fathers in non-manual occupations is 2.96 points higher than for those with fathers in skilled manual occupations, who in turn have a mean 4.63 IQ points increase over those with fathers in semi-skilled or unskilled manual occupations. Two neonatal problems, low birth weight and long hospital stay after birth, both had reductions in adjusted mean IQ of around 4 points. The lower adjusted mean IQ in females is of borderline

Table 4 Results of the optimal regression of child IQ on log(tooth lead) and ten confounding variables

Variable	Regression coefficient*	t-statistic	p value
Log(tooth lead)	−0.77	−1.23	0.22
Mother's IQ	+3.74	5.35	0.0001
Marital relationships	−1.35	−2.05	0.04
Family characteristics	−1.02	−1.60	0.11
Parental interest	−1.09	−1.52	0.13
Family size 3	−3.77	−2.81	0.005
Non-manual social class	+2.96	2.06	0.04
Social class IV and V	−4.63	−2.53	0.01
Low birth weight	−3.71	−1.96	0.05
Long hospital stay after birth	−4.42	−2.04	0.04
Female sex	−2.10	−1.68	0.09

*For each continuous variable (i.e. the first five listed), we present the standardized regression coefficient = the change in child IQ for a one standard deviation increase in the variable. For each binary variable (i.e. the next six listed) we present the change in child IQ for the feature being present compared with it being absent. In each case this is done after allowance for all other variables in the model

significance, and this unexpected finding may perhaps be attributed to chance.

The standardized regression coefficient for log (tooth lead) in this optimal model is not statistically significant ($p = 0.22$) and is much smaller than the standardized coefficients for the quantitative confounders. Nevertheless this coefficient means that a doubling of tooth lead in a child is associated with an estimated mean decrease in IQ of 0.65 points, with 95% confidence limits = −1.70 and +0.41 points. Hence, one cannot dismiss the possibility of a weak negative relationship between tooth lead levels and child IQ, but these data provide no evidence of such a relationship. An alternative approach is to revert to the eight ordered groups presented in Figure 2. An analysis of covariance allowing for the ten confounders listed in Table 4 resulted in adjusted mean IQs shown in Figure 4. Allowance for confounders has considerably reduced the group differences in IQ by lowering the means for the lowest two lead groups and raising the means for the highest three lead groups, and there remains no tangible lead–IQ relationship after allowance for confounders.

Exploring for interactions between lead and confounders

It has been hypothesized that any lead–IQ association may not apply uniformly to all young children, but may be more pronounced in certain social groups. It is difficult to explore such statistical interactions between lead and confounding variables because of the large number of ways of classifying children into social subgroups. Nevertheless, some tentative observations may be of value.

Since social class is widely used for classifying people into social groupings

160

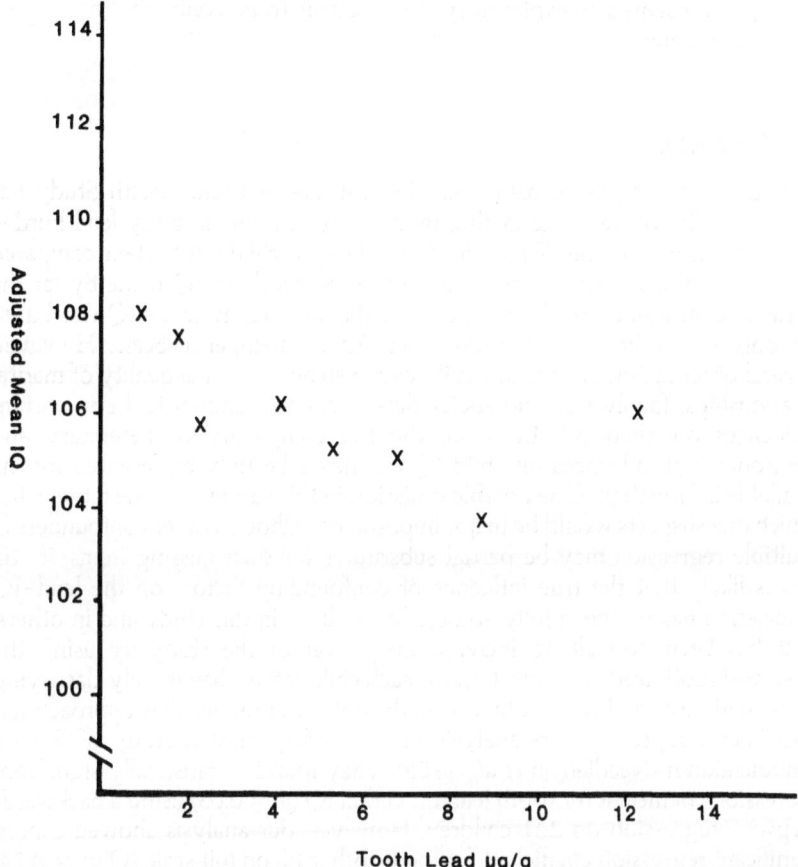

Figure 4 Mean IQ adjusted for confounding variables for children in eight ordered groups of tooth lead

it is sensible to see if the regressions of child IQ on log (tooth lead) would vary across the social classes. In fact the (unstandardized) regression coefficients ± standard error for log (tooth lead) for non-manual classes, class III manual and classes IV and V are −1.46 ± 1.13, −1.48 ± 1.20 and 0.82 ± 2.39 respectively. This provides no evidence for the impact of lead on IQ being more marked in the lower social classes.

A similar analysis of any sex differences in the lead–IQ association produced unstandardized regression coefficients ± standard errors of log (tooth lead) equal to −2.95 ± 1.09 for boys and +0.84 ± 1.02 for girls. The statistical test for interaction, comparing these lead regression coefficients for boys and girls, is significant ($p = 0.01$). This unexpected finding implies a negative association between tooth lead and IQ for boys only, which remains significant after allowance for confounders, whereas for girls the association is positive though non-significant. Since there was no prior hypothesis to support such a sex difference in the lead–IQ relationship, this finding is presented as exploratory data analysis to be confirmed (or refuted) by other studies.

DISCUSSION

This detailed analysis of data from the Institute of Child Health Study has reinforced the overall finding that moderate elevations in body lead burden play only a minor role, if any, in determining a child's IQ when compared with parental and socio-environmental factors. Mother's IQ made by far the greatest contribution to child IQ, despite the fact that mother's IQ was based on only two subtests of the Wechsler Adult Intelligence Scale. However, several other factors reflecting family circumstances, e.g. the quality of marital relationships, family size and social class, were also shown to be important influences on child IQ. Even so, the full complexity of hereditary and environmental influences on child IQ can never be fully represented by the available information. One notable omission in this survey was the father's IQ, which one suspects would be major importance. Alhough other confounders in multiple regression may be partial substitutes for such missing items, it still seems likely that the true influence of confounding factors on the lead–IQ association has not been fully accounted for, both in this study and in others.

It has been possible to increase the power of the study by using the observed tooth lead concentration for each child rather than merely classifying each child into the low, medium or high tooth lead range. This approach has also been adopted in a re-analysis of the widely quoted study of Boston schoolchildren (Needleman et al., 1985). They found a statistically significant regression coefficient for tooth lead on verbal IQ ($p = 0.03$) using a backwards stepwise regression on 221 children. However, our analysis showed a non-significant regression coefficient for log (tooth lead) on full-scale IQ ($p = 0.24$) using an 'optimal' regression procedure on 377 children. The two studies have a broadly similar design except that the Institute of Child Health Study has added a middle group of tooth leads and includes more children.

Slight differences in statistical analysis techniques are unlikely to matter, and the different choice of confounders is inevitable since the interviews of parents used different techniques. One major difference is that the Boston children had much higher body lead burdens than the London children (Medical Research Council, 1984), so that it is plausible that while moderate elevations in body lead burden for London school children may be of no consequence, the markedly higher lead exposures in the Boston study may enter the realm of detrimental effects on IQ.

However, such a positive assertion is not the only interpretation. A valid argument exists for 'reverse causality', whereby relatively poor children of lower IQ may, either by their behaviour or their social environment, be more prone to lead exposure during their earlier years. Cross-sectional studies can never account for such effects of low IQ on lead uptake; a fruitful development has been to undertake prospective studies of birth cohorts which can relate a longitudinal assessment of lead exposure from birth to subsequent measures of neuropsychological development. Unfortunately, many of the longitudinal studies now under way may not be large enough to have adequate power, particularly as investigators continue to explore many different measures of neuropsychological development.

One problem in studies based on tooth lead measurement is that one is dependent on children donating shed milk teeth. Even with an enthusiastic research team some 30–40% of eligible children are excluded from the results. Hence, any inconsistency between different studies of tooth lead and IQ could possibly be attributed to biases in sample selection. For instance, children of lower intelligence may be less likely to donate teeth; and it is uncertain what potential bias this could have. A comparison of tooth-givers with non-givers in this study was described previously (Smith *et al.*, 1983).

Some exploration of statistical interactions has been made to see if the lead–IQ relationship may be more or less pronounced in certain subgroups of the children. Data from previous British studies (Harvey *et al.*, 1984; Yule and Lansdown, 1973) had suggested that lead's association with IQ might be confined to more socially deprived children, but our investigation of different social classes has found no evidence to support this hypothesis.

A more curious subgroup finding is that for boys there is a statistically significant negative association between tooth lead and IQ which could not be accounted for by confounding factors, whereas for girls the association, although non-significant, is actually slightly positive. Whilst one cannot dismiss the possibility that boys may be more sensitive to neurotoxins such as lead, we are unaware of any previous scientific evidence for such a sex difference, and therefore suggest this unexpected finding be viewed with a healthy scepticism. Nevertheless, this issue merits further investigation. Another possible explanation relates to the 'reverse causality' mentioned earlier. The behaviour patterns of young boys and girls tend to be quite different – to put it bluntly boys have a tendency to be grubbier and are more frequently engaged in play activities of a dirtier nature. Perhaps such sex differences in play activities become more pronounced amongst less intelligent children, which might enhance lead uptake amongst boys (but not girls) of lower IQ.

Another relevant issue is that the boys in this study had a higher mean IQ than girls, which contradicts the intended design of the full-scale Revised Wechsler Intelligence Scale for Children to have no sex difference. This anomaly may be due to the type of children donating teeth; more girls donated teeth than boys, and perhaps the less intelligent boys were less likely to donate teeth, thus biasing upwards the mean IQ in the boys available for neuropsychological testing. However, a study of black American children has also found higher IQ scores in boys using the WISC-R (Vance and Engin, 1978).

This paper has emphasized the need to specify a clearly defined analysis strategy for this kind of epidemiological study. Multiple regression analysis can be employed in many different ways, so that it is important to lay down one's criteria for selecting variables for inclusion in a final model. The use of 'optimal' regression based on minimizing Mallow's C_p has proved of value in this study, and in particular the sequence of models in Table 3 helped one to appreciate how the negative association between lead and IQ could be diluted to non-significance by adding further relevant confounders into the model.

In general, the investigation of possible neurotoxic effects of low-level lead exposure has been hampered by the small size of most studies. The Institute of Child Health Study is one of the largest studies of lead and IQ, but still is not as large as one would like. For instance, recent studies of lead and blood pressure in adults have been on several thousand subjects (Shaper and Pocock, 1985), whereas the total evidence on lead and IQ is much less substantial. Perhaps the prime reason for this lack of extensive data is the practical difficulty in measuring body lead burden and obtaining reliable neuropsychological assessments in young children. From this relative paucity of information, and the interpretive limitations of observational studies, one cannot provide definitive proof that moderate body burdens of lead have no effect on children's intelligence. However, the available findings from other recent British studies (Harvey *et al.*, 1984; Lansdown *et al.*, 1986), combined with our own overall lack of association, enables one to conclude that there is no evidence to support the hypothesis that lead exposure as currently experienced by British children is of any relevance to their intellectual development.

ACKNOWLEDGMENTS

We greatly appreciate the cooperation of Professor Barbara Clayton, Professor Philip Graham, Dr Trevor Delves and Dr Richard Lansdown, and also the Department of the Environment in enabling us to undertake further analyses of their Institute of Child Health/Southampton Study. Dr Ashby is supported on a special project grant from the Medical Research Council.

REFERENCES

Environmental Protection Agency (1985) *Air Quality Criteria for Lead*: Chapter 13, Evaluation of human health risk associated with exposure to lead and its compounds (Research Triangle Park, USA: EPA)

Gower, J.C. and Ross, G.J.S. (1969) Minimum spanning trees and single linkage cluster analysis *Appl. Stat.*, **18**, 54–64

Great Britain Office of Population Censuses and Surveys (1970) *Classification of occupations* (London: HMSO)

Harvey, P.G., Hamlin, P.W., Kumar, R. and Delves, H.T. (1984) Blood lead, behaviour and intelligence test performance in pre-school children. *Sci. Total Env.*, **40**, 45–60

Lansdown, R., Yule, W., Urbanowicz, M-A. and Hunter, J. (1986) The relationship between blood-lead concentrations, intelligence, attainment and behaviour in a school population: the second London study. *Int. Arch. Occup. Env. Health*, **57**, 225–235

Mallows, C.L. (1973) Some comments on C_p. Technometrics, **15**, 661–675

Medical Research Council (1984) *The Neuropsychological Effects of Lead in Children: a review of recent research 1979–1983* (London: MRC)

Needleman, H.L., Geiger, S.K. and Frank, R. (1985) Lead and IQ scores: a reanalysis. *Science*, **227**, 701–704

Pocock, S.J. and Ashby, D. (1985) Environmental lead and children's intelligence: a review of recent epidemiological studies. *Statistician*, **34**, 31–44

Shaper, A.G. and Pocock, S.J. (1985) Blood lead and blood pressure (editorial). *Br. Med. J.* **291**, 1147–1149

Smith, M., Delves, T., Lansdown, R., Clayton, B. and Graham, P. (1983) The effects of lead exposure on urban children: The Institute of Child Health/Southampton Study. *Dev. Med. Child Neurol.*, **25** (Suppl. 47)

Vance, H. and Engin, A. (1978) Analysis of cognitive abilities on black children's performance on WISC-R. *J. Clin. Psychol.*, **34**, 452–456

Wechsler, D. (1974) *Wechsler Intelligence Scale for Children*, rev. edn (New York: Psychological Corporation)

Yule, W. and Lansdown, R. (1973) Lead and children's development: recent findings. Proceedings of 4th International Conference: *Heavy Metals in the Environment*, Heidelberg, Germany, 6–9 Sept.

3.2
Child–Caregiver Environmental Factors Related to Lead Exposure and IQ

S. R. SCHROEDER

SUMMARY

From 1975 to 1985 the authors conducted a series of interdisciplinary research studies of lead effects on cognitive functioning and other aspects of neurobehavioural development in children identified as part of a statewide lead screening programme sponsored by the North Carolina Division of Health Services. The research strategy employed involved both evaluation of paediatric subjects using only traditional psychometric measures, such as IQ; and the use, in assessing other subjects, of longitudinal observations of children's behaviour and electrophysiological parameters, as well as other factors (e.g. home observations, parent–child interactions, etc.), that might be related to low-level lead exposure and its developmental effects. This paper describes three such studies of lead effects on IQ and other neuropsychological measures among very low socioeconomic (SES) children residing in rural areas of the State of North Carolina (USA). In general, the results of the studies demonstrate that the quality of the caregiving environment is an important determinant of lead burdens in young children, i.e. caregiving environment deficiencies were associated with increased lead burdens. Significant relationships between blood lead (PbB) levels and child's IQ found in the studies were complicated by an intricate interweaving of social factors. Nevertheless, in a uniformly low SES Black paediatric population, IQ deficits were significantly associated with PbB levels across a range of 6.3 to 47.4 μg/dl ($x = 20.8\,\mu$g/dl), even after controlling for the influence of important covariates.

A major challenge is better understanding of interrelationships between social factors, lead, and child IQ. Most studies have attempted to control for possible covariates such as social class, age, maternal IQ, pica, and parents' attitude towards education, but not for quality of the caregiving environment. Studies of relationships between socioeconomic status (SES) and intelligence and academic achievement have yielded mixed results. In a meta-analysis of 200 studies relating SES to academic achievement, White (1982) found that home atmosphere correlated much higher with academic achievement than any other combination of SES indicators. The most important variables were childrearing practices and stimulation of learning at home and school, not parents' occupation, income, or education. SES, then, appears to be a broad but crude measure of a cluster of factors, e.g. caregiving practices, resources, etc., that may be better examined separately. Results of previous studies suggest that there might be deficiencies in the caregiving environment of children who evidence increased lead burden (Chatterjee and Gettman, 1972; Lansdown et al., 1974; Millican et al., 1956; Rennert et al., 1970; Rummo et al., 1979).

Milar et al. (1980) compared two groups of children, 12 to 30 months and 31–78 months, showing increased lead burden with another group matched for age, sex, and SES, but with no increased lead burden. The quality of the caregiving environment of these children was assessed with the Home Observation for Measurement of the Environment (HOME) Inventory (Caldwell et al., 1966), and maternal intelligence was also measured. For the younger children, significant deficits in maternal IQ and quality of the caregiving environment were associated with increased lead burden. Subscales of the HOME Inventory assessing maternal emotional and verbal responsivity and maternal involvement with the child showed significant deficiencies in the caregiving environment of the children with increased lead burden. For the older children the HOME Inventory also showed deficiencies in the caregiving environment with increased lead burden, but not at $p \leqslant 0.05$.

Traditionally, interpretation of research on lead effects in humans holds that increased lead burden directly results in deficits in cognitive functioning. However, several alternative hypotheses are also plausible. First, the Milar et al. (1980) results suggest the possibility that cognitive deficits in children exposed to lead may be a direct result of deficiencies in the caregiving environment, rather than being due to lead per se. The research of Bradley and Caldwell (1976a, b) tends to support this conclusion.

Second, it is possible that caregiving environment deficiencies are responsible for increased lead burden and the cognitive deficits are due to lead. A child in a lead-contaminated environment would be much more likely to ingest significant amounts of lead if left unsupervised by his/her caregiver. The poor caregiving environment may be an antecedent to lead exposure, but lead-induced neurotoxic effects may be responsible for observed cognitive deficits. This situation may be analogous to malnutrition in children. Severe malnutrition can lead to cognitive deficits (Dobbing, 1970), but Cravioto and DeLicardie (1972) have also shown that aspects of the caregiving environment may place children at risk for malnutrition.

A third hypothesis is that the caregiving environment and lead combine to affect intellectual development adversely, similar to the relationship found by Werner et al. (1968) between perinatal complications and later psychological development. At 20 months of age, IQ differences between children with and without perinatal complications were only 5–7 points for children from a favourable social background; but for low-SES infants the IQ differences ranged from 19 to 37 points. Apparently, perinatal insult and the quality of the child's environment both affected development. Similarly, even with low lead levels, it might be anticipated that combined effects of SES, maternal IQ, the caregiving environment, inadequate nutrition, and lead may pose an increased cumulative risk of handicaps in cognitive and adaptive behaviour development.

In our research on low-level lead exposure we adopted a strategy of cross-sectional and longitudinal study of the intellectual, social, and neurobehavioural development of preschool children exposed to low or moderate blood lead (PbB) levels. We asked two questions: (a) Does cross-sectional comparison show a significant interaction between age and PbB levels, between age and type of exposure (occupational versus non-occupational), or between age and the important behavioural covariates of lead exposure (SES level, maternal IQ, and quality of the caregiving environment); and (b) Upon regular 5-year re-evaluations, can changes in these children's intellectual, social, and neurobehavioural development be related to current PbB levels or to cumulative previous PbB levels after removal of lead from their home environment?

GENERAL METHODOLOGY

Several sources were used to recruit subjects, including: (1) referrals from the North Carolina statewide Early and Periodic Screening, Diagnosis, and Treatment (EPSDT) Program; (2) referrals from local lead screening programmes in Wake, Lenoir and New Hanover counties, NC and (3) direct recruitment of children from families employed or residing near lead-related industries. Direct contact, recruitment, and scheduling of subjects were done by a Patient Coordinator through local or county health departments under the aegis of the North Carolina Statewide Lead Screening Advisory Committee.

Experimental design and statistical methodology

The present research used a cross-sectional observational epidemiological design and did not manipulate independent variables. For purposes of hypothesis testing the recruited subjects were assumed to be a random sample representative of children likely to be considered for screening for lead exposure in the EPSDT population.

The principal statistical analysis approach involved multiple-regression modelling, with age and PbB as predictors for central nervous system (CNS) outcomes. When considering IQ as the outcome, the regression models controlled for age, SES, home environment score and maternal IQ. The general strategy for determining the best model paralleled the approach by Kleinbaum *et al.* (1982).

168

Lead analysis procedures

An essential part of this research was accurate assessment of indices of body lead burden; PbB concentration was the key predictor variable studied. Measurements of PbB levels, as well as lead in house paint and house dust, were done by the Heavy Metals Analysis Laboratory, Department of Pathology, UNC-Chapel Hill.

Lead in blood

The Delves cup microprocedure (Delves, 1970) with the modification of Ediger and Coleman (1972) was employed for whole blood (and plasma) lead determinations. Direct insertion of blood samples into Delves cups followed by drying, preignition and atomization of the contained lead, was rapid and relatively free of contamination problems. Special precautions were taken to minimize sample contamination prior to analysis. All glassware coming into contact with samples was washed and chemically debrided of metal contaminants by low-metal acid washing, followed by repeated deionized water rinsing. Reagents, solvents for reagents, and other assay materials were selected for very small or undetectable metal contaminant content. With human subjects, blood was collected via venepuncture into B-D low-lead vacutainer tubes.

Quality control was maintained by both internal and external means. Frequent preparation and testing of aqueous and matrix-matched standards on a daily or weekly basis was used to assess changes in day-to-day precision and accuracy. External monitoring of laboratory performance was done via participation in the Center for Disease Control's (CDC) proficiency testing for PbB determinations. The laboratory's performance has been quite good over the range of PbB levels encountered in the CDC proficiency survey. Further evaluation was done using certified blood samples of known metal content, either from a commercial source (Kaulson Laboratories) or the NY State Health Department.

Instrument and test battery development

This project had several unique features: (1) the development of a mobile neurotoxicity testing laboratory that permitted assessment of children in remote catchment areas with sophisticated behavioural and electrophysiological measures; (2) a cooperative arrangement with Federal, State, county, and local health agencies and private industry that permitted coordinated screening and assessment of 'at-risk' children across the state; and (3) an opportunity to obtain valuable longitudinal data on long-term effects of early lead exposure on neurobehavioural and cognitive development. Behavioural and medical evaluations were carried out by professional staff from the Division for Disorders of Development and Learning (DDDL), a clinical training facility of the University of North Carolina Child Development Research Institute and Biological Sciences Research Center (BSRC).

169

Daily test protocol and home visit
Electrophysiological data were collected at the DDDL or in the field mobile laboratory. Demographic, psychometric and medical data were obtained in an auxiliary trailer or space provided by local health agencies. Families were seen for a testing protocol that took about 4 h to complete, and informed consent was obtained from the parent(s). At testing, the examiner was blind as to the child's lead exposure. A maximum of four children per day were evaluated in the mobile laboratory.

After evaluation day, a home visit was made for several reasons. If behaviour problems are assumed to be related to lead exposure, then control assessments have to be made of the home environment to estimate its contribution to the child's cognitive or other behavioural problems. The Caldwell HOME Inventory was used for this purpose. Each home was also evaluated as a vehicle for continued lead exposure; and the lead, if discovered, was removed by cleaning supervised by the county health department. Dust samples from the living-room carpet, bedroom, and inside the front door were obtained by suction on preweighed glass filters and analysed for lead by X-ray fluorescence using a portable unit. Home water supply was also analysed for lead by AAS. These analyses led to the clean-up of several homes, with resultant reductions of PbB levels of exposed children (Milar and Mushak, 1982). Once all the clinical data were gathered and evaluated, each case was reviewed at a staffing conference and any problems discovered, whether lead-related or not, were referred to appropriate local community resources for follow-up.

Medical, psychometric, and behavioural measures
Table 1 summarizes the PbB, other blood chemistry, medical, electrophysiological, psychometric, behavioural and demographic measures collected from participating children and parents. These measures were chosen to provide convergent information from several different perspectives to elaborate more clearly the subtle and complex effects of asymptomatic lead exposure on CNS development. Several tests were selected on the basis of guidelines later adopted at an International Symposium on Neurobehavioral Methodology in Pediatric Lead Research (Cincinnati; OH; September 1981). These guidelines included: (1) use of standardized, age-normed tests with documented validity and reliability when available; (2) use of experimental measures to evaluate areas of function for which standardized measures are not available, and (3) use of instruments with cross-cultural comparison data.

An extensive medical history was taken on each child to rule out a variety of problems related to mental retardation, but not attributable to lead, and to evaluate lead exposure history. The instrument used was the *Lead Poisoning Study Questionnaire* developed at the Fantus Lead Screening Clinic at Cook County Hospital in Chicago. This 28-page questionnaire examines pertinent demographic history, prenatal history, child development milestones, past medical history, lead poisoning symptomatology, dietary history, family history, immunizations, illnesses, vital signs, chelation therapy and side-effects.

Table 1 Summary of evaluations conducted

I. *Exposure evaluation*
  A. Fantus lead poisoning questionnaire
  B. Blood lead (PbB): flameless atomic absorption spectrometry
  C. Free erythrocyte protoporphyrin (FEP)

II. *Medical evaluation*
  A. Medical history
  B. Pediatric neurological examination
  C. Growth: height, weight, head circumference
  D. Laboratory tests: BDS, WBC, RBC, Hgb, HCT, MCV, MCH, MCHC

III. *Electrophysiological evaluation*
  A. Slow cortical potentials during sensory conditioning
  B. Brainstem auditory evoked potentials
  C. Pattern-reversal visual evoked potentials

IV. *Psychometric–behavioural evaluation*
  A. Stanford-Binet intelligence test – revised
  B. Bayley Scales of Infant Development ($<$30 months of age)

V. *Demographic covariate evaluation*
  A. Maternal IQ: Ammons quick test or Peabody picture vocabulary test revised (PPVT-R)
  B. Socioeconomic status: Hollingshead two-factor index
  C. Quality of caregiving environment: Caldwell's home observation for measurement of the environment
  D. Chronological age
  E. Sex

STUDY 1: COMPARISON OF CHILDREN OCCUPATIONALLY AND NON-OCCUPATIONALLY EXPOSED TO LEAD

A North Carolina Memorial Hospital case report of lead poisoning in a family from Raleigh, NC, uncovered a highly stable and cooperative population associated with a battery plant in Wake County where their relatives were employed. The children were exposed to lead-contaminated dust brought home on workers' clothing and deposited in house dust and carpets, which placed toddlers at the crawling stage at risk (Dolcourt, 1977; Dolcourt *et al.*, 1978). From 1977 to 1979 we evaluated over 115 children, 42 of whom were children of employees in that plant and 104 of whom met the criteria for study; the children were then followed longitudinally.

Methods

Subjects
One hundred and four children in Wake County, NC, aged 10 months to 6.5 years at the time of initial testings, and who met inclusion criteria, served as subjects. They were mostly Black (94%) from lower social classes – i.e., $\bar{x} = 4.5$ on the Hollingshead Two-Factor Index (Hollingshead, 1957). Children previously evidencing CNS disease or insult, having undergone chelation therapy for lead poisoning, or with prediagnosed language delay or mental retardation, were excluded from data analysis. Approximately half of the children were less than 30 months old. Half were EPSDT children and half

were children of battery factory workers referred from a local county health department to the Lead Screening Program at North Carolina Memorial Hospital.

Procedures

Subjects were evaluated at DDDL in the protocol described above under General methodology, except that the only electrophysiological measures obtained were slow cortical potentials during sensory conditioning (see Otto *et al.*, 1981).

Results and discussion

A preliminary forward stepwise regression analysis of the relationship of lead to IQ and 18 of their covariates showed no effect of occupational exposure among the present cohort of children (Hawk and Schroeder, 1983). Therefore, further analysis of occupational exposure was dropped, and the number of confounding variables was reduced to HOME, SES, maternal IQ, age, sex, test (Bayley vs. Stanford-Binet), presence of father in the home, and number of siblings, in order to avoid overcontrol and type II errors. The main statistical model used a multivariate regression analysis, in which a set of all the interaction terms was tested first. If the set was non-significant, all interactions were dropped from the model. The second step was to test the main effects of the confounding variables. Then, finally, the test for the main effects of lead was performed. Any significant result was then further reduced in a stepwise manner for individual or linear combinations of variables for inclusion into the final model (Kleinbaum, *et al.*, 1982).

The main result was a significant linear relationship between PbB level (range 6–59 μg/dl) and IQ ($F = 7.689$; d.f. 1,96; $p < 0.01$) (Figure 1). None of the interaction terms or any of the quadratic or cubic effects was significant. Of the confounding variables, only SES was significant ($F = 20.159$; d.f. 1,96; $p < 0.001$) and remained in the model. Nevertheless the main effect of lead on IQ remained significant.

The failure of HOME, maternal IQ, and age to reach significance, as they usually have in other studies, was likely the result of multicollinearity with SES. Table 2 shows that the intercorrelation of these variables was high. It appears that whichever of these variables enters the regression equation first is likely to render the effects of the others less significant. While SES and HOME shared much variance, one would ordinarily expect a direct measure of caregiving environment (like the HOME) to be a more accurate measure than an indirect one based on parental occupation and education (like SES). Order of entry of multicollinear covariates into the regression equation was important in determining which were significant and which were not. The matter of separating the effects of social factors on the relationship between lead and IQ is addressed below in the Replication Study.

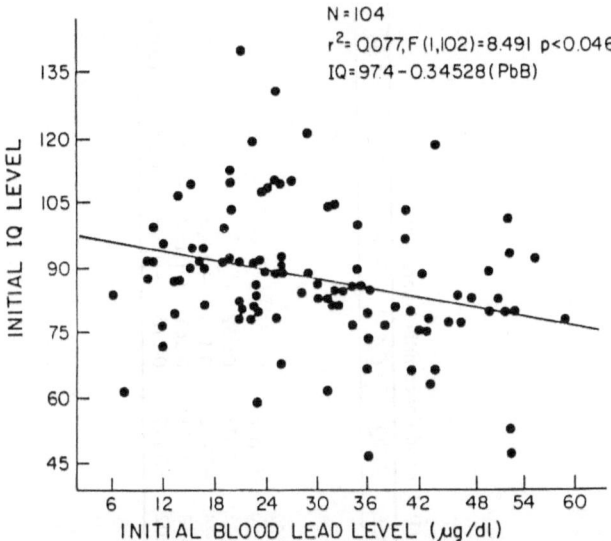

Figure 1 Initial IQ as a function of initial blood lead levels of children screened from 1977 to 1979

STUDY II: FIVE-YEAR FOLLOW-UP STUDY

The objective of this study (Schroeder *et al.*, 1985) was to determine if asymptomatic lead exposure in early childhood resulted in residual altered CNS function in children when they reached school age. There might be latent or cumulative effects, even though their PbB levels would typically be lower because of having grown out of the toddler stage.

Methods

Subjects
Eighty of the 104 children from Study I were located through county health department and school records 5 years later in 1983. Of the 80, 50 agreed to re-evaluation.

Procedures
Children were seen at the Wake County Health Department in the mobile laboratory using the same protocol as Study I described under General methodology, except that the home visit was not repeated. Most of their PbB levels had come down (Figure 2).

Results and discussion

The same backward multiple-regression analysis was used as in the initial study except that initial PbB level was used as the independent variable,

Table 2 Correlation matrix of blood lead level and child IQ (1977) and concomitant variables

Variables	PbB	IQ	HOME	MIQ	CA	Sex	SES	FaPr
Blood lead level (PbB)								
Child IQ	-0.276							
Caldwell HOME	-0.269	0.451						
Maternal IQ (MIQ)	-0.193	0.379	0.522					
Chronological age (CA)	-0.068	0.254	0.089	0.029				
Sex	-0.072	0.130	0.123	-0.028	0.062			
Socioeconomic status (SES)	0.183	-0.449	-0.624	-0.475	-0.143	-0.064		
Father present (FaPr)	-0.010	0.165	0.433	0.178	0.161	0.054	-0.495	
Number of siblings (Sibs)	0.314	-0.284	-0.202	-0.177	0.116	-0.003	0.161	-0.064

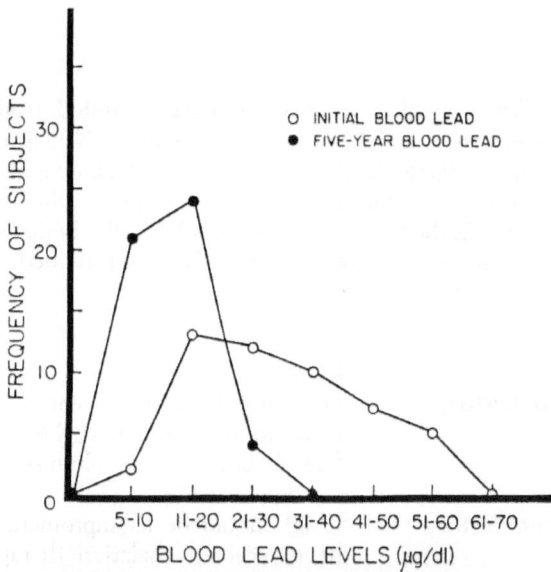

Figure 2 Frequency distribution of blood lead levels of children seen from 1977 to 1978 and follow-up 5 years later

current PbB level was added to the list of covariates, and 'test' and 'age' were dropped as covariates, since all children received the Stanford-Binet IQ test this time. The two PbB measures were highly correlated ($r = 0.74$); the correlation of initial PbB to follow-up IQ was also significant ($r = 0.34$, $p < 0.05$).

The main result in this study was that lead was no longer a significant effect in the regression analysis after the confounding variables were added to the model ($F < 1$). Apparently the decline in PbB levels, while not appreciably disturbing the relation of social factors to lead and IQ, did negate lead's relation to IQ when confounding factors were controlled. This was not due to self-selection bias as follow-up, since the demographic characteristics of the families who participated were very similar to those who did not.

In conclusion, it appeared that, in the present cohort of mainly low-SES Black families, the covariance matrix among social factors and the relationship of lead to IQ were fairly stable over a 5-year period. SES appeared to capture much of the variance related to the other covariates due to multicollinearity with HOME, maternal IQ, and age.

STUDY III: REPLICATION STUDY

The primary objectives of this study were to replicate the previous studies in a more homogeneous group (all-Black, low-SES children aged 3–7 years) and to find the best regression model based on both accuracy and precision that described the relationship of lead and IQ (Hawk *et al.*, 1986).

Methods

Subjects
Eighty Black children aged 3 to 7 years were recruited from high-risk neighbourhoods in Lenoir and New Hanover counties, NC, in cooperation with county health agencies and the Environmental Epidemiology Branch (EEB) of the North Carolina Division of Health Services. Most of the New Hanover sample were in the Headstart Program. A list of criteria for eligibility of individual children for inclusion in the study was provided to referring health agencies, as specified below:

1.	Age	3–7 years.
2.	Race	Black.
3.	Health status/history	No current acute or chronic illness or medication of any sort. Perinatal history free of complications. No history of neuro-biological insults.
4.	Lead-exposure history	Child should be asymptomatic and never have received chelation therapy or been treated for lead poisoning. A range of PbB levels from 5 to 60 μg/dl was desired.
5.	Socioeconomic status	Low-income families defined as Class IV or V (Hollingshead scale). EPSDT families were included in this group.
6.	IQ	In order to exclude any children who were clearly mentally retarded, a minimum subject IQ of 60 was required.

Procedures
The same procedures as outlined in the General methodology section were performed. Based on the results of our previous studies, covariates were restricted here to HOME, SES, maternal IQ, age, and gender. Of the 80 children screened, 75 met the inclusion criteria and were used for analysis; their demographic characteristics are given in Table 3.

Results

Statistical analysis strategy for assessing interaction and confounding of social factors
The main objective of the statistical analysis strategy was to find the best model that described the relationship between lead and IQ. The principal approach involved multiple-regression modelling, with PbB level as a predictor variable; child IQ as the outcome variable; and age, SES, HOME score, gender, and maternal IQ (MIQ) as control variables. The control variables were restricted to those five which had proven significant in our earlier studies to reduce type II errors due to over-control (Kleinbaum *et al.*, 1982). Type I errors were controlled by focusing on one confirmatory hypothesis: that PbB levels would be significantly related to child IQ, while controlling for SES,

176

Table 3 Demographic characteristics of children in the replication study

Demographic characteristics	Mean score	SD	Range
Mean blood lead level (μg/dl)	21.80	9.76	6.00–39.00
High blood lead level (μg/dl)	26.71	14.11	6.20–56.00
Most recent blood lead level (μg/dl)	20.65	9.73	6.20–47.40
Most recent FEP (μg/dl)	32.74	14.03	8.0–193.0
Home caregiver practices (Caldwell, 1976, 1979)	59.84	15.08	20–87
Maternal IQ (PPVT-R, 1983)	63.41	11.29	40–94
Chronological age (months)	58.40	11.74	39–94
Socioeconomic class (Hollingshead two-factor index)	4.91	0.20	4–5

MIQ, HOME (caregiving environment), gender, and age. Exploratory analyses were performed to find the most accurate and precise model that described the relationship between lead, IQ, and their covariates. The general strategy for determining the best regression model was the hierarchical modelling strategy of Kleinbaum *et al.* (1982). This strategy incorporated the assessment of confounding variables, interactions between lead and the other variables, and precision (i.e. which set of variables accounted for the most variation) into the selection of variables for the final model. A backward stepwise multiple-regression approach was used in which the set of interaction terms (PbB × age, PbB × SES, PbB × sex, PbB × MIQ, PbB × HOME) was tested first in one overall test (chunk test), followed by a chunk test of the set of possible confounding covariate effects, followed by examination of main effects of lead and IQ.

Results of the confirmatory analysis
Chunk tests for interaction variables ($F = 0.55$; d.f. 5,63; $p < 0.74$) and for the control variables after dropping interactions ($F = 1.82$; d.f. 2,58; $p < 0.12$) were not significant, although the latter approached significance (Table 4). The terms were therefore dropped from the final model, which included only lead and IQ. In the final model there was a highly significant relationship between PbB level and IQ ($F = 12.31$; d.f. 1,23; $p < 0.0008$). Similar results were also found if maximum PbB levels (historically highest level available from public health records for each child) ($p < 0.0018$) or mean PbB levels ($p < 0.002$) were used instead of current PbB levels. The average number of PbB determinations by the state laboratory prior to the current study for these children was three (range 1–14). No quadratic or cubic effects were

Table 4 Summary table of the confirmatory analysis of the relation of blood lead and IQ (Univariate F, p)

	Stanford-Binet IQ test					
	Using current PbB		Using mean PbB		Using highest PbB	
Effect	F	p	F	p	F	p
Interactions	0.55	0.74	1.01	0.42	1.34	0.26
Control	1.82	0.12	1.86	0.11	1.76	0.13
Lead PbB	12.31	0.0008	10.08	0.002	10.55	0.0018
R	0.144		0.121		0.126	

significant, but rather a linear relationship was found between PbB levels and IQ. This trend and the confidence intervals are shown in Figure 3.

Results of the exploratory analyses
The multiple-regression analysis for the interaction terms using the overall chunk test was not significant, so all interaction terms were dropped from the model. However, the chunk test for control variables, keeping PbB in the model, approached significance, suggesting that a more accurate and precise model could be found. Furthermore, inspection of Table 5 shows that, while the regression model with lead and IQ alone, considering no covariates, was the most precise (i.e. had the smallest confidence interval), the coefficient for lead differed considerably from that of the 'gold standard', i.e. the model

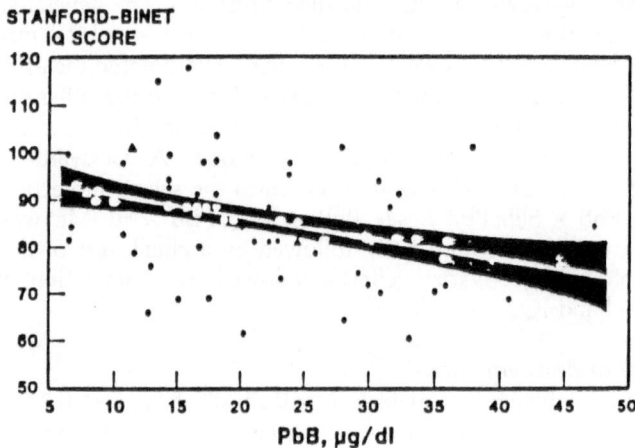

Figure 3 Child IQ as a function of blood lead levels of children screened in the replication study

Table 5 Accuracy and precision of different models of regression of blood levels on IQ including different combinations of variables as candidates for control variables

Candidate subset	β Coefficient [a]	95% Confidence interval $[\beta \pm ({}^t 64,975)(S_\beta)]$		
1. Age,SES,Gender,HOME,MIQ,PbB,IQ[e]	−0.254	0.049[b]	−0.558[c]	0.607[d]
2. Age, Gender,HOME,MIQ,PbB,IQ	−0.248	0.051	−0.548	0.598
3. SES, HOME,MIQ,PbB,IQ	−0.282	0.021	−0.585	0.606
4. Gender,HOME,MIQ,PbB,IQ[f]	−0.255	0.043	−0.554	0.597
5. HOME,MIQ,PbB,IQ	−0.273	0.026	−0.572	0.598
6. MIQ,PbB,IQ	−0.396	−0.102	−0.637	0.535
7. PbB,IQ	−0.456	−0.196	−0.715	0.520

[1] This is the β coefficient for lead
[b] Lower bound of the confidence interval
[c] Upper bound of the confidence interval
[d] Absolute difference between the lower and upper bounds of the confidence interval
[e] The baseline model or 'gold standard' with all control variables included
[f] The match to the gold standard with least confounding (β coefficient for lead that is closest to that in the 'gold standard') while maintaining good precision (small confidence interval)

which included lead, IQ, SES, HOME, MIQ, age and gender. Therefore, regression analyses were performed in which each control variable was considered. Using the strategy recommended by Kleinbaum *et al.* (1982) for considering confounding and precision, a number of alternative models were developed, as presented in Table 5. The model that best controlled for confounding with the greatest precision (i.e. the most accurate *and* precise model) contained lead, MIQ, HOME, and gender. Nevertheless, two other models (IQ, PbB, age, gender, HOME, and MIQ; IQ, PbB, gender, HOME, and MIQ) gave very similar accuracy and precision. All the models in Table 5 were significant beyond the $p < 0.01$ level, whether social factors were controlled or not. Table 6 gives the correlation coefficients of the predictor, outcome, and control variables.

DISCUSSION

The highly significant relationship between lead and IQ found in this study is important because of the relatively low levels of lead burden in our sample (mean = 20.8 μg/dl, range = 6.3–47.4 μg/dl). Of the children in this study, 72% had PbB levels below 25 μg/dl, the Center for Disease Control's currently accepted lead toxicity screening criterion for children, and yet PbB level was still significantly related to child IQ. This result, combined with statistical significance even when controlling for confounding variables, strengthens the consensus of current research concerning lead's effect on child IQ, at least in low-SES populations.

The results of exploratory analyses suggest that the most precise regression model may not always be the most accurate model in dealing with the issue of confounding variables in child lead studies. In the past, Milar *et al.* (1980), and Perino and Ernhart (1974), found maternal IQ to be a significant covariate of child IQ. But when Milar's data were reanalysed by Hawk and Schroeder (1983) using regression analysis, it was found that, once the HOME score was entered, MIQ no longer was significantly related to child IQ. That is, quality of caregiving environment and MIQ shared a great deal of covariance. In the Hawk and Schroeder (1983) sample it appeared that caregiving environment accounted for more variance in the model than did the MIQ. In the present study, while MIQ was included in the precision model, this covariate was collinear with quality of caregiving environment in the model that controlled for confounding. This finding is consistent with the results of

Table 6 Correlation coefficients of predictor, outcome, and control variables

	CA	SES	MIQ	HOME	Gender	CIQ
Blood lead level (PbB)	−0.098	0.397*	−0.314*	−0.526*	−0.129	−0.380*
Age (CA)		0.043	−0.076	0.124	0.135	0.152
Socioeconomic status (SES)			−0.404*	−0.576*	−0.011	−0.223
Maternal IQ (MIQ)				−0.414	0.125	0.326*
Caregiver environment (HOME)					−0.087	0.377*
Gender						0.207

* $p < 0.01$

Longstreth *et al.* (1981) where MIQ was the more significant covariate relative to caregiving environment in the regression equation based on precision. The present results are also consistent with other studies (Ramey *et al.*, 1979; Elardo *et al.*, 1975; White and Watts, 1973; Dietrich *et al.*, 1985), which have demonstrated a great deal of heterogeneity in quality of caregiving environments among lower-SES families. Thus, while caregiving environment may be confounded with MIQ, it also appears to be a more complex and intricate entity that requires further study.

It also appears that caregiving environment was confounded with SES. Once one of these variables was entered into the general linear model (i.e. precision model), the other was no longer significant enough to remain in the model. The order in which these variables were eliminated suggests that quality of the caregiving environment was actually the more precise and valid of the two in the present study. The fact that SES was not a significant covariate in the present study is likely due to the greater homogeneity of the SES variable in this sample compared to previous studies. Thus, the range of SES was restricted by sampling in the present study.

On the other hand, in a sample more heterogeneous with regard to SES (104 Wake County children, part of the initial North Carolina Lead Screening Program), Schroeder *et al.* (1985) found that lead and SES were the only significant variables in relation to child IQ. Schroeder *et al.* (1985) concluded that controlling for SES under such circumstances appeared to capture much of the variance related to other covariates due to multicollinearity, e.g., caregiver practices, MIQ, number of siblings, and lead exposure history. We cautioned, however, that it is important initially to consider all major covariates (i.e., SES, caregiver environment, MIQ, and lead exposure history).

Although PbB level was significantly related to child IQ in the present study, this relationship was complicated by an intricate interweaving of social factors. Future studies might ideally employ a prospective design to capitalize on the use of statistical techniques such as path analysis to understand better how these factors interact across time. Early results of ongoing prospective studies in Boston by Bellinger *et al.* (1984) and in Cincinnati by Bornschein *et al.* (1985) suggest that there is much to be learned from such an approach. For example, these latter investigators have found that both the total HOME and three subscales (Maternal Involvement with Child, Provision of Appropriate Play Materials, and Emotional and Verbal Responsivity of Mother) were negatively correlated with cumulative lead, with the strength of these associations increasing dramatically between 9 and 15 months of age. They suggest that infants who receive less than adequate physical and social stimulation may engage in more mouthing behaviour, which has been shown to be a major source of lead exposure in infants and young children. Further, Bornschein's hypothesized exposure pathway from housing quality to dust lead to hand lead to PbB was supported, with the Maternal Involvement with Child HOME subscale being a significant modifier of hand lead. This type of information, as it evolves over time, will provide valuable guidance in determining how and when to intervene most effectively, and will shape future research directions.

ACKNOWLEDGMENTS

I wish to acknowledge the many people who collaborated on this project: (1) My co-investigators, Dr David Otto of the Neurotoxicology Division of the USEPA; Dr Paul Mushak, PhD, head of the Heavy Metals Laboratory in the Department of Pathology, UNC, whose staff did all of the blood analyses; (2) Dr David Kleinbaum, PhD, Department of Biostatistics, UNC, who served as our statistical consultant to our data analysis group at EPA, consisting of Keith Muller, PhD and Curtis Barton, MA; (3) to the members of the Lead Screening Mobile Unit Team: Lois Boone, LPN, clinical coordinator, Sally Robinson, PhD aand Donna Arendhorst, PhD, psychologists who did IQ testing, Barbara Hawk, PhD, who did home visitations, George Robinson, PhD, Stephen Baumann, PhD, James Williford, BS, and Angela Duprée, who did the electrophysiological testing; (4) local paediatricians who did the paediatric examinations, Betsy Coulson, MD, Joanna Dalldorf, MD, Charles Hicks, MD, William Keiter, MD, Ave Lachiewicz, MD, Mihtili Rajan, MD, Orvil Reece, MD, Frank Reynolds, MD, William Stewart, MD, Mary Sugioka, MD; (5) heads of county health departments who cooperated: Helen Cannon, MD, Marian Duggan, RN, Christine Maroules, RN, Robert Parker, BA; (6) public health nurses who are heads of lead screening programmes in these county health departments: Virginia Bonar, RN, Jo Glick, RN, Margaret King, RN and members of their staff, Susan O'Brian, Patricia Stephenson and Beth Barnes; (7) the Environmental Epidemiology Branch of the NC Statewide Lead Screening Program who did the screening probes: John Freeman, DVM, Linda Brinkley, MPH, and Claudette Simpson, RN.

Finally, we wish to acknowledge the Neurophysiology Branch, Neurotoxicology Division, Health Effects Research Laboratory of USEPA, MCH Project 916, which funds the Division for Disorders of Development and Learning; and HD03110, which funds the Biological Sciences Research Center, all of whom provided invaluable logistic and administrative support, especially Judy Perry, Deborah Sparrow, Jo Nichols, and C. Rodriguez.

REFERENCES

Bellinger, D.C., Needleman, H.L., Leviton, A., Waternaux, C., Rabinowitz, M.B. and Nichols, M.L. (1984) Early sensory-motor development and prenatal exposure to lead. *Neurobehav. Toxicol. Teratol.*, **6**, 387–402

Bornschein, R.L. (1985) Influence of social factors on lead exposure and child development. *Environ. Health Perspect.*, 343–351

Bradley, R. and Caldwell, B. (1976a) Early home environment and changes in mental test performance in children from 6 to 36 months. *Dev. Psychol.*, **12**, 93–97

Bradley, R. and Caldwell, B. (1976b) The relation of infants' home environments to mental test performance at fifty-four months: a follow-up study. *Child Dev.*, **47**, 1172–1174

Caldwell, B., Heider, J. and Kaplan, B. (1966) The inventory of home stimulation. Paper presented at the meeting of the American Psychological Association

Chatterjee, P. and Gettman, J.H. (1972) Lead poisoning: subculture as a facilitating agent? *Am. J. Clin. Nutr.*, **25**, 324–330

Cravioto, J. and DeLicardie, E. (1972) Environmental correlates of severe malnutrition and language development in survivors from Kwashiorkor and Marasmus, In *Nutrition: The nervous system and behavior*, Scientific Publication No. 251 (Washington, DC: Pan American Health Organization)

Delves, H. (1970) A micro sampling method for the rapid determination of lead by atomic absorption spectrometry. *Analyst*, **95**, 431–438

Dietrich, K.N., Krafft, K.M., Pearson, D.T., Harris, L.C., Bornschein, R.L., Hammond, P.B. and

Succop, P.A. (1985) The contribution of social and developmental factors to lead exposure during the first year of life. *Pediatrics*, **75**, 1114–1119

Dobbing, J. (1970). Undernutrition and thea developing brain. In W. A. Hamwick (ed.), *Developmental Neurology*. (Springfield, Ill.: Charles C. Thomas)

Dolcourt, J. (1977) Lead poisoning in children of battery plant employees in North Carolina. *Morbid. Mortal. Weekly Rep.*, 30 September

Dolcourt, J., Hamrick, H., O'Tuama, L., Wooten, J. and Baker, E.L. (1978) Increased lead burden in children of battery workers. *Pediatrics*, **62**, 563–571

Ediger, R.D. and Coleman, R.L. (1972) Modified Delves cup atomic absorption procedure for determination of lead in blood. *Atomic Absorpting Newsletter*, **11**, 33

Elardo, R., Bradley, R. and Caldwell, B.M. (1975) The relation of infants' home environments to mental test performance from six to thirty-six months: a longitudinal analysis. *Child Dev.*, **46**, 71–76

Hawk, B. and Schroeder, S.R. (1983) Factors interactive with IQ and blood lead levels in children. Paper presented at the XVIth Annual Conference on Mental Retardation and Developmental Disabilities, Gatlinburg, TN, March

Hawk, B.A., Schroeder, S.R., Robinson, G., Otto, D., Mushak, P., Kleinbaum, D. and Dawson, G. (1986) Relation of lead and social factors to IQ of low-SES children: a partial replication. *Am. J. Mental Def.*, **91**, 178–183

Hollingshead, A.B. (1957) Two-factor index of social position. Unpublished manuscript (available from A.B. Hollingshead, 1965 Yale Station, New Haven Connecticut)

Kleinbaum, D., Kupper, L. and Morgenstern, H. (1982) *Epidemiologic Research: Principles and Quantitative Methods* (London: Lifetime Learning Publications)

Lansdown, R.G., Sheperd, J., Clayton, R.E., Delves, H.T., Graham, P.J. and Turner, W.C. (1974) Blood lead levels, behavior, and intelligence: a population study, *Lancet*, **1**, 538–541

Longstreth, L.E., Davis, B., Carter, L., Flint, D., Owen, J., Rickert, M. and Taylor, E. (1981) Separation of home intellectual environment and maternal IQ as determinants of child IQ. *Dev. Psychol.*, **12**, 532–541

Milar, C. and Mushak, P. (1982). Lead-contaminated housedust: hazard, measurement, and decontamination, in Chisholm, J. and O'Hara, D. (eds), *Management of Increased Lead Absorption in Children: Clinical, Social and Environmental Aspects* (Baltimore, Maryland: Urban & Schwarzenburg)

Milar, C.R., Schroeder, S.R., Mushak, P., Dolcourt, J.L. and Grant, L.D. (1980) Contributions of the caregiving environment to increased lead burden in children. *Am. J. Mental Def.*, **84**, 339–344

Millican, F.K., Lourie, R.S. and Layman, E.M. (1956) Emotional factors in the etiology and treatment of lead poisoning. *Am. J. Dis. Child.*, **91**, 144–149

Otto, D.A., Benignus, V.A., Muller, K.E. and Barton, C.N. (1981) Effects of age and body lead burden on CNS function in young children. I. Slow cortical potentials. *EEG Clin. Neurophysiol.*, **52**, 229–239

Perino, J. and Ernhart, C.B. (1974) The relation of subclinical lead level to cognitive and sensorimotor impairment in black preschoolers. *J. Learn. Disabil.*, **7**, 26–30

Ramey, C.T., Farran, D.C. and Campbell, F.A. (1979) Predicting IQ from mother–child interactions. *Child Dev.*, **50**, 804–814

Rennert, O.M., Weiner, P. and Madden, J. (1970) Asymptomatic lead poisoning in 85 Chicago children. *Clin. Pediat.*, **9**, 9–13

Rummo, J.H., Routh, D.K., Rummo, H.J. and Brown, J.F. (1979) Behavioral and neurological effects of symptomatic and asymptomatic lead exposure in children. *Arch. Environ. Health*, **34**, 120–124

Schroeder, S., Hawk, B., Otto, D., Mushak, P. and Hicks, R. (1985) Separating the effects of lead and social factors on IQ. *Environ. Research*, **38**, 144–154

Werner, E., Honzik, M. and Smith, R. (1968) Prediction of intelligence and achievement at ten years from twenty months pediatric and psychological examinations. *Child Dev.*, **39**, 1063–1075

White, B. and Watts, J.C. (1973) *Experience and Environment: Major influences on the development of the young child* (Englewood Cliffs, NJ: Prentice-Hall)

White, K.R. (1982) The relation between socioeconomic status and academic achievement. *Psychol. Bull.*, **91**(3), 461–481

3.3

Blood Lead and Other Influences on Mental Abilities – Results from the Edinburgh Lead Study

G. M. RAAB, M. FULTON, G. O. B. THOMSON, D. P. H. LAXEN*, R. HUNTER and W. HEPBURN

SUMMARY

The influence of blood lead on ability and attainment was studied in a sample of children aged 6–9 years in central Edinburgh. The geometric mean blood lead was 10.4 μg/dl. A stratified subsample of 501 children completed individual tests of ability and attainment (number skills and reading) from the British Ability Scales (BAS). An interview with a parent probed the social and family background. There were statistically significant negative relationships between log blood lead and BAS combined score ($p = 0.003$), number skills ($p = 0.04$) and reading ($p = 0.001$) after control for social and family background. The size of the effect was small compared to that of other factors.

The Edinburgh Lead Study was set up in 1983 at the instigation of the Medical Research Council with support from the Scottish Home and Health Department. Its main aim was to investigate the association between blood lead levels and mental abilities in a population of Edinburgh school children, taking into account a wide range of other influences.

Most of the centre of Edinburgh was built in the nineteenth century. Many homes still retain some of their original lead plumbing, and the water is plumbosolvent. Thus water lead makes a substantial contribution to some children's lead intake (Raab et al., 1987). Unlike other inner-city areas, central Edinburgh is more affluent than the rest of the city with a high proportion of owner-occupiers and of people in professional and managerial occupations (SASPAK, 1983).

---

* Present address: London Scientific Services, County Hall, London SE1 7PB, UK

DESIGN AND PROCEDURES

The basic design was a cross-sectional study of children in their third and fourth years of primary schooling (6–9-year-olds) at local-authority schools in a defined area of central Edinburgh. The schools were approached in random order, with all stages of the study in each school being completed within 2–3 months. The field work lasted from August 1983 to June 1985. A total of 18 schools were studied (excluding two pilot schools) to attain the target of 500 children in the final sample.

The first step in each school was the compilation of a list of eligible children, and requests to the parents for their children's participation. From the total of 1210 eligible children parental consent was obtained for 948 (78%) to take part. Further details of the eligibility criteria and other aspects of the design have been published (Raab *et al.*, 1985; Fulton *et al.*, 1987). A medical team then visited the school to obtain venous blood samples which were assayed for lead. A satisfactory blood sample and a successful lead assay were obtained for 855 children (90% of those whose parents agreed). A main study sample was then selected by blood lead levels, which included all children in the top quartile of the blood-lead distribution in each school, and a one-in-three (approximately) sample of the remainder.

The selected children were tested by a psychologist who visited the school. The test battery consisted of measures of inspection and reaction time, and ability and attainment tests. The latter were all taken from the British Ability Scales (BAS) (Elliott *et al.*, 1983; Elliott, 1983) which have been recently validated and standardized on a United Kingdom population. The attainment tests were of reading and number skills. Five ability tests were used, which together give a combined score (BASC score), standardized on the same scale as the WISC-R IQ score (Wechsler, 1974). Subsequently, an extensive home interview with one parent (usually the mother) collected data on the child's home and family background. This included tests of the parent's vocabulary and spatial ability (Raven *et al.*, 1978). Behaviour ratings (Rutter, 1976) for each child were completed by parents and teachers. Only the BAS results are presented here. In addition, an attempt to obtain some information about early exposure to lead was made by collecting information on residential history, and by asking the children to donate their shed milk teeth. These data will be presented at a later date.

RESULTS

Blood lead levels and BAS scores

The geometric mean blood lead (PbB) for the 855 children was 10.4 μg/dl (mean of natural logs 2.34, SD 0.37) and the distribution appeared normal after log transformation. There were considerable differences in the average PbB values in the 18 schools with geometric means ranging from 8.6 to 13.9 μg/dl. These PbB levels are comparable with other recent UK studies (Quinn, 1985; Smith *et al.*, 1983) and are lower than have been found in inner-city populations in the USA (Needleman *et al.*, 1979; Schroeder *et al.*,

1985). They are somewhat higher than the populations recently studied by Bellinger *et al.* (1984) and Hansen *et al.*, this volume).

The mean results for the BAS tests are given in Table 1. The children performed considerably better than the national population on which the tests were standardized, except on basic-number skills where their performance was comparable to that of the standardization population. Again, there were large differences between schools with the school means for the BASC score ranging from 98 to 122.

Interview data

Many factors in the social and family background are potentially related to a child's performance in ability or attainment tests and these factors may also influence exposure to lead. A large part of the parent's interview was devoted to questions which probed these areas, and this information was combined into a set of 33 scores for potential confounding variables. These variables were chosen because of their potential relationship with children's performance rather than for any direct association with exposure to lead. Our selection was based on the experience of long-term child development studies (Douglas, 1964; Douglas *et al.*, 1971; Davie *et al.*, 1972; Kellmer-Pringle *et al.*, 1966), reports in the psychological literature (Rutter and Madge, 1976; Fogelman *et al.*, 1978) and experience in other lead studies, particularly the Institute of Child Health/Southampton study (Smith *et al.*, 1983). It was made *before* we examined the relationship in our own data between these variables and the children's ability test results or blood lead levels.

Some confounding variables are simple factual items, e.g. age, sex of child, family size and birth order; some are based on well-established classifications, e.g. social class and educational qualifications; and some have been measured

Table 1 Means and standard deviation of BAS tests ($n = 501$)

Ability tests		
T scores *(standardized mean = 50; SD = 10)*	*Mean*	*SD*
Matrices	54	8.8
Similarities	58	8.4
Block design		
level	54	8.7
power	57	8.9
Digit span	56	10.2
Word definitions	56	9.5
BASC score *(standardized mean = 100; SD = 15)*	112	13.4
Attainment tests		
T scores *(standardized mean = 50; SD = 10)*	*Mean*	*SD*
Basic number skills	51	7.6
Word reading	56	9.3

by standardized tests, e.g. parent's ability. We also constructed more complex confounding variables by combining a number of related items in the data collected at interview and scoring them. Examples are: parent's general and mental health scores, family structure score, and child's interest score. The items used in these scores are shown in the Appendix. Scores for each variable were obtained for all children. For one-parent families we imputed values for a second parent.

The univariate associations between the BASC score, blood lead levels and the confounding variables are shown in Table 2. As expected, there is a clear relationship between the BASC score and many of the confounding variables including parents' qualifications, social class and scores in the vocabulary and matrices tests. Several of the derived scores, including the child's interest score, the parent's participation score, and the parent–child communication score, are strongly related to the ability score, as are the child's height and the index of overcrowding (persons/room). Most confounding variables are not strongly associated with PbB levels. The most marked relationships are with height, qualifications and social class and the parent's performance in the vocabulary test. Significance levels are not quoted on this table because a p value does not assess a variable's confounding potential (Dales and Ury, 1978).

Table 2 Univariate associations of BASC score and blood lead with confounding variables

Confounder	Categories	No. of children	BASC score mean	r	Blood lead (µg/dl) geometric mean	r
Parent's vocabulary score score (PVOC)	<30	5	89.4	0.52	10.89	−0.13
	30–39	69	102.4		11.90	
	40–49	144	106.5		12.51	
	50–59	142	114.7		11.01	
	60–69	86	120.0		10.67	
	70+	55	121.1		11.21	
Mother's qualifications (MQUAL)	None	88	101.6	0.52	11.82	−0.15
	Commercial/apprent.	111	108.1		12.37	
	Ordinary school cert.	85	109.2		11.67	
	Higher school cert.	41	116.2		12.65	
	Further education	79	118.3		10.83	
	Degree	97	121.5		10.28	
Father's qualifications (FQUAL)	None	87	102.2	0.49	11.70	−0.12
	Commercial/apprent.	92	107.2		11.99	
	Ordinary school cert.	91	110.9		12.25	
	Higher school cert.	35	109.9		12.18	
	Further education	36	116.8		11.27	
	Degree	160	120.0		10.65	
Parent's matrices score (PMAT)	<20	12	96.3	0.46	11.87	−0.01
	20–29	35	98.6		11.73	
	30–39	100	107.2		11.51	
	40–49	214	113.0		11.22	
	50+	140	118.7		11.86	

continued

Table 2 *continued*

Confounder	Categories	No. of children	BASC score mean	r	Blood lead (µg/dl) geometric mean	r
Child's interest	0–<1	16	95.7	0.40	11.60	−0.06
score (CHILDINT	1–<2	53	102.3		12.74	
	2–<3	119	111.4		11.52	
	3–<4	138	112.3		11.34	
	4–<5	116	114.0		11.25	
	5–<6	51	121.0		11.26	
	6–<7	8	126.9		11.23	
Mother's	I, II	198	118.4	−0.39	10.80	0.08
social class	III non-manual	227	109.0		12.14	
(MSOC)	III manual	36	106.7		11.27	
	IV, V	40	101.9		11.79	
Father's	I, II	217	117.9	−0.37	10.78	0.15
social class	III non-manual	56	109.0		11.69	
(FSOC)	III manual	181	107.5		12.14	
	IV, V	47	105.7		12.42	
Parental	1–<2	14	98.6	0.33	11.90	−0.06
participation	2–<3	22	102.9		12.32	
with child	3–<4	33	107.6		12.41	
(PARPART)	4–<5	77	109.2		11.71	
	5–<6	162	111.9		11.06	
	6–<7	193	116.0		11.52	
Occupancy ratio	<0.5 persons/room	5	122.4	−0.32	13.99	0.05
(OCCUPAT)	0.5–0.65	56	117.2		11.51	
	0.66–0.99	134	115.8		11.52	
	1	143	112.3		11.03	
	>1–1.5	111	108.1		11.57	
	>1.5	52	103.1		12.40	
Standardized	<−2.00	6	94.8	0.26	17.50	−0.20
height	−2.00 to −1.01	35	105.3		12.18	
(STHEIGHT)	−1.00 to −0.01	160	110.4		12.15	
	0.00 to 0.99	206	113.0		11.24	
	1.00 to 1.99	77	115.2		10.77	
	>2.00	17	119.6		9.40	
Parent/child	Bad 1–4	59	103.9	0.24	11.88	−0.05
communication	5	77	108.1		11.71	
(PARCHCOM)	6	133	113.8		11.69	
	7	163	114.5		11.26	
	Good 8	69	113.8		11.17	
Cigarettes	None	246	114.6	−0.22	11.48	0.08
smoked per day	1–10	58	113.9		10.57	
(both parents)	11–20	88	107.2		11.37	
(TOTCIGS)	21–40	87	110.0		11.89	
	41–80	22	105.0		13.42	
Age (AGEINT)	<7:0	16	121.0	−0.18	12.43	−0.09
	7:0–7:5	99	114.4		12.03	
	7:6–7:11	120	112.4		11.82	
	8:0–8:5	130	110.7		11.18	
	8:6–8:11	105	112.1		11.18	
	>9:0	31	103.0		10.66	

continued

187

Table 2 *continued*

Confounder	Categories	No. of children	BASC score mean	r	Blood lead (μg/dl) geometric mean	r
Parental involvement with school (PARSCHL)	Bad 0	5	101.6	0.16	16.42	0.02
	1	39	107.1		11.43	
	2	96	108.6		10.72	
	3	157	113.1		11.99	
	4	130	114.7		11.25	
	5	56	112.0		11.44	
	Good 6	18	114.2		12.75	
Car/telephone ownership (CARPHONE)	Neither	28	101.6	0.15	11.82	−0.05
	Either	148	111.9		11.83	
	Both	325	112.9		11.33	
Absence from school in last year (OFFSCHL)	0 days	39	113.8	−0.15	11.62	−0.05
	1–10	306	113.0		11.59	
	11–20	119	111.1		11.28	
	21–30	25	103.5		11.43	
	>30	12	107.7		11.06	
Birth weight (BIRTHWT)	>2500 g	473	112.4	−0.14	11.47	0.03
	<2500 g	28	104.4		12.02	
Handedness (HANDED)	right	441	112.7	−0.14	11.48	0.02
	left	60	107.1		11.70	
Gestation (GESTAT)	38+ weeks	455	112.5	−0.12	11.42	0.05
	34–37	43	107.7		12.41	
	<34	3	101.7		11.55	
Class year (CLASSYR)	P3	249	113.3	−0.10	11.69	−0.04
	P4	252	110.7		11.33	
Family size (FAMSIZE)	1 child	74	108.9	0.08	11.08	0.02
	2	289	112.5		11.62	
	3+	138	112.6		11.49	
Birth problem score (BIRTHSCO)	Good 0	307	112.5	−0.07	11.27	0.05
	1	138	111.7		11.92	
	2	41	110.4		11.77	
	Bad 3	15	107.7		11.72	
Medical history score	Good 0	399	112.4	−0.07	11.67	−0.08
	Bad 1	102	110.3		10.86	
Parent's health score (PARHLTH)	Good 0	376	112.6	−0.06	11.31	0.02
	1	76	109.9		12.70	
	2	37	109.9		11.64	
	Bad 3+	12	112.9		10.17	
Birth order (BIRTHORD)	1st	241	112.6	−0.04	11.69	−0.06
	2nd	182	111.7		11.54	
	3rd+	78	111.0		10.85	
Working mother (or single father) (WORKMUM)	No paid employment	185	112.1	0.03	11.52	−0.02
	Part-time	249	111.4		11.58	
	Full-time	67	114.1		11.16	

continued

Table 2 *continued*

Confounder	Categories	No. of children	BASC score mean	r	Blood lead (μg/dl) geometric mean	r
Family	0	411	112.0	−0.03	15.5	−0.04
structure score	0.5–2.5	40	113.1		15.56	
(FAMSTRUCT)	3.0–5.0	50	110.7		11.09	
Employment of	Seeking work	23	110.5	0.02	12.74	−0.06
father or	Employed or other	478	112.1		11.44	
single mother						
(UNEMPLOY)						
Parent's mental	0 (good)	384	11.9	0.02	11.57	−0.01
health score	1	68	112.8		10.98	
(PARMENT)	2	26	110.8		12.15	
	3 + (bad)	23	112.3		11.12	
Recent change	Not within last year	476	112.1	−0.02	11.58	−0.08
of school	Within last year	25	110.6		10.15	
(MOVESCHL)						
Time of day	a.m.	294	112.1	−0.1	11.71	−0.06
of tests	p.m.	207	111.8		11.22	
(TIMEDAY)						
Consumer goods	None	8	111.0	0.01	11.56	0.03
(CONSUMER)	1 item	67	112.9		10.71	
	2	209	111.8		11.79	
	3	171	111.4		11.41	
	All 4 items	46	114.3		11.73	
Sex	Male	261	112.1	−0.00	11.85	−0.08
(SEX)	Female	240	111.9		11.14	

The confounding variables are ordered by their correlation with BASC score. The correlation (r) of each covariate with log blood lead and BASC score is also shown.

As expected, many of the confounding variables were strongly related to each other. Figure 1 shows McQuitty's elementary linkage analysis (McQuitty, 1957) for the confounding variables. This procedure links each variable with the variable to which it is most highly correlated (shown by an arrow), thus forming clusters of related variables. The confounding variables form five groups; four small groups contain items on the age of the child, variables relating to birth, family size and parent–child communication. The fifth and largest group includes those variables which relate to the social and educational background of the family. There appear to be two sub-branches within this group, one of which relates to the social situation of the family, centred on the social class measures and the other relating to the quality of the child's home life centring on the child's interest score.

Regression analysis of test scores on confounding variables and lead

The relationships between the test scores (as dependent variables), log PbB and the confounding variables were investigated by multiple-regression analysis using BMDP programs (Dixon, 1985). The school which the child

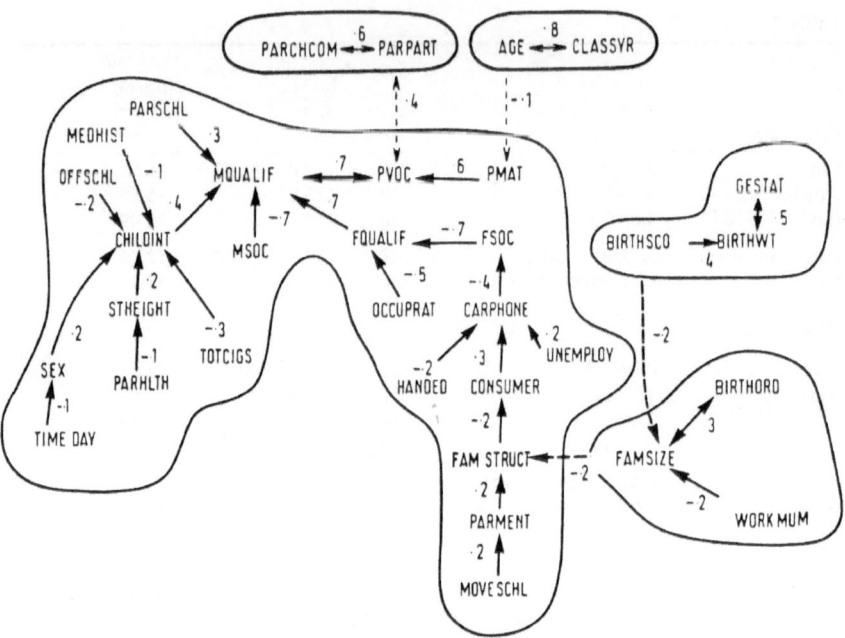

Figure 1 McQuitty's elementary linkage analysis of the covariates. Mnemonics are as in Table 2. A solid arrow points from each variable to the other variable with which it is most highly correlated. The dotted arrows show the highest correlation from one cluster of variables to a variable in another cluster

attended was included as a factor in the analysis, thus restricting the analysis to within-school differences. The significance of the PbB coefficients are assessed by one-sided tests, because a beneficial effect of lead on test scores would not be credible.

The coefficients of PbB for the various test scores are shown in Table 3. There are significant negative relationships between log PbB and the three test scores after adjusting for all the confounding variables. The effect is strongest for the reading score and the BASC score, but for the number score the p value is only 0.04 on a one-sided test. For all three scores the relationships between lead and test scores are stronger before adjusting for the confounding variables. The lead coefficients for the optimal regressions (Mallows, 1973) are very similar to those for the full model. These optimal regressions are intended to give accurate predictions over the range of the data by excluding confounding variables which add little to the predictive value of those already in the model. They are used below in the calculation of adjusted means.

Although the coefficients of PbB are significant (highly so for reading and BASC score), the size of effect is small compared with the influence of other factors on the scores. For BASC score only 0.9% of a total of 44.7% variance explained by all the predictors can be attributed to the effect of lead after controlling for other covariates. Detailed results are shown in Table 4.

To look at the dose–response relationship of PbB on the ability scores,

190

Table 3 Blood lead coefficients for ability and attainment tests

	BASCS		NUMBERS		READING	
Regression model	Log* blood lead coeff. (SE)	p Value†	Log* blood lead coeff. (SE)	p Value†	Log* blood lead coeff. (SE)	p Value†
All covariates	−3.79 (1.37)	0.003	−1.47 (0.83)	0.039	−3.16 (1.05)	0.001
Optimal regression	−3.70 (1.31)	0.003	−1.45 (0.78)	0.032	−2.92 (1.00)	0.002
Lead only	−5.45 (1.54)	<0.001	−2.00 (0.82)	0.012	−5.00 (1.06)	<0.001

* All logs are natural logs
† One-tailed test

Table 4 Variance explained for various regression models

	Dependent variable		
	BASC score	Numbers	Reading
Model	R^2 (%)*	R^2(%)*	R^2(%)*
Schools + covariates + lead (full model)	44.7	36.6	32.0
Schools + covariates	43.8	36.3	30.8
Difference due to lead	0.9	0.3	1.2
Lead alone	2.2	0.8	4.1

* The corrected R^2 is calculated from the raw value R^2_{RAW} by $R^2 = 1 - (1 - R^2_{RAW})\,(n - p - 1)/(n - 1)$ where n is the number of observations and p the degrees of freedom for covariates. This gives an unbiased estimate of the population R^2. The raw R^2 values would be slightly higher

the children were ordered by their PbB values and put into 10 groups of approximately 50 children each. For each group the average difference from the school mean score was calculated, after adjusting the scores for the influence of the covariates. The group mean adjusted BASC scores are plotted against the group mean PbB values in Figure 2, which also shows the fitted regression line. The outlines of the plot show the range of the individual data points which vary from $+29$ to -24. Between the 1st and 10th groups there is a difference in the adjusted combined score of -5.8 points and between the 1st and 3rd quartiles of PbB, a difference of -1.8 points. The data show a dose–response relationship with no evidence of a threshold. Similar plots were made for the two attainment tests. In the number-skills test the difference between the 1st and 10th groups was -2.3 points and in the word reading test it was -5.1 points.

The covariates which were included in the optimal regression models are

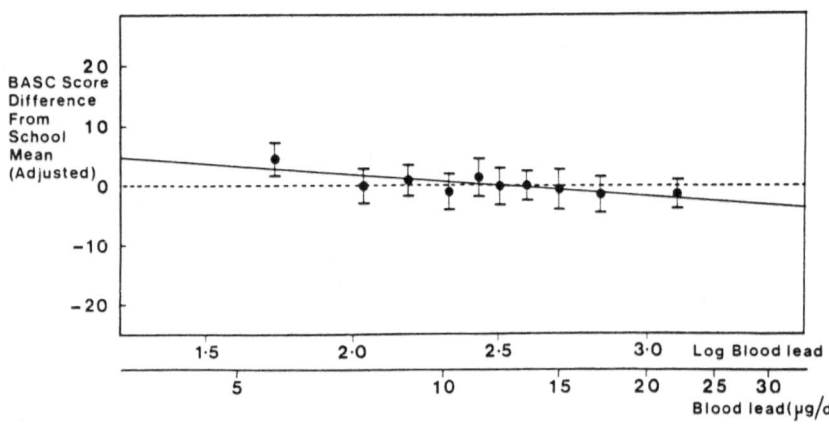

Figure 2 BASC score (means and 95% confidence limits) for groups ordered by log blood lead. The BASC scores have been adjusted for the covariates in the optimal regression

shown in order of importance in Table 5. For the BASC score the most important covariates are the parents' vocabulary and matrices scores (PVOC and PMAT) and the child interest score (CHILDINT). The effect of the covariates on the scores can be examined in the same way as we looked at the lead effect. For the ability score the children were grouped by the value of a combined score which measured the joint effect of PVOC, PMAT and CHILDINT on ability. The test scores were then adjusted for lead, and the other covariates. The plot for the BASC score is shown in Figure 3. The effect of the selected covariates is opposite in direction and much larger than that of lead. The difference between the 1st and 10th groups is $+23.5$ points and between the 1st and 3rd quartiles it is $+8.3$ points. Similar relationships were found for the number skills test where the difference between the 1st and 10th groups was $+9.9$ points and for the word reading test it was $+12.2$ points.

The PbB coefficients for the individual tests making up the BASC score are shown in Table 6 after adjustment for confounding variables. The full model has been used in this analysis. All coefficients are negative and go in the expected direction. The number and reading scores have been included for comparison. The tests most strongly related to lead levels are reading, followed by matrices and digit span.

Interactions

We have investigated the interactions with lead for the covariates in each of the regression models to test whether the effect of lead appears to be similar at different values of the covariates – for example, for boys and girls, and for all social groups. Because we are examining a total of 33 possible

Table 5 Covariates in optimal regression model (Mallow's C_p) Lead and schools forced into model

BASC score	Numbers score	Reading score
Parent's vocabulary score	Age	Parent's vocabulary score
Parent's matrices score	Class year	Birth order
Child's interest score	Child's interest score	Child's interest score
Age	Parent's matrices score	Age
Father's qualifications	Parental involvement with school score	Class year
Length of gestation	Parent's vocabulary score	Parental involvement with school score
Parental involvement with school score	Standardized height	Number of cigarettes smoked by parents
Class year	Parents' mental health score	Father's social class
Days absent from school	Birth order	Standardized height
Sex	Family structure score	Car/telephone ownership
Standardized height		
Car/telephone ownership		
Father unemployed		
$R^2 = 45.5\%^*$	$R^2 = 38.2\%^*$	$R^2 = 33.6\%^*$

Variables are listed in the order in which they are entered and remained in the model during the search procedure.
* Corrected R^2 – see Table 4.

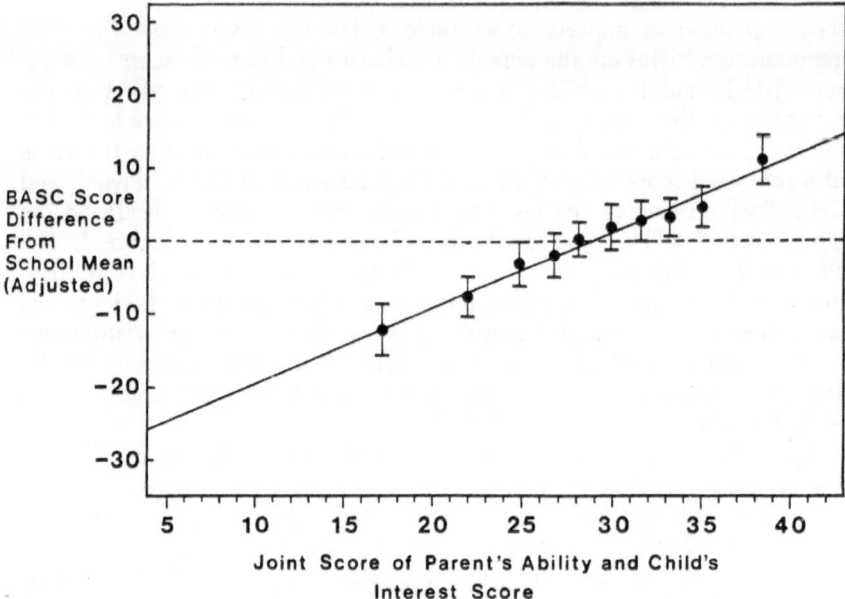

Figure 3 BASC score (means and 95% confidence limits) for groups ordered by the joint effect of parent's ability and child's interest score. The BASC scores have been adjusted for lead and the other covariates in the optimal regression model

Table 6 Log blood lead coefficients for individual tests making up BASC score and for attainment tests for the 501 study children

Test	Log blood lead coeff. (SE)	p Value, one-tailed test
BASC score		
Matrices	−2.4 (1.10)	0.02
Similarities	−1.4 (0.89)	0.05
Block design		
level	−0.9 (1.05)	0.19
power	−1.5 (1.13)	0.10
Digit span	−3.0 (1.28)	0.01
Word definitions	−1.0 (1.07)	0.17
Attainment tests		
Numbers	−1.5 (0.83)	0.04
Reading	−3.2 (1.05)	0.001

These coefficients are derived from the full model.

interactions for the three tests the results must be interpreted with caution. There was no evidence of any interaction with lead for any of the covariates with the BASC score. The reading score shows some evidence of interaction between lead and the child's interest score (test for interaction p value = 0.04) and between lead and the age or stage of the child (p value = 0.06). The interactions are such that the effect of lead appears to be greatest when the children are younger and when there has been a low score for child's interest.

The slope of the PbB/reading score relationships is still negative over the range of the data, although it becomes fairly shallow for the oldest children and for those with the best score on child's interests.

The only variable to appear to show an interaction with lead for the numbers score is parent's mental health (interaction test p value = 0.04), with the effect of lead appearing to be greatest when the parent has evidence of mental health problems.

Other studies have suggested that the effect of lead may be greater in certain subgroups of children such as the socially disadvantaged (Yule *et al.*, 1981; Harvey *et al.*, 1984; Schroeder *et al.*, 1985; Bellinger *et al.*, 1984). We have not confirmed this, but it may gain some support from our results, in that the relationship between lead and the attainment scores appears to be strongest in the youngest group and where the child's interest score is low. We have not replicated Pocock *et al.*'s (1987) result for the reanalysis of the London study data (Smith *et al.*, 1983) where an effect of lead was found for boys but not for girls.

DISCUSSION

Influence of lead on test scores

We have demonstrated a significant negative relationship between lead and ability tests in children with a mean PbB level of 10.1 μg/dl. As Grant and Davis (this volume) point out, the evidence for IQ decrement at PbB levels below 30 μg/dl is mixed, with recent British and German studies giving negative results. Our study was larger than any of these studies and was comprehensive in its control of confounding variables. It has many features in common with the tooth lead study of Smith *et al.* (1983), where the relationships between lead and IQ failed to attain statistical significance at the 5% level after control for confounding variables. Comparing Smith *et al.*'s results with ours, we appear to have found a stronger influence of lead on ability, but the difference could be the result of chance variations between the two samples. This is illustrated in Figure 4a, where we show the estimated difference due to lead between the lowest and highest 10% of the lead distribution in this study compared with a similar difference in Smith *et al.* (1983). The results differ in that one refers to the PbB distribution and the other to that of tooth lead, and the ability tests differ. However, this approach allows at least a crude comparison of the relative size of the effects. We can see that there is considerable overlap between the 95% confidence intervals, indicating that the results from the two studies are not incompatible.

We have found the apparent effect of lead on attainment tests to be greater for reading and lower for the numbers test. This is in line with other studies where reading tests have more often shown an association with lead than have number tests (Smith, this volume). The same reading test was used by Smith *et al.* (1983) as was used in this study. Smith *et al.* report results as raw scores, whereas our results are presented in terms of the standardized t scores, because this improved the normality of their distribution and made the measurement scale equivalent to those of the other tests. For comparison

195

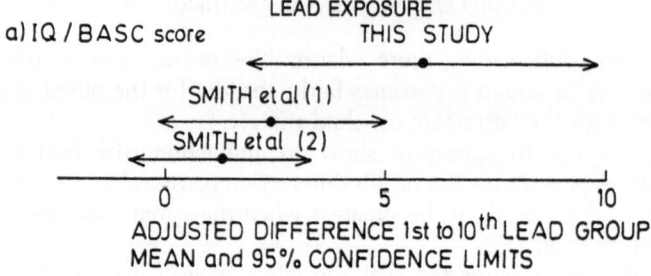

a) IQ / BASC score

LEAD EXPOSURE

THIS STUDY

SMITH et al (1)

SMITH et al (2)

0   5   10

ADJUSTED DIFFERENCE 1st to 10th LEAD GROUP
MEAN and 95% CONFIDENCE LIMITS

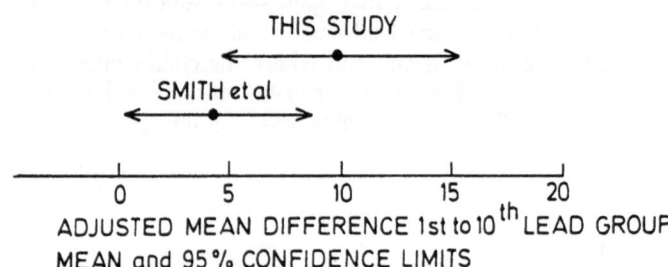

b) WORD READING

THIS STUDY

SMITH et al

0   5   10   15   20

ADJUSTED MEAN DIFFERENCE 1st to 10th LEAD GROUP
MEAN and 95% CONFIDENCE LIMITS

Figure 4 Covariate adjusted differences in (a) IQ/BASC score and (b) word reading raw score, for this study and Smith *et al.* (1983). The results from Smith *et al.* are taken from their Table XXIX for IQ (1) and reading, and thus may be slightly inaccurate. The reanalysis of the IQ data by Pocock *et al.* (2) is also illustrated

with Smith *et al.* we repeated the analysis of the reading test using the raw scores and obtained the results which are shown in Figure 4b. Again we can see considerable overlap between the two confidence intervals. It is interesting to note that the reading test in Smith *et al.*'s study showed the strongest association with tooth lead, coming close to 5% significance on a one-sided test (Smith M, personal communication).

Our study also shares many design features with that of Hatzakis *et al.* (this volume), who studied a population with much higher blood leads. Their study suggests that there may be a threshold for the effect of lead at a level of 15–25 μg/dl, which is in contradiction to our results. At present we can only speculate on the possible reasons for this difference. It may be related to the different routes of exposure, and the relationships between present lead levels and those which affected the children as infants. We hope that our data on tooth lead and residential history may help us to interpret the Edinburgh results further.

There has been considerable discussion about the choice of confounding variables and the problems of under-control and over-control in lead studies. We excluded certain covariates where the possibility of over-control seemed likely. For example, the family cleanliness scale, (Davie *et al.*, 1983) assessed on the home visit has not been used, as it may be controlling out an effect of lead. There are other covariates which *are* included in the regressions which may have resulted in over-control. By using school as a covariate we may be controlling out an exposure to lead which is common to all the pupils at

196

a given school. Similarly, by controlling for birth weight we may be over-controlling if a low birth weight has been caused by lead exposure *in utero*, as has been suggested by Bornschein *et al.* (this volume). These examples of over-control would have caused us to *underestimate* the effect of lead. More serious is the possibility that we may have omitted important covariates. We have measures of ability for only one parent, and perhaps controlling for the other parent's abilities would change the lead coefficient. However, we do have other information about the second parent's education and social class which is controlled for in the analysis. Also, the inclusion of further social variables into the regressions after schools and the first one or two covariates alters the lead coefficients very little.

The apparent influence of lead on children's ability identified in this study is open to interpretations other than the direct influence of lead. Blood lead levels reflect recent exposure to lead, and in this study were measured on one occasion only. Alternative explanations for the observed associations must therefore be considered. As mentioned above, the association could be the result of some confounding variable for which we have not controlled in our analysis. This seems unlikely because of the relatively weak associations in our data between lead levels and the important correlates of the ability tests. A more serious problem for studies of lead exposure is reverse causation. We may be observing an association because children who get low scores on ability tests are more likely to have behaviour which would result in increased lead intake. Examples would be outdoor play in dirty places, lack of hand-washing, and thumbsucking. We cannot rule this out as a contribution to the association we have found. However we might expect that it would be of lesser importance for water, which is an important source in Edinburgh (Raab *et al.*, 1987), than for some other sources of lead.

The influence of factors other than lead on test scores

The interrelationships between the confounding variables (Figure 1) and their association with ability (Table 2) are consistent with other published work, and with our expectations when we derived the scores. For the attainment tests the fact that the parent's vocabulary score is the best predictor of the reading test, and the matrices test is a strong predictor of the numbers test (Table 5) is reassuring. The relationship between age and all of the test scores, which are age-standardized, was unexpected, and the data were examined to seek some explanation of this. For all the tests the younger children performed better than their older classmates on the age-standardized tests. The explanation probably lies in the fact that we tested all the children in a school within a few days of each other, and restricted the sample to two class-year groups. The Scottish school system enforces the dates of starting school fairly rigidly, so that each class contains a group of children with a 1-year range of ages. Thus, within each class the younger children will have more years of schooling than children of the same age in the standardization population, and the opposite will be true for the older children. We found that the negative relationship between test scores and age held within the two year-groups (P3 and P4). Another covariate with an unexpected relationship with the outcome measures was 'parental involvement with school'. The univariate analyses showed small positive correlations with outcome, but after control for other social variables the sign of this coefficient reversed so that a high score on parental interest was predicting poor performance. In deriving this score we were aware of the possibility that a child's poor school performance might result in greater contact between the home and the school. We excluded visits which were initiated by the school, when deriving the score, to avoid this effect. However, these results suggest that we may not have been entirely successful. The consequences for the lead results are not likely to be serious because our inclusion of such a variable would be likely to produce over-control which would diminish the apparent effect of lead.

We have seen that the effect of lead on ability is much less than that of the most important covariates. It is interesting to look for covariates whose influence on ability is of the same order of magnitude as that of lead. One such example is gestation at birth. Children with gestation <38 weeks had BASC scores which averaged 4.5 points lower than those born later, after controlling for other variables. This result was statistically significant ($p = 0.01$) although, as for lead, the proportion of variance explained by gestation was small. It is in good agreement with other published work on prematurity (Illsley and Mitchell, 1984).

Although there is clear evidence of an association between ability and both lead and gestation across the population, neither a high lead level nor a premature birth need preclude a very high level of ability in an individual child.

CONCLUSION

Our results add to the evidence that lead at low levels of exposure has a small harmful effect on the performance of children in ability and attainment tests. The effect of lead is much smaller than that of other influences on the tests, such as the parent's ability and social background variables. An observational study can never prove causality, and so our results must be interpreted with some caution. However, the level of lead in the environment, unlike some of the other influences on the test scores, is amenable to alteration by appropriate policies. We consider that our study suggests that such policies should be strengthened. Further analysis of our environmental data will, we hope, give guidance as to the most appropriate policy measures.

ACKNOWLEDGMENTS

We are grateful to the study team for their enthusiasm and hard work on the project: Mrs L. Kirkwood and Mrs J. Kennedy (organization and secretarial support); Mrs F. Ferguson and Mrs P. Jeffrey (psychologists); Mrs D. Sinfield, Mrs M. Walker and Ms M. Harvey (interviewers); Mrs F. Lindsay (technical assistant for environmental data); Drs J. Knight, A. Elliman, H. Macdonald, B. Innes, J. Leitch, and J. Murray (medical practitioners); Mrs A. Pugh and Mrs P. Ross (nurses); Mr A. Keating and Mrs L. Keating (laboratory technicians); Mrs L. Boyd (statistician/programmer); Ms A. Brackenridge and

Mrs C Maguire (coders). Our thanks are also due to our laboratory colleagues: Dr G.S. Fell and Dr D. Halls, Departments of Pathological Biochemistry, University of Glasgow and Mr S.J. Davis, Strathclyde Water Board. The Education Department of Lothian Regional Council kindly allowed us access to schools. Finally we must thank all the children, their families and teachers, without whose time and willing cooperation the study would not have been possible. We gratefully acknowledge the financial support of the Medical Research Council and the Scottish Home and Health Department.

APPENDIX: SUMMARY OF ITEMS WHICH HAVE BEEN USED IN DERIVING SCORES

Unless otherwise stated, higher scores indicate more problems

Birth problems score   Type of delivery, admission to a special care baby unit, duration of hospital stay.

Medical history score (child)   Hospital admission for head injury, history of fits, presence of chronic or recurrent illness.

Parents' health score   History of chronic illness or accident, general practitioner, outpatient or inpatient care, scored for both parents and combined. Single-parent score is doubled.

Parents' mental health score   History of depression, anxiety or other psychiatric problem, general practitioner, outpatient or inpatient hospital care, prescription of psychotropic drugs, chronic mental illness in last 10 years. Scored for both parents and combined. Single-parent score is doubled.

Family history score   Measures departure from nuclear family using loss of natural parent(s), most recent disruption in carers, age of child when these events occurred, current carers, father working away from home.

Child's interest score   Assesses child's regular activities based on number of books in the home, use of library, attendance at organized activities including recreational/sporting, artistic/musical and instructional/educational activities, frequency of these activities. A higher score indicates a wider range or higher frequency of activity.

Parent–child communication score   Talking with parent(s) about school or study tests and games, supervision of homework, read stories by parents. A higher score indicates a higher degree of communication.

Parental participation with child score   Joint activities with a parent, in sports, outings, indoor games, reading stories, annual holiday, meals together. A higher score indicates a higher degree of parental participation.

Parental involvement with school score   Self-initiated parental visits to school, attendance at interviews and parents' meetings, child's visit to school with parent before starting, discussing child's progress at school. A higher score indicates more parental involvement.

REFERENCES

Bellinger, D.C., Needleman, H.L., Leviton, A., Waternaux, C., Rabinowitz, M.B. and Nichols, M.L. (1984) Early sensory-motor development and prenatal exposure to lead. *Neurobehav. Toxicol. Teratol.*, **6**, 387–402

Dales, L.G. and Ury H.K. (1978) An improper use of significance testing in studying covariables. *Int. J. Epidemiol.*, **7**, 373–375

Davie, C.E., Hutt, S.J., Vincent, E. and Mason, M. (1983) The family cleanliness scale, in: *The Young Child at Home* (London: NFER/Nelson)

Davie, R., Butler, N.R. and Goldstein, H. (1972) *From Birth to Seven: a report of the National Child Development Study* (London: Longman for the National Children's Bureau)

Dixon, W.J. (ed.) (1985) *BMDP Statistical Software* (Berkeley, California: University of California Press)

Douglas, J.W.B. (1964) *The Home and the School* (London: MacGibbon & Kee)

Douglas, J.W.B., Ross, J.M. and Simpson H.R. (1971) *All our Future* (London: Panther)

Elliott, C.D. (1983) *British Ability Scales Manual 2 – Technical Handbook* (Windsor: NFER)

Elliott, C.D., Murray, D.J. and Pearson, L.S. (1983) *The British Ability Scales* (Windsor: NFER/Nelson)

Fogelman, K.R., Goldstein, H., Essen, J. and Ghodsian, M. (1978) Patterns of attainment. *Educ. Stud.*, **4**(2), 121–130

Fulton, M., Raab, G.M., Thomson, G., Laxen, D., Hunter, R. and Hepburn, W. (1987) Influence of blood lead on the ability and attainment of children in Edinburgh. *Lancet*, **1**, 1221–1226

Harvey, P.G., Hamlin, M.W., Kumar, R. and Delves, H.T. (1984) Blood lead, behaviour and intelligence test performance in preschool children. *Sci. Total Environ.*, **40**, 45–60

Illsley, R. and Mitchell, R.G. (eds) (1984) *Low Birth Weight: a medical, psychological and social study* (Chichester: John Wiley)

Kellmer-Pringle, M.L., Butler, N.R. and Davie, R. (1966) *11,000 Seven-year-olds* (London: Longman for the National Children's Bureau)

Mallows, C.L. (1973) Some comments on C_p. *Technometrics*, **15**, 661–675

McQuitty, L.L. (1957) Elementary linkage analysis for isolating orthogonal and oblique types and relevances. *Educ. Soc. Meas.*, **17**, 207–215

Needleman, H.L., Gunnoe, C., Leviton, A., Reed, R., Peresie, H., Maher, C. and Barrett, P. (1979) Deficits in psychologic and classroom performance of children with elevated dentine lead levels. *N. Engl. J. Med.*, **300**, 689–695

Pocock, S.J., Ashby, D. and Smith, M.A. (1987) Lead exposure and children's intellectual performance. *Int. J. Epidemiol.*, **16**, 57–67

Quinn, M.J. (1985) Factors affecting blood level concentrations in the United Kingdom: Results of the EEC blood lead surveys 1979–81. *Int. J. Epidemiol.*, **14**, 420–431

Raab, G.M., Fulton, M., Laxen, D.P.H. and Thomson, G.O.B. (1985) The Edinburgh lead Study: aspects of design and progress. *Statistician*, **34**, 45–57

Raab, G.M., Laxen, D.P.H. and Fulton, M. (1987) Lead from dust and water as exposure sources for children, in Thornton, I. and Culbard, E, (ed.), *Lead in the Home Environment*, pp. 127–139. (London: Science Reviews Ltd; in press)

Raven, J.C., Court, J.H. and Raven, J. (1978) *Manual for Raven's Progressive Matrices and Vocabulary Scales* (London: H.K. Lewis)

Rutter, M. (1967) A children's behaviour questionnaire for completion by teachers: preliminary findings. *J. Child Psychol. Psychiatry*, **8**, 1–11

Rutter, M. and Madge, M. (1976) *Cycles of Disadvantage* (London: Heinemann)

SASPAK User Manual, Release 3 (1983). (London: Local Authority Management Services & Computer Committee)

Schroeder, S.R., Hawk, B., Otto, D.A., Mushak, P. and Hicks, R.E. (1985) Separating the effects of lead and social factors on IQ. *Environ. Res.*, **38**, 144–154

Smith, M., Delves, T., Lansdown, R., Clayton, B. and Graham, P. (1983) The effects of lead exposure on urban children: the Institute of Child Health/Southampton study. *Dev. Med. Child Neurol.*, **25** (suppl. 47)

Wechsler, D. (1974) *Wechsler Intelligence Scale for Children*, rev. edn (New York: Psychological Corporation) (English edition, Windsor: NFER/Nelson)

Yule, W., Lansdown, R., Millar, I.B. and Urbanowicz, M-A. (1981) The relationship between blood lead concentrations, intelligence and attainment in a school population: a pilot study. *Dev. Med. Child Neurol.*, **23**, 567–576

3.4
The Birmingham Blood Lead Studies

P. G. HARVEY, M. W. HAMLIN, R. KUMAR, J. MORGAN,
A. SPURGEON and T. DELVES

SUMMARY

Two separate studies are described in which young children (one sample aged 2.5 years and one aged 5.5 years) were assessed on a wide variety of cognitive, neuropsychological and behavioural parameters. Blood lead concentration, derived from a single sample of venous blood, was the indicator of lead body-burden. Extensive measures of family characteristics were also taken.

The results show that both samples had generally low blood lead concentrations with means of $15.6\,\mu g\,dl^{-1}$ and $12.8\,\mu g\,dl^{-1}$ for the younger and older sample respectively. In general, there were few significant relationships between blood lead and the outcome measures on initial analysis and those that did arise were small. Multivariate analysis showed that even fewer remained significant after accounting for confounding variables.

Caution is expressed at interpreting and generalizing these results to other populations.

This paper summarises the two neurobehavioural studies carried out during the years 1979 to 1985 in Birmingham. This is England's second largest city with a population of just over 1 million inhabitants. It does not have any specific actual or potential lead hazard and its environmental lead levels are comparable with those in the UK generally. This paper will review briefly the major features of the studies prior to addressing some methodological and interpretive issues.

GENERAL BACKGROUND

In both studies, young children were investigated – in general, taking 'young' to mean aged at the first year primary level or below (that is, under 6 years old). This was decided upon because of the relative lack of data about such children compared with that available for older ones. In the light of the evidence that blood lead concentrations tend to be higher at these ages (e.g. Quinn, 1985), such information would be of considerable value. In every case, the guiding principle was to provide data which would be as generalizable as possible to the relevant age group. Thus, samples of subjects from particular social groupings or institutional settings would not be appropriate, and subjects were selected at random from the general population. Because the studies were concerned with young children, however, it was felt appropriate to choose age homogenous samples, thus avoiding the problem of having to account, and control, for age-linked developmental factors in the final analyses.

SAMPLING AND SUBJECTS

There is no unified database for all children in Birmingham. The only single source of relevant information is that contained on the City's birth records. These records contain details of the child, their home address at time of birth and sparse sociodemographic details of the parents. Subjects were selected from these records using the following criteria:

(1) The child had to live in a prespecified ward of the inner city of Birmingham;
(2) The child had to be of a specific age (see below);
(3) The parents both had to be of European origin;
(4) The child had to be legitimate;
(5) The child had to be born in hospital;
(6) The child had to weigh at least 2500 g at birth;
(7) The mother had to be aged between 20 and 29 years of age when the child was born.

These criteria were applied to the birth records data and randomized lists of names were created. Standard personalized letters were sent to the parents after checking with the Electoral Register whether they were still resident. All letters were carefully checked for readability prior to being sent out. Initial letters were followed up by personal calls to explain the project and to recruit subjects. At least one call-back was made if the family was not at home.

In general, the recruitment rates were satisfactory. In Study 1, where the age of the children was 30 months, 788 families were contacted initially. Of this number, 44.4% had moved out of the area since the birth of the child. Of the remaining 438, contact was made with 284. The remaining 154 were not contacted because each child was tested within the calendar month of their birthday and thus, for some months, there were more children available than testing periods. Sixty-five families refused to take part, and, of the 194 children remaining, seven agreed but were not tested owing to illness or moving. Thus, the final sample for Study 1 was made up of 102 boys and 85 girls (187 in total).

In Study 2, the length of time that had elapsed between the birth and the time of testing was much greater; thus, a higher removal rate was expected.

In this study, the children were all aged 66 months. Of the 1218 names on the birth records, 881 (72%) were unavailable because the family had moved, the child had died or had some serious mental or physical handicap. Of the remaining 337 families, 38 were not contacted for the same reasons as outlined for Study 1. Of the remaining 299 families, 23 were not in when the recruiter called back, 8 had children who were ill when testing was to have taken place, and 67 refused to take part. Of these refusers, 34 were interviewed and no significant differences were shown between them and the families who chose to take part. The final sample of 201 was made up of 110 boys and 91 girls.

MEASUREMENT OF LEAD BODY-BURDEN

As the children were under six years of age, the only practical means of assessing body-burden of lead was that of lead concentration in the blood (PbB). After obtaining clearance from the Ethics Committee of the Queen Elizabeth Medical Centre, it was decided to take samples of venous blood. These samples were always taken by an experienced medical practitioner with skilled nursing support.

A single 2.5 ml sample of venous blood was taken no later than 48 hours after testing by a consultant paediatric haematologist at the Birmingham Children's Hospital. Samples were collected in standard tubes (Labco to BS 4581 with EDTA) and sent to the laboratory of the Department of Chemical Pathology and Human Metabolism at the University of Southampton. Blood lead analyses were performed using flame microsampling atomic absorption spectroscopy (Delves, 1970) with minor modifications to the original procedure: sample volumes were reduced to $6 \mu l$, the wavelength was 217.0 nm, Al_2O_3 absorption tubes were used and absorption signals were integrated. Two internal quality control (IQC) blood specimens of known lead concentration were analysed singly before and after each set of five duplicate measurements of survey specimens. The results of the survey specimens were only accepted if they were bounded by results of both IQC specimens that were all within predetermined accepted limits. These limits were 5.8–7.3 $\mu g\, dl^{-1}$ and 14.9–17.6 $\mu g\, dl^{-1}$. Assessments of analytical competence of the laboratory were made from participation in national and international quality assessment programmes (Department of the Environment, 1983). The coefficient of variation of analyses ranged from 7.7% at 5.8 $\mu g\, dl^{-1}$ to 2.4% at 25.1 $\mu g\, dl^{-1}$. External quality control procedures (Department of the Environment, 1983 (Appendix B)) demonstrated a high level of agreement between four UK laboratories (including the one used in these studies) and the CEC reference laboratory: 95% of samples were within $\pm 2.0 \mu g\, dl^{-1}$ and 99.5% were within $\pm 4.0 \mu g\, dl^{-1}$.

BEHAVIOURAL AND COGNITIVE MEASURES

Each of the studies used different measures and these are tabulated in Tables 1 and 2. In the case of Study 1 (Table 1), the age of the children (30 months)

203

mitigated against using long tests, and, at that age, the range of measurable abilities is itself small. Thus, in this project, cognitive performance was assessed using parts of a recently standardized UK-developed IQ test as well as items from an older test.

In Study 2 (Table 2), because the children were older, a wider range of measures could be employed. As well as a standard IQ test (the Wechsler Pre-School and Primary Scale of Intelligence – WPPSI), measures of reaction time and vigilance performance were also taken. This was the first time that this latter measure had been used in studies of this kind. Another unique feature was the use of a comprehensive neuropsychological test battery. A large range of other measures was also taken, including behaviour ratings by both parents and teachers.

A common (and unique) procedure to both studies was the direct observation of the child's behaviour. This was done using videorecordings of the child in standard settings at the project offices (either a playroom or the testing situation). The tapes were analysed using sophisticated standardized behavioural ratings.

Extensive measures of sociodemographic and family characteristics were taken. The interview schedules used in both studies contained enough questions in common to ensure comparability of each study with the other.

The measurement process itself was assessed as part of the routine data collection. While the concepts of quality control are both established and expected in, for example, biochemical analysis, such procedures are rarely (if ever) properly accounted for in the measurement of behavioural or cognitive

Table 1 Study 1 – complete list of measures

Child

Cognitive

Four tests from the British Ability Scales:
- naming ability;
- recall of digits;
- verbal comprehension;
- visual recognition.

Three tests from the Stanford–Binet:
- shapes (time and performance);
- blocks (tower, bridge performance and time);
- beads (performance and time).

Behavioural

Structured behaviour rating of videotape of one 9 minute play period;
Structured behaviour rating of videotape of complete test period;
Tester rating scale;
PIP Developmental Charts completed by parents.

Body burden of lead

Single 2.5 ml venous blood sample.

Parents Structured 68-item interview;
Modified Locke–Wallace Marital Questionnaire;
Holmes and Rahe Life Events Schedule;
General Health Questionnaire (mothers only);
Ravens Progressive Matrices (mothers only);
Mill Hill Vocabulary Scale (mothers only).

Table 2 Study 2 – complete list of measures

Child

Cognitive
Wechsler Preschool and Primary Scale of Intelligence.

Neuropsychological
Wisconsin Motor Battery;
Reitan Indiana Test Battery;
Bender Gestalt Test without and with the Canter Background Interference Procedure.

Attentional
Visual reaction time;
Continuous performance test.

Behaviour – directly observed
Playroom with mother;
Playroom alone;
During WPPSI testing;
During CPT.

Behaviour – teacher rating
Needleman Scale;
Infant Rating Scale.

Behaviour – parent rating
Rutter Scales;
Werry–Weiss–Peters

Behaviour – tester rating
Sattler Rating Scale.

Body burden of lead
Single 2.5 ml venous blood sample.

Parents Structured Interview;
Dyadic Adjustment Scale;
Schedule of Recent Events;
General Health Questionnaire;
Ravens Progressive Matrices (mothers only);
Mill Hill Vocabulary Scale (mothers only).

parameters. In the light of the importance of such procedures, there was an explicit commitment to build in reliability checks throughout all stages of each project.

DATA ANALYSIS

Meticulous care was taken to ensure that the data were sound. Not only were extensive reliability checks made during the measurement process itself, but also the raw data were subjected to accuracy checks at all stages.

Statistical analyses were chosen systematically and multiple regression procedures were used throughout after preliminary univariate analyses. Decisions about the statistical procedures and analytical strategies were decided before the data collection was complete rather than being derived by an *ad hoc* process afterwards. Throughout the analyses, blood lead was treated as a continuously distributed variable and children were not grouped on the basis of their blood lead concentrations. Covariates were selected on the basis of their empirically demonstrated relationship with the outcome measures and on theoretical grounds. Collinearity was dealt with by using a single variable most representative of the set of related variables. Multivariate analyses were carried out on significant univariate associations between blood lead and outcome. The phrase 'statistically significant' was interpreted liberally and all values of $p \leqslant 0.10$ were regarded in this way.

RESULTS

Results from **Study 1** have been presented both in a conference paper (Harvey, Hamlin and Kumar, 1983) and in the scientific press (Harvey et al., 1984). The mean blood lead concentration of the group was $15.6 \, \mu g \, dl^{-1}$. Essentially, there was a small significant correlation between PbB and IQ ($r = -0.17$; $p < 0.05$; $n = 133$). On further analysis, this coefficient was found to be of a different value depending on the father's social class. In the non-manual social group, the correlation was a non-significant $+0.16$, while, in the manual social grouping, it was -0.32 ($p < 0.01$). The multivariate analyses showed that the contribution that PbB made to the explained variance in IQ was less than 1%. There were no significant relationships between the behavioural measures and PbB.

Results from **Study 2** have been presented briefly at a conference (Harvey et al., 1985), in greater detail in a thesis (Harvey, 1986) and in Harvey et al., 1988. In this group, the mean blood lead concentration was $12.8 \, \mu g \, dl^{-1}$. In essence, the results show that, for IQ, no significant associations exist between PbB and any of the three IQ parameters (see Table 3). If the sample is divided as before, the only correlation coefficient greater than 0.09 is that between PbB and verbal IQ ($r = -0.22$; $n = 38$) in the non-manual social grouping – the converse of the previous finding. This figure is marginally significant ($p = 0.09$), and, on multivariate analysis, it is clear that PbB makes no significant contribution to the explained variance in IQ.

A small positive correlation ($r = +0.27$; $p < 0.01$) was found between PbB and one of the six reaction time parameters (the first non-cued block) which remained significant on multivariate analysis, showing that PbB accounted for about 9% of the variance. The relationship between PbB and vigilance performance was small ($r < 0.2$) and non-significant.

There were no associations between parent ratings of behaviour and PbB, and small ($r < 0.2$) associations between three of the seven teachers' ratings and PbB. However, PbB does not appear in the final regression equation in

Table 3 Parametric correlations between blood lead and IQ by father's social grouping

Social grouping	n	Verbal	IQ performance	Full scale
Non-manual	38	−0.22(0.093)	0.09(0.302)	−0.05(0.383)
Manual	111	−0.03(0.382)	0.07(0.218)	0.02(0.417)
Unemployed	24	0.08(0.332)	−0.09(0.332)	0(0.500)
Overall	177*	−0.05(0.219)	0.04(0.280)	−0.01(0.460)

* This figure is greater than the sum of the three above as 4 social class ratings were missing
p values in brackets after the correlation coefficients

these cases. Similarly, there were no significant associations at all between PbB and any of the parameters derived from the behavioural observation procedure. Ratings by the testers showed an inconsistent relationship with PbB, with higher PbB being associated with 'worse' ratings. However, there were differences between testers and interactions with other child characteristics which make these findings difficult to interpret.

In the case of the neuropsychological battery, few significant relationships occurred. For psychomotor skills, there is an increase in speed on maze performance with increasing PbB but no associated increase in errors. A similar finding was noted for the tactual performance test. In both cases, the relationship held after multivariate analysis with PbB accounting for between 3% and 6% of the variance. In the Bender Gestalt test of visuomotor skill, increasing PbB lead to a worsening of performance. This effect did not remain after multivariate analysis.

The clear majority of outcome measures, however, show no relationship at all with PbB.

DISCUSSION

Rather than discuss these results in detail three more general points will be raised concerning generalizability, measures and interpretation.

The issue of generalizability relates to the sampling procedure and sample characteristics. As was noted earlier, the samples in both studies were homogeneous both as to age and ethnicity. In one way, this is a strength as the lack of variability on these dimensions means that the 'noise' of influential variables is reduced. Conversely, this very homogeneity means that the application of these results to children of other ages or ethnic groupings may not be advisable. While there are no strong reasons to suppose that the samples were not typical of their base populations, it is not being suggested that these base populations are necessarily representative of the whole population. A further issue is relevant here. The mean blood lead concentration is comparable with other UK neurobehavioural studies and major national surveys. The distribution is fairly narrow with few subjects having blood lead levels above $25\,\mu\mathrm{g}\,\mathrm{dl}^{-1}$. In fact, in both these studies and a further one in Birmingham (which between them cover a total of nearly 600 children under 6), only 8% of the children had blood lead concentrations above $21\,\mu\mathrm{g}\,\mathrm{dl}^{-1}$ and all but one of these was below $30\,\mu\mathrm{g}\,\mathrm{dl}^{-1}$. These results are not untypical of UK samples, but the question of their typicality internationally is perhaps more doubtful. The concentrations of body burdens of lead reported by most US studies, for example, are generally higher than their UK counterparts. Therefore, when neurobehavioural studies are being compared, we may not be comparing like with like. Similarly, with the age issue, it may not be wise to compare results of studies using different aged children, either because lead may affect children differentially at different ages, or the measures (and the behaviours/skills) may be different. Having said that, however, and raised these cautions, the present data are felt to be reasonably representative of urban white young children in the UK.

The first methodological issue concerns the process of measurement itself. Psychological testing is unique in that it both requires and demands that there is an interaction between the tester and the subject. Thus, the quality of that relationship can influence the test results. There are few studies that explicitly assess tester reliability both within and between testers. In the present studies, inter- and intratester agreements were high, ranging from above 80% between testers to about 95% within testers. The expectation that is held for say, biochemical analyses, is that both internal and external quality control procedures are built in, carried out and reported upon. The fact that such an expectation is not held for psychometric testing is surprising considering the large number of sources of variability to which this procedure is subject.

The second methodological issue relates to the comparability of techniques. While most studies use measures that are broadly comparable (e.g. teacher rating scales), often such comparability is assumed rather being based on empirical data. There are some measures, however, where there is marked lack of comparability which may in turn lead to interpretive problems. The reaction time (RT) data are a good example of this. All the studies reporting the use of this measure have used paradigms that differ – sometimes quite significantly – on almost every parameter. So, while the present results show that there is a significant lead effect on one of the six blocks, this differs from results of other studies showing an effect (although the majority of studies show no relationship between RT and lead). Whether the differences are a reflection of an underlying lead effect or due to technical differences is unresolvable at present. Overall, the inconsistency shown in the results could be due to an inconsistency of procedures.

This leads on to the third issue concerning the problem of interpreting the results. Many studies (these included) have proceeded in a largely atheoretical manner. There are good reasons for following this course but there are also problems. To return to the reaction time finding noted above, the fact that there may be a slowing of reaction time in some children is in and of itself, an interesting finding. However, if we attempt to find *post hoc* explanations, then our interpretations of the result can be misleading. To attempt to explain these data outside of some theoretical or empirically derived predictive framework is more likely to confuse than to clarify. This is further compounded when the performance deficits are given labels (such as 'distractibility') to explain the findings on measures not explicitly designed to measure the phenomenon. While such explanations may be correct, this cannot be assumed until corroborative data are available from other measures included primarily to assess the particular set of behaviours. The point at issue here is not to question the reality of the findings, but rather to allow them to stand as they are, devoid of extraneous labels. Until the phenomena are better measured and described, such caution may allow a more systematic approach to be followed, linking previous data with predictive models. There is a problem in that there is a variety of competing theoretical structures available which in turn leads to difficulties in choosing the appropriate one(s). However, it would appear that there are now enough data from a variety of sources (both within and outside of lead research) which could allow for the creation of coherent testable models, if not full-blown theories.

There is a further point regarding interpretation. Because of the social and political interest in data arising from studies such as these, there is a danger that the interpretive process may become confused. The understanding of a particular set of results and drawing conclusions from them is not the same as drawing policy conclusions. The fact that the present studies give no support for a consistent lead effect does not mean that there is no effect, nor does it mean that it is unnecessary to follow environmentally appropriate action. That there is little evidence of a lead effect at the PbB concentrations found in this study should not lead to generalizations about the effects of lead at higher levels. Furthermore, the fact that the majority of children in these studies had relatively low PbB concentrations does not mean that we can afford to be complacent about ensuring that these levels go no higher.

Finally, in focussing on the effects of lead on the present and future well-being of our children, it may be important not to see the results of these and other studies in isolation and outside of the wider context of influences on the developing child.

ACKNOWLEDGMENTS

These studies were funded by the UK Department of the Environment. Many individuals and groups contributed to the projects in various ways. These include Jenny Targett who was Project Assistant throughout; Frank Hill and his staff at the Department of Haematology at the Birmingham Childrens Hospital; Gill Haines and Richard Illman of the City of Birmingham Statistical Office; the analytical staff of the Department of Chemical Pathology and Human Metabolism, especially Mrs S. Diaper and Mrs J. North; at various times the following people gave advice on particular aspects of design, methodology or statistical analysis: Mick Archer, Donald Broadbent, Gerry Giltrow, Mike Hewitt, John Mackintosh, Sandy MacRae, Mike Quinn, Michael Rutter, Roy Tomlinson, Tony Waldron and Allan White; some additional data were collected by Mary Buckles, Anne Carr and Heather Storr; finally, we owe a considerable debt to the families who gave of their time and patience freely and generously.

REFERENCES

Delves, H.T. (1970). A microsampling method for the rapid determination of lead in blood by atomic absorption spectrophotometry. *Analyst*, **95**, 431–438

Department of the Environment (1983). *European Community Screening Programme for Lead: United Kingdom Results for 1981*. (Pollution Report 18). (London: Department of the Environment)

Harvey, P.G. (1986). The relationship between blood lead level and various measures of intelligence, performance and behaviour in young children. *Unpublished Doctoral Thesis*, University of Birmingham

Harvey, P.G., Hamlin, M.W. and Kumar, R. (1983). The Birmingham blood lead study. Paper presented at the *Annual Conference of the British Psychological Society*, York

Harvey, P.G., Hamlin, M.W., Kumar, R. and Delves, H.T. (1984). Blood lead, behaviour and intelligence test performance in preschool children. *Sci. Total Environ.*, **40**, 45–60

Harvey, P.G., Hamlin, M.W., Kumar, R., Morgan, J., Spurgeon, A. and Delves, H.T. (1985). Blood lead, behaviour and intelligence test performance in young children. In T.D. Lekkas (ed.) *Proceedings of the Fifth International Conference on Heavy Metals in the Environment*, Athens. (Edinburgh: CEP Consultants)

Harvey, P.G., Hamlin, M.W., Kumar, R., Morgan, J., Spurgeon, A. and Delves, H.T. (1988). Relationships between blood lead, behaviour, psychometric and neuropsychological test performance in young children. *Br. J. Dev. Psychol.*, **6**, 145–156

Quinn, M.J. (1985). Factors affecting blood lead concentrations in the UK: results of the EEC blood lead surveys, 1979–1981. *Int. J. Epidemiol.*, **14**, 420–431

3.5
Psychometric Intelligence Deficits in Lead-exposed Children

A. HATZAKIS, A. KOKKEVI, C. MARAVELIAS,
K. KATSOUYANNI, F. SALAMINIOS, A. KALANDIDI,
A. KOUTSELINIS, C. STEFANIS and D. TRICHOPOULOS

SUMMARY

The psychometric intelligence and the blood lead (PbB) of 509 children living near a lead smelter in Lavrion, Greece, were evaluated. The mean PbB was 23.7 μg/dl and the range 7.4–63.9 μg/dl. After controlling for 17 variables, including parent IQ, with a multiple linear regression model, it was found that PbB was significantly associated with full-scale IQ of the WISC-R ($b = -0.270, p = 0.000069$). Verbal and performance IQs were almost equally affected. The adjusted full-scale IQ difference between 'high' (> 45 μg/dl) and 'low' PbB children was 9.1 units. The dose–response curve showed evidence of a threshold at the level of about 25 μg/dl PbB.

The lasting neurotoxic sequelae of overt lead intoxication in children, in the presence of acute encephalopathy, are well documented in this volume (Grant and Davies; Smith). These sequelae include intellectual impairment, visual–perceptual problems, short attention span, sensorimotor deficits, poor academic achievement and behaviour disorders. Evidence derived from the early studies prompted more recent research efforts during the 1970s and 1980s exploring the neurotoxic effects of non-overt lead intoxication in children. The clinic-type studies of the mentally retarded or behaviourally deviant children with elevated blood (PbB) levels cannot be interpreted causally because the lead exposure may be the effect, and not the cause, of the mental retardation. The clinic-type studies overall, despite their short-comings and inconsistencies, were sufficient to document that increased lead body burden, denoted as PbB > 40–50 μg/dl, is associated with cognitive and behavioural impairments (De la Burde and Choate, 1972, 1975; Rummo et al., 1979; Kotok et al., 1977;

Perino and Ernhart, 1974; Ernhart *et al.*, 1981). The studies of children drawn from the general paediatric population, or living in the proximity of lead smelters, seem to have a more desirable epidemiological design to explore the question of the neurobehavioural effects of low levels of lead exposure, but since the potential effect is expected to be small, the methodological issues of the study design are of paramount importance. Needleman *et al.* (1979) summarized these issues as: adequate markers of the lead exposure, unbiased ascertainment of the subjects, adequate identification and handling of the confounding variables, sensitive markers of the neurobehavioural performance and adequate statistical power. Overall, the evidence from the general population studies – even though they include some of the most rigorous studies in the field (Needleman *et al.*, 1979; Smith *et al.*, 1983) – has been frustratingly mixed (Needleman *et al.*, 1979; Yule *et al.*, 1981; Smith *et al.*, 1983; Harvey *et al.*, 1984; Yule *et al.*, 1984; Hansen *et al.*, 1985; Lansdown *et al.*, 1986). The smelter area studies present some theoretical strengths – e.g. a wide range of lead exposure permitting a more thorough dose–response evaluation – but their generalizability is usually inferior to general population studies. In theory, also, these studies may provide a satisfactory alternative in the argument of reverse causality, since the lead exposure of the children is clearly extrinsic and less dependent on their behaviour (Rutter, 1983). However, the earlier reported smelter area studies did not provide consistent evidence for neurobehavioural deficits in the lead-exposed children (Landrigan *et al.*, 1975; McNeil and Ptasnik, 1975; Ratcliffe, 1977). The more recent studies (Winneke *et al.*, 1982, 1983, 1984) provide better assessments of the exposure and the neurobehavioural outcomes, but they also failed to detect significant effects on the cognitive function and behaviour. An obvious problem of the reported smelter studies is the small sample size resulting in inadequate statistical power.

In the present paper we report on a cross-sectional smelter study of the neurobehavioural effects of lead, addressing many of the methodological issues which have been identified in earlier studies.

METHODS

The Athens University Medical School Lead Study was conducted in Lavrion, a town of 10 000 inhabitants, 60 km southeast of Athens. Earlier studies in Lavrion had shown a heavy background lead pollution due to a lead mining and smelting industrial complex (Nakos, 1979). Lavrion mines were known as silver mines since 600 BC. The contemporary mining and smelting complex has been established since 1864, primarily as a lead–zinc smelting plant. Studies of the soil and plants collected in and around the town had shown an unusually heavy lead pollution with lead levels ranging from 1300 to 18 000 ppm, compared to a range of 20–500 ppm measured in the soil of other industrial areas of Greece (Nakos, 1979). The studies by our group in Lavrion started in 1983 (Figure 1). In April 1983 blood, hair and nails were collected from children attending all the primary schools of the area. At the same time the behaviour, and school attainment, of the children were

212

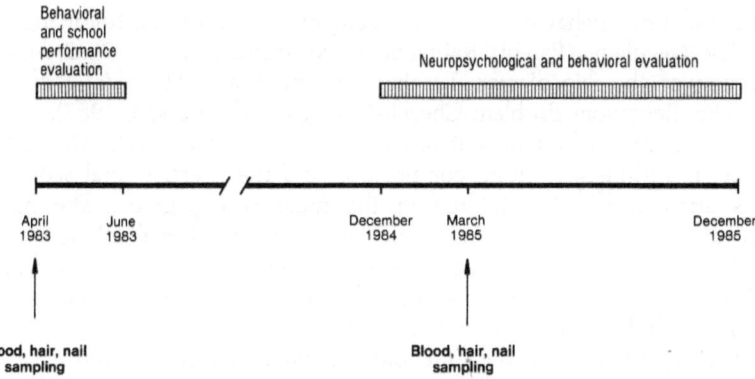

Figure 1 Timetable of the neurobehavioural and lead exposure studies conducted on Lavrion children during the 1983–85 period

evaluated. Blood, hair and nails were collected again in March 1985, and more detailed neuropsychological studies and children's behavioural evaluation were conducted during 1985.

Sample selection and neurobehavioural evaluation

The study population consisted of children attending the four primary schools of the town during the academic year 1984–85. The parents' agreement for blood, hair and nail sampling was requested in letters emphasizing the benefits of the children's participation in a health survey, including estimation of the lead burden and their neurobehavioural status. In order to sustain the participation rate at acceptable levels, the children were tested in an appropriately equipped psychological laboratory which was established in Lavrion. The children were brought by a parent, usually the mother. While the child completed the neuropsychologic evaluation the parent filled out questionnaires on the social and family background and the child's behaviour and medical history. Parents' intelligence was assessed by means of a short form of the 'Wechsler's Adult Intelligence Scale' (Wechsler, 1958), consisting of the Vocabulary and Block Design subtests (Kokkevi et al., 1979).

The neuropsychological evaluation of the children comprised assessment of:

1. Psychometric intelligence, using the Wechsler Intelligence Scale for Children (WISC-R) (Wechsler, 1974).
2. Visual motor integration, using two tests: (a) the Bender Gestalt test scored according to a German scale (Schlange et al., 1972) and (b) the trail-making test of the Reitan Indiana Battery (Reitan, 1966).
3. Attentional performance using four tests: (a) reaction time under intervals of delay (Hunter et al., 1985); (b) reaction–performance test known as the 'Wiener reaction device' (Winneke et al., 1983); (c) symbol cancellation task (Pieron, 1929) and (d) a digit ordering test (Dornbush and Kokkevi, 1977).

213

The children's behaviour was evaluated by means of the following scales: (1) The 'Needleman Parents' Rating Scale' (Needleman et al., 1979); (2) a modified version of the 'Needleman Teachers' Rating Scale' (Hatzakis et al., 1985); (3) The 'Behaviour Problem Checklist' (Quay and Peterson, 1967).

The educational attainment of children was evaluated using the children's score in arithmetic, writing composition and the average total score which was attained by the children in the most recent grade. The modified 'Needleman Teachers' Rating Scale' and the educational attainment were evaluated in the 1983 studies (Hatzakis et al., 1985). Most of the neurobehavioural tests administered, and the quality control procedures, conformed to the WHO/UNDP Protocol (WHO, 1984).

This report refers to the psychometric intelligence evaluation.

Lead measurements

Venous blood samples (approximately 5 ml) were collected in heparinized tubes and analysed in duplicate by atomic absorption spectometry (Stoeppler et al., 1978) in Dusseldorf University, Institute of Environmental Hygiene. The mean lead values from the duplicate samples have been used in the statistical analyses. The lead in hair and nails are not as yet determined.

Statistical methods

Our strategies for evaluating the association between lead exposure, indicated by PbB, and the neurobehavioural outcomes involved the following steps. First, bivariate analyses were carried out in order to identify the degree of association of the non-lead variables with the outcome (full-scale IQ, etc.). Thirty-six non-lead variables were screened by means of one-way analysis of variance or Pearson correlation coefficients. Second, the associations of the non-lead variables with PbB were evaluated by means of one-way analysis of variance and Pearson correlation coefficients. The variables which reached $p \leqslant 0.10$ were considered significantly associated with the full-scale IQ or PbB. Based on these analyses the 36 non-lead variables were classified as those associated with full-scale IQ and PbB (potential confounders), those associated with full-scale IQ only (full-scale IQ correlates), those associated with PbB (PbB correlates) and those not associated with either full-scale IQ or PbB. The last group was not considered in any of the subsequent analyses. Third, multiple linear regression analyses were carried out in order to obtain a valid estimation of the PbB–IQ association. Computations were performed using the Statistical Package for the Social Sciences (Nie et al., 1975).

RESULTS

Of the total population of 1038 eligible children comprising the total number of children attending the four primary schools of the Lavrion area, 644 (62%)

donated venous blood while the remainder have not participated in the blood sampling, either because their parents had not consented, or because the children refused. Among the 644 children who donated blood samples, 533 (51.3%) were neuropsychologically evaluated (Figure 2); 111 children were not tested because they had moved, were not located, were not interested or did not consent. Twenty-four children who were tested were excluded from the analysis because their blood samples were lost in a laboratory accident.

The mean (SD) PbB was 23.7 (9.2) μg/dl, and the range was 7.4–63.9 μg/dl. The median PbB was 21.5 and the 90% and 10% points of the PbB cumulative frequency distribution were 13.9 μg/dl and 36.0 μg/dl respectively (Figure 3). The mean (SD) full-scale, verbal and performance IQ scores were: 87.2 (14.8), 93.3 (14.9) and 83.2 (15.0), respectively. The frequency distribution of the full-scale IQ is shown in Figure 4.

Twenty-four non-lead variables were classified as potential confounders or full-scale correlates, or PbB correlates according to their association with the full-scale IQ and PbB. The potential confounders were: parent IQ, birth order, family size, father's age, father's education, mother's education and alcoholic mother. Full-scale IQ correlates were the variables age, bilingualism, birth weight, length of child's hospital stay after birth, walking age, history of CNS disease, history of head trauma, illness affecting sensory function, parents' divorce. Blood lead correlates were the variables sex, Lavrion resident since birth, history of chronic disease, pica, nail-biting and thumb-sucking.

Various regression models were tested in order to describe the PbB–IQ association (Table 1). In the first model the PbB effect on full-scale IQ without adjustment for confounders was tested. The regression coefficient was $b = -0.376$, and $p = 0.000\,000\,23$. In the next model, allowing for the covariates which were indicated as actual or potential confounders, the b

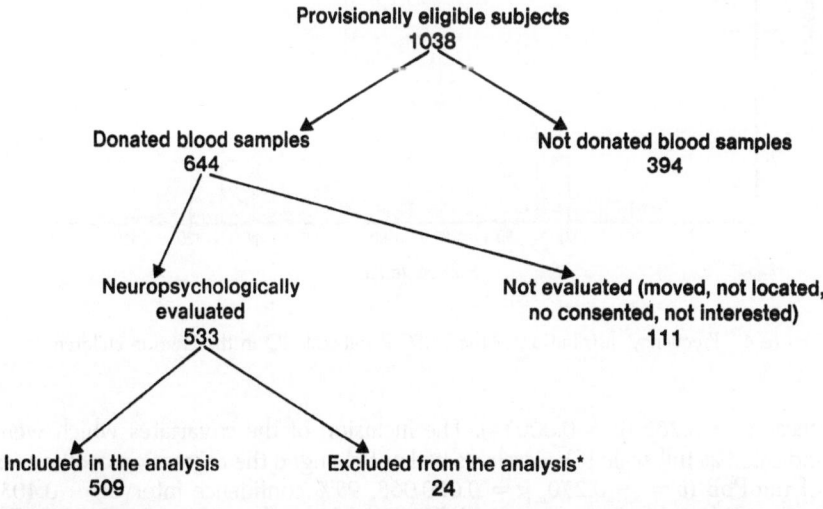

Figure 2 Selection of the sample included in the analysis from the eligible children attending the primary schools of Lavrion (* 24 blood samples were lost in a laboratory accident)

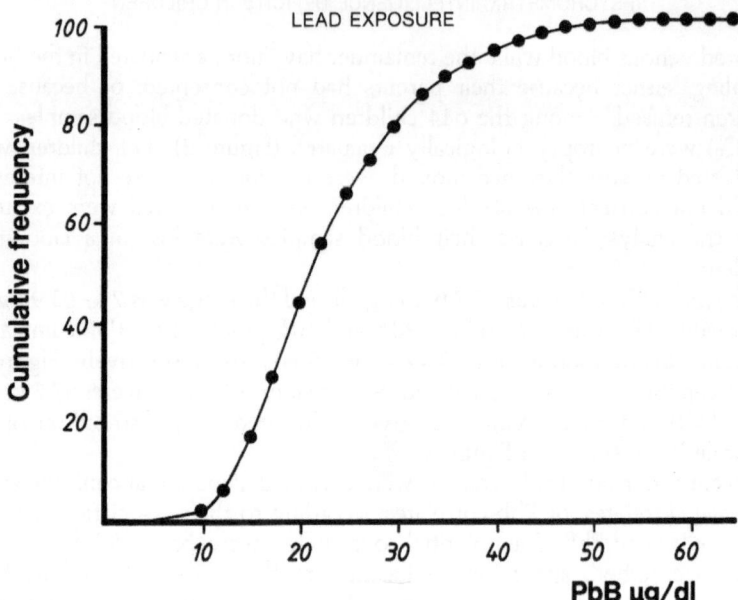

Figure 3 Cumulative frequency (percentage) distribution of PbB values in the Lavrion children

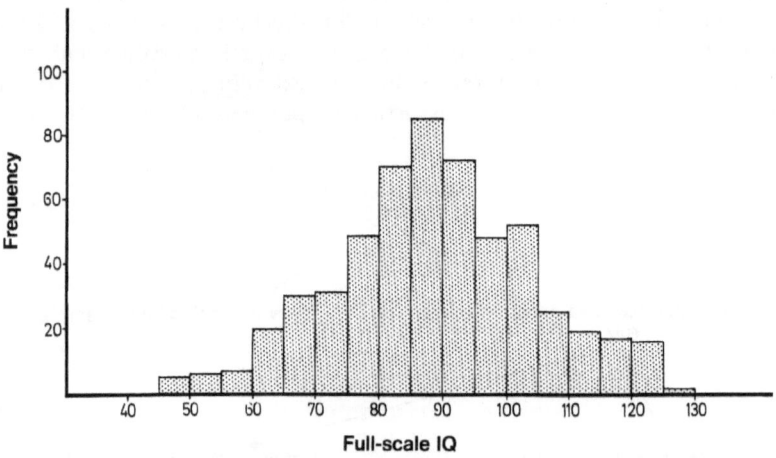

Figure 4 Frequency distribution of the WISC-R full-scale IQ in the Lavrion children

became -0.266 ($p = 0.00014$). The inclusion of the covariates which were indicated as full-scale IQ correlates had not changed the regression coefficients of the PbB ($b = -0.270$, $p = 0.000\,068$; 95% confidence interval -0.403, -0.137) but the improvement of the model fit – indicated by changes in R^2 – was substantial (Table 1). The alternative inclusion in the regression model

216

Table 1 Results of various multiple linear regression models evaluating the full-scale IQ, PbB association in the children of Lavrion

Full-scale IQ on	No. of independent variables	b_{PbB}	95% C.I. of b_{PbB}	p value	R^2
(a) PbB	1	-0.376	-0.519,-0.234	2.3×10^{-7}	0.056
(b) PbB 'Potential confounders'[1]	9	-0.266	-0.403,-0.129	1.4×10^{-4}	0.250
(c) PbB 'Potential confounders' 'Full-scale IQ correlates'[2]	18	-0.270	-0.403,-0.137	6.9×10^{-5}	0.312
(d) PbB 'Potential confounders' 'Full-scale IQ correlates' 'PbB correlates'[3]	24	-0.260	-0.399,-0.120	2.7×10^{-4}	0.321
(e) PbB 'Potential confounders' 'Full-scale IQ correlates' School attended	19	-0.240	-0.382,-0.098	9.3×10^{-4}	0.322

[1] Parent IQ, birth order, family size, father's age, father's education, mother's education, father's occupation, alcoholic mother.
[2] Age, bilingualism, birth weight, length of child's hospital stay after birth, walking age, history of CNS disease, history of head trauma, illness affecting sensory function, parents' divorce.
[3] Sex, Lavrion resident since birth, history of chronic disease, pica, nail-biting, thumb-sucking.

of the PbB correlates or the variable 'school attended by the children' did not considerably change the PbB regression coefficients, the p values or the R^2. Blood lead explained 8.1% of the total variance when it was included in the last step. The model with the 17 non-lead variables which were introduced as potential confounders and full-scale IQ correlates, plus the PbB ('optimal model') was used in the subsequent analyses.

Table 2 lists the remaining variables used in the 'optimal model'. Parent IQ, mother's and father's education, illness affecting sensory function, birth weight, walking age and parent's divorce reached the level of significance.

The 'optimal' model was also used in the analysis of the verbal IQ, performance IQ and WISC-R subtests. The verbal and performance part of the WISC-R were almost equally associated with the PbB levels (Table 3). In the analyses of the association of WISC-R subtests with PbB, most of them reached the level of significance, with the exception of arithmetic and object assembly.

In order to explore the dose–response pattern of the full-scale IQ–PbB association we have used PbB as categorical variable with five levels (< 14.9, 15.0–24.9, 25.0–34.9, 35.0–44.9, and > 45.0 $\mu g/dl$). The full-scale IQ difference between the two extreme PbB levels was 11.1 units (Figure 5). After allowance for the covariates of the 'optimal' model the full-scale IQ difference was 9.1 units. A consistent decrease of the IQ by PbB was noted in levels higher than 25.0 $\mu g/dl$.

DISCUSSION

This is a 'second-generation' cross-sectional study addressing the neurobehavioural effects of lead exposure in children. Since the study was designed after the publication of similar studies which were conducted in the 1970s and early 1980s, attention was paid to the issues of sample size, assessment of the neurobehavioural outcome and control of the confounding variables. The study was large enough to demonstrate a highly significant association ($p = 0.000\,069$) of PbB on the full-scale IQ of the WISC-R. An extensive number of confounding variables – including parent IQ – was controlled. Attention was also paid to the unbiased ascertainment of the subjects. All the children attending the primary schools of the area were eligible to participate, and 62% of them donated blood samples; there was no evidence of lead-related selection for participation. Preliminary analyses showed that the children who did not participate were similar to the ones who participated in 16 out of 18 items of a behavioural questionnaire (Hatzakis et al., 1985). In addition to the study design considerations, the environmental conditions presented a unique opportunity to estimate lead effects in the neurobehavioural outcomes, since the range of PbB values was broad, and the lead exposure relatively stable over time, permitting the reliable use of PbB as a measure of long-term exposure to lead. The PbB levels were similar in successive cohorts of school-aged Lavrion children at least since the late 1980s (Hatzakis et al., 1985; Benetou-Marantidou et al., 1985).

The full-scale IQ–PbB association was fairly robust using various models

Table 2 Direction of association and p values of the regression coefficients of the full-scale IQ on the PbB, 'potential confounders'[1] and 'full-scale IQ correlates'[2]

Variable	Explanation	Direction of the association with full-scale IQ	p value for regression coefficients
PbB	Continuous variable (μg/dl)	↓	0.000069
Parent IQ	Two subtests of WAIS	↑	10^{-13}
Birth order	A dummy variable for a birth order $\geqslant 3$	↓	NS[3]
Family size	A dummy variable for number of children $\geqslant 3$	↓	NS
Age	Continuous variable (months)	↑	NS
Father's age	Continuous variable (years)	↑	NS
Father's education	Continuous variable (years of schooling)	↑	0.032
Mother's education	Continuous variable (years of schooling)	↓	0.021
Skilled workers	Four dummy	↑	NS
Clerical workers	variables defining	↓	NS
Intermediate occupations	father's occupation[4]	↑	0.013
Professionals		↓	NS
Alcoholic mother	Dummy variable (no = 0, yes = 1)	↓	NS
History of CNS disease	Dummy variable (no = 0, yes = 1)	↓	NS
Illness affecting sensory function	Dummy variable (no = 0, yes = 1)	↓	0.043
History of head trauma	Dummy variable (no = 0, yes = 1)	↓	NS
Bilingualism	Dummy variable (no = 0, yes = 1)	↓	NS
Birth weight	Dummy variable (> 2000 g = 0 $\leqslant 2000$ g = 1)	↓	0.008
Length of child's hospital stay after birth	Dummy variable ($\leqslant 10$ days = 0 > 10 days = 1)	↓	NS
Walking age	Continuous variable (months)	↓	0.034
Parents' divorce	Dummy variable (no = 0, yes = 1)	↓	0.011

[1] See footnote 1 of Table 1
[2] See footnote 2 of Table 1
[3] NS denotes a p value $\geqslant 0.10$
[4] Unskilled workers is the reference category

with eight to 23 covariates, resulting in a decrease of 2.4–2.7 units of IQ for every 10 μg/dl increase in PbB. Alternatively, the adjusted full-scale IQ difference between 'high' PbB (> 45 μg/dl) and 'low' PbB ($< 15\mu$g/dl) groups was 9.1 units. This difference is one of the highest ever reported within a lead study (Smith, this volume) and it may be attributed to the unusual range

Table 3 Associations of verbal IQ, performance IQ and WISC-R subtests with PbB using a model including PbB, 'potential confounders'[1] and 'full-scale IQ correlates'[2]

WISC-R	b_{PbB}	95% C.I. of b_{PbB}	p value	R^2
Verbal IQ	−0.252	−0.391, −0.113	0.0004	0.274
Information	−0.061	−0.090, −0.032	0.00004	0.235
Similarities	−0.049	−0.079, −0.019	0.001	0.166
Arithmetic	−0.016	−0.049, +0.016	0.326	0.136
Vocabulary	−0.046	−0.081, −0.012	0.009	0.278
Comprehension	−0.036	−0.065, −0.007	0.015	0.224
Performance IQ	−0.230	−0.374, −0.086	0.002	0.235
Picture completion	−0.034	−0.067, −0.0003	0.048	0.109
Picture arrangement	−0.045	−0.076, −0.014	0.004	0.155
Block design	−0.030	−0.058, −0.002	0.036	0.162
Object assembly	−0.005	−0.038, +0.029	0.787	0.125
Coding	−0.053	−0.086, −0.020	0.002	0.180

[1] See footnote 1 of Table 1
[2] See footnote 2 of Table 1

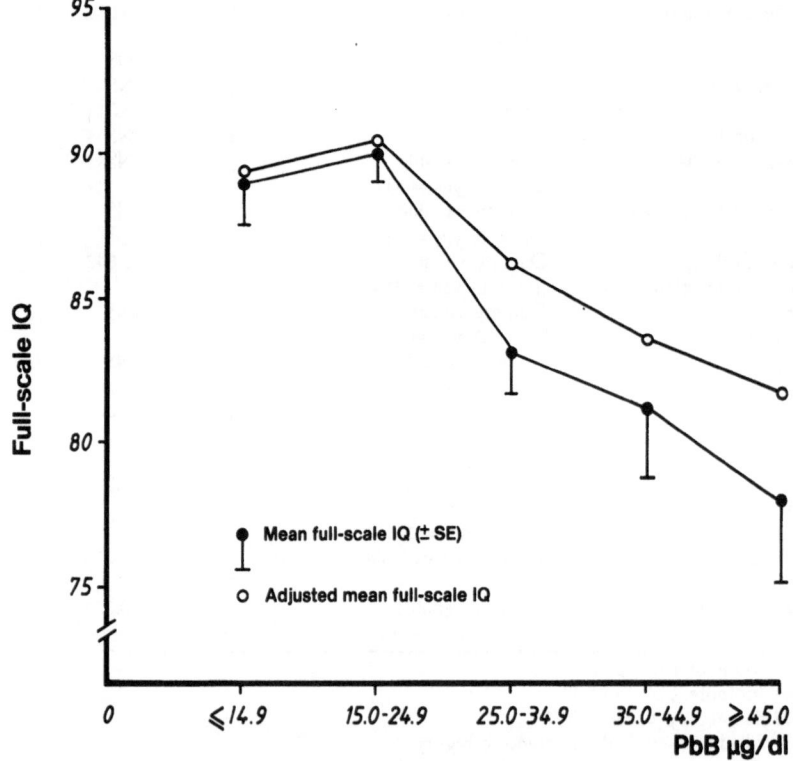

Figure 5 Adjusted and unadjusted mean WISC-R full-scale IQ values by PbB levels in the Lavrion children

of PbB exposure observed in the children living in Lavrion. The plausibility of the 'optimal' model used as indicated in Table 2 was in concordance with our prior beliefs for the association of the remaining covariates used in the model. The verbal and performance parts of the WISC-R were almost equally associated to the PbB. In most of the studies reporting a significant association of PbB with intelligence, the effects on the verbal part were predominant (Needleman et al., 1979; Yule et al., 1981; Hansen et al., chapter 00 in this volume). This finding was considered as inconsistent with the clinical experience where performance IQ is more vulnerable to neurotoxic insults (Smith, 1985). The present study demonstrates that performance abilities are clearly affected, and this may be attributed to the higher levels of lead exposure which are noted in the studied population.

The WISC-R subtest analyses showed that eight out of 10 subtests administered were significantly associated with PbB. The overall pattern suggests that a wide range of abilities are influenced by lead, but it is difficult to draw firm conclusions about specific insults attributed to lead based on the WISC-R subtests profile (Kaufman, 1979). Moreover, it is not possible to speculate on the underlying neurological mechanisms by which lead affects brain function based on the data derived from this or similar studies.

The wide range of lead exposure, and the large number of tested children, gave us the opportunity to examine the dose–response curve by using five levels of PbB values. The lead effects were evident at PbB levels higher than 25 μg/dl. The existence of a threshold of lead effects on IQ was also suggested by Bellinger and Needleman (1983), who found a sharp decrease in IQ for dentine lead levels higher than 30 ppm. Recently, Raab et al. (chapter 00 in this volume) have completed a study of 501 children in Edinburgh with mean PbB 10.4 μg/dl and a range 2.9–34.0 μg/dl. After controlling for confounding variables a highly significant decrease in the abilities score for increased PbB values was observed. However, their data showed a dose–response relationship with no evidence of threshold.

The results of the present study, in the light of evidence published earlier, suggest that lead has a definite detrimental effect on the psychometric intelligence of children. This study indicates that lead effects are evident at PbB levels higher than 25 μg/dl. Children with subthreshold levels may be at low, if any, risk of adverse effects on intelligence. Further research is needed in order to explore this issue thoroughly.

ACKNOWLEDGMENTS

This research was supported by grants from the EEC (contract no ENV-795-GR), the Ministry of Physical Planning, Housing and Environment and the Ministry of Youth and Sports. We are indebted to M. Hatzibirou, A. Kokolodimitraki, M. Korvesi and C. Theologou who performed the psychological tests, and to P. Drogari, I. Argyropoulou and T. Chassapladakis for their administrative and secretarial support. Our thanks are also due to Drs A. Brockhaus, U. Ewers and W. Collet in the Institute of Environmental Hygiene of the Dusseldorf University for the PbB analysis and the quality control of our neuropsychologic battery. Finally we are grateful to D. Poggas, Mayor of Lavrion, for his invaluable help and encouragement, and to the children, their families and teachers for participation and willing cooperation.

REFERENCES

Bellinger, D.C. and Needleman, H.L. (1983) Lead and relationship between maternal and child intelligence. *J. Pediatr.*, **102**, 523–527

Benetou-Marantidou, A., Nakou, S. and Micheloyiannis, I. (1985) The use of a battery of tests for the estimation of neurological effects of lead in children. In Lekkas, T.D. (ed.), *Heavy Metals in the Environment* (Edinburgh: CEP Consultants)

De la Burde, B. and Choate, M.S. (1972) Does early asymptomatic lead exposure in children have latent sequelae? *J. Pediatr.*, **81**, 1088–1091

De la Burde, B. and Choate, M.S. (1975) Early asymptomatic lead exposure and development at school age. *J. Pediatr.*, **87**, 638–642

Dornbush, R. and Kokkevi, A. (1977) Withdrawal from cannabis: psychological test performance. In Stefanis, C., Dornbush, R. and Fink, M. (eds.), *Hashish: Studies of Long-term Use* (New York: Raven Press)

Ernhardt, C.B., Landa, B. and Schell, N.B. (1981) Subclinical levels of lead and developmental deficit – a multivariate follow-up reassessment. *Pediatrics*, **67**, 911–919

Hansen, D.N., Lyngbye, T., Trillingsgaard, A., Beese, I. and Grandjean, P. (1985) A neuropsychological and behavioural assessment of children with low level lead exposure. In Lekkas, T.D. (ed.), *Heavy Metals in the Environment.* (Edinburgh: CEP Consultants)

Harvey, P.G., Hamlin, M.W., Kumar, R. and Delves, H.T. (1984) Blood lead, behaviour and intelligence test performance in preschool children. *Sci Total Env.*, **40**, 45–60

Hatzakis, A., Salaminios, F., Kokkevi, A., Katsouyanni, K., Maravelias, K., Kalandidi, A., Koutselinis, A., Stefanis, K. and Trichopoulos, D. (1985) Blood lead and classroom behaviour of children in two communities with different degree of lead exposure: evidence of a dose-related effect? In Lekkas, T.D. (ed.), *Heavy Metals in the Environment* (Edinburgh: CEP Consultants)

Hunter, J., Urbanowicz, M.A., Yule, W. and Lansdown, R. (1985). Automated testing of reaction time and its association with lead in children. *Int. Arch. Occup. Env. Health*, **57**, 27–34

Kaufman, A.S. (1979) *Intelligent Testing with the WISC-R*, (New York: John Wiley & Sons)

Kokkevi, A., Repapi, M., Adamou, N. and Stefanis, C. (1979) Adjustment and standardization of a WAIS short form in two Greek samples. *Iatriki*, **35**, 512 (in Greek)

Kotok, D., Kotok, R. and Heriot, J.T. (1977) Cognitive evaluation of children with elevated blood lead levels. *Am. J. Dis. Child.*, **131**, 791–793

Landrigan, P.G., Whitworth, R.H., Baloh, R.W., Staehling, M.W., Barthel, W.F. and Rosenblum, B.F. (1975) Neuropsychological dysfunction in children with chronic low-level lead absorption. *Lancet*, **1**, 708–712

Lansdown, R., Yule, W., Urbanowicz, M.A. and Hunter, J. (1986) The relationship between blood-lead concentrations, intelligence, attainment and behaviour in a school population: the second London study. *Int. Arch. Occup. Env. Health*, **57**, 225–235

McNeil, J.L. and Ptasnik, J.A. (1975) Evaluation of long-term effects of elevated blood lead concentration in asymptomatic children. In *Recent Advances in the Assessment of the Health Effects of Environmental Pollution*. Proceedings, Vol. 2, pp. 571–590 (Paris: CEC)

Nakos, G. (1979) Lead pollution: the fate of lead in the soil and its effects on *Pinus halepensis*. *Plant and Soil*, **53**, 427–433

Needleman, H.L., Gunnoe, C., Leviton, A., Reed, R., Peresie, H., Maher, C. and Barret, P. (1979) Deficits in psychologic and classroom performance of children with elevated dentine lead levels. *N. Engl. J. Med.*, **300**, 689–695

Nie, N.H., Hull, C.H., Jenkins, J.E., Steinbrenner, K. and Bent, D.H. (1975) *Statistical Package for the Social Sciences* (New York: McGraw-Hill)

Perino, J. and Ernhart, C.B. (1974) The relation of subclinical lead level to cognitive and sensorimotor impairment in black preschoolers. *J. Learn Disorders*, **7**, 26–30

Pieron, H. (1929). Etalonage d'un test d'attention. *BINOP*, No. 4, Paris

Quay, H.C. and Peterson, D.R. (1967) *Behavior Problem Checklist* (Champaign, Ill.: Children's Research Center, University of Illinois)

Ratcliffe, J.M. (1977) Development and behavioural functions in young children with elevated blood lead levels. *Br. J. Prev. Soc. Med.*, **31**, 258–262

Reitan, R.M. (1966) A research program on the psychological effects of brain lesions in human beings. In Ellis, N.R. (ed.), *International Review of Research in Mental Retardation*, Vol. 1, pp. 153–218 (New York: Academic Press)

Rummo, J.H., Routh, D.K., Rummo, N.J. and Brown, J.F. (1979). Behavioural and neurological effects of symptomatic and asymptomatic lead exposure in children. *Arch. Env. Health*, **34**, 120–124

Rutter, M. (1983). Scientific issues and state of the art in 1980. In Rutter, M. and Russel Jones, R. (eds.). *Lead versus Health*, (Chichester: John Wiley & Sons)

Schlange, H., Stein, B., Boetticher, J. and Taneli, S. (1972) *Goettinger Formreproductions test* (G-F-T) (Hogrefe: Goettingen)

Smith, M., Delves, T., Lansdown, R., Clayton, B. and Graham, P. (1983) The effects of lead exposure on urban children: the Institute of Child Health/Southampton study. *Dev. Med. Child Neurol.* (Suppl. 47)

Smith, M. (1985) Recent work on low-level lead exposure and its impact on behaviour, intelligence and learning: a review. *J. Am. Acad. Child Psychiatry*, **24**, 24–32

Stoeppler, M., Brandt, K. and Rains, T.C. (1978) Contributions to automated trace analysis. II. Rapid method for the automated determination of lead in whole blood by electrothermal atomic absorption spectrophotometry. *Analyst*, **103**, 714–722

Wechsler, D. (1958). *The Measurement and Appraisal of Adult Intelligence* (Baltimore: Williams & Wilkins)

Wechsler, D. (1974) *Wechsler Intelligence Scale for Children*, rev. edn. (New York: Psychological Corporation)

WHO (1984) *Consultation on Monitoring of Lead Neurotoxicity in Children*. Executive Summary, European Regional Programme on Chemical Safety, Dusseldorf (June)

Winneke, G., Hrdina, K.G. and Brockhaus, A. (1982) Neuropsychological studies in children with elevated tooth-lead concentrations. I. Pilot study. *Int. Arch. Occup. Env. Health*, **51**, 169–183

Winneke, G., Kraemer, U., Brockhaus, A., Ewers, U., Kujanek, G., Lechner, H. and Janke, W. (1983) Neuropsychological studies in children with elevated tooth-lead concentrations. II. Extended study. *Int. Arch. Occup. Env. Health*, **51**, 231–252

Winneke, G., Beginn, U., Ewert, T., Havestadt, C., Kraemer, U., Krause, C., Thon, H.L. and Wagner, H.M. (1985) Comparing the effects of perinatal and later childhood lead exposure on neuropsychological outcome. *Env. Res.*, **38**, 155–167

Yule, W., Lansdown, R., Millar, I. and Urbanowicz, M.A. (1981). The relationship between blood lead concentrations, intelligence and attainment in a school population: a pilot study. *Dev. Med. Child Neurol.*, **23**, 567–576

Yule, W., Urbanowicz, M.A., Lansdown, R. and Millar, I.B. (1984). Teachers' ratings of children's behaviour in relation to blood lead levels. *Br. J. Dev. Psychol.*, **2**, 295–305

3.6
Evaluation of Different Biological Indicators of Lead Exposure Related to Neuropsychological Effects in Children

G. VIVOLI, M. BERGOMI, P. BORELLA, G. FANTUZZI, L. SIMONI,
D. CATELLI, N. STURLONI, G. B. CAVAZZUTI, R. MONTORSI,
R. CAMPAGNA, A. TAMPIERI and P. L. TARTONI

SUMMARY

The present study was designed to evaluate the relationship between different biological indicators of body lead burden and some neuropsychological functions in 7–8-year-old children, living in an industrial area polluted by lead. The neuropsychological functions were estimated by a battery of 6 psychometric tests. Lead was measured in blood, hair and teeth, and mean levels of 11.45 μg dl^{-1}, 9.94 μg g^{-1} and 6.80 μg g^{-1}, respectively, were obtained.

The mean ALA-D activity was also measured, and a mean of 51 mU ml^{-1} RBC was obtained.

By analysis of covariance, after regressing out the variance accountable to confounding variables (age, sex, occupation and education level of parents) the total and verbal scale of WISC IQ and Toulouse–Piéron tests were significantly associated with teeth lead levels. ALA-D values appeared to be related to vocabulary subtests of WISC and to delayed reaction time (12 s delay) after backward regression analysis was applied.

On the basis of published studies, it is not yet possible to establish whether lead exposure at current environmental levels can induce neuropsychological impairment in children (Needleman et al., 1979, 1984; Smith et al., 1983; Harvey et al., 1984; Winneke and Kraemer, 1984; Pocock and Ashby, 1985). There are several critical points which seem to influence the conflicting results obtained to date: the various criteria used in the selection of samples and the characteristics of the population studied; the choice of lead exposure indicators, and of psychometric tests for assessing neuropsychological functions; the selection of confounding variables, and the statistical methods used in the analyses of data.

In our study, the children recruited had been exposed to unstable conditions of lead exposure, with high levels at birth, decreasing after the first years of life. Four biochemical indicators were analysed: three exposure parameters (lead in blood, hair, and teeth) and one parameter of effect (ALA-D activity). The possible relationship between current and long-term indicators was evaluated in our exposure conditions. Numerous standardized psychometric tests, selected for their sensitivity and ability to assess different cognitive functions, were carried out.

The aims of our present study are: to establish which of the lead indicators are better correlated with the scores on psychometric tests; to define the minimum level which is associated with deficits in psychological performance for each of the lead indicators; to determine the most suitable neurological tests for evaluating the early effects of low lead exposure.

MATERIALS AND METHODS

The town near Modena (Northern Italy) where we collected our samples is a lead-polluted industrial zone with 193 ceramic factories located in few square kilometers.

In Table 1, we report measurements of lead content in blood from children living in this area, taken during different periods. The mean value in 1979 was $17.7 \, \mu g \, dl^{-1}$ against a mean value of 11.3 observed this year, a 36% decrease in six years. Lead pollution in the town studied (Sassuolo) has been steadily decreasing since 1978, mainly due to severe legal provisions; therefore the children studied had been exposed to decreasing levels of lead.

Only children born in 1977 were considered, as shown in Table 2. In the area studied there were 682, attending the second grade of 15 elementary schools. We selected 11 of these schools, excluding the other four because they were located in residential zones with low levels of lead pollution. All 532 children in these schools were informed about the research; 77 children were excluded following criteria proposed by WHO (1984) (Table 3).

A total of 237 children were included in the study. The numbers of males and females were almost equal; the group was subdivided into two socioeconomic categories with respect to both parents' education and occupation. A score was assigned to both mothers and fathers according to education level (0 = no schooling, 1 = eight years or less of education,

Table 1 PbB ($\mu g \, dl^{-1}$) in children living in Sassuolo sampled in different periods

Date	n	Mean	SD
1979	107	17.7	4.7
1981	366	14.0	5.4
1986 (this study)	314	11.3	3.3
Difference 1979–1986 = -36% ($6.4 \, \mu g \, dl^{-1}$)			

Table 2 Characteristics of studied population

TOTAL SCHOOLS IN THE AREA = 15 with   682 Children (2th Class only)
↓   ↓ −22%
Examined Schools   = 11 with   532 Children
↓ −41% (parents' agreement)
Entering children   314
↓ −24.5% (exclusion criteria)
INCLUDED CHILDREN   237

Sex: males 131 (55.3%);   females 106 (44.7%)

Age: mean = 7 years and 8 months;   range = 7−8.5 years

Parents' status (Education/Occupation) = lower level 106 (44.7%); upper level 118 (49.8%)

Table 3 Criteria for exclusion

− Birthweight less than 2000 g
− The mother reports the child was blue at birth
− The child was discharged from hospital at least 10 days after the mother
− Evidence of heavy alcohol consumption or drug abuse by the mother during pregnancy, or epilepsy of the mother
− Rubella infection during pregnancy
− The mother reports that the child has suffered from a central nervous system disease (e.g. meningitis, epileptic seizure)
− The child has ever suffered severe head injury
− The child suffers from obvious motor or sensory deficits or any diagnosed chronic disease
− The child's parents have been divorced or if either has died in the last year
− Children who have not lived in the area all their lives

2 = senior highschool, 3 = university degree) and occupational status (0 = unemployed, 1 = unskilled, 2 = skilled/craftsmen, 3 = white collar/ manager). The first group included parents with a sum of points less than seven, and the second category those with higher total score.

Lead in whole blood (PbB) was measured for each of the 237 children, following the procedure of Fernandez (1975), with slight modifications. The accuracy of the analyses was ascertained by regular participation in the quality control programme organized by the United Kingdom (UKEQAS) and by the Italian Istituto Superiore di Sanita' (Morisi et al., 1984).

Whole incisors were collected from 111 children, and the lead content (PbT) of these was measured using the method of Ewers et al. (1982). Quality control samples of tooth powder were provided by WHO within the Euro Research Project on Monitoring of lead neurotoxicity in children. In addition, about 10% of real samples were sent to the Hygiene Institute of Düsseldorf for an interlaboratory comparison of results.

Hair samples taken from the nape of the neck near the scalp were washed with a non-ionic detergent (7X-OMatic), as proposed by Harrison, Yurachek and Benson (1969). After drying, they were wet ashed utilizing strong acids (nitric−sulphuric and perchloric acid mixture). Calibration curves were assayed both in hair and in aqueous solutions (PbH).

ALA-D activity was measured with the standardized European method (Berlin and Schaller, 1974).

All analyses of lead were measured by atomic absorption spectroscopy using a Perkin Elmer mod. 5000 instrument equipped with a graphite furnace system mod. 400.

A battery of neuropsychological tests were administered to each child by one of four trained psychologists. With the exception of the delayed reaction time test, all other tests were carried out in a fixed order, during a single morning session at school, with a short midmorning break. The delayed reaction time was administered a few days later to avoid tiring the children.

The battery of tests covered several different aspects of intellectual performance:

(1) *"Intelligence"* was assessed by means of two verbal and two performance subtests of the Wechsler Intelligence Scale for Children (WISC: Wechsler, 1974). The subtests used were Vocabulary and Comprehension, and Block Design and Picture Completion.

(2) *"Scholastic attainment"* was evaluated with the teachers' help according to a protocol planned out by our team, in which four different scores (mathematics, reading, drawing, writing) were obtained.

(3) *"Visual motor performance"* was assessed by means of the Bender Gestalt test, using the German scoring system of the Goettinger Form Reproduction Test (GFT) (Schlange et al., 1972).

(4) *"Visual–motor and visual sequential ability"* was assessed by the Trail Making Test carried out in agreement with the Danish study group as proposed during the WHO consultation of monitoring of lead neurotoxicity in children (WHO, 1984). In the protocol, only the time score for part A was considered.

(5) *"Symbol memory and attention"* was evaluated by means of Toulouse–Piéron Cancellation Test, according to the method proposed by the Belgian group in the WHO consultation.

(6) *"General attentional performance"* was studied with a delayed reaction time task, using the computed program of Hunter et al. (1985). Only results obtained in 3rd block (12 s delay) were recorded.

Statistical analysis

Our data were submitted to descriptive analysis in terms of mean values, range and frequency distributions. Since the distributions of lead exposure parameters were skewed, a $\log_{10}$ transformation of values was applied. Pearson's correlation coefficients were calculated to evaluate the association between neuropsychological impairments and lead exposure. The level of significance assumed was $p < 0.05$ (one-tailed). To evaluate the influence of potential confounding variables on measured parameters, analysis of variance (ANOVA) was performed. In addition, we estimated the variance of psychometric tests explained by covariates (ALA-D, PbB, PbH, PbT) after regressing out the effects of demographic variables (ANCOVA).

227

RESULTS

The arithmetic and geometric means, the medians and ranges of lead found in the biological matrices investigated are shown in Table 4.

Figures 1 and 2 show the frequency distributions of ALA-D and other lead exposures parameters. As expected, lead distributions in blood, hair and teeth are skewed. 12.2% of blood lead measures, 33.7% of hair lead measures, and 33.3% of tooth lead measures show values higher than 15 μg dl^{-1}, 15 μg g^{-1} and 5 μg g^{-1}, respectively. ALA-D and PbT values are significantly affected when the influence of sex and parents' status was investigated by analysis of covariance. However, as shown in Figure 3, the influence of parents' status on mean values of ALA-D and PbT exists only for males.

In Table 5, the linear correlation coefficients between the biological parameters are reported. Overall the correlation coefficients obtained are low, but blood lead levels are significantly related to ALA-D and lead in hair, although not with teeth. Furthermore, lead in teeth is significantly correlated with lead in hair and ALA-D. In order to determine whether the degree of association is increased at different levels, we computed the linear correlations dividing the values of biochemical parameters according to percentile distribution.

As shown in Table 6, the inverse relationship between PbB and ALA-D is stronger ($r = -0.487$; $p = 0.000$) for blood lead values higher than 12.88 μg dl^{-1} ($>$75th percentile).

Furthermore, it is interesting to note that the correlation between PbT and PbB increases to a significant level in the group of children characterized by the highest tooth lead levels (PbT higher than 8.71 μg g^{-1}).

First-order correlations between lead exposure parameters and WISC-R and Scholastic Attainment measures are shown in Table 7. A significant relationship was found between ALA-D values and WISC-R full scale IQ, and this is manifest in both the verbal and performance components of the full scale.

For children with levels of ALA-D lower than 25th percentile

Table 4 Means, medians and ranges of the biochemical parameters

Biochemical parameters	n	Arithmetic mean	SD	Geometric mean	Median	Range
PbB (μg dl^{-1})	216	11.46	3.44	10.99	11.00	3.80–28.40
PbH (μg g^{-1})	212	9.94	8.57	6.79	7.66	0.47–59.97
PbT (μg g^{-1})	115	6.80	3.42	6.05	5.93	1.60–21.92
ALA-D (mU ml^{-1} RBC)	214	50.58	8.03	—	50.60	24.80–74.90

Table 5 Linear correlations between the biochemical parameters

	ALA-D			Log_{10} PbB			Log_{10} PbH		
	n	r	p	n	r	p	n	r	p
Log_{10} PbB	213	−0.280	0.000	—	—	—	—	—	—
Log_{10} PbH	207	−0.108	0.059	210	0.125	0.035	—	—	—
Log_{10} PbT	111	−0.192	0.021	113	0.122	0.097	111	0.208	0.014

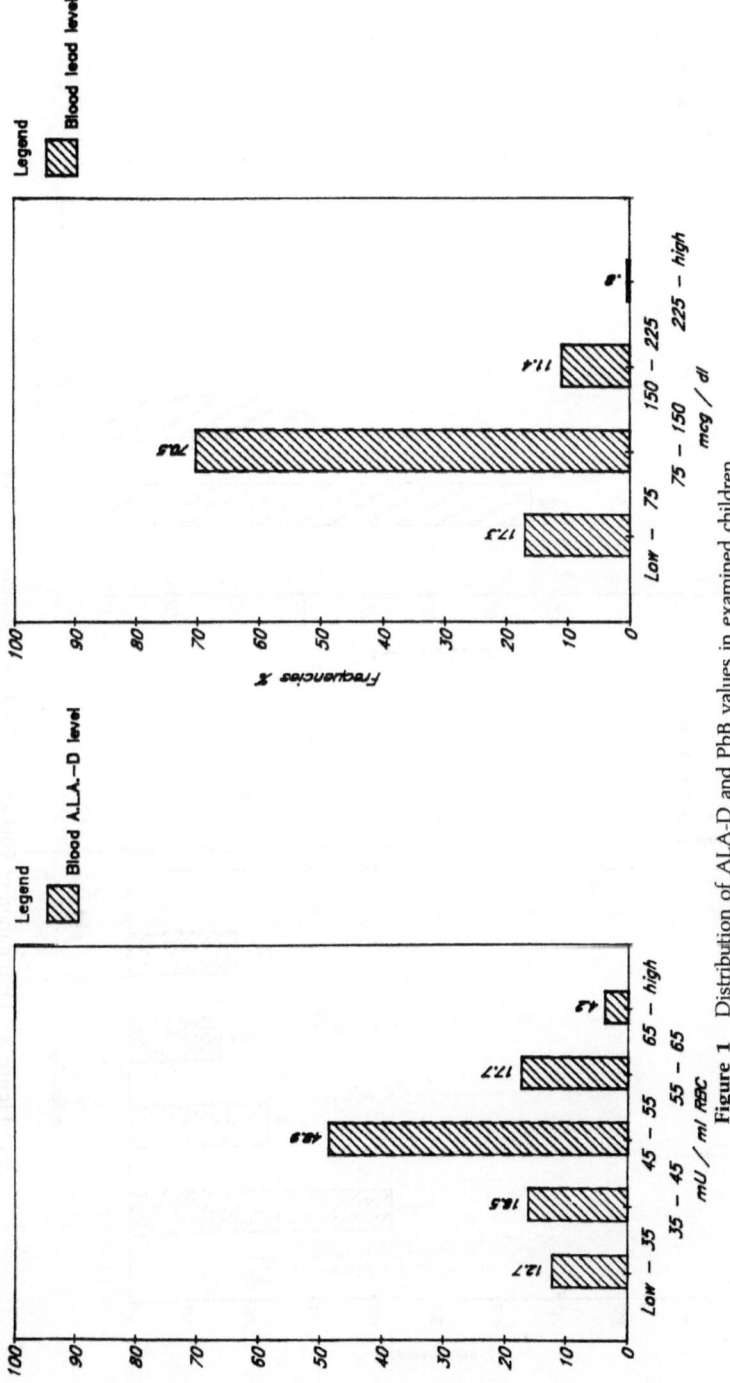

Figure 1 Distribution of ALA-D and PbB values in examined children

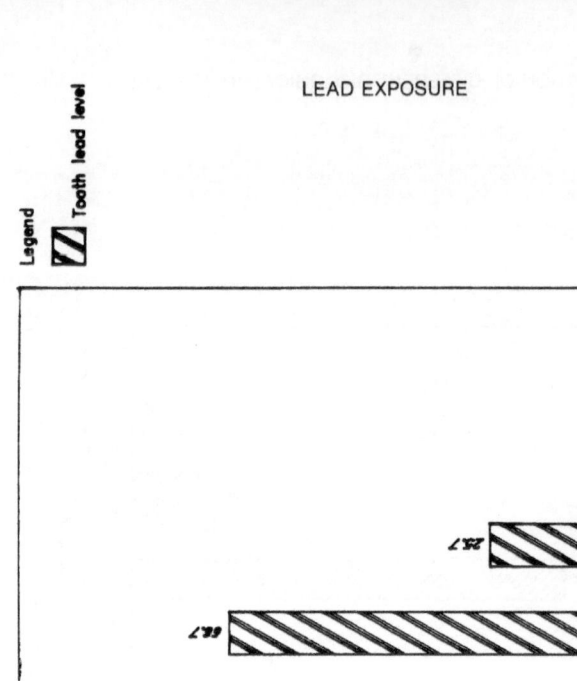

Figure 2   Distribution of PbH and PbT values in examined children

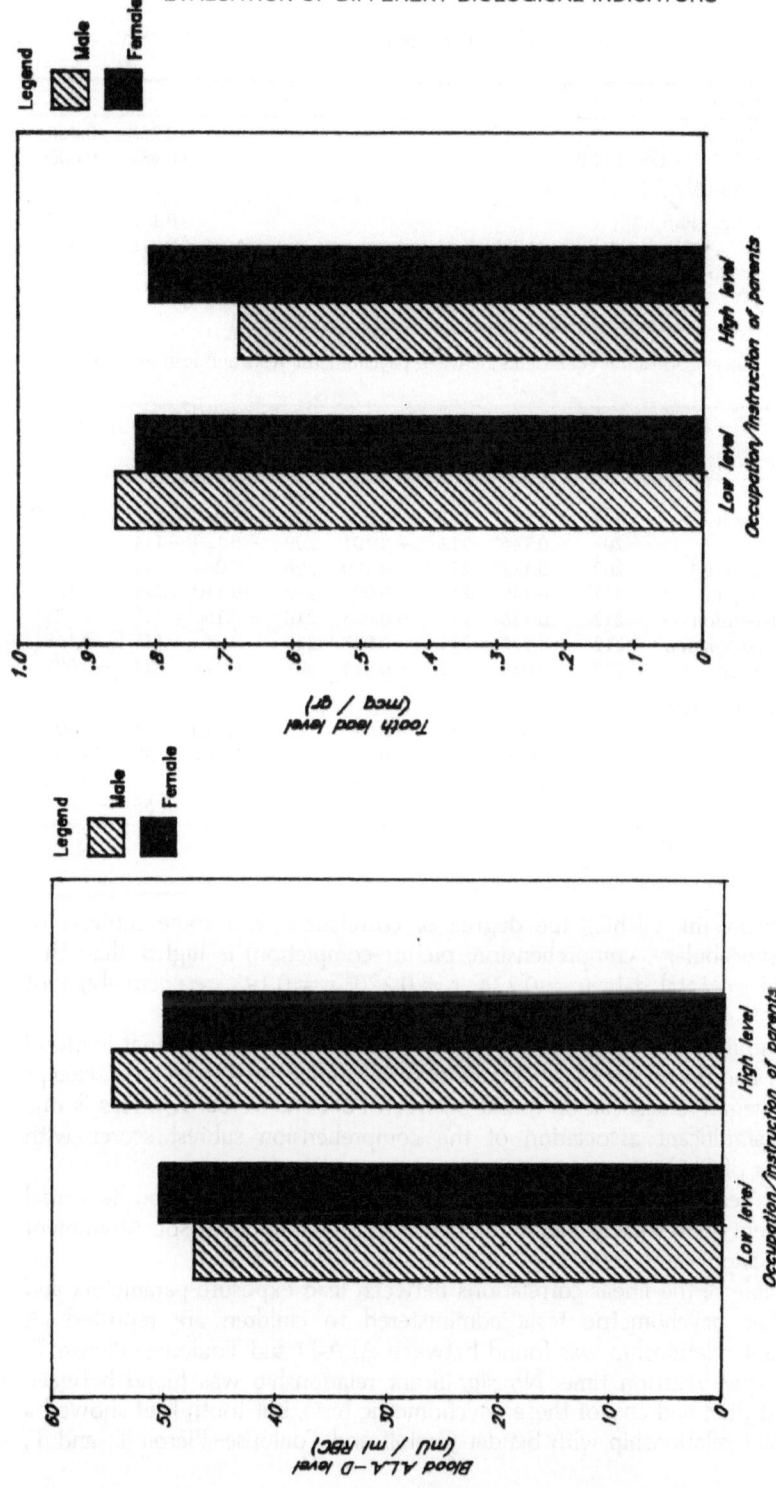

Figure 3 ALA-D and PbT values divided by sex and parents' status

Table 6 Increase of correlation coefficients in upper classes of exposure (> 75th percentile)

Linear correlations	r	p
Log$_{10}$ PbB/ALAD	−0.280	0.000
12.88 μg dl^{-1} Log$_{10}$ PbB/ALA-D	−0.487	0.000
(> 75th percentile)		
Log$_{10}$ PbT/Log$_{10}$ PbB	0.122	0.097
8.71 μg g^{-1} Log$_{10}$ PbT/Log$_{10}$ PbB	0.318	0.049
(> 75th percentile)		

Table 7 Linear correlation coefficients between psychometric tests and lead exposure indicators

	ALA-D		Log$_{10}$ PbB		Log$_{10}$ PbH		Log$_{10}$ PbT	
Psychometric tests	n	r	n	r	n	r	n	r
WISC-R								
Total scale IQ	208	0.155*	211	−0.064	208	−0.057	113	−0.219**
Verbal IQ	209	0.146*	212	−0.101	209	−0.129*	114	−0.237**
Performance IQ	208	0.132*	211	−0.100	208	0.063	113	−0.135
Vocabulary IQ	212	0.159*	214	−0.093	210	−0.110	115	−0.189*
Comprehension	212	0.128*	214	−0.063	210	−0.168*	115	−0.185*
Picture completion	212	0.177*	214	0.022	210	0.051	115	−0.145
Block design	210	0.059	212	−0.035	208	0.023	114	−0.077
Scholastic attainment								
Mathematics	86	−0.164	87	−0.017	86	−0.133	58	−0.201
Reading	86	−0.127	87	−0.009	86	−0.091	58	−0.193
Writing	86	−0.040	87	−0.066	86	−0.167	58	−0.232*
Drawing	86	−0.035	87	0.005	86	−0.053	58	−0.086

*$p < 0.05$; **$p < 0.01$

(< 46.05 mU ml^{-1} RBC), the degree of correlation with some subtests of WISC (vocabulary, comprehension, picture-completion) is higher than that obtained on total data ($r = 0.224$; $r = 0.270$; $r = 0.193$, respectively) (not shown).

No significant relationship was found between lead concentrations in blood and hair and the scores of psychometric tests administered to children, except for the negative association found between PbH and verbal IQ. This is due to the significant association of the comprehension subtest scores with measures of PbH.

Tooth lead levels correlate significantly with full scale IQ (and its verbal component subtests and verbal IQ). Writing scores of Scholastic Attainment are also significantly correlated with measures of tooth lead.

In Table 8, the linear correlations between lead exposure parameters and the other psychometric tests administered to children are reported. A significant relationship was found between ALA-D and Toulouse–Piéron T$_1$ and delayed reaction time. No significant relationship was found between PbB and PbH and any of these psychometric tests, but tooth lead showed a significant relationship with Bender Gestalt and Toulouse–Piéron T$_1$ and T$_2$ scores.

Table 8 Linear correlation coefficients between psychometric tests and lead exposure indicators

Psychometric tests	ALA-D n	r	Log_{10} PbB n	r	Log_{10} PbH n	r	Log_{10} PbT n	r
Bender GT (n.v.)	209	−0.096	211	0.046	207	0.048	114	0.161**
Bender GT (i.v.)	208	−0.075	210	0.012	206	0.021	113	0.139
Trail making test (B)	208	0.052	205	0.039	201	0.058	112	0.119
Toulouse–Piéron T_1	208	−0.146*	210	−0.044	206	−0.010	113	0.155*
Toulouse–Piéron T_2	208	−0.079	210	−0.017	206	0.014	113	0.248†
Toulouse–Piéron E_1	197	0.018	198	0.045	195	0.101	107	0.075
Toulouse–Piéron E_2	200	0.052	201	0.027	199	0.096	107	0.098
Delayed reaction time	192	−0.170**	195	0.063	193	0.074	104	−0.058

*$p < 0.05$;   **$p < 0.01$;   †$p < 0.005$

The degree of association found between lead in teeth and scores of Toulouse–Piéron (T_1 and T_2) was greater in children with PbT levels higher than 8.61 μg g^{-1} (> 75th percentile) ($r = 0.393$; $r = 0.395$, respectively).

When we considered hair lead levels higher than 13.18 μg g^{-1} (> 75th percentile), a significant relationship was found with the Toulouse–Piéron test (especially with the scores E_1 and E_2, $r = 0.302$ and $r = 0.276$ respectively). Trail making scores were also significantly related to the highest levels of PbB and PbT ($r = 0.380$; $r = 0.366$, respectively).

By analysis of covariance (ANCOVA), we evaluated the effects of sociodemographic variables on psychometric tests.

In almost all tests (with exception of the WISC-R), no influence of sociodemographic variables was observed. All four subtests of WISC-R were affected by parents' occupation–education status whereas only some subtests (comprehension and block design) were affected by sex.

We estimated the variance of psychometric tests explained by covariates (ALA-D, PbB, PbH, PbT) after regressing out the effects of demographic variables.

Since the analysis of covariance was calculated using all the biochemical measures as covariates, only the children who provided teeth were included in these statistics. No significant difference for the biochemical parameters investigated was found between tooth givers and non-givers (Table 9), and sex and parents' status did not differ between the two groups. Thus, this subsample can be considered representative of the total population studied.

In Figures 4, 5 and 6, the results of analysis of covariance (for the psychometric tests significantly associated with the lead exposure parameters)

Table 9 Results of the exposure parameters for tooth givers and non-givers

	With teeth 115 (48.5%) n	Mean	SD	Without teeth 122 (51.5%) n	Mean	SD
ALA-D (mU ml^{-1} RBC)	111	51.23	7.68	102	49.88	8.37
PbB (μg dl^{-1})	113	11.61	3.58	103	11.29	3.29
PbH (μg g^{-1})	111	9.38	7.75	102	10.14	9.40

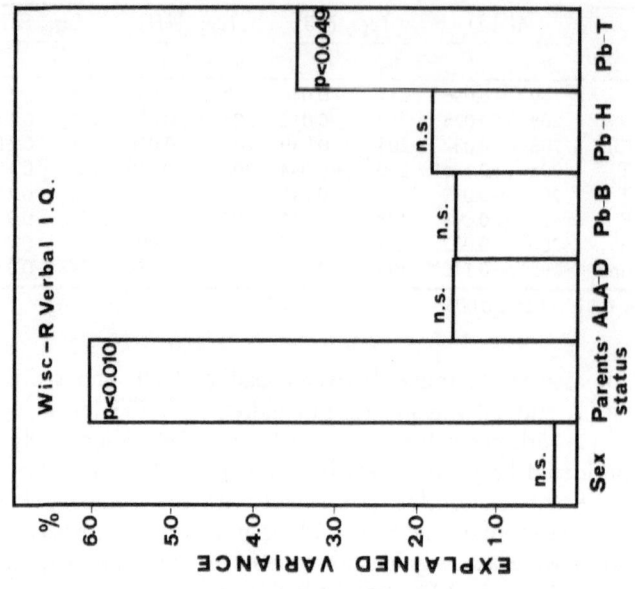

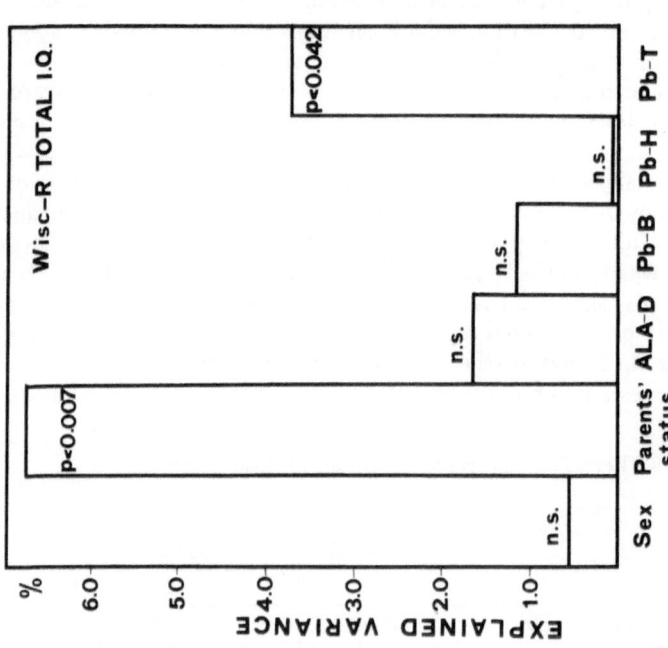

Figure 4 Effects of sociodemographic variables and lead exposure parameters on WISC-R total IQ and verbal IQ evaluated by ANCOVA

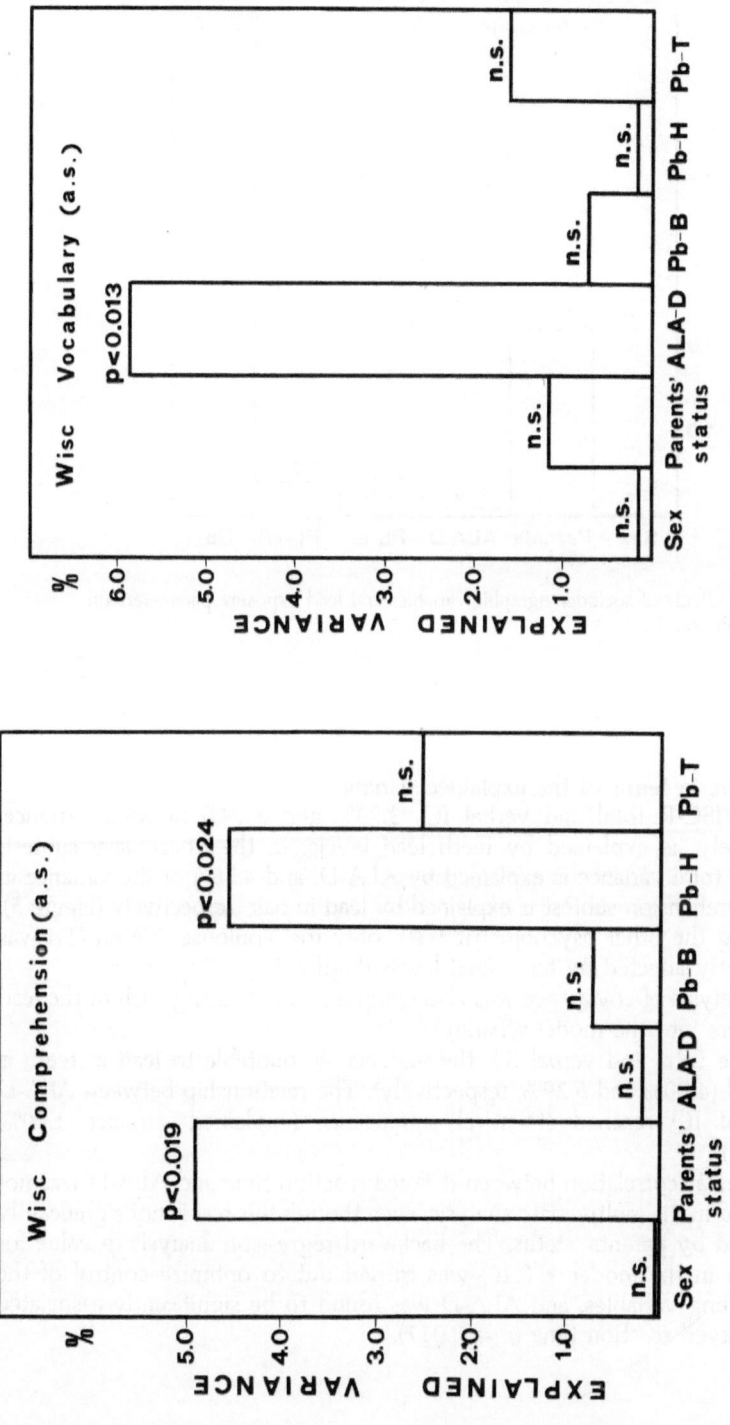

Figure 5 Effects of sociodemographic variables and lead exposure parameters on WISC-R verbal subtests

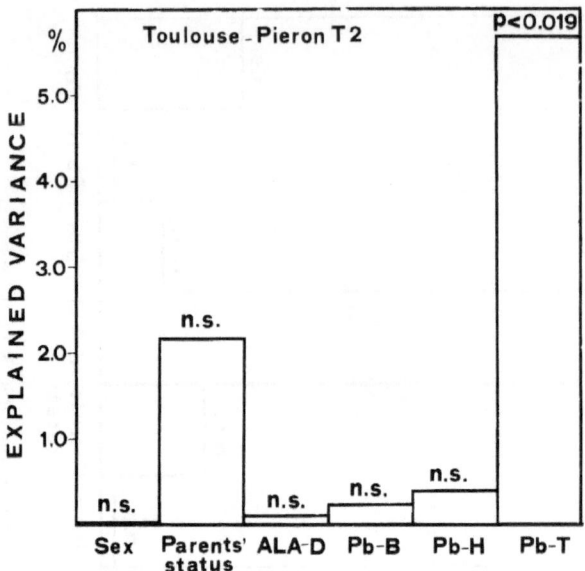

Figure 6 Effects of sociodemographic variables and lead exposure parameters on Toulouse–Piéron T$_2$

are shown, in terms of the explained variance.

For WISC-R total and verbal IQ, 3.73% and 3.49% of total variance, respectively, is explained by teeth lead levels. In the vocabulary subtest, 5.88% of total variance is explained by ALA-D, and 4.58% of the variance in the comprehension subtest is explained by lead in hair, respectively (Figure 5).

Among the other psychometric tests, only the Toulouse–Piéron (T$_2$) was significantly affected by teeth lead levels (Figure 6).

An analysis of covariance was also computed, introducing each of the lead parameters into the model separately.

For the total and verbal IQ, the variance accountable to lead in teeth is increased (4.80% and 5.29%, respectively). The relationship between ALA-D and total IQ reached statistical significance (explained variance 1.80%; $p = 0.05$).

The linear correlation between delayed reaction time and ALA-D was not confirmed in the multivariate analysis, even though this test is not significantly influenced by parents' status. The backward regression analysis (p value for retention in the model <0.10) was carried out to optimize control of the confounding variables, and ALA-D was found to be significantly associated with delayed reaction time ($p = 0.017$).

DISCUSSION

In terms of current lead exposure, lead values for this population fall within the range found by several authors in urban areas (Smith *et al.*, 1983; Silva *et al.*, 1984; Lansdown *et al.*, 1986). The slightly higher PbT levels found in our children compared with other groups having similar PbB values, and the lack of significant correlation between these two markers, may be explained by the unstable conditions of lead exposure which were a feature of the area studied. The low level of correlation between PbB and ALA-D can be attributed to the relatively low PbB levels of our sample, according to a similar finding of Hurst and Hughes (1985). In fact, a stronger association between these two parameters was found in those children with higher blood lead levels.

With respect to neuropsychological effects of the metal exposure, lead was found to be associated with impairments on the cognitive functions evaluated by WISC-R. After regressing out the variance attributable to confounding factors, the total and verbal scale of IQ was related to lead in teeth, in agreement with findings of other workers (Bellinger *et al.*, 1984; Hansen *et al.*, 1985). Furthermore, the two verbal subtests of WISC (vocabulary and comprehension) were associated with ALA-D and PbH, respectively.

Some superior functions, such as perception and symbol memory, estimated by Toulouse–Piéron, were found to be associated with lead levels in teeth.

By contrast, after control for confounding variables, our results did not show any influence of lead exposure on visual motor performance, evaluated by Bender Gestalt Test, by the Trail Making Test, and on scholastic attainment.

General attentional performance, estimated by delayed reaction time (12 s delay), was significantly related to ALA-D activity when backward regression analysis was applied.

Among the four biochemical indicators investigated, tooth lead had the highest predictive value of impairment of some neuropsychological functions. Our results suggest that current (PbB) and short-term (PbH) indicators of lead exposure have little or no value as predictors of neuropsychological performance. The significant relationship found with long-term exposure indicators (PbT) supports the hypothesis that some neurological functions were affected in the first years of life, when the levels of lead pollution were higher.

To conclude, it is worth noting the relationship between ALA-D and the two independent neuropsychological functions: the WISC-R vocabulary subtest and delayed reaction time, neither of which was significantly associated with PbB levels. One possible hypothesis is that this indicator of effect is more sensitive at monitoring early impairments of intellectual performance than a measure of current exposure. Another hypothesis is that small quantities of biologically active lead might be released from storage organs. This would have relatively little effect on total blood lead levels but would influence ALA-D activity or induce a partial inhibition of ALA-D synthesis in the bone marrow. A third possible explanation is that ALA-D activity is related to intellectual performance, as observed in mentally retarded children (Telisman, Prpic-Majic and Beritic, 1983), with no relation to lead exposure.

ACKNOWLEDGMENT

Supported by a grant from the EEC (contract no. ENV-812-I).

REFERENCES

Bellinger, D., Needleman, H., Leviton, A., Watenaux, C., Rabinowitz, M. and Nichols, M. (1984). Early sensory-motor development and prenatal exposure to lead. *Neurobehav. Toxicol. Teratol.*, **6**, 387−402

Bender, L. (1983). A visual motor gestalt test and its clinical use. Research Monograph n.3, American Orthopsychiatric Association

Berlin, A. and Schaller, K.H. (1974). European standardized method for the determination of delta-aminolevulinic acid dehydratase activity in blood. *Z. Klin. Chem. Klin. Biochem.*, **12**, 389−390

Ewers, V., Brockaus, A., Winneke, G., Freier, I., Jermann, E. and Kramer, U. (1982). Lead in deciduous teeth of children living in a non-ferrous smelter area and a rural area of the FRG. *Int. Arch. Occup. Environ. Health*, **50**, 139−151

Fernandez, F.J. (1975). Micromethod for lead determination in whole blood by atomic absorption with use of the graphite furnace. *Clin. Chem.*, **21**, 558−561

Hansen, O.N., Lyngbye, T., Trillingsgaard, A., Beese, I. and Granjean, P. (1985). A neuropsychological and behavioral assessment of children with low level lead exposure. In Lekkas, T.D. (ed.) *Heavy Metals in the Environment*. (Edinburgh: CEP Consultans)

Harrison, W.W., Yurachek, J.P. and Benson, C.A. (1969). The determination of trace elements in human hair by atomic absorption spectroscopy. *Clin. Chim. Acta*, **23**, 83−91

Harvey, P.G., Hamlin, M.W., Kumar, R. and Delves, H.T. (1984). Blood lead, behaviour and intelligence test performance in preschool children. *Sci. Total Environ.*, **40**, 45−60

Hunter, J., Urbanowicz, M.A., Yule, W. and Lansdown, R. (1985). Automated testing of reaction time and its association with lead in children. *Int. Arch. Occup. Environ. Health*, **57**, 27−34

Hurst, P.L. and Hughes, P.M. (1985). Poor correlation between erythrocytic 5-aminolevulinic acid dehydratase activity and blood lead concentration in a group of eleven-year old children. *Clin. Chem.*, **31**, 1244−1245

Lansdown, R., Yule, W., Urbanowicz, M.A. and Hunter, J. (1986). The relationship between blood-lead concentrations, intelligence, attainment and behaviour in a school population: the second London study. *Int. Arch. Occup. Environ. Health*, **57**, 225−235

Morisi, G., Patriarca, M., Bortoli, A., Mattiello, G., Gelosa, L., Fortuna, E., Vivoli, G., Borella, P., Bergomi, M., Piovano, V., Rampa, P., Pallotti, G., Consolino, A., Alessio, L., Grilli, G., Baston, W., Leyendecker, W., Chiarotti, F. and Taggi, F. (1984). Un programma di sicurezza di qualita' per la determinazione del piombo nel sangue, svolto nell'ambito dell'attuazione della direttiva CEE sulla sorveglianza biologica della popolazione contro il rischio di saturnismo. *Biochim. Clin.*, **8**, 157−158

Needleman, H.L., Gunnoe, C., Leviton, A., Reed, R., Peresie, H., Maher, C. and Barrett, P. (1979). Deficits in psychologic and classroom performance of children with elevated dentine lead levels. *N. Engl. J. Med.*, **300**, 689−695

Needleman, H.L., Rabinowitz, M., Leviton, A., Linn, S. and Schoenbaum, S. (1984). The relationship between prenatal exposure to lead and congenital anomalies. *J. Am. Med. Assoc.*, **251**, 2956−2959

Pocock, S.J. and Ashby, D. (1985). Environmental lead and children's intelligence: a review of recent epidemiological studies. *Statistician*, **34**, 31−44

Schlange, H., Stein, B., Boetticher, J. and Taneh, S. (1972). Goettinger formreproduktionstest (G.F.T.). Hogrefe, Goettingen

Silva, P.A., Hughes, P., Crosado, B. and Faed, J. (1984). A pilot study of blood lead levels, cognitive development and behaviour problems in 579 Dunedin eleven year old children. Presented at *Workshop on Lead Research*, University of Auckland

Smith, M., Delves, T., Lansdown, R., Clayton, B. and Graham, P. (1983). The effects of lead exposure on urban children: the Institute of Child Health/Southampton study. *Dev. Med. Child Neurol.*, Suppl. 47

Telisman, S., Prpic-Majic, D. and Beritic, T. (1983). Pb-B and A.L.A.-D in mentally retarded and normal children. *Int. Arch. Occup. Environ. Health*, **53**, 361–369

Wechsler, D. (1974). *Wechsler Intelligence Scale for Children*, revised ed. (New York: Psychological Corporation) (English edition, NFER/Nelson, Windsor)

WHO (1984). Consultation on monitoring of lead neurotoxicity in children. *Executive Summary, European Regional Programme on Chemical Safety*, Dusseldorf (June)

Winneke, G. and Kraemer, U. (1984). Neuropsychological effects of lead in children: interactions with social background variables. *Neuropsychobiology*, **11**, 195–202

3.7
Neuropsychological Profile of Children in Relation to Dentine Lead Level and Socioeconomic Group

O. N. HANSEN, A. TRILLINGSGAARD, I. BEESE, T. LYNGBYE and
P. GRANDJEAN

INTRODUCTION

The adverse effects of lead intoxication on neuropsychological development
were first systematically studied by Byers and Lord (1943) in their follow-up
of 20 children who had been hospitalized previously because of lead
intoxication. They reported that 19 of the children later made unsatisfactory
progress in school, presumably due to sensorimotor deficits, short attention
span, and behavioural disorders. Since that time, many studies have assessed
cognitive and behavioural variables in children with varying degrees of low-
level lead exposure. Some studies have reported general intellectual or specific
cognitive impairment among affected children (de la Burde and Choate, 1972,
1975; Perino and Ernhart, 1974; Landrigan et al., 1975; Needleman et al.,
1979; Thatcher et al., 1983; Winneker et al., 1982a, b; Yule et al., 1981; Shapiro
and Marecek, 1984), while others have failed to replicate these findings (Kotok
et al., 1977; Lansdown et al., 1974; McNeil et al., 1975; Ernhart et al., 1981
and Smith et al., 1983). Rutter (1980) pointed out that the interpretation of
a number of these studies is obscured by methodological limitations, including
inadequate markers of exposure to lead, insensitive measures of performance,
bias in selection of subjects and inadequate handling of confounding covariates.
   The study reported here has examined the neuropsychological function of
children exposed to low levels of environmental lead. In the study design,
account was taken of the limitations noted by Rutter (1980). Thus, we selected
children for our study by screening a well-defined population of normal
school children from the town of Aarhus, Denmark. We collected extensive
medical and demographic information about these children to control
adequately the confounding variables. Also, the battery of neuropsychological
tests that we used was selected to detect subtle levels of impairment across

a broad range of functions. Finally, we used an index of cumulative rather than current exposure to lead, by measuring the lead retained in shed deciduous teeth. The circumpulpal dentine, which is formed after the eruption of the tooth, continues to accumulate lead until the tooth is shed. Analysis of lead in this dental tissue was used as an integrated measure of the total exposure during early life.

MATERIALS AND METHODS

The study was carried out in the municipality of Aarhus, a town of 250 000 inhabitants. The population is very homogeneous with very small ethnic and language minorities. The standard of housing is high in this area, and no major point source of lead pollution is present.

We conducted a cross-sectional cohort study of school children in first grade in 1982–83. We contacted 2412 children and asked them to submit their shed teeth to the teacher. A special badge was awarded to each child who had donated a tooth. A total of 1291 children delivered at least one usable tooth, a response rate of 54% among all eligible children. For each tooth the teacher filled in a small slip with the date, name and address of the child, the occupation of the father and mother, and position in the jaw of the tooth. Subsequently, a children's dentist identified the type of each tooth using specific morphological criteria.

The lead level was determined according to procedures described in detail elsewhere (Grandjean et al., 1984, 1986). In short, each tooth is split into two halves. The exposed pulp chamber is then thoroughly cleaned, and about 0.5–1 mg of the soft circumpulpal dentine from one of the two tooth segments is removed by a wolfram-carbide rosette burr. The powder is weighed and dissolved in 100 μl concentrated HNO_3 which is subsequently diluted by 400 μl redistilled water in a sample cup. The detection of lead takes place by electrothermal atomic absorption spectrometry. This method has shown excellent reproducibility.

The average of dentine lead for all teeth was 10.7 μg/g, with extremes ranging from 0.40 to 168.5 μg/g. The dentine lead concentrations were not normally distributed but transformed to a log normal distribution. Eight per cent of the children ($n = 110$) had a lead level above 18.7 μg/g. These children were selected as a 'high' lead exposure group. We matched the high-lead children for sex and parental social group with children with a dentine lead level below 5 μg/g. The risk of misclassification between the high-lead and low-lead group was minimal because the tooth lead concentrations of both groups represented non-overlapping distributions, with mean values of 3.25 μg/g and 26.8 μg/g for the two groups. Subsequent blood analysis showed a total average blood-lead level of 5.1 μg/100 ml, thus confirming the generally low-level lead exposure (Lyngbye et al., 1988a) of this population.

The paediatrician of the team, who was blind to the lead data, interviewed the parents to obtain basic demographic, medical and exposure data. Since the interview phase started a year later than the collection of the teeth, some children had changed their address or even family name during this period.

241

However, all children who had donated teeth were identified by name, date of birth, address and names of their parents. With this information it was possible to retrieve former addresses and change of family name at the central municipal register. Consequently, all children selected were identified, even when they had moved away from the area.

During this procedure both drop-out and exclusion took place. We had selected 213 families for interview, but 13 were non-responders. The 200 interviewed were further reduced by 14 drop-out cases where parental consent for participation could not be obtained, and one child was missed due to administrative error. The drop-out children were predominantly high-lead, and the non-responding families of low socioeconomic status (SES). Table 1 shows the distribution of SES among the children eligible, the 1302 children donating teeth and the 200 children interviewed. No major bias of SES was found (Lyngbye et al., 1988b), and there were no differences in the distribution of SES between the whole population and children tested.

Children with neurological syndromes or abnormalities, with impact on neuropsychological function such as birth complication, and well-defined risk factors were excluded from the study group. Furthermore, we decided to exclude children whose social conditions were atypical and also known to be risk factors for subnormality (Lyngbye et al., 1988c). After excluding children with risk factors, the experimental group consisted of 162 children, who were tested in the school as soon as the interview had been carried out.

The clinical psychologist, also blind to the lead data, administered the tests in a fixed sequence, the first part given to the child one day and the second part on the following day at the same time. The battery included the following tests: Part I, Bender Visual Motor Gestalt Test, Wechsler Intelligence Scale for Children; Part II, Seashore Rhythm Test, Visual Sequential Memory (ITPA), Trail-making Test, part A and B, Sentence Repetition Test, Continuous Performance Test and a behavioural rating. These tests were chosen either because they had shown a relationship to lead exposure in similar studies or

Table 1 Distribution of socioeconomic status (SES) in the total cohort of children and the three groups studied

SES	Children eligible		Tooth-givers		Children interviewed		Children tested	
	n	%	n	%	n	%	n	%
I	229	10.3	138	11.3	21	10.5	15	9.6
II	294	13.3	191	15.6	22	11.0	15	9.6
III	462	20.9	292	23.7	46	23.0	40	25.6
IV	766	34.6	404	33.0	69	34.5	56	35.9
V	422	19.1	187	15.3	42	21.0	30	19.2
Unknown	41	1.8	13	1.1	0	0	0	0
Total	2214	100.0	1225	100.0	200	100.0	156	100.0
Not stated	156	0	77	0	0	0	0	0
Total	2370		1302		200		156	

because they were known to be sensitive to minimal neuropsychological dysfunction.

Wechsler Intelligence Scale for Children (WISC)

This is the most recent test of general intelligence devised by Wechsler, and it has been in use since the early 1940s. Ten short subtests are given to each child individually. Five of the tests are predominantly 'verbal' in nature and five are predominantly non-verbal, or 'performance'. Raw scores are transformed into age-adjusted standard scores (mean of 10), and these scaled scores are added to yield estimates of intelligence – Verbal IQ, Performance IQ and Full Scale IQ. The Danish version is standardized for use with children aged 6 to 17 years (Wechsler, 1974).

Bender Visual Motor Gestalt Test

This test first appeared in 1938 and is said to be suitable for children aged 5 years and above. Children are asked to look at a design and reproduce it. Children with neurological disorders, learning difficulties and behaviour problems perform less adequately than normal children. In this study we used a more recent, detailed, objective scoring system (Schlange et al., 1972).

Seashore Rhythm Test

The Rhythm Test is a subtest of the Seashore Test of Musical Talent. The child is instructed to respond with a 'same' or 'different' to indicate which of 30 pairs of rhythmic beats are the same and which are different. This test appears to measure alertness to nonverbal auditory stimuli, sustained attention, and the ability to perceive and compare different rhythmic sequences.

Trail-making Test

This test consists of two parts. Part A consists of 15 numbered circles distributed over a white sheet of paper. The child is required to connect the circles with a pencil line as quickly as possible, beginning with circle 1 and proceeding in numerical sequence. Part B consists of 15 circles numbered from 1 to 8 and lettered from A to G. The child is required to connect the circles, alternating between sequences of numbers and letters. Two scores are recorded – the number of seconds required to finish each part and the number of errors. This test appears to require immediate recognition of the symbolic significance of numbers and letters, ability to scan the page continuously to identify the next number or letter in sequence, flexibility in integrating the numerical and alphabetical sequence, and completion of these requirements under the pressure of time.

Visual Sequential Memory from Illinois Tests of Psycholinguistic Abilities

The child has a 5-s look at a sequence of figures, and is required to remember and reproduce the correct sequence.

Continuous Performance Test

This test measures the child's ability to sustain attention. The child is seated in front of a screen with a response box. The test starts with a practice session to make sure that the child understands the task. The stimulus for this test is 12 letters. One letter at a time appears on the screen, with a stimulus duration of 0.2 s and a interstimulus interval of 1.5 s. The stimulus to which the child is instructed to respond is the letter H when it is immediately following the letter S. The 12 letters are randomized over a series of 100 stimuli, with 15 significant stimuli (S followed by H). The total run of 100 stimuli is repeated six times. A session of the task lasts about 15 min. The test is controlled by a computer which also collects data.

Behavioural Rating

At the same time as the child was doing the Continuous Performance Test a psychologist measured the on- and off-task behaviour of the child. Every 10 s the psychologist made a time sampling. The behavioural rating was based on 90 samples over 15 min.

Statistical analysis

The data processing was performed at the UNI-C centre for education and research. The statistical packages used were BMDP and SPSS. T-tests with two-tailed probabilities were used in crude statistical analyses of the results. Two more detailed analytical strategies were used. In the first model, cases and controls were treated as matched pairs and analysed by the paired t-test. In the second model a systematic search for confounding was performed bivariately and by multi-variate methods for 60 variables. The behavioural group of possible confounders consisted of pica, thumb-sucking and nail-biting. The exposure data included mother's smoking during pregnancy and at present, and the father's smoking. The seven social variables were: socioeconomic status of the family, educational status of the mother (MES) rated on the length of education, mother's age standardized for parity, proband's number in the sibship, number of siblings, single parent family and employment status. Finally, 47 medical variables were analysed, according to a detailed strategy to be described elsewhere (Lyngbye et al., 1988d).

A logistic multivariate regression with lead groups as the dependent variable was performed for each group of possible confounders. The variables showing association with lead ($p < 0.2$), were then analysed in a multivariate regression with the respective effect measures as dependent variables. The possible confounders identified by this approach, and sex of the child and SES were entered into a stepwise multiple-regression analysis with the different outcome measurements as the dependent variables. In this model, we used a conservative analysis by entering the dentine lead level as the last step after partialling out all the covariates.

RESULTS

In the crude analysis the high-lead children scored lower on the WISC when compared to low-lead children, especially on the Verbal IQ ($p < 0.001$) and Full Scale IQ ($p < 0.01$). There was no significant difference between the high- and low-exposure groups on the Performance IQ or on the different experimental tests. However, impaired function associated with lead exposure was also found on the Bender Visual Motor Gestalt Test ($p < 0.001$) and on the behavioural rating ($p < 0.03$).

To relate neuropsychological differences between the matched groups to environmental lead exposure, similarity of the groups in terms of confounding variables had to be demonstrated. The children in the two groups were already matched in terms of age and sex of the child, and rematching according to SES and MES was carried out. For occupational and educational status a misfit of 1 point up or down was accepted. Successful matching was obtained for 156 cases or 78 pairs. In the next step of statistical analysis the matched-sample t-test was used. The results from these analyses may be summarized as follows (Table 2): The main results shown are the same as those found for WISC, Bender-Gestalt test and behaviour in the pooled statistical analysis, as well as a borderline-significant deficit of Visual Sequence ($p < 0.1$) and a borderline effect on attentional performance as measured by the Continuous Performance Test, where the high-lead children made more errors ($p < 0.1$) and had fewer correct responses ($p < 0.2$).

The effects of lead in groups of children with different social backgrounds were then examined. In this analysis the Bender scores and the verbal IQ were broken down by socioeconomic status, and the different social strata were then analysed separately with the matched-sample t-test (Table 3). The results show a clear effect of lead in the different socioeconomic groups, despite the small number of pairs.

In the final model we entered the confounding variables which showed an association with dentine lead: normal pregnancy, home from hospital later than the mother, left-handedness, jaundice, phototherapy, SES, birth order, age of the mother adjusted for parity and number of siblings, together with MES, sex of the child and previous pica. These data were entered into a stepwise multiple-regression analysis with the different outcome measurements as the dependent variables. The three multiple regression analyses are summarized in Table 4. The final model for the Bender test accounted for 42% of the observed variance with a highly significant relationship between dentine lead level and Bender errors ($F = 56.74$, d.f. $= 0.64$, $p < 0.001$), the confounding variables only explaining a minimal portion of the variance. The final model for Verbal IQ accounted for 26% of the variance observed; in

245

Table 2 Matched-sample *t*-test for neuropsychological test performance in high- and low-lead children

Matched pair 78	Low lead mean	High lead mean	p Value, two-tailed
WISC			
Full scale IQ	114.23	108.30	<0.01
Verbal IQ	110.94	102.37	<0.001
Information	12.43	10.84	<0.01
Comprehension	10.74	8.43	<0.001
Arithmetic	11.41	11.05	N.S.
Similarities	12.38	11.67	<0.1
Vocabulary	10.98	9.75	<0.01
Digit Span	10.64	10.10	N.S.
Performance IQ	116.80	114.16	N.S.
Picture Completion	11.76	11.83	N.S.
Picture Arrangement	12.23	12.05	N.S.
Block Design	13.33	12.72	N.S.
Object Assembly	12.51	12.07	N.S.
Coding	11.49	10.98	N.S.
Bender Errors	16.56	21.56	<0.001
Behavioural Score	4.52	7.43	<0.01
Sentence Repetition	15.42	15.36	N.S.
Rhythm Test	22.66	22.33	N.S.
Visual Sequence	23.71	21.18	<0.1
Trail-making A	30.05	29.33	N.S.
Trail-making B	59.33	64.36	N.S.
Continuous performance			
Errors	3.83	6.41	<0.1
Correct	85.49	84.01	<0.2

Table 3

Status	Number of matched pairs	Low-lead mean	High-lead mean	p Value, two-tailed
(a) Number of errors in the Bender test, as broken down by socioeconomic status (paired *t*-test)				
I–II	15	14.87	20.27	<0.01
III	20	15.80	21.55	<0.001
IV	28	17.57	22.39	<0.001
V	15	17.27	21.33	<0.01
(b) Verbal IQ broken down by socioeconomic status (paired *t*-test)				
I–II	15	119.73	106.47	<0.02
III	20	113.55	102.55	<0.001
IV	28	106.36	101.07	<0.05
V	15	108.4	103.6	<0.20

Table 4 Summary of stepwise regression analyses

Variable	Order	Regression coefficient	Standard error	F	p	R change
Bender	1 Dentine lead	5.11	0.65	62.52	0.001	
	Constant	11.28				
	R square	0.294				
Bender	1 Family size	−0.45	0.37	1.47	0.227	0.091
	2 Photo-therapy	4.04	1.91	4.48	0.036	0.024
	3 MES (mother)	0.71	0.31	5.25	0.023	0.024
	4 Sex of the child	−1.67	0.61	7.55	0.007	0.023
	5 Pregnancy normal	1.74	0.85	4.17	0.043	0.013
	6 Left-handedness	0.32	0.69	0.21	0.648	0.007
	7 Pica earlier	1.25	1.06	1.41	0.237	0.003
	8 Dentine lead	4.80	0.64	56.74	0.001	0.232
	Constant	8.57				
	R square	0.42				
Verbal IQ	1 Dentine lead	−8.57	2.22	14.98	0.001	
	Constant	119.52				
	R square	0.091				
Verbal IQ	1 Birth order	2.63	1.23	4.53	0.035	0.120
	2 Mother's age	−3.35	1.26	7.11	0.009	0.032
	3 MES (mother)	−1.98	1.19	2.75	0.1	0.029
	4 Sex of the child	−3.70	2.08	3.17	0.077	0.015
	5 Home from hospital later than mother	−9.54	9.30	1.05	0.307	0.008
	6 Jaundice	−3.35	2.42	1.91	0.170	0.003
	7 SES (father)	−0.77	1.04	0.54	0.463	0.000
	8 Dentine lead	−6.66	2.21	9.07	0.003	0.047
	Constant	148.81				
	R square	0.26				
Full Scale IQ	1 Dentine lead	−5.51	1.91	8.35	0.004	
	Constant	119.44				
	R square	0.053				
Full Scale IQ	1 Birth order	1.98	1.07	3.41	0.067	0.105
	2 MES (mother)	−1.58	1.05	2.30	0.132	0.025
	3 Mother's age	−2.37	1.09	4.77	0.030	0.026
	4 Home from hospital later than mother	−8.77	8.02	1.20	0.276	0.008
	5 Jaundice	−3.19	2.10	2.30	0.131	0.006
	6 SES (father)	−0.74	0.91	0.67	0.415	0.001
	7 Dentine lead	−4.27	1.91	4.98	0.027	0.028
	Constant	139.95				
	R square	0.20				

this model birth order, and mother's age adjusted for parity, together accounted for more of the variance than did dentine lead level, but dentine lead level still accounted for a significant portion of the variance ($F = 9.07$, d.f. $= 2.21$, $p < 0.003$). The final model for Full Scale IQ accounted for 20% of the observed variance; as expected, birth order, mother's age adjusted for parity and MES together accounted for more of the variance than did dentine lead, but dentine lead still explained a significant portion of the variance ($F = 4.98$, d.f. $= 1.91$, $p < 0.027$). However, variation in lead levels accounted for only 2.8% of the total variance found in the Full Scale IQ.

Each of the outcome measures proved to have an individual profile of confounding. The WISC was mainly influenced by social factors, but not by medical factors, while 3% of the variance in the Bender was explained by medical factors. Within the group of social factors the profile also varied according to the measure. Thus, WISC was mostly influenced by mother's age, SES and birth order, whereas the Bender test was mostly influenced by MES and sex of the child.

DISCUSSION

The significant relationship between lead and the performance on Bender, Verbal WISC and Full Scale WISC found in this study is important because of the low level of lead absorption in our cohort. This result remains statistically significant even when controlling for confounding variables, and supports the emerging consensus of current research concerning the effect on children's visuomotor performance and IQ. In our study the effect of lead was not limited to a group of socially disadvantaged children; the results show a clear effect of lead in all socioeconomic groups.

Several recent studies have determined the lead level in whole tooth or crown (Ewers et al., 1982; Smith et al., 1983; Winneke et al., 1982b), although a tooth contains at least three different lead compartments: enamel, primary dentine, and circumpulpal dentine. Thus, the physiological interpretation of a whole-tooth lead concentration may be difficult. If long-term, postnatal lead exposure is supposed to be the main problem, then lead levels should be measured in the circumpulpal dentine (Grandjean et al., 1986). In our study we used the circumpulpal dentine as previously suggested by Needleman et al. (1979) and Shapiro and Marecek (1984), who found that the lead concentration in circumpulpal dentine was a better predictor of neuropsychological impairment than was the lead concentration in primary dentine. The reason for this finding could be that circumpulpal dentine is in constant contact with the bloodstream and retains lead for the entire time that the tooth is functional. In contrast, primary dentine is in direct contact with the bloodstream only prior to the eruption of the tooth. Indeed, lead levels in circumpulpal dentine of permanent teeth increase with the age of the individual (Grandjean et al., 1979). For this reason, the best predictor of chronic childhood lead exposure would be the lead level in circumpulpal dentine.

The most clear-cut results of our study relate to the Bender Gestalt test. This test has been included in the test batteries of a number of studies. Significant differences in the error scores for this test have been found in five (de la Burde and Choate, 1975; Winneke et al., 1982a, b; Shapiro and Marecek, 1984; Harvey et al., 1984) while two studies did not identify any lead-related difference. The Bender Gestalt test which requres a number of skills should be particularly sensitive to the presence of mild cerebral dysfunction. The decreased performance on this test could be due to a dysfunction in fine motor coordination (Trillingsgaard et al., 1985).

The picture which emerges from epidemiological studies of children is that children with higher levels of lead generally perform slightly worse on psychometric tests. The results from our study may indicate that, if present, the threshold must be very low for lead-related neuropsychological deficits. This conclusion is conceivable because present-day, so called 'low' lead exposures are much higher than prehistoric lead levels (Grandjean et al., 1979). Even in a minimally polluted area some children appear to be at risk for neuropsychological developmental deficits due to long-term lead exposure.

ACKNOWLEDGMENTS

This study was supported by grants from the Commission of the European Communities (contract no. ENV-786-DK) and the Danish Medical Research Council.

REFERENCES

Byers, R.K. and Lord, E.E. (1943) Late effects of lead poisoning on mental development. Am. J. Dis. Child., 66, 471–494

de la Burde, B. and Choate, M.S. (1972) Does early asymptomatic lead exposure in children have latent sequelae? J. Pediatr., 81, 1088–1091

de la Burde, B. and Choate, M.S. (1975) Early asymptomatic lead exposure and development at school age. J. Pediatr., 87, 638–642

Ernhardt, C., Landa, B. and Schell, E. (1981) Subclinical levels of lead and developmental deficit: a multivariate followup reassessment. Pediatrics, 67, 911–919

Ewers, U., Brockhaus, A., Winneke, G., Freier, I., Jermann, E. and Kramer, U. (1982) Lead in deciduous teeth of children living in a non-ferrous smelter area and a rural area of the FRG. Int. Arch. Occup. Environ. Health, 50, 139–151

Grandjean, P., Nielsen, O.V. and Shapiro, I.M. (1979) Lead retention in ancient Nubian and contemporary populations. J. Environ. Pathol. Toxicol., 2, 781–787

Grandjean, P., Hansen, O.N. and Lyngbye, K. (1984) Analysis of lead in circumpulpal dentin of deciduous teeth. Ann. Clin. Lab. Sci., 14, 270–275

Grandjean, P., Lyngbye, T. and Hansen, O.N. (1986) Lead concentration in deciduous teeth: variation related to tooth type and analytical technique. J. Toxicol. Environ. Health, 19, 437–445

Harvey, P.G., Hamlin, M.W., Kumar, R. and Delves, H.T. (1984) Blood lead, and intelligence test performance in preschool children. Sci. Total Environ., 40, 45–60

Kotok, D., Kotok, R. and Heriot, J.T. (1977) Cognitive evaluation of children with elevated blood lead levels. Am. J. Dis. Child., 131, 791–793

Landrigan, P.J., Whitworth, R.H. and Baloh, R.W. (1975) Neuropsychological dysfunction in children with chronic low-level lead absorption. Lancet, 1, 708–712

Lansdown, R.G., Shepherd, J., Clayton, B.E., Delves, H.T., Graham, P.J. and Turner, W.C. (1974) Blood lead levels, behaviour, and intelligence: population study. Lancet, 1, 538–541

Lyngbye, T., Hansen, O.N., Jørgensen, P.J. and Grandjean, P. (1988a) Validity and interpretation of blood lead levels: a study of Danish school children (in preparation)

Lyngbye, T., Hansen, O.N. and Grandjean, P. (1988b) Bias from non-participation: a study of low-level lead exposure. Scand. J. Med. (in press)

Lyngbye, T., Hansen, O.N. and Grandjean, P. (1988c) Neurological deficits in children: medical risk factors. Neurotoxicol. Teratol. (in press)

Lyngbye, T., Hansen, O.N., Trillingsgaard, A., Beese, I. and Grandjean, P. (1988d) The significance of low-level lead-exposure for the need for special teaching in school children:

an evaluation of confounding factors (in preparation)

McNeil, J.L., Ptasnik, J.A. and Croft, D.B. (1975) Evaluation of long-term effects of elevated blood lead concentrations in asymptomatic children. *Arch. Ind. Hyg. Toxicol.*, **26**, suppl 27

Needleman, H.L., Gunnoe, L.A., Leviton, A., Reed, R., Peresie, H., Maher, C. and Barrett, P. (1979) Deficits in psychologic and classroom performance of children with elevated dentine lead levels. *N. Engl. J. Med.*, **300**, 689–695

Perino, J. and Ernhart, C.B. (1974) The relation of subclinical lead level to cognitive and sensorimotor impairment in black preschoolers. *J. Learn. Dis.*, **7**, 26–30

Rutter, M. (1980) Raised lead levels and impaired cognitive/behavioural functioning: a review of the evidence. *Dev. Med. Child Neurol.*, **22**, suppl. 42

Schlange, H., Stein, B., Boetticher, J. and Taneli, S. (1972) *Göttinger Form-reproduktons test (G-F-T) Handbuch.* (Göttingen: Hogrefe)

Shapiro, I.M. and Marecek, J. (1984) Dentine lead concentration as a predictor of neuropsychological functioning in inner-city children. *Biol. Trace Elem. Res.*, **6**, 69–78

Smith, M., Delves, T., Lansdown, R., Clayton, B. and Graham, P. (1983) The effects of lead exposure on urban children: The Institute of Child Health/Southampton study. *Dev. Med. Child Neurol.*, **25**, 1–54

Thatcher, R.W., Lester, M.L., McAlaster, R. and Ignasias, S.W. (1983) Intelligence and lead toxins in rural children. *J. Learn. Dis.*, **16**, 355–359

Trillingsgaard, A., Hansen, O.N. and Beese, I. (1985) Environmental Health Document 3, *Neurobehavioural Methods in Occupational and Environmental Health* (Copenhagen: World Health Organization), pp. 189–193

Wechsler, D. (1974) *Wechsler Intelligence Scale for Children, Danish version* (Copenhagen: Dansk Psykologisk Forlag)

Winneke, G., Hrdina, K.G. and Brockhaus, A. (1982a) Neuropsychological studies in children with elevated tooth-lead concentrations, I: Pilot study. *Int. Arch. Occup. Environ. Health*, **51**, 169–183

Winneke, G., Kramer, U., Brockhaus, A., Ewers, U., Kujanek, G., Lechner, H. and Janke, W. (1982b) Neuropsychological studies in children with elevated tooth-lead concentrations. II: Extended study. *Int. Arch. Occup. Environ. Health*, **51**, 231–252

Yule, W., Lansdown, R., Miller, I.B. and Urbanowicz, M.A. (1981) The relationship between blood lead concentrations, Intelligence and attainment in a school population: a pilot study. *Dev. Med. Child Neurol.*, **23**, 567–576

3.8

A Regression Analysis Study of the Brussels Lead and IQ Data

R. J. G. CLUYDTS and A. STEENHOUT

SUMMARY

This paper presents the results of a stepwise regression analysis on the tooth lead and psychological data of 41 children living in the greater Brussels area.

Age, gender and socioeconomical status were treated as confounding variables.

The increase in the explained variance due to whole tooth lead level was only limited and reached a 10% significance level only for the number of errors in the simple visual reaction time test, the WISC-R performance test, more specificly for the block design and picture arrangement subtest, as well as for the number of errors in the Toulouse–Piéron attention task.

In this paper, we present the results of a regression analysis which was performed on the data gathered in the Brussels lead and behaviour study. Preliminary results, not controlling for confounding variables, were reported at the Heavy Metals Conference in Athens in 1985 (Cluydts *et al.*, 1985).

A stepwise multiple regression analysis entering successively the most important confounders, with the lead exposure measure entered as the last explanatory variable, was chosen because it allows us to assess its additional contribution and its importance.

SUBJECTS AND METHODS

Forty-one children (21 girls and 20 boys) with a mean age of 9.52 years (range 8.42–11.03 years) were tested with a (neuro-)psychological test battery. Most of the testing was carried out in schools during normal teaching periods.

251

The subjects were selected from a group of 90 eligible children as parents' written agreement to testing had been obtained.

Exclusion criteria included: problematic pregnancy, premature or abnormal delivery, birth weight under 2.5 kg, perinatal complications, severe childhood diseases with or without hospitalization, (residual) fine motor or perceptual problems, attendance at special 'task' classes for extra teaching, and also some familial factors, such as parental divorce, or psychiatric disease or subnormal intelligence in one of the parents.

The sample was thus a very homogeneous one, made up of children attending primary school, having no educational problems, and living in the vicinity of Brussels. The homogeneity is further evidenced by the socioeconomic status data; this factor was assessed using an occupational prestige scale and showed our sample to be in the middle and upper classes.

As an index of lead exposure, the whole tooth lead level was used. This was measured by the Department of Sciences under the responsibility of Dr A. Steenhout. The median value of our sample was $7.125\ \mu g\ g^{-1}$ with a range of $0.2-23.44\ \mu g\ g^{-1}$. The 10th percentile was at 2.07 and the 90th percentile at $11.90\ \mu g\ g^{-1}$. For the whole sample of Dr Steenhout's epidemiological study in Brussels ($n = 337$), from which our study sample was drawn, the median was at 6.33, the 10th percentile was at 2.03 and the 90th at $15.18\ \mu g\ g^{-1}$ (Steenhout, 1983).

Psychological testing was carried out by two trained clinical child psychology students in their final year. They were 'blind' to the lead level when testing the children. The testing was done on Tuesdays to Fridays, always in the morning, in two sessions with a 20-minute break in between. The tests used were: (in a fixed order) the full WISC-R, alternating verbal and performance subtests, the Bender Gestalt test in its GFT-form, a visuomotor test, a simple visual reaction time test and a sustained attention test, the Toulouse–Piéron.

RESULTS

A stepwise multiple regression analysis (SPSS-X) was run on the data, entering successively age, gender, socioeconomic class, and whole tooth lead. In the table below we present the equation coefficients with their corresponding T-value and its significance. The (variance) explained after each step in the analysis is shown on the right hand side.

DISCUSSION

As can be inferred from this overview of some important psychological variables, few increases in the explained variance due to the tooth lead level reach the 5% level of significance; only the number of errors in the simple reaction time test is significantly related to the lead level. However, the relationship is a discordant one which needs further exploration. On the other hand, if a 10% level of statistical significance is accepted, there is some indication of a relationship between the tooth lead level and the WISC-R

Table 1 Equation coefficients and explained variance by the independent variables for some selected psychological test results

	Coefficient	T	p	R^2 incr. (%)	Total R^2	p
1/reaction time (speed)						
Age	3.41E−04	2.89	0.006	18.98	18.98	0.004
Gender	8.96E−06	0.06	0.95	00.01	18.99	0.99
SES	3.60E−07	0.07	0.94	00.03	19.01	0.91
PbT (log)	−1.47E−04	−0.53	0.60	00.63	19.64	0.60
Cte	−1.23E−04					
Number of errors in RT test (log)						
Age	0.70	1.27	0.21	04.22	04.22	0.20
Gender	0.50	0.78	0.44	00.48	04.70	0.66
SES	−8.37E−04	−0.37	0.72	00.04	04.74	0.90
PbT (log)	−0.39	−3.06	0.004	19.63	24.37	0.004
Cte	−0.08					
Total WISC-R IQ						
Age	−3.05	−1.02	0.31	02.78	02.78	0.30
Gender	−3.27	−0.89	0.38	03.11	05.89	0.27
SES	0.10	0.77	0.44	01.75	07.64	0.41
PbT (log)	−5.62	−0.80	0.43	01.62	09.26	0.43
Cte	133.59					
Verbal WISC-R IQ						
Age	−3.03	−1.09	0.28	03.39	03.39	0.25
Gender	−2.84	−0.83	0.41	02.57	05.96	0.31
SES	0.14	1.21	0.24	03.65	09.61	0.23
PbT (log)	0.35	0.05	0.96	00.01	09.62	0.96
Cte	123.43					
Performance WISC-R IQ						
Age	−2.87	−0.88	0.38	01.87	01.87	0.39
Gender	−3.04	−0.76	0.45	02.42	04.29	0.33
SES	0.03	0.22	0.83	00.27	04.56	0.75
PbT (log)	−11.28	−1.48	0.15	05.47	10.03	0.15
Cte	141.82					
Block design subtest WISC-R						
Age	−0.85	−1.00	0.33	02.29	02.29	0.35
Gender	−0.27	−0.28	0.78	00.76	03.05	0.59
SES	0.16	0.44	0.66	00.79	03.84	0.58
PbT (log)	−3.49	−1.73	0.09	07.40	11.24	0.09
Cte	21.09					
Number of errors in the Toulouse–Piéron test (log)						
Age	−0.13	−1.02	0.32	02.71	02.71	0.30
Gender	−2.23E−04	0.00	0.99	00.24	02.95	0.76
SES	0.00	−0.73	0.47	01.82	04.77	0.41
PbT (log)	0.50	1.74	0.09	07.40	12.17	0.09
Cte	1.73					
Bender Gestalt (GFT scoring)						
Age	2.18	1.29	0.21	03.77	03.77	0.22
Gender	−3.63	−1.74	0.09	07.34	11.11	0.08
SES	−0.02	−0.22	0.83	00.12	11.24	0.82
PbT (log)	0.36	−0.09	0.93	00.02	11.26	0.93
Cte	32.88					

performance IQ, in the picture arrangement (not shown on the table), block design and coding subtests, and with the number of errors in the Toulouse–Piéron test. In the reaction time test the total number of errors is very limited (only 1 to 2 errors), whereas on the Toulouse–Piéron test more errors (a mean of 6–10 errors) were made.

In conclusion, our data suggest that a small, but clinically significant, effect of lead is detectable on some cognitive measures, although it does not reach the accepted 5% level of statistical significance. The size of this very homogeneous low-exposure group must be increased to confirm the suggested relationship.

REFERENCES

Cluydts, R., Steenhout, A. and Vandenbreede, S. (1985). Explorative study on the neuropsychological effects of lead in Belgian urban children. In Lekkas, T.D. (ed.) *Heavy Metals in the Environment*, Vol. 1. (Edinburgh: CEP Consultants)

Steenhout, A. (1983). *L'exposition Cumulative au Plomb dans la Population Bruxelloise.* (Brussels: University Press (PUB))

3.9
The Sydney Study of Health Effects of Lead in Urban Children

W. G. McBRIDE, C. J. CARTER, J. R. BRATEL, G. COONEY and A. BELL

SUMMARY

The overall objective of this longitudinal study is to examine the relationship between low to moderate levels of lead in the environment and the neuropsychological and behavioural development of children from newborn to age five years. Children ($n = 440$) born in Sydney, Australia, hospitals to mothers of widely varying socioeconomic backgrounds were recruited into the study, starting in 1982. A variety of physical and psychological development measures, e.g. the Bayley Scales of Infant Development, were administered at 6, 12 and 24 months of age, and the McCarthy Scales of Children's Abilities were administered at 3, 4 and 5 years. Measures of several potential confounding variables (e.g. parental IQ, occupation, age of parents, birth order, HOME scores) were also obtained for use in statistical analyses of possible relationships between the physical and psychological development measures and maternal, cord, and postnatal (6, 12, 18, 24, 30, 36 month) blood lead levels. Preliminary analyses to date have shown no statistically significant associations between any of the Bayley cognitive, psychomotor or behavioural measures and blood lead levels, averaging 9.74 µg/dl (maternal), 8.36 µg/dl (cord), and 13 to 18 µg/dl (postnatal).

There is no argument that excessively high blood lead (PbB) levels adversely affect the neuropsychological development of children. However, despite the considerable research conducted in this area there is still considerable controversy on what constitutes 'excessively high blood lead levels'. In his survey of the research prior to 1980, Rutter (1980) concluded that 'The evidence suggests that persistently raised blood lead levels in the range of 40 µg/dl may cause slight cognitive impairment and, less certainly, may increase the risk of behavioural difficulties.'

Research in the early 1980s did not fully clarify the issue further, as results from several published studies were ambiguous (Harvey, 1984; Rutter, 1983; Bornschein et al., 1980; Medical Research Council, 1984). The ambiguous results stemmed partly from the different designs and methodologies used, and partly from the complexity of the relationship itself.

The Sydney study was one of several longitudinal studies commenced in the early 1980s designed to investigate the effects of lead in children from birth to 5 years and to help resolve earlier ambiguities in the literature on low-level lead exposure effects. This report presents information on the design of the Sydney study and preliminary results from initial data analyses.

DESIGN AND SUBJECTS

The Sydney study commenced in April 1982 with the recruitment of 318 children, over a 12-month period, from three Sydney hospitals. There was considerable range in the demographic characteristics of the parents and in the type of socioeconomic areas in which they lived. A second cohort of 123 children was recruited to increase the number of children in the total study.

The study was designed to monitor the infants' development over a 5-year period with 6-monthly blood samples being taken from each infant to determine PbB levels, and a variety of physical and psychological measures taken at 6 months, 12 months and hence at 12-month intervals.

Measures chosen were comparable with those used in the other longitudinal studies being conducted: The Bayley Scales of Infant Development (1969) were used to measure mental and psychomotor development at 6 months, 12 months and 24 months; the Bayley Infant Behaviour Record and the Toddler Temperament Questionnaire (Fullard et al., 1978) to monitor behavioural problems. At 3 years the McCarthy Scales of Children's Abilities (1972) replaced the Bayley Scales, and this test was employed also at 4 years and, currently, at 5 years. At 5 years a special computer vigilance task is being employed to assess attention span and attain reaction time measures. (This task was written by Jacobson and Jacobson at Wayne State University, Detroit, USA.)

Because the neuropsychological development of children is determined by many factors, including health, heredity, maternal IQ, diet, socioeconomic factors, and quality of the home environment, data were collected on these aspects as well.

Standard demographic measures (parental IQ, education, occupation, age of parents, birth order, the Family Cleanliness Scale, etc.) have been employed, together with the HOME Inventory (Caldwell and Bradley, 1984), and questions on diet, pica and health. These variables are being used, where appropriate, as covariates to control for confounding factors and hence isolate the portion, if any, of the observed neuropsychological relationships which can be regarded as genuinely attributable to effects of lead, as illustrated in Figure 1.

Neither parents nor the research psychologists were aware of the actual PbB levels of the children. Where PbB levels are regarded as high (originally

256

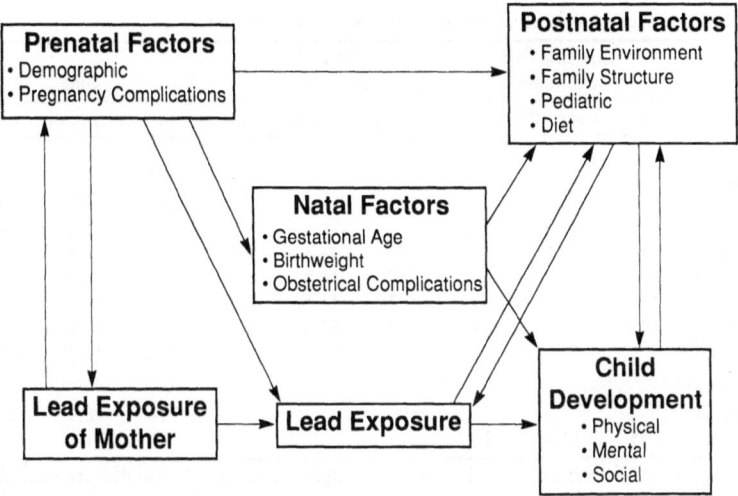

Figure 1 Modelled relationships between sets of variables being evaluated in the Sydney Study

equal to or greater than 30 μg/dl, now 25 μg/dl) a second blood sample is taken and analysed. If this also is high, appropriate clinical tests are carried out on the child. All blood collections and testing were carried out in the children's homes.

DATA COLLECTION

Table 1 details the attrition figures with associated reasons from the initial cohort of 318 children recruited into the study.

Table 1 Reasons for attrition of subjects from original cohort

Moved – cannot trace	24
Personal reasons	9
Blood tests	13
Moved overseas, interstate, or out of metropolitan area	28
No phone – letter unanswered	6
English not first language	10
No phone (initially it was decided not to include subjects without a phone)	1
Not followed up from pilot study	6
Premature baby	1
Mother thinks baby is doing OK	1
Baby is chronically ill – cannot be bled	2
Baby has severe developmental delay	1
Several appointments made, but not kept by mothers	1
Total remaining	211

Table 2 Blood lead levels obtained for both cohorts of children

	Capillary PbB concentrations			Venous PbB concentrations			Total		
	n	$\bar{x}$ (μg/dl)	SD	n	$\bar{x}$ (μg/dl)	SD	n	$\bar{x}$ (μg/dl)	SD
First cohort									
Maternal							299	9.47	2.73
Cord							298	8.36	3.08
6 months	245	16.8	9.1				245	16.71	9.07
12 months	154	18.1	6.5	99	14.4	6.5	253	16.65	6.78
18 months	132	19.2	8.3	120	16.8	8.2*	252	17.99	8.34
24 months	107	17.7	6.7	132	15.5	7.5*	239	16.52	7.22
30 months	43	17.5	6.0	184	13.4	5.5	227	14.22	5.86
36 months				218	12.95	5.1	218	13.75	5.86
Second cohort									
Maternal							114	8.9	2.40
6 months	85	11.4	3.73				85	11.4	3.73

* The large standard deviations for the venous samples at 18 and 24 months are caused by two outliers, one at 18 months (79 μg/dl) and one at 24 months (59 μg/dl). With these removed the standard deviations are 5.9 and 6.4 respectively

ANALYSIS OF DATA

From the initial cohort of 318 subjects a total of 211 remained in the study as at the completion of collection of 4-year data. From the second cohort of 123 children a total of 117 remained as at the completion of collection of the 12-month data. In addition to calculating summary statistics, preliminary regression analyses have been conducted to assess relationships between measures of physical and neuropsychological development and PbB or the other above-mentioned types of potentially confounding covariates.

BLOOD LEAD LEVELS

Table 2 shows the basic descriptive statistics for PbB levels over time for both cohorts, classified by method of collection.

RELATIONSHIPS BETWEEN BLOOD LEAD LEVELS AND NEUROPSYCHOLOGICAL MEASURES

The preliminary analyses completed at this stage show no significant relationship between the PbB levels and any of the Bayley cognitive, psychomotor or behavioural measures. There are the expected correlations between these and maternal characteristics such as maternal IQ, and between the Bayley scales and parenting characteristics as measured by the HOME Inventory at 6 months and 12 months. The relationships between the Bayley M.D.I. and the HOME Inventory are stronger at 12 months than 6 months. Correlations between parenting characteristics and PbB levels are small and also not significant.

REFERENCES

Bayley, N. (1969) *Manual for the Bayley Scales of Infant Development*, (Ohio: Psychological Corporation)

Bornschein, R., Pearson, D. and Reiter, L. (1980) Behavioural effects of moderate lead exposure in children and animal models. *CRD Rev. Toxicol.*, November

Caldwell, B.M. and Bradley, R.H. (1984) *Administration Manual, Revised Edition, H.O.M.E.* (Little Rock, Ark: University of Arkansas)

Fullard, W., McDevitt, S.C. and Carey, W.G. (1978) *The Toddler Temperament Questionnaire.* (available from the authors)

Harvey, P.G. (1984) Lead and children's health: recent research and future questions, *J. Child Psychol. Psychiatry*, **25**, 517–522

McCarthy, D. (1972) *Manual: McCarthy Scales of Children's Abilities*, (Ohio: Psychological Corporation)

Medical Research Council (1984) *The Neuropsychological Effects of Lead in Children, a review of recent research; 1979–1983*

Rutter, M. (1980) Raised lead levels and impaired cognitive/behavioural functioning: a review of the evidence. *Dev. Med. Child Neurol.*, **22** (Suppl. 42)

Rutter, M. (1983) Low level lead exposure: sources, effects and implications. In Rutter, M. and Russell-Jones, R. (eds), *Lead versus Health* (Chichester: Wiley)

3.10
Follow-up Studies in Lead-Exposed Children

G. WINNEKE, W. COLLET, U. KRÄMER, A. BROCKHAUS,
T. EWERT and C. KRAUSE

SUMMARY

Seventy-six children out of 114 first tested at age 6 in 1982 were retested in 1985 at age 9. The range of blood lead values had been 3.9–22.8 μg/dl in 1982 ($x_g = 8.2$) and was 4.4–21.4 μg/dl ($x_g = 7.8$) in 1985; tooth lead concentrations were also available ($x_g = 4.68\,\mu$g/g; 1.8–28.2). Neuropsychological testing (WISC-R, Bender Gestalt test, Vienna Reaction Device and Delayed Reaction Times) and neurophysiological testing (sensory nerve conduction velocities = NCV and visual evoked potentials = VEP) was repeated in this group of children. Consistent associations with lead exposure (blood and teeth) after correction for confounding were, again, established for performance on the Vienna Reaction Device and for VEP latencies. Few significant but inconsistent associations were found for intelligence, delayed reaction times and NCV. These results are compatible with the hypothesis that some effects of lead on the CNS do not disappear with ageing over 3 years, if exposure remains unchanged.

Lead-induced neurobehavioural deficit has been found to be persistent in several animal species, if exposure occurs during the early stages of brain maturation (Winneke, 1986; Lilienthal et al., 1986). Little evidence exists, however, to show that this holds true for children as well. Follow-up studies provide a means to test this possibility. Few such studies have been performed so far: Otto and co-workers, using event-related brain potentials as the endpoint, found some persistence of lead-related alteration upon re-testing of the same children after 2 years (Otto et al., 1982) but not after 5 years (Otto et al. (1985). Likewise Schroeder et al. (1985) were unable to replicate exposure-related IQ deficit in a 5-year follow-up study. In both studies blood lead (PbB) values had declined during the test–retest interval from markedly elevated initial levels, to rather low levels at retesting.

The present study represents another effort to test the hypothesis of the persistence of lead-related neurobehavioural deficit by retesting a group of children after an interval of 3 years, using a broad spectrum of neuropsychological and neurophysiological end-point measures. The results of the initial testing at age 6 have been published elsewhere (Winneke *et al.*, 1985; Ewert *et al.*, 1986).

MATERIAL AND METHODS

The follow-up study resembled the first study as closely as possible. This was true for the general procedure, the set of outcome measures and confounding variables, the methodology and laboratory of blood lead (PbB) determination, as well as for the statistical evaluation. Some changes in terms of testing personnel, as well as place and time of testing, were unavoidable, however. Whereas the initial study was conducted in September/October 1982, the follow-up testing and blood sampling took place in June 1985.

Study area

The city of Nordenham is a seaport of about 33 000 inhabitants, located on the mouth of the river Weser, in the northern part of the Federal Republic of Germany. A large lead–zinc smelter is the source of airborne lead pollution in the area. Since about 1974 different strata of the population have been screened for indications of undue lead absorption by the Federal Health Office (Berlin). One such screening programme represents the basis of both the initial and the follow-up study.

Sample

The basic sample consisted of those 122 children first tested in 1982. Seventy-six of these (62%) agreed to participate in the follow-up testing. In order to check for possible self-selection bias, participating and non-participating children were compared for all available variables. Binary variables, tested by means of the chi^2-statistic, included social and biological–medical background information as follows: sex, social status, occupation, education and income, family size and birth order, marital status of mother, pregnancy and delivery information, such as infections, smoking, alcohol consumption and drug intake, anaemia, prematurity, and the Apgar score, as well as mouthing behaviour during childhood. Continuous variables, tested by means of the t-test, included age, perinatal and 1982 blood and tooth lead values, as well as outcome variables from the initial study, such as IQ values, errors and hits on the Vienna Reaction Device, Bender test scores, and delayed reaction times. None of these comparisons yielded significant differences, thus allowing the conclusion that self-selection bias cannot be considered important.

Markers of lead exposure

Blood lead concentrations from venous samples were measured in the same laboratory of the Federal Health Office (Berlin) using the Delves cup method (Delves, 1970) with atomic absorption spectrophotometry (AAS). For 50 out of the 76 children for whom shed incisor teeth were available from the 1982 sample, lead concentrations were measured by the AAS method described elsewhere (Ewers et al., 1982). This will be considered as a second marker of cumulative long-term lead exposure.

Outcome measures

The complete set of data included neuropsychological as well as neurophysiological measures, most of which had already been taken in our previous study (Winneke et al., 1985). The test procedures were the same, unless otherwise stated.

General intelligence was, again, estimated from only four subtests of the Wechsler Intelligence Scale for Children (WISC), the German version of which is the 'Hamburg Wechsler Intelligenztest für Kinder (HAWIK)'. In contrast to the previous study, however, the revised and restandardized German version, called HAWIK-R (Tewes, 1983), was available this time. The same four subtests – vocabulary, comprehension, picture completion and block design – were again selected. For the assessment of visual-motor integration the Bender Gestalt test with the German scoring system of the 'Göttinger Form Reproduktionstest (GFT)' (Schlange et al., 1972) was used again. Delayed reaction times (RT) were, as before, measured using the modified 'Leeds Psychomotor Tester' (Zak GmbH, Simbach/Inn, FRG) as follows: after 3 (RT-3) or 10 (RT-10) seconds delay following a tone signal, one predetermined light from a semicircular arrangement of lights was switched on, and this had to be switched off by touching the corresponding response button. Lift-off as well as push-button latencies were measured across 10 signal presentations.

Complex reaction performance was measured by means of the Vienna Reaction Device (Klebelsberg, 1960). This is a serial reaction test, in which subjects are given a quasi-random sequence of 180 light or tone signals in a row, which have to be responded to by pressing the appropriate button. Hits, late responses, and errors are recorded for a given signal sequence (Winneke et al., 1985). Two levels of task difficulty, namely slow vs. fast signal speed, were chosen, the task being more difficult than in the former study in order to account for the age increase. The slow signal sequence had inter-stimulus intervals (ISI) of 1.39 s (version 9), and the faster sequence (version 7) intervals of 1.08 s.

Neurophysiological measures were taken as described elsewhere (Ewert et al., 1986). Distal sensory nerve conduction velocities (NCV) were recorded by means of a two-channel-1500 digital-EMG-system (DISA) for N. radialis and N. medianus, and skin temperatures at the recording site were kept between 36 and 37°C by infrared heating. Visual evoked potentials (VEP) were measured for electrode positions OZ-FZ (10–20 system), using checkerboard reversal-stimulation at 2 Hz frequency and averages across 128 sweeps.

Latencies of components N_2, P_2 and N_3, as well as amplitudes N_2–P_2, were evaluated (Figure 1).

General procedure

Two psychologists and a medical technician were responsible for the psychological and neurophysiological testing, respectively. Blood sampling by venepuncture was done by a physician at the end of a test session; none of the testing-staff was aware of the individual child's previous PbB values. One test session lasted for about 120 min and was subdivided into three blocks of outcome variables, namely intelligence and RT assessment, reaction and Bender Gestalt performance, and neurophysiological testing. Three children were examined simultaneously; each of them was assigned to one out of six possible block sequences according to a systematic plan of permutations.

Data analysis

For reasons of comparability the statistical procedures, as well as the set of confounders, were identical to our previous study (Winneke et al., 1985). As before a forced stepwise multiple-regression analysis with the lead exposure

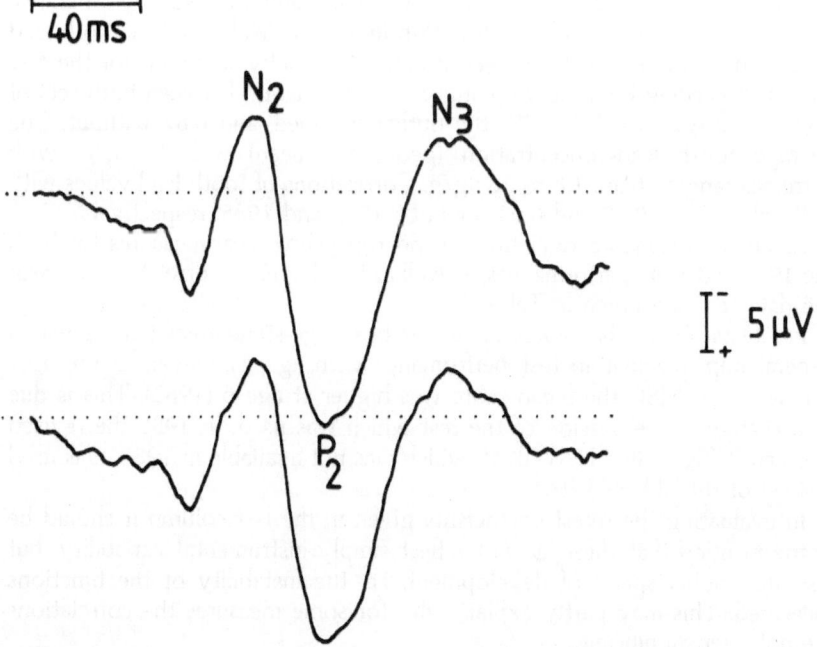

Figure 1 Typical VEP traces with definition of components N_2, P_2 and N_3

variable entered as the last step was the statistical tool. Again, one-tailed probabilities were chosen throughout, because lead-induced neurobehavioural deficit was the directional hypothesis to be tested. Age, sex and social hereditary background (SHB) were entered as confounders. This latter SHB variable had resulted from a large set of 59 potential confounders tested for association with PbB; only occupational status and qualification of the father had been found to exhibit significant and consistent association with the exposure variable. Since, however, there was almost complete overlap for these two variables, occupational status of the father alone was taken to represent the SHB variable. A child was given a score of 1 if the father was classified as an unskilled worker; otherwise he or she was given the SHB score of 0.

RESULTS

The following statistical considerations are based on the subset of 76 children who participated in both the 1982 and the 1985 studies.

Descriptive statistics

Geometric means and standard deviations of the 1985 PbB values were 7.8 $\pm$ 1.4 μg/dl, with extremes ranging from 4.4 to 21.4 μg/dl. The cumulative frequency distributions of the 1985 and 1982 PbB values, as well as the correlation diagram, are given in Figure 2. The outlier, marked by an empty circle in the diagram, had had a low PbB in 1982 as well as a low tooth lead level, and was found to have been involved in hobby soldering for the few months preceding the follow-up study. The correlation between both sets of PbB values was $r = 0.76$ with the outlier included, and 0.82 without. The average tooth lead-concentration (geometric mean) was 4.7 μg/g, with extremes ranging from 1.8 to 28 μg/g. Correlations of tooth lead values with PbB values were 0.57 and 0.63 for PbBs 1982 and 1985, respectively.

Means and standard deviations of neuropsychological measures for both the 1982 and 1985 performances, as well as the degree of correlation between the data sets, are given in Table 1.

For tests where the scores have not been age-standardized there was a general improvement in test performance with age. However, in the age-standardized WISC the mean score was higher at age 6 (1982). This is due to a change in the version of the test which was used. In 1985 the revised German WISC, called HAWIK-R, which was not available in 1982, was used instead of the old HAWIK.

In evaluating the retest coefficients given in the last column it should be borne in mind that these do not reflect simply instrumental variability, but also differential speed of development, i.e. the instability of the functions measured. This may partly explain why for some measures the correlations are not even significant.

Means and standard deviations of neurophysiological measures taken in 1982 and 1985, as well as the stability coefficients, are given in Table 2;

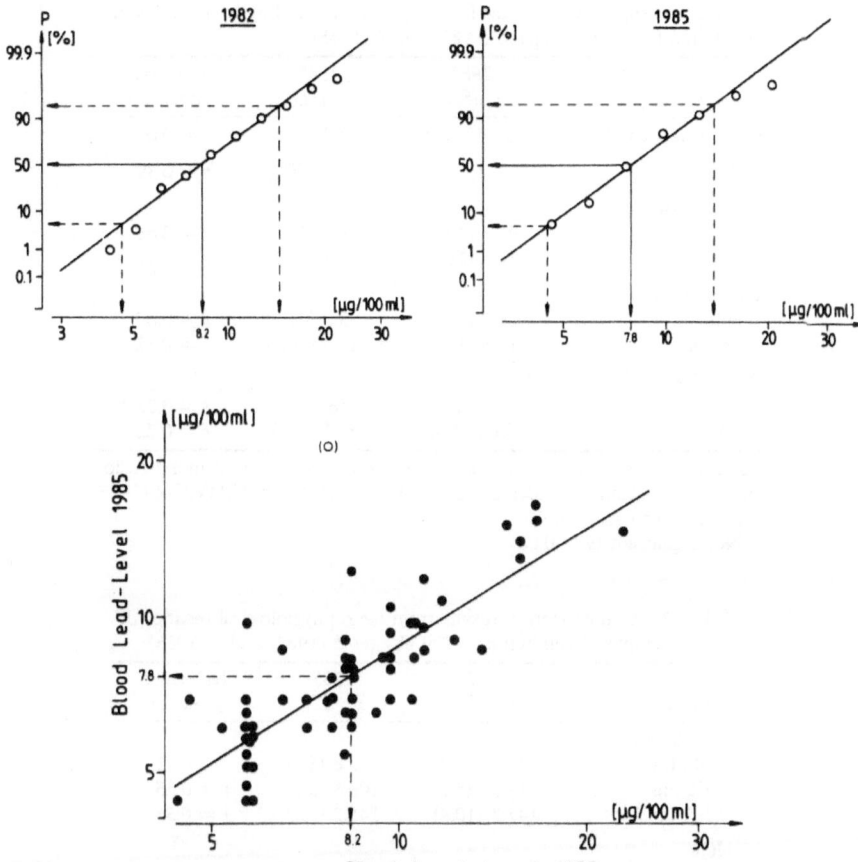

Figure 2 Frequency distributions of PbB concentrations at age 6 (1982) and age 9 (1985), as well as the correlation diagram

definition of VEP components may be taken from Figure 1.

Contrary to the psychological test scores (Table 1) there was no pronounced age-related change of mean values between 1982 and 1985. Test–retest correlations for VEP latencies and sensory nerve conduction velocities (NCV) are, again, only low to moderate, and even insignificant for sensory NCV of the radial nerve.

Inferential statistics

The main results from stepwise multiple-regression analysis for the lead exposure variables are given in Tables 3 (neuropsychological measures) and 4 (neurophysiological measures). The information given in these tables is the percentage variance additionally explained by the lead exposure variable after correction for confounding. Downward and upward arrows, taken from the sign of the regression coefficient, indicate the direction of covariation, namely

Table 1 Comparison of results from psychological testing for the subsample of children ($n = 76$) at ages 6 (1982) and 9 (1985)

Variable	1982 $\bar{x}_g$ (SD)	1985 $\bar{x}_g$ (SD)	Test–retest correlation
WISC total score*	51.4 (8.6)	36.7 (7.3)	$r = 0.60$
GFT errors	30.1 (4.0)	17.0 (5.2)	$r = 0.39$
Vienna (slow)			
Hits	95.3 (29.5)	139.9 (33.3)	$r = 0.65$
Errors	16.5 (15.1)	6.3 (7.3)	$r = 0.28$
Vienna (fast)			
Hits	65.2 (30.8)	75.0 (41.7)	$r = 0.69$
Errors	19.6 (17.6)	10.6 (10.2)	$r = 0.32$
Delayed RT (ms)			
3 s	561 (213)	368 (62.0)	$r = 0.23$**
10 s	864 (404)	532 (195)	$r = 0.22$**

* Sum of age-standardized scores from subtests vocabulary, comprehension, picture completion and block design of HAWIK (1982) or HAWIK-R (1985). Expected mean score is 40
** Not significant ($p > 0.05$)

Table 2 Comparison of results from neurophysiological testing for the subsample of children ($n = 76$) at ages 6 (1982) and 9 (1985)

Variable	1982 $\bar{x}_g$ (SD)	1985 $\bar{x}_g$ (SD)	Test–retest correlation
VEP (latencies)			
N2 (ms)	77.3 (4.4)	77.8 (5.4)	$r = 0.41$
P2 (ms)	111.9 (5.6)	109.5 (5.7)	$r = 0.55$
N3 (ms)	147.7 (10.4)	145.2 (8.2)	$r = 0.33$
NCV			
N. med. (m/s)	53.4 (5.5)	53.8 (5.0)	$r = 0.47$
N. rad. (m/s)	54.5 (5.2)	52.4 (4.8)	$r = 0.23$*

* Not significant ($p > 0.05$)

an increase (upward) or decrease (downward) of the respective variable with increasing lead exposure. Markers of lead exposure considered here are the PbB values measured in 1982 and 1985, as well as tooth lead concentrations (PbT) being available for only 50 children from the subsample of 76. Teeth were collected in 1982/83.

Neuropsychological measures
As for intelligence estimated from the four subtests of the WISC-R (HAWIK-R) significant negative association with lead exposure was observed at age 9 (1985) with respect to the earlier but not to the current PbB; at age 6 (1982) no such association was found. With respect to PbT the reverse was true: a negative association at age 6, no such finding at age 9.

Deficit of visual motor integration, as assessed by means of the Bender test (GFT), was found to be associated in a significant manner with PbB and PbT at age 6, but not at age 9. In general, however, the error score increased

Table 3 Results of stepwise multiple-regression analysis of neuropsychological measures for the lead exposure variables after correction for confounding

Testing: Lead marker:	1982 PbB–1982	1985 PbB–1982	1985 PbB–1985	1982 PbT–82/83	1985 PbT–82/83
WISC: Four subtests	↓0.3	↓4.4**	↑1.3	↓8.5**	0.0
GFT: Errors	↑6.6***	↑1.6	↑0.8	↑13.4***	↑2.2
Vienna (LS): Hits	↓1.9	↓0.9	↓0.1	↓6.4**	↓3.4*
Vienna (LS): Errors	↑4.3**	↑4.2**	↑1.3	↑4.3*	↑1.7
Vienna (HS): Hits	↓3.7**	↓4.3**	↓2.3*	↓3.3*	↓3.3*
Vienna (HS): Errors	↑14.3***	↑6.8***	↑6.0**	↑9.9**	↑3.6*
Delayed RT (3 s): lift-off latencies	0.0	↑2.6*	↑1.2	↑10.9**	↑19.3***
Delayed RT (10 s): lift-off latencies	↑0.4	↑4.9**	↑1.3	↓0.4	12.5***

$* \ p < 0.10; \quad ** \ p < 0.05; \quad *** \ p < 0.01$ (one-tailed)

Percentage additional variance explained by lead exposure is given; ↑ or ↓, taken from the regression coefficients, indicate the direction of change

with increasing levels of lead exposure. As for reaction performance on the Wiener Reaction Device for slow (LS) and high (HS) signal speed, significant disruption was associated with lead exposure for both hits and errors at ages 6 (1982) and 9 (1985), with respect to PbB and PbT levels. Hits decreased and errors increased with increasing values of the exposure variables, although the degree of association was typically higher for errors than for hits. In addition the effects were typically more pronounced for the difficult (HS) as opposed to the easier version (LS), and somewhat smaller at age 9 (1985) than at age 6 (1982).

As for the outcome of neurophysiological testing (Table 4) fewer significant associations with lead exposure were observed for sensory nerve conduction velocities (NCV) of peripheral nerves as opposed to measures of central visual processing taken from characteristics of the visual evoked potential (pattern reversal). Generally speaking VEP latencies decreased with increasing lead

Table 4 Results of stepwise multiple-regression analysis of neurophysiological measures for the lead exposure variables after correction for confounding

Testing: Lead marker:	1982 PbB–1982	1985 PbB–1982	1985 PbB–1985	1982 PbT–82/83	1985 PbT–82/83
VEP					
N_2 Latency	↓7.3*	↓3.5	↓1.9	↓3.0	↓1.4
P_2 Latency	↓5.4*	↓3.9*	↓3.4	↓3.4	↓1.4
N_3 Latency	↓2.5	↓0.1	↓0.4	↓7.5*	↓1.5
N_2/P_2 Amplitude	↑0.5	↓0.5	↓0.3	–	↓3.4
NCV					
N. medianus: velocity	↑1.2	↑0.9	↑0.9	↑0.6	↑0.3
N. radialis: velocity	↑6.4*	↑1.8	↑1.7	↑4.9	0.0

$* \ p < 0.10; \quad ** \ p < 0.05$ (two-tailed)

Percentage additional variance explained by lead exposure is given; arrows were taken from the regression coefficients

exposure, and this was true for ages 6 (1982) and 9 (1985), at least for components N_2 and P_2. In partial agreement with this finding sensory nerve conduction velocities increased with increasing lead exposure, significant only at age 6 (1982) for the radial nerve.

DISCUSSION

Testing for the persistence of neurobehavioural effects of lead exposure, strictly speaking, requires retesting of the same cohort of children after discontinuation of exposure and concomitant substantial decline of PbB concentrations. This can hardly be achieved in an epidemiological study design, but is typically done in experimental approaches using animal models (e.g. Munoz et al., 1986). In our cohort PbB concentrations had not changed markedly between 1982 and 1985. If, under these circumstances, similarity of outcome is demonstrated for retesting at age 9 as compared to initial testing at age 6, the hypothesis of constant lead damage for both ages is supported. A demonstration of constant lead damage must be considered a minimum requirement for assuming persistent lead damage. Statistical significance of the observed associations and consistency of effects both across ages, as well as across markers of exposure, will be considered in evaluating outcome and implications of this follow-up study.

As for intelligence the observed associations, although significant for some comparisons, do not seem to be consistent. If the improved psychometric quality of the German WISC-R (HAWIK-R) is considered responsible for the significant findings at age 9 (1985) with respect to PbB, the reverse tendency with respect to PbT levels clearly cannot be explained along these same lines. These findings thus seem to agree more closely with recent observations suggesting lead-related IQ deficit to be associated with PbB levels exceeding 25 μg/dl (Hatzakis et al., this volume).

Although there was a general tendency for GFT errors to increase with increasing lead exposure, which corresponds to previous experience of our group (Winneke et al., 1982, 1983), this effect was no longer observed at age 9 (1985). It should, furthermore, be added that for the total group of 114 children no significant association between GFT errors and lead exposure was shown for PbB at age 6, and only a borderline one for PbT levels (Winneke et al., 1985). These findings are thus difficult to explain within the framework of the reversibility issue. It should be remembered, however, that Bender Gestalt performance is most likely to reflect complex perceptual, attentional and fine motor skills, and that the developmental improvement of the fine motor component might well compensate for a persistent deficit of the perceptual–attentional component.

This tentative argument is partly supported by the findings related to performance at the Vienna Reaction Device. For this set of outcome measures a high degree of consistency of associations was observed at ages 6 and 9, as well as for PbB and PbT levels as markers of past and recent exposure, respectively. In an effort to elucidate the functional validity of performance at the Vienna Device factor analysis of hits, variability of hits and total number of reactions was done within the context of other performance and personality measures (Kallina, 1964). It was shown that performance measures from the Wiener task had highest loadings on a factor identified as 'ability to pay attention'.

In the framework of such findings the conclusion is drawn that low levels of childhood lead exposure as encountered in our sample of Nordenham children are most likely to be associated with subtle attention deficit, and that this deficit does not disappear until age 9 if exposure remains unchanged.

The results from delayed reaction time testing do not exhibit a consistent pattern of associations with the lead exposure variables. Although, generally speaking, reaction times tended to increase with increasing lead exposure, thus supporting similar findings of Needleman *et al.* (1979), this was only true at age 9 (1985) and not at age 6 (1982); a detailed discussion in terms of persistent lead effect for these findings is therefore irrelevant. The outcome may, perhaps, be taken to reflect more reliable reaction time testing at age 9 as opposed to age 6, although additional evidence would be needed to support this hypothesis.

The findings from neurophysiological testing, although internally consistent, are at variance with results from studies based on experimental or occupational lead exposure. Whereas in the present study VEP latencies for components N_2 and P_2 tended to decrease with increasing lead exposure, both at ages 6 and 9, longer VEP latencies and associated amplitude decreases, in a dose-dependent manner were recently observed in lead-exposed monkeys (Lilienthal *et al.*, this volume). This discrepancy is hard to explain, although it should be mentioned that experimental lead exposure was associated with PbB levels around $50\,\mu g/dl$, which is far in excess of the values encountered in the children of our follow-up study. Independent replication of these findings would be necessary, therefore, in order to support the hypothesis of disinhibitory effects at low and inhibitory effects at high levels of lead exposure. This is also true for the unexpected findings regarding sensory nerve conduction velocities, which tended to increase with increasing lead exposure, although significantly so only at age 6 (1982). Studies conducted in lead-exposed workers have typically shown increased PbB levels to be associated with decreasing motor nerve conduction velocities (e.g. Seppaelaeinen *et al.*, 1979). Since, however, this effect did not prove stable in our follow-up study after 3 years, despite essentially unchanged exposure conditions, its validity needs to be checked in larger samples across a wider range of PbB levels.

ACKNOWLEDGMENTS

This work was partly supported by CEC (Brussels) within contract No. ENV 733-D.

REFERENCES

Delves, H.T. (1970) A microsampling method for the rapid determination of lead in blood by atomic absorption spectrophotometry. *Analyst*, **93**, 431–437

Ewers, U., Brockhaus, A., Winneke, G., Freier, I., Jermann, E. and Krämer, U. (1982) Lead in deciduous teeth of children living in a nonferrous smelter area and a rural area of the FRG. *Int. Arch. Occup. Environ. Health*, **50**, 139–151

Ewert, T., Beginn, U., Winneke, G., Hofferberth, B. and Jörg, J. (1986) Sensible Neurographie, visuell und somatosensorisch evozierte Potentiale (VEP und SEP) an bleiexponierten Kindern. *Nervenarzt*, **57**, 465–471

Kallina, H. (1964) 'Validitätsuntersuchung und Faktorenanalyse verkehrspsychologischer, diagnostischer Methoden.' *Z. Exp. Ang. Psychol.*, **9**, 56–70

Klebelsberg, D. (1960) Wiener Determinationsgerät. *Diagnostica*, IV/Heft 4

Lilienthal, H., Winneke, G., Brockhaus, A. and Molik, B. (1986) Pre- and postnatal lead-exposure in monkeys: Effects on activity and learning set formation. *Neurobehav. Toxicol. Teratol.*, **8**, 265–272

Munoz, C., Garbe, K., Lilienthal, H. and Winneke, G. (1986) Persistence of retention deficit in rats after neonatal lead exposure. *Neurotoxicology*, **7**, 569–580

Needleman, H.L., Gunnoe, C., Leviton, A., Reed, R., Peresie, H., Maher, C. and Barrett, P. (1979) Deficits in psychologic and classroom performance of children with elevated dentine lead levels. *N. Engl. J. Med.*, **300**, 689–695

Otto, D., Benignus, V., Muller, K., Barton, C., Seiple, K., Prah, J. and Schroeder, S. (1982) Effects of low to moderate lead exposure on slow cortical potentials in young children: Two-year follow-up study. *Neurobehav. Toxicol. Teratol.*, **4**, 733–737

Otto, D., Robinson, G., Baumann, S., Schroeder, S., Mushak, P., Kleinbaum, D. and Boone, L. (1985) Five-year follow-up study of children with low-to-moderate lead absorption: Electrophysiological evaluation. *Environ. Res.*, **38**, 168–186

Seppaellaeinen, A.M., Hernberg, S. and Kock, B. (1979) Relationship between blood lead-levels and nerve conduction velocities. *Neurotoxicology*, **1**, 313–332

Schlange, H., Stein, B., Boetticher, J. and Tanelli, S. (1972) *Göttinger Formreproduktionstest (G-F-T)*. (Göttingen: Hogrefe)

Schroeder, S., Hawk, B., Otto, D., Mushak, P. and Hicks, R. (1985) Separating the effects of lead and social factors on IQ. *Environ. Res.*, **38**, 144–154

Tewes, U. (1983) HAWIK-R. Hamburg Wechsler Intelligenztest für Kinder. Revision 1983. *Handbuch und Testanweisung*. (Bern u.a. Huber)

Winneke, G. (1986) The effects of lead: animal studies, in: Lansdown, R. and Yule, W. (eds), *The Lead Debate: the environment, toxicology and child health*, (London–Sydney: Croom Helm)

Winneke, G., Hrdina, K.G. and Brockhaus, A. (1982) Neuropsychological studies in children with elevated tooth lead-levels. I. Pilot study using a pair-matching approach. *Int. Arch. Occup. Environ. Health*, **51**, 169–183

Winneke, G., Krämer, U., Brockhaus, A., Ewers, U., Kujanek, G., Lechner, H. and Janke, W. (1983) Neuropsychological studies in children with elevated tooth lead-levels. II. Extended study. *Int. Arch. Occup. Environ. Health*, **51**, 231–252

Winneke, G., Beginn, U., Ewert, T., Havestadt, C., Krämer, U., Krause, C., Thron, H.L. and Wagner, H.M. (1985) Comparing the effects of perinatal and later childhood lead exposure on neuropsychological outcome. *Environ. Res.*, **38**, 155–167

3.11
Automated Assessment of Attention, Vigilance and Learning in Relation to Children's Lead Levels

W. YULE, R. LANSDOWN, M. URBANOWICZ, D. MUDDIMAN
and J. HUNTER

SUMMARY

Earlier studies of the effects of low-level lead exposure in children suggested that attention and activity levels may be adversely affected. A recent study from our group (Hunter et al., 1985) replicated Needleman's finding that reaction time under delayed conditions was related to increased blood levels, especially in younger children. Building on this work, and seeking to develop measures of more subtle effects, six tests have been developed for presentation on microcomputers. As far as possible, tests are administered and scored automatically to reduce tester bias.

Standardization data were collected on 500 children aged 6–11 years, along with measures of general intelligence, educational attainment and classroom behaviour. Immediate, short-term and long-term (3-month or 6-month) test–retest data were obtained on subsamples. The battery is also being used with 78 children whose blood lead levels have recently been assayed. This paper describes the tests, the developmental trends they reveal and their test–retest stability.

The main aim of our studies over the past 3 years has been to develop and standardize tests of attention, vigilance and learning for use with children aged 6 to 11 years – tests which are sensitive to alterations in CNS functioning.

The starting point was an assessment of the then current literature, from which it was concluded that moderately high levels of body lead burden may be associated with an overall lowering of cognitive functioning – equivalent to about 5 IQ points between extreme groups – and with a variety of behavioural deficits, notably in attention and activity level (Lansdown and Yule, 1986).

Unfortunately, both in the lead research area in particular and child development in general, there is little agreement as to what constitutes 'attention' (Taylor, 1980) or how best to measure it. It has been operationalized in a variety of ways, and few paradigms have been properly standardized and normed. For example, it is not immediately obvious what scores on a reaction time task have in common with a test to match familiar figures or a teacher's global rating of 'attending well in class', let alone with auditory evoked potentials or other derived scores from EEGs.

There is interest in developing tests of attention for a further reason. One of the main methodological problems facing studies of the health effects of low-level lead exposure is that of dealing appropriately with confounding social variables (Yule and Rutter, 1985; Yule, 1986). It is recognized that general measures of intelligence and global ratings of children's behaviour are influenced by a variety of social factors, some of which are also related to lead exposure. The aim of studies in this area ought not to be to 'explain away' common variance, but rather to explain it, in the sense of understanding the causal mechanisms, no matter how complicated they are. In the absence of agreed models of the effects of lead on the CNS, there is still little agreement on how best to deal with common variance − the four 'Cs' which get used interchangeably in discussion are Controlling, Confounding, Concomitants and Covariates. Ideally, confounding factors should be dealt with identically in different studies if one is really measuring a biological effect. The move towards more precisely replicated studies is to be welcomed. Replication should help to disentangle which 'confounds' are universal and which are specific to a particular sample, thus paving the way for a better understanding of the effects of social factors on general intelligence and other relevant dependent measures. As was demonstrated at the Imperial College meeting (Urbanowicz et al., 1988) despite using closely similar methods to measure social factors, it was found that they related differently to lead burden and IQ in our samples than they did in the Institute of Child Health/Southampton study (Smith et al., 1983). This questions the interpretation of all unreplicated studies.

Another approach to dealing with this problem is to employ criterion measures which are less influenced than IQ by social factors. Hence the interest in measuring neuropsychological functions such as attention, vigilance, reaction time, evoked potential and power spectral EEG analysis. These are presumably less influenced by social factors, but they probably are influenced by factors such as diet, and by whether the child is tense or relaxed.

A further reason for developing tests in this area is that microcomputers can be used in both administration and scoring. Given that one may be trying to explain less than 5% of the variance in the criterion measure, then the more errors of measurement can be reduced, the greater the probability of identifying a true effect. Individual testing, even by well-trained psychologists, is expensive and introduces inter-tester variability. Microcomputers can reduce the source of error.

Thus, the aim was to develop a battery of tests which would discriminate well across the 6–11-year age band, which would have adequate floor and ceiling at all ages; which would be robust and have good short-term test–retest reliability. This latter point was particularly important for monitoring the effects of drug and diet interventions in the treatment of conditions such as epilepsy and phenylketonuria. A well-standardized battery of tests of attention would have immediate applicability in such clinical areas, provided additional psychometric data were available.

Initially, two paradigms were of interest – reaction time and continuous performance test. Both are widely used in developmental psychology, but both exist in many different forms. Other tests were added and we were fortunate to be able to spend some time piloting them to emerge with a battery of six. The battery was given to 25 boys and 25 girls in each 6-month age band from 6 years 0 months to 10 years 11 months; some 500 children in all. In addition, children were tested individually on the WISC-R and tests of reading, spelling, arithmetic and letter cancellation. Teachers' ratings of children's behaviour were also obtained.

Because of problems with equipment, standardization testing was delayed so that it is not yet possible to report how the tests interrelate – i.e. whether there is an identifiable factor of 'attention' and how it relates to general intelligence and teachers' ratings. What can be commented on are the developmental trends and the test–retest stability of the measures.

CLAVIER – COMPUTERIZED ASSESSMENT OF LEARNING, ATTENTION AND VIGILANCE

The automated battery runs on a small home computer with disc drives, a portable television monitor and a specially built switch. The six tests are delivered in a fixed sequence, although this can be overridden by the tester.

Children were tested in school in as quiet a room as was available, seated in front of the console and a portable TV screen. The operator is prompted on how to administer the tests and the child's responses are recorded on to disc. Summary scores are calculated automatically.

The test battery

1. Paired associate learning
This test requires the child to learn associations between abstract symbols and numbers. Presentation is random and the tester can choose to present 4, 6, 8 or 10 pairs to be learned. Criterion is reached when the child makes no errors on two consecutive trials of each set. The task is abandoned after 12 trials.

A number of measures could be obtained to characterize the child's performance. At present we are using the total number of errors made. This shows a highly significant negative correlation with age ($r = -0.43$, $p < 0.001$) – older children making fewer errors.

2. Serial simple visual reaction time – with distractor

The child presses a button while watching the TV screen. As soon as a visual signal – a '0' between two marks – appears, the finger is removed to press another button. On 50% of trials a distractor – a moving spaceman – appears.

Reaction times are significantly related to chronological age: -0.20 ($p < 0.001$) with distractor; -0.22 ($p < 0.001$) without distractor. The presence of the distractor significantly increases the reaction time. Reaction time appears to reach asymptote between 9 and 10 years, and this may explain why some investigators obtain different results in younger than in older samples.

3. Speed of information processing

Five two-digit numbers are displayed on the screen and the child has to indicate which is the largest by touching it with a stylus.

Performance on this task yields a number of different measures. First, the number of errors made indicates the child's accuracy. Second, since the computer automatically records the time between presenting the stimulus and the child making a response, it is possible to quantify the relationship between speed and accuracy and use these results to characterize the child's style of responding.

Of the measures examined to date, the number of errors made in 20 trials correlates highly (-0.52, $p < 0.001$) with age.

The correlation between scores on the microcomputer task and a standardized paper and pencil version ranges from 0.7 to 0.9.

4. Reaction time with delay

This is an automated version of the Rodnick and Shakow's (1940) paradigm used by Needleman et al. (1979) in the Boston studies. In an earlier study of 302 children (Hunter et al., 1985) it was shown that scores were related to age and that our higher lead group (mean PbB = 17 μg/dl) had slower reaction times than our lower lead group (mean PbB = 7.4 μg/dl).

The current standardization data show that reaction time after 12 s delay is more strongly related to age ($r = 0.38$, $p < 0.001$) than reaction time after 3 s delay ($r = -0.16$, $p < 0.001$), but these differences may alter when the data have been fully analysed to take account of possible differences between computers used (see below).

Test–retest at one week and three months on a sample of 26 children aged 8 years showed that while the mean reaction time of the group remains stable, there is considerable indidvidual variation. The test–retest correlation is satisfactory at 3 seconds delay (0.66) but less so at 12 seconds delay (0.42–0.51).

5. Finger tapping

Children are asked to tap a button, first with their right index finger and then their left index finger. The number of taps in 10 second periods is recorded. These are highly related to age ($+0.40$, $p < 0.001$ for left hand $+0.52$. $p < 0.001$ for right hand), and good reliability is obtained ($r = 0.66$–0.74) with fairly similar rates of tapping occurring in retest. Data will be analysed

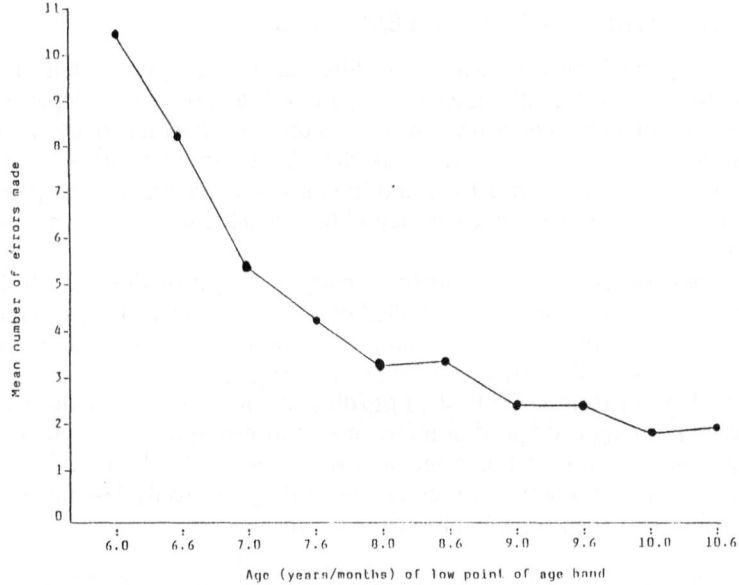

Figure 1 Speed of information processing – mean errors at each age group

according to preferred versus non-preferred hand, and spontaneous rest pauses can be calculataed on the latest version of the programme.

6. Continuous performance test
Despite its wide usage, this task gave more trouble than any other. Originally, a 30 minute version was used, but this was far too demanding for the children. A ten minute version in which the sequence of stimuli is predetermined was then developed. Children have to press a response key only when a letter X follows a letter A.

Eight-year-olds made few errors of omission or commission on the task. Test–retest correlations are in the region of +0.6. Few other studies have reported test–retest correlations and these data suggest that the test may be much less stable than hitherto assumed.

DISCUSSION

The whole battery takes from 43 min to $1\frac{1}{2}$ h per child. The greatest variation in time comes from different times to complete the Paired Associate Learning Test. Only one child out of over 500 could not complete the battery, and that was because he had an asthmatic attack. Children aged under 7 found some difficulty with the speed of information processing task; this may be because they did not fully understand the instruction to point to the largest number. Otherwise, there is confidence that this battery is age-related and suitable for the intended age range. Scores still have to be related to other psychometric and behavioural rating data in order to establish the construct validity of the measures.

RELATIONSHIP WITH BODY LEAD BURDEN

The battery has been used with 78 children aged 6–6½ years whose body lead burdens were recently assessed as part of the current UK Department of the Environment monitoring exercise. PbB was determined by venous sample analysed by Dr T. Delves at the University of Southampton. In addition to the automated battery and the psychometric assessment, parents are being interviewed so that we may obtain detailed information on social factors.

The range of PbB is 4.9–16.7 µg/dl; average = 9.5 µg/dl (SD = 2.58). This is very similar to the total group studied by the Department, and much lower than any of our earlier studies. The probability of obtaining interesting results in a small sample with restricted range of PbB is slight, but there are indications that the highest quartile (PbB ⩾ 11 µg/dl) make more errors on the Paired Associate Learning and Speed of Information Processing tests. It is premature to say more than that at this stage, and we are not yet able to address the crucial question of whether scores on the battery are really less influenced by social factors than from traditional measures.

CONCLUDING COMMENTS

In the attempt to solve some old problems, many new ones have been encountered. For example, there are clear sex differences in the extent to which boys and girls play with computers at home. Within each sex group some children are much more 'keyboard-wise' than others. Sex differences and familiarity must therefore be controlled in critical studies.

Such problems are easily managed. Of greater concern is the question of equipment reliability. Psychologists are not used to the notion of an intelligence test breaking down. They may give the wrong instructions or look up the wrong table, but the test manual and material are simple and robust; not so an automated test battery.

During our development work there were a number of mechanical problems. It was necessary to use a larger computer than that employed for an earlier reaction time study as the latter had insufficient memory to run the full battery. The next machines proved unreliable as they overheated, and data were lost. Currently, the battery is run on a BBC computer which is proving very satisfactory. However, in the course of moving from one computer to another it became evident that different machines are calibrated differently. This does not matter where a study uses only one machine, at least as far as within-study results are concerned, but it clearly complicates across-study comparisons.

Electronic equipment can be sensitive to temperature and humidity, as well as to being moved around. This study was conducted in schools in order to reduce the burden put on children and their parents. However, if it proves crucial to standardize for brightness of television screens and so on, such testing can then only be undertaken in specially equipped laboratories (mobile or not), thereby adding to the expense. Care had to be taken when transporting computer tapes and discs as these can be degraded if passed through powerful

276

electromagnetic fields, as has happened on the London underground and at airport security checks.

Finally, the speed with which computer technology is developing is such that there is a real danger that by the time a battery such as this is properly standardized, the computer used is obsolete. Already two of the small computers we have used in the past 5 years are out of production. Again, this makes it hard to develop methodologies which can be used in comparative studies. Larger-scale investment in the development of hardware, software and their application to clinical problems is needed. More attention must be paid to the calibration of instruments used in studies of the effect of lead so that international collaboration can be facilitated.

During the past 3 years these six tests have been developed and applied to 500 children in the 6–11-year age range. Scores on the tests are often strongly related to age, although the variation at each age remains very large. If the battery measures psychological functioning in ways that are less susceptible to social influences than traditional psychometric tests, then it will have exciting applications in the investigation of central nervous system functioning in children.

ACKNOWLEDGMENTS

The work reported in this paper was supported by the Commission of the European Community (Contract ENV 780 UK(H)) and the United Kingdom Medical Research Council (SPG 831763). We are grateful to the Inner London Education Authority and the many teachers, parents and children who participated in the studies. We are grateful to the Department of the Environment, and especially to Mr M. Quinn and Mr P. Cooney for allowing us access to part of the sample involved in the UK Department of the Environment monitoring exercise.

REFERENCES

Hunter, J., Urbanowicz, M.A., Yule, W. and Lansdown, R. (1985) Automated testing of reaction time and its association with lead in children. *Int. Arch. Occup. Environ. Health*, **57**, 27–34

Lansdown, R. and Yule, W. (eds) (1986) *The Lead Debate: the environment toxicology and child health* (Beckenham: Croom Helm)

Needleman, H., Gunnoe, C., Leviton, A., Reed, R., Peresie, H., Maher, C. and Barrett, P. (1979) Deficits in psychological and classroom performances of children with elevated dentine lead level. *N. Engl. J. Med.*, **300**, 689–695

Rodnick, E.H. and Shakow, D. (1940) Set in the schizophrenic as measured by a composite reaction time index. *Am. J. Psychiatry*, **97**, 214–225

Smith, M., Delves, T., Lansdown, R., Clayton, B.E. and Graham, P. (1983) The effects of lead exposure on urban children. Institute of Child Health/University of Southampton Study. *Dev. Med. Child Neurol.*, **24**, (Suppl. 47)

Taylor, E. (1980) Development of attention. In Rutter, M. (ed), *Scientific Foundations of Developmental Psychiatry*, (London: Heinemann)

Urbanowicz, M.A., Hunter, J., Yule, W. and Lansdown, R. (1988) Social factors in relation to lead on the home environment. *Lead in the Home Environment*. Northwood, Middlesex, UK: Science Reviews Ltd.

Yule, W. (1986) Methodological and statistical issues. In Lansdown, R. and Yule, W. (eds) *The Lead Debate: the environment toxicology and child health* (Beckenham: Croom Helm)

Yule, W. and Rutter, M. (1985) Effect of lead on children's behaviour and cognitive performance: A critical review. In Mahaffey, K.R. (ed), *Dietary and Environmental Lead* (Amsterdam: Elsevier), Chap. 8

3.12
Electrophysiological Assessment of Sensory and Cognitive Function in Children Exposed to Lead: A Review*

D. A. OTTO

SUMMARY

Sensory evoked and event-related slow brain potentials have been used to study the effects of lead exposure on central nervous system function in man and animals. Most human data derive from a series of studies carried out in North Carolina (Otto et al., 1981, 1982, 1985; Hawk et al., 1986; Robinson et al., 1985; Schroeder et al., 1985). Electrophysiological results have been reviewed previously (Otto, 1987). An updated review with some previously unreported observations is presented below.

SENSORY CONDITIONING

The challenge that guided the author's initial selection of tests was the need for an electrophysiological index of cognitive function that could be obtained in children as young as 1 year of age. The available measures included the contingent negative variation (CNV), a slow negative shift in the electrical baseline of the brain that occurs during the reaction-time foreperiod (Walter et al., 1964), and the late positive component (LPC), a slow wave (SW) that occurs 300–900 milliseconds (ms) after the presentation of an infrequent stimulus (Sutton et al., 1965). These are the best known and most widely studied members of the event-related slow brain potential family (Otto, 1978). The existing literature, however, was based primarily on *homo sophmorionus in collegio*, the backbone of experimental psychology in the United States.

* This article has been reviewed by the Health Effects Research Laboratory, U.S. Environmental Protection Agency and approved for publication. Approval does not signify that the contents necessarily reflect the views and policies of the Agency.

Both CNV and LPC tests require either a motor response or a mental decision beyond the capability of a 1-year-old. Passive tests were clearly needed.

Meager evidence existed that the CNV and LPC could both be elicited passively (Otto *et al.*, 1980). Walter *et al.* (1964) long ago demonstrated that the CNV could be elicited by a conditioned stimulus (tone) paired with an unconditioned stimulus (air puff), although a more robust waveform occurred when a voluntary motor response was required after the 'unconditional' stimulus. Roth (1973) had also reported that a 'rare' stimulus embedded in a sequence of 'frequent' stimuli elicited an LPC even when subjects were instructed to ignore the stimuli.

Based on these findings, the present investigators designed a classical conditioning test that would engage the attention of a 1-year-old child. The test consisted of pairing a brief tone (conditioned stimulus – CS) with the blackout of a cartoon (unconditioned stimulus – UCS) that the child was watching. The investigators then measured the slow potential shift during the interval between the tone (CS) and cartoon blackout (UCS); this measure was operationally defined as an index of sensory conditioning (Figure 1). In the absence of any behavioural measure, however, the relationship of SW voltage and conditioning remains speculative.

The results of our initial study (Otto *et al.*, 1981) indicated a systematic linear relationship of SW voltage and blood lead (PbB) concentrations. The

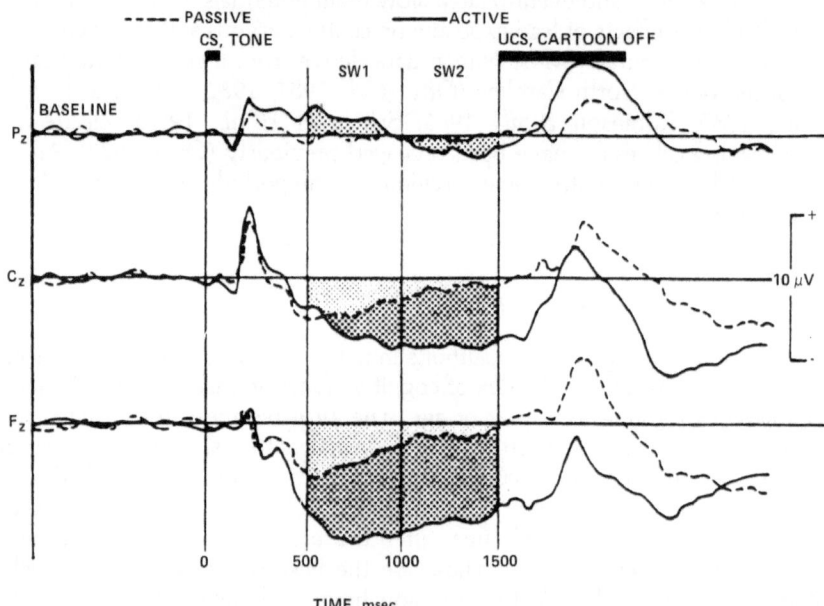

Figure 1 Summary averages of slow brain potentials recorded over the frontal (Fz), central (Cz), and parietal (Pz) cortex in children during active and passive sensory conditioning. The horizontal bars above the averages indicate intervals during which conditioned (CS) and unconditioned (UCS) stimuli were presented. Slow wave measurement intervals (SW1 and SW2) are designated by vertical lines. Larger slow waves were obtained during active conditioning than during passive conditioning

slope of the SW–PbB function, moreover, varied with age. A similar age × PbB interaction of SW voltage was observed in a 2-year follow up evaluation (Otto *et al.*, 1982). Although the functional significance of the SW measure remained uncertain, the partial replication of the earlier finding suggested that SW voltage was a sensitive index of lead-induced change in the central nervous system (CNS) function of children.

When a 5-year follow up evaluation of 49 children was completed (Otto *et al.*, 1985), no significant age × PbB interaction of SW voltage recorded during passive conditioning was found in the older children. The average PbB (14 μg/dl) of the children at 5-year follow up, however, was only half the original level (28 μg/dl). The original study had shown that the passive test did not elicit SW in adults. The passive conditioning test, therefore, may be ineffective in older children, or insensitive at PbB levels below 30 μg/dl.

Since the children now ranged from 6 to 12 years of age, and were quite capable of making sophisticated motor and mental responses, an active sensory conditioning test and a frequent–rare auditory test were added to the protocol. Comparisons of waveforms averaged across subjects for the active and passive conditions clearly demonstrated the superiority of the active test in eliciting a larger SW (see Figure 1). Futhermore, results of the active conditioning test indicated a linear relationship of SW voltage and current PbB levels at all three scalp recording sites (Figure 2). The active test thus appears to be more sensitive than the passive test as an index of lead effects in older children. Reaction time, recorded during active conditioning, was not significantly related to PbB.

Results of a subsequent study in children from North Carolina raised another red flag regarding the passive sensory conditioning test. No tests of SW voltage revealed any lead-related effects at frontal or vertex recording sites. A recent analysis of SW data recorded over the occipital lobe in 21 of these children, however, revealed a surprising finding: SW voltage in this group of children was inversely related to maximal PbB. This preliminary

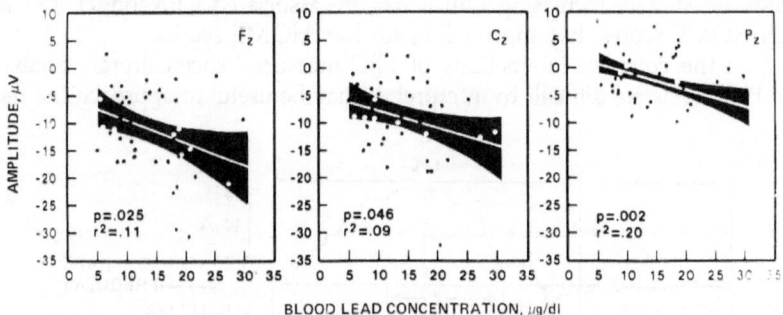

Figure 2 Slow potential amplitude was recorded at three scalp locations during active sensory conditioning and plotted as a function of current blood lead (PbB) levels of children in the 5-year follow up study. Negativity increased linearly with current PbB. Measurements were obtained during the SW2 epoch as shown in Figure 1. Individual data points and 95% confidence limits for derived regression lines are plotted. (Redrawn from *Environ. Res.*, 1985, **38**, 176)

result raises the possibility that an important part of the brain may have been ignored in previous SW analyses.

FREQUENT–RARE AUDITORY TEST

The frequent–rare auditory test, affectionately known in psychophysiology as an 'oddball' test, consisted of presenting a series of tones at 1.5 s intervals. A low-pitch frequent tone was presented on 75% of the trials, and a high-pitch rare tone (or oddball) was presented randomly on 25% of the trials. Children in the 5-year follow up study (Otto et al., 1985) were instructed to press a button as rapidly as possible when the rare tone occurred. This test is a simple variant of the continuous performance test widely used in studies of developmental disorders.

An electroencephalogram (EEG) was recorded at standard midline scalp locations over the frontal (Fz), central (Cz), and parietal (Pz) cortex. Figure 3 shows summary averages across 39 subjects for frequent and rare stimuli. The maximal positive peak latency and amplitude were measured during a window of 250–600 ms after stimulus onset. The LPC was largest in amplitude at Pz following rare stimuli. The LPC is not clearly defined following frequent stimuli in summary averages but could be identified in many individual averages. Table 1 summarizes the results of exploratory regression analyses. Significant age effects were found for reaction time (RT) and several LPC measures. Consistent with other developmental studies, RT and LPC latency decreased with age.

No significant relationship was found between original PbB levels and RT or LPC measures. Regression analyses using current blood lead levels (PbB5), however, revealed complex interactions of PbB, RT, Home Observation for Measurement of the Environment (HOME) caregiving scores, and maternal IQ. Figure 4 illustrates the interactive effects of HOME scores, RT, and PbB. Predicted regression lines for children with low (20) and high (70) HOME scores are shown. Increasing PbB levels are associated with longer RTs for high HOME scores, but shorter RTs for low HOME scores.

Since the complex interactions of LPC measures, sociocultural variables, and PbB levels are difficult to interpret, it may be useful to approach the data

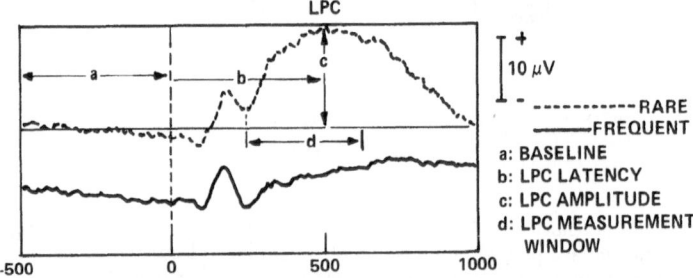

Figure 3 Summary averages of slow potentials elicited by frequent (solid line) and rare (dashed line) stimuli recorded over parietal cortex in 6–12-year-old children. The latency and amplitude of a late positive component (LPC) were measured during time window *d*

Table 1 LPC Exploratory regression analysis, p-values

		Cz		Pz		Reaction time
		Rare	Frequent	Rare	Frequent	
Omnibus interactions	Amplitude	0.45	0.004	0.13	0.049	0.005
	Latency	0.65	0.47	0.51	0.20	
Significant interactions	PbB × HOME		0.0002*		0.004*	0.0001
	PbB × MIQ		0.0231*			0.003
Omnibus main effects	Amplitude	0.85	0.59	0.42	0.21	0.008
	Latency	0.10	0.10	0.81	0.12	
Significant main effects	Age***	0.016**	0.011**	0.045*	0.029**	0.0001
PbB effects	Amplitude	0.25	0.18	0.92	0.041	0.26
	Latency	0.64	0.99	0.87	0.88	

*LPC Amplitude;   **LPC Latency;   ***A separate analysis was done for age effects, controlling for PbB, sex, SES, MIQ, and HOME scores

MIQ = maternal IQ
HOME = Home Observation for Measurement of the Environment
LPC = late positive component
SES = socioeconomic status

from a different perspective. Another analysis of the LPC data was undertaken to examine the relationship of LPC measures and child IQ, including current PbB as a control variable. Results of this analysis, shown in Table 2, suggest that LPC latency during frequent trials varies inversely with PbB at central and parietal recording sites. That is, LPC latency decreases as PbB increases, as shown in Figure 5.

Interpretation of these results must be made very cautiously owing to the exploratory nature of the analysis and the confusing interactions noted above. The inverse relationship of LPC latency and PbB, nonetheless, has intriguing implications. In the first place, shorter LPC latencies are normally considered to reflect more efficient information processing (Kutas et al., 1977). This interpretation would be inconsistent with extensive literature (U.S. EPA, 1986) that associates low to moderate lead exposure with intellectual impairment in children. This finding also appears to be inconsistent with brainstem auditory evoked potentials recorded in the same children (see below), in which latencies increased with higher PbBs.

On the other hand, the LPC result is consistent with results of the active sensory conditioning test in which slow wave negativity increased with PbB. Increased negativity, like decreased LPC latency, is generally associated with improved cognitive function (Otto, 1978). Winneke et al. (1984) have also reported faster peripheral nerve conduction velocity and shorter visual evoked potential latency in children with increasing PbB levels. The electrophysiological findings of Winneke et al. also appear to be inconsistent with behavioural results in the same children, i.e. reaction times increased directly with PbB levels.

The apparent contradictions of electrophysiological and behavioural measures, however, could be manifestations of a common underlying problem resulting from lead absorption. Learning disorders, poor performance, develop-

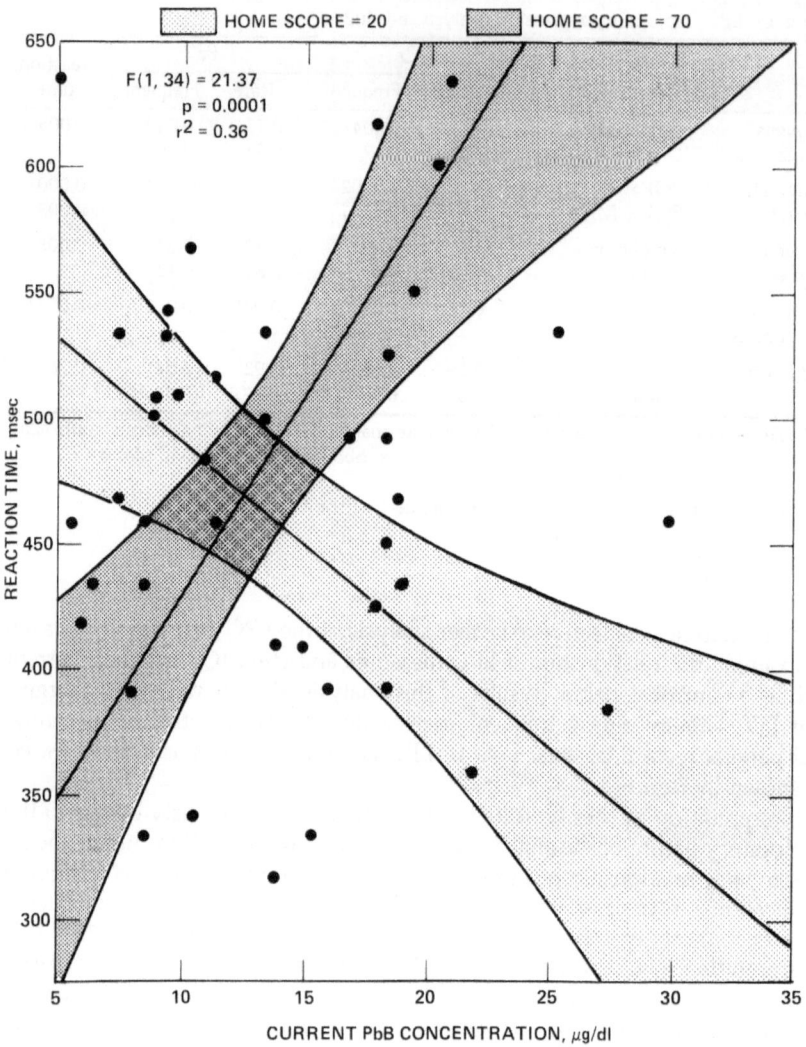

Figure 4 Interaction of current PbB levels and HOME caregiving evaluation scores with reaction times to rare stimuli. 95% confidence bands for regression lines are shown

mental delays, and hyperexcitability of the peripheral and central nervous system are all compatible with attention deficit disorder (DSM-III: American Psychiatric Association, 1980). Increased nervous system excitability and cognitive impairment viewed as common symptoms of attention deficit disorder could thus be observed in the same children as a consequence of lead exposure.

Table 2 Exploratory multivariate regression analysis of late positive component (LPC), IQ, and control* variables (p-values)

		Rare		Frequent	
		Cz	Pz	Cz	Pz
Omnibus	Amplitude	n.s.	n.s.	n.s.	n.s.
interactions	Latency	n.s.	n.s.	n.s.	n.s.
Omnibus	Amplitude	n.s.	n.s.	n.s.	n.s.
main effects	Latency	0.052	n.s.	0.019	0.001
	IQ	n.s.	n.s.	n.s.	0.046
Significant	Age	0.015	n.s.	0.006	0.001
Latency	PbB	n.s.	n.s.	0.017	0.001
Main effects	SES	n.s.	n.s.	0.023	0.001

* Control variables were age, sex, maternal IQ, HOME, SES, PbB
Abbreviations as in Table 1

VISUAL EVOKED POTENTIALS

The effects of lead exposure on visual evoked potentials have been studied in man and animals, but the results of these studies are quite inconsistent. Flash evoked potentials (FEP) have been used in animals, whereas pattern-reversal visual evoked potentials (PREP) have been used in humans. Fox *et al.* (1977) reported increased latencies, Feeney *et al.* (1979) found decreased latency, and Winneke (1979) found no latency differences in lead-exposed rats compared with controls. Similar differences were noted in FEP amplitude measures: Winneke reported depressed amplitudes, but Fox *et al.* (1979) found increased amplitude recovery (cortical excitability) to paired flashes in lead-exposed rats relative to controls. Fox *et al.* added to the confusion by interpreting the increased latencies as evidence of decreased CNS recovery (1977) and the amplitude effects as evidence of increased CNS recovery (1979). Both Fox *et al.* reports, moreover, were based on the same animals in the same experiment!

FEPs have also been used in two studies of neonatally lead-exposed monkeys. Bowman and Bushnell (1980) reported no lead effects on FEPs, but Lilienthal *et al.* (this volume) found a dose-dependent decrease in amplitude and an increase in latencies.

Similar disparities are evident in human studies. Sborgia *et al.* (1983) reported increased P1 latency* in PREPs of lead workers compared to controls, but Winneke *et al.* (1984) found decreased P1 latency with increasing PbBs of Nordenham children. The mean PbB level of workers in the Sborgia *et al.* study, however, was 62.5 μg/dl, while PbB levels in the Nordenham children were considerably lower (4–23 μg/dl). These findings raise the possibility of biphasic effects on visual function wherein lead might exert an excitatory effect at low levels, but an inhibitory effect at higher levels.

PREP evaluations of North Carolina children yielded similar discrepant

---

* PREP measures are labelled on the bases of the polarity and sequence of peaks in the waveforms, e.g., P1 is the first positive peak, N2 is the second negative peak, and P1N2 amplitude is the voltage difference between the P1 and N2 peaks.

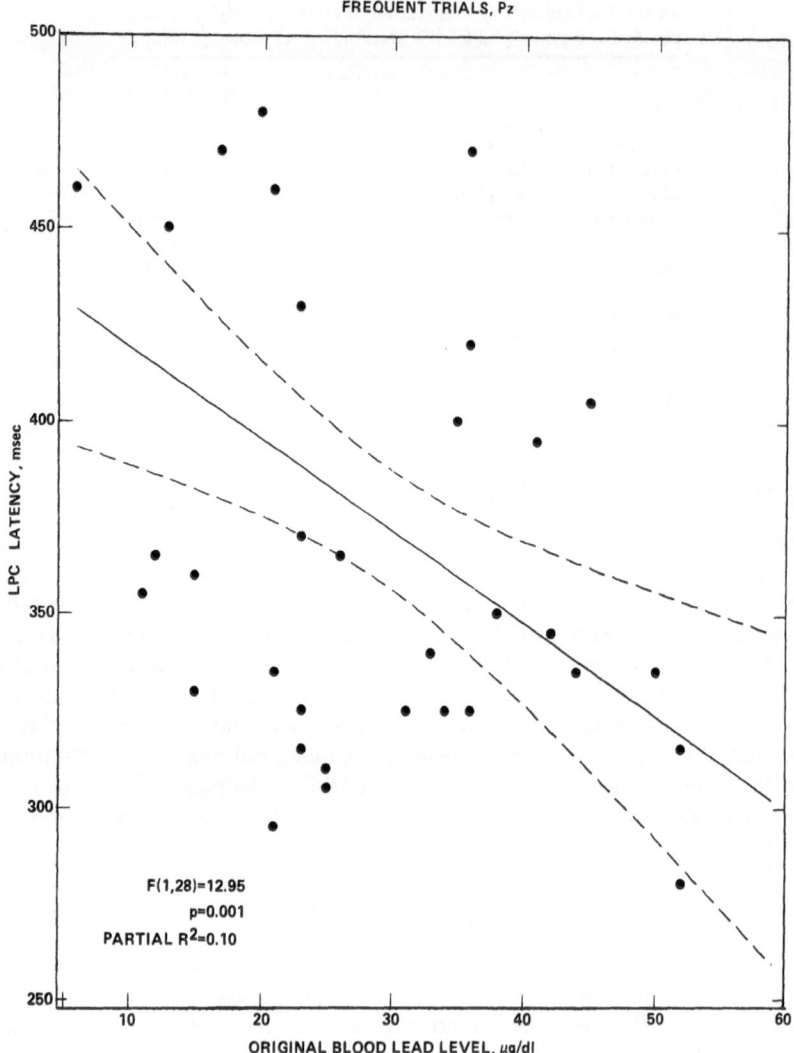

FREQUENT TRIALS, Pz

F(1,28)=12.95
p=0.001
PARTIAL R^2=0.10

Figure 5 Relationship of late positive component latency following frequent stimuli over parietal cortex and PbB levels obtained 5 years earlier in children aged 6–12 years. Dashed lines indicate 95% confidence bands for regression lines

results. Older children in the 5-year follow up study (Otto *et al.*, 1985) showed increased N1P1 amplitude, decreased N2 latency, but no change in P1 amplitude or latency with increasing PbB levels. The only lead-related effect observed in younger children in a subsequent study was a decrease in P1N2 amplitude with increasing PbB (Figure 6). Results of the 5-year follow up study were consistent with Winneke *et al.* (1984) but contrary to prediction. Results of the later study were inconsistent with the authors' earlier findings and those of Winneke *et al.* The mean PbB level of the older children was 14 µg/dl and the mean PbB level of the younger children was higher

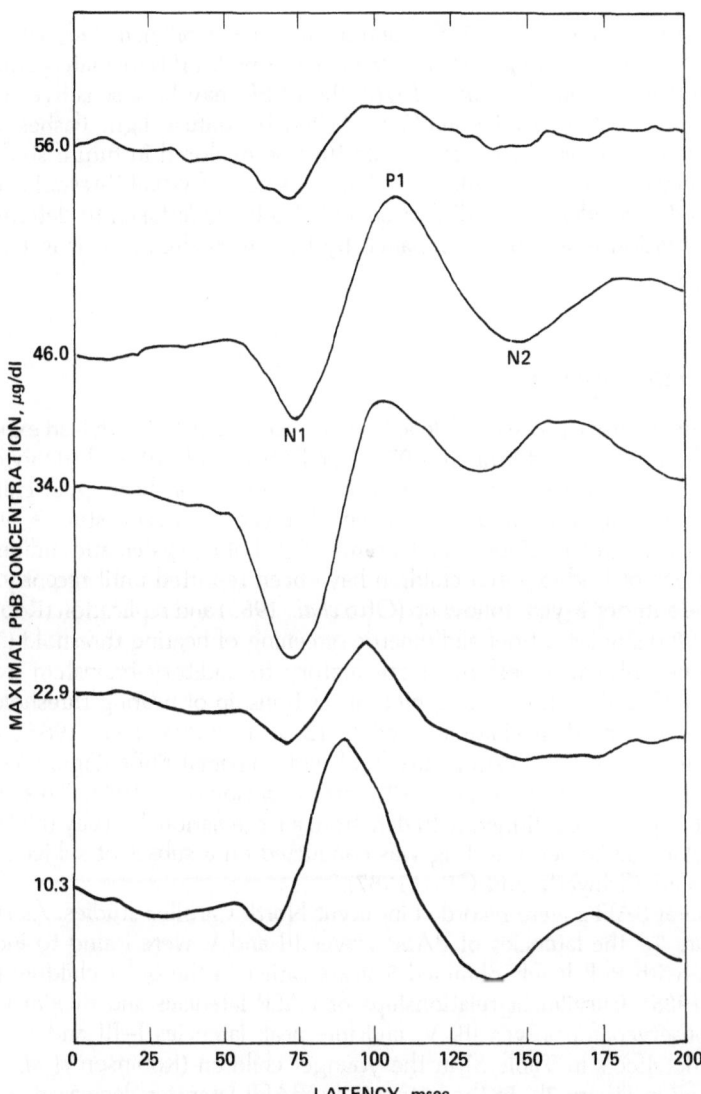

Figure 6 Pattern-reversal visual evoked potentials recorded binocularly in five girls aged 3 to 7 with varying PbB levels. PIN2 peak-to-peak amplitude decreased significantly with increasing PbB. (Redrawn from Otto *et al.*, 1985)

(20.6 µg/dl) at the time of testing. Further study of the dose–response relationship of PbB levels and visual evoked potential measures in children is needed to determine if the relationship is biphasic.

Another aspect of visual function that requires further study in children in relation to lead exposure is light and dark adaptation. Several animal studies suggest that rods (which mediate scotopic, dark-adapted vision) are more susceptible than cones (which mediate photopic, light-adapted vision) to lead toxicity (Bushnell *et al.*, 1977; Fox and Sillman, 1979; Sillman *et al.*, 1982; Fox *et al.*, 1985; Tessier-Lavigne *et al.*, 1985). Since the PREP is mediated primarily by foveal (cone) vision (Sokol, 1976), the PREP may be insensitive to lead absorption. Flash evoked potentials, elicited by diffuse light flashes which stimulate both rods and cones, should thus be explored in future studies of lead exposure effects in children. Systematic study of visual thresholds under light- and dark-adapted conditions should also be undertaken to determine if scotopic vision is selectively impaired by lead in children as it is in rats and monkeys.

AUDITORY FUNCTION

Although auditory processing deficits have been associated with lead exposure in children (Perino and Ernhart, 1974; Needleman *et al.*, 1979), little evidence is available concerning the effects of lead exposure on hearing in children. Elevated hearing thresholds have been observed in several studies of lead workers (reviewed by Repko and Corum, 1979), but no systematic audiometric evaluations of lead-exposed children have been reported until recently.

In the authors' 5-year follow up (Otto *et al.*, 1985) and replication (Robinson *et al.*, 1985) studies, a brief audiometric screening of hearing threshold (2 kHz pure tone only) was performed preparatory to auditory brainstem evoked potential (BAEP) testing. No significant relationship of hearing threshold and PbB was observed in children aged 6–12 years (Otto *et al.*, 1985), but a significant increase in hearing threshold with maximal PbBs (Figure 7a) was found in younger children aged 3–7 years (Robinson *et al.*, 1985). This finding was subsequently confirmed with data from a large national survey (NHANES II) in which audiometric testing was conducted on a subset of subjects aged 4–19 years (Schwartz and Otto, 1987).

Binaural BAEPs were recorded in recent North Carolina studies. As shown in Figure 7c, the latencies of BAEP waves III and V were found to increase linearly with PbB levels obtained 5 years earlier in the older children (Otto *et al.*, 1985). Curvilinear relationships of BAEP latencies and maximal PbBs were observed for waves III, V, and interpeak latencies I–III and I–V (see quadratic effects in Table 3) in the younger children (Robinson *et al.*, 1985) as shown in Figure 7b. In the latter study, BAEP latencies decreased as PbBs increased from 5 to about 25 μg/dl PbB, but then increased with PbBs above 25 μg/dl as observed previously in older children.

Results of the replication study in the younger children indicated a problem in the BAEP methodology employed in both North Carolina studies. Click intensity (based on audiometric screening) was adjusted so that all subjects would hear clicks at the same sensation level. While this procedure is used widely in psychophysical research, it is not advisable in BAEP testing because wave I latency is very sensitive to click intensity. That is, wave I latency varies inversely with click intensity, an effect that does not necessarily correlate directly with hearing threshold.

Although hearing threshold increased directly with PbB in the younger chidren, a seemingly paradoxical linear *decrease* in BAEP wave I latency was

288

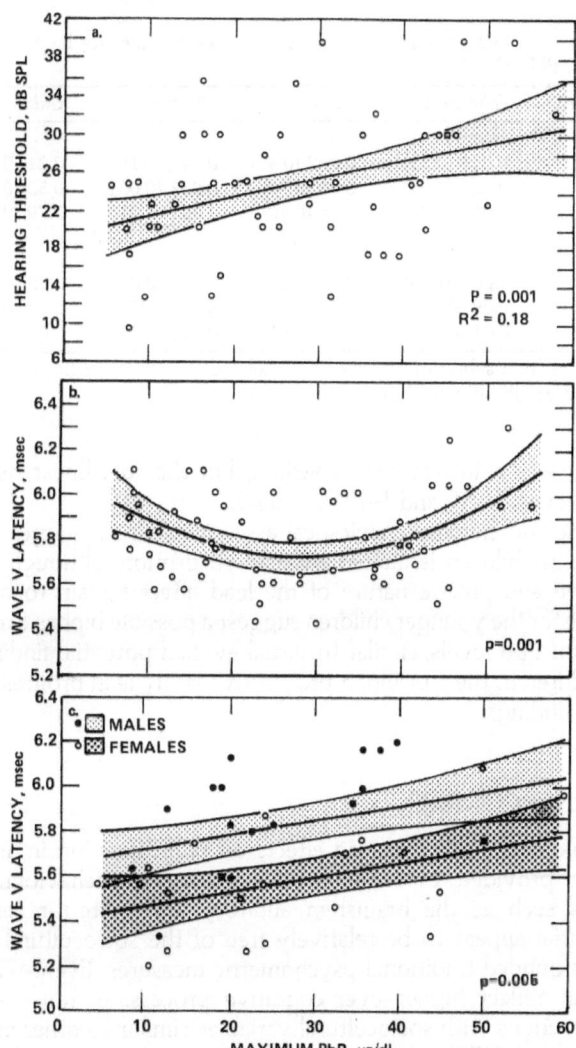

Figure 7 Scatter plots, regression lines, and 95% confidence limits of (a) 2 kHz hearing thresholds in children aged 3 to 7, (b) BAEP wave V latencies in children aged 3 to 7, and (c) in children aged 6 to 12 as functions of maximal PbB levels. Linear relationships of PbB and hearing threshold in younger children and wave V latency in older children were found, while a curvilinear relationship of PbB and wave V latency was observed in younger children

observed. In view of the known latency–intensity relationship of wave I, the latter effect was more likely due to increasing click intensity than to increasing PbB level. This hypothesis was confirmed by reanalysis of BAEP data from a subset of children ($n = 49$) from whom BAEPs were recorded within a limited click intensity range of 77.5–85 dB sound pressure level (SPL). Results of this reanalysis are shown in Table 3 (p values shown in parentheses). The significant linear relationship of wave I latency and PbB disappeared when

Table 3 Exploratory analysis of BAEP measures: p-values for higher-order maximal PbB effect*

Dep. var.	Polynomial	Linear	Quadratic	Cubic
Latency				
I	0.013 (0.32)	0.007 (0.37)	0.14 (0.11)	0.21 (0.84)
III	0.021 (0.011)	0.41 (0.70)	0.003 (0.001)	0.50 (0.44)
V	0.015 (0.09)	0.75 (0.40)	0.001 (0.018)	0.79 (0.87)
Interpeak latency				
I–III	0.06 (0.048)	0.15 (0.24)	0.022 (0.014)	0.76 (0.47)
III–V	0.09 (0.71)	0.08 (0.33)	0.08 (0.97)	0.62 (0.95)
I–V	0.01 (0.18)	0.038 (0.16)	0.008 (0.09)	0.64 (0.95)

* p Values for a subset of 49 children stimulated at click intensities between 77.5 and 85 dB SPL are shown in parentheses

click intensity was held relatively constant, but the curvilinear relationships of PbB and waves III, V, and I–III remained.

Audiometric and electrophysiological assessments both suggest that auditory function in children is altered by lead absorption, although the dose–response curve and precise nature of the lead effect remain to be clarified. BAEP findings for the younger children suggest a possible biphasic relationship of latencies and PbB levels, similar to visual evoked potential findings. BAEP testing of children in the Cincinnati prospective study is in progress to clarify our previous findings.

CONCLUDING COMMENT

Electrophysiological studies of lead effects on brain function in animals and humans have provided evidence complementary to behavioural studies. Sensory tests such as the brainstem auditory and pattern-reversal visual evoked potential appear to be relatively free of the sociocultural influences that have confounded traditional psychometric measures. Event-related brain potentials that reflect higher-level cognitive processing, however, exhibit complex interactions with sociocultural variables similar to other measures of cognitive function. While some electrophysiological measures have varied systematically with PbB levels in each of the studies in which they have been employed, numerous inconsistencies among studies are apparent. Suggestions of biphasic lead effects on both visual and auditory evoked potentials were noted. More human and animal evoked potential studies are needed to clarify the existing evidence.

ACKNOWLEDGMENTS

Support for the North Carolina paediatric lead studies was provided by NIEHS Grant ES-01104, EPA Contract 68-02-1702, and EPA Collaborative Agreement CR809992 with the University of North Carolina. A large and dedicated staff was required to collect and analyse the data. Co-principal investigator was Stephen Schroeder, PhD, University of North Carolina

School of Medicine. Major contributors included V. Benignus, S. Baumann and G. Robinson (electrophysiology); C. Milar and B. Hawk (psychometrics); P. Mushak (analytical chemistry); K. Muller, D. Kleinbaum, and C. Barton (statistics). The assistance of Lenoir, New Hanover, and Wake County Health Departments in recruiting subjects, and K. Jares and Vickie Worrell for manuscript preparation is gratefully acknowledged.

REFERENCES

American Psychiatric Association (1980) *Diagnostic and Statistical Manual of Mental Disorders*, 3rd ed, DSM-III. (Washington, DC)

Bowman, R. and Bushnell, P. (1980) Scotopic visual deficits in young monkeys given chronic daily low levels of lead. In Merigan, W. and Weiss, B. (eds), *Neurotoxicity of the Visual System* (New York: Raven Press), pp. 219–231

Bushnell, P., Bowman, R., Allen, J. and Marlar, R. (1977) Scotopic vision deficits in young monkeys exposed to lead. *Science*, **196**, 333–335

Feeney, D., Longo, J., Cosden, M., Zenick, H. and Padich, R. (1979) Detection of the effects of lead exposure by visual evoked response latency. *Physiol. Psychol.*, **7**, 143–145

Fox, D. and Sillman, A. (1979) Heavy metals affect rod, but not cone, photoreceptors. *Science*, **206**, 78–80

Fox, D., Lewkowski, J. and Cooper, G. (1977) Acute and chronic effects of neonatal lead exposure on the development of the visual evoked response in rats. *Toxicol. Appl. Pharmacol.*, **40**, 449–461

Fox, D., Lewkowski, J. and Cooper, G. (1979) Persistent visual cortex excitability alterations produced by neonatal lead exposure. *Neurobehav. Toxicol.*, **1**, 101–106

Fox, D., Farber, D., Chu, L. and Stein, J. (1985) Rod photoreceptors are selectively altered by lead: electrophysiological, biochemical and morphological studies. *Toxicologist*, **5**, 81 (abstr).

Hawk, B., Schroeder, S., Robinson, G., Otto, D., Mushak, P. and Barton, C. (1986) Relation of lead and social factors to IQ of low-SES children: A partial replication. *Am. J. Ment. Defic.*, **91**, 178–183

Kutas, M., McCarthy, G. and Donchin, E. (1977) Augmenting mental chronometry: The P300 latency on stimulus evaluation processes. *Psychophysiology*, 21: 171–186

Needleman, H.E., Gunnoe, C., Leviton, A., Reed, R., Peresie, H., Maher, C. and Barrett, P. (1979) Deficits in psychologic and classroom performance of children with elevated dentine lead levels. *N. Engl. J. Med.*, **300**, 689–695

Otto, D. (ed.) (1978) *Multidisciplinary Perspectives in Event-related Brain Potential Research*. EPA-600/9-77-043, (Washington, DC: US Government Printing Office)

Otto, D. (1987) The relationship of event-related brain potentials and lead absorption: a review of current evidence. In Goldwater, L., Wysocki, L. and Volpe, R. (eds), *Lead Environmental Health: The Current Issues*. (Duke University, Durham, NC: Division of Occupational Medicine), pp. 151–164

Otto, D., Benignus, V., Seiple, K., Loiselle, D. and Hatcher, T. (1980) ERPs in young children during sensory conditioning. *Brain Res.*, **54**, 574–578

Otto, D., Benignus, V., Muller, K. and Barton, C. (1981) Effects of age and body lead burden on CNS function in young children. I. Slow cortical potentials. *Electroenceph. Clin. Neurophysiol.*, **52**, 229–239

Otto, D., Benignus, V., Muller, K., Barton, C., Seiple, K., Prah, J. and Schroeder, S. (1982) Effects of low to moderate lead exposure on slow cortical potentials in young children: two-year follow-up study. *Neurobehav. Toxicol. Teratol.*, **4**, 733–737

Otto, D., Robinson, G., Baumann, S., Schroeder, S., Mushak, P., Kleinbaum, D. and Boone, L. (1985) Five-year follow-up study of children with low-to-moderate lead absorption: Electrophysiological evaluation. *Environ. Res.*, **38**, 168–186

Perino, J. and Ernhart, C.B. (1974) The relation of subclinical lead level to cognitive and sensorimotor impairment in Black preschoolers. *J. Learn. Disorders*, **7**, 616–620

Repko, J. and Corum, C. (1979). Critical review and evaluation of the neurological and behavioural sequelae of inorganic lead absorption. *CRC Crit. Rev. Toxicol.*, **6**, 135–187

Robinson, G., Baumann, S., Kleinbaum, D., Barton, C., Schroeder, S., Mushak, P. and Otto, D. (1985) Effects of low-to-moderate lead exposure on brainstem auditory evoked potentials in children. *Environmental Health*, Doc. 3 *Neurobehavioral Methods in Occupational and Environmental Health*) (Copenhagen: World Health Organization), pp. 177–182

Roth, W.T. (1973) Auditory evoked responses to unpredictable stimuli. *Psychophysiology*, **10**, 125–138

Sborgia, G., Assennato, G., L'Abbate, N., DeMarinis, L., Paci, C., DeNicolo, M., Demarinis, G., Montrone, N., Ferrannini, E., Specchio, L., Masi, G. and Olivieri, G. (1983) Comprehensive neurophysiological evaluation of lead-exposed workers. In Gilioli, R., Cassito, M. and Foa, V. (eds), *Neurobehavioral Methods in Occupational Health* (Oxford: Pergamon Press), pp. 283–294

Schroeder, S., Hawk, B., Otto, D., Mushak, P. and Hicks, R. (1985) Separating the effects of lead and social factors on IQ. *Environ. Res.*, **38**, 144–154

Schwartz, J. and Otto, D. (1988) Blood lead, hearing thresholds and neurobehavioral development in children and youth. *Arch. Environ. Health*, **42**, 153–160

Sokol, S. (1976) Visually evoked potentials: theory, techniques and clinical applications. *Surv. Ophthalmol.*, **21**, 18–44

Sillman, A., Bolnick, D., Bosetti, J., Haynes, L. and Walter, A. (1982) The effects of lead and of cadmium on the mass photoreceptor potential: the dose-response relationship. *Neurotoxicology*, **3**, 179–194

Sutton, S., Braren, M. and Zubin, J. (1965) Evoked potential correlates of stimulus uncertainty. *Science*, **150**, 1187–1188

Tessier-Lavigne, M., Mobb, P. and Attwell (1985) Lead and mercury toxicity and the rod light response. *Invest. Ophthal. Vis. Sci.*, **26**, 1117–1123

U.S. Environmental Protection Agency (1986) *Air Quality Criteria for Lead*, Vol. IV, EPA-600/8-83-028dF

Walter, W.G., Cooper, R., Aldridge, V.J., McCallum, W.C. and Winter, A.L. (1964) Contingent negative variation: an electric sign of sensorimotor association and expectancy in the human brain. *Nature (Lond.)*, **203**, 380–384

Winneke, G. (1979) Modification of visual evoked potentials in rats after long term blood lead elevation. *Activ. Nerv. Sup. (Praha)*, **21**, 282–284

Winneke, G., Beginn, U., Ewert, T., Havestadt, C., Kramer, U., Krouse, Ch., Thron, H. and Wagner, H. (1984) Studie zur Erfassung subklinischer Bleiwirkungen auf das Nervensystem von Kindern mit vekannter pranataler Exposition in Nordenham. *Schr.-Reine Verein Wabolu*, **59**, 215–229

3.13
Type II Fallacies in the Study of Childhood Exposure to Lead at Low Dose: A Critical and Quantitative Review

H. L. NEEDLEMAN and D. C. BELLINGER

SUMMARY

Scientists, justifiably conservative in their approach to causal inference, emphasize avoiding Type I errors. Less attention is given to avoiding Type II errors. Many of the recent reviews and studies of lead at low dose and children's neurodevelopment have committed Type II errors in evaluation. Among the more common errors encountered are the following: (1) treating the criterion $p = 0.05$ as a sacrament; (2) positing phantom confounders; (3) constructing false causal models; (4) making no-effect inferences from samples too small to give adequate power; (5) underestimating the importance of 'small' differences between groups; (6) examining each study in isolation; and (7) requiring proof of causality.

We review all 14 of the recent informative studies of lead at low dose, estimate effect sizes for each study, estimate power to find an effect and, uing Fisher's method of aggregation, calculate a joint probability that the effects reported were due to chance under the null hypothesis.

The power of many studies was surprisingly small, due to sample size and the number of covariates controlled. The effect sizes of the differences between exposed and non-exposed groups was 0.4 standard deviations. The joint probability of the effects found in the 14 studies occurring by chance was 3×10^{-12}. These findings converge strongly on the conclusion that lead at low dose is neurotoxic. They also provide guidelines for future studies of the question.

Studies of lead at low dose and neurocognitive function are appearing at an exponentially increasing rate, and the issue has produced almost as many review articles as original papers. In an area where methodological changes

293

are rapid (compare, for example, the biostatistical and neurobehavioural methods in lead papers published between 1974 and 1985), scientists seeking to make causal judgements are compelled to balance the risk of Type I and Type II errors.

Minimizing Type I errors (that is, accepting spurious relationships as real) is widely regarded as appropriate scientific behaviour. But scepticism towards causal claims is sometimes purchased at the price of leniency towards the commission of Type II errors (rejecting valid associations as spurious). In examining the current lead literature we have observed a marked increase in the sophistication and rigour displayed in the majority of modern studies. At the same time we have noted in some relatively recent papers the uncritical employment of tactics which tend to increase the risk of Type II errors in interpretation. We first focus our attention on these tactical solecisms and then proceed to present a quantitative integrative review of the more recent studies of lead exposure. In doing this we calculate a mean effect size, and a joint probability of the effect found occurring by chance. We then examine the 'file drawer problem', and estimate the number of unpublished 'no-effect' studies required to dilute out the published evidence for lead's toxicity at low dose.

In earlier publications (Needleman *et al.*, 1979; Bellinger and Needleman, 1982), we called attention to four common experimental problems encountered in studying the neurobehavioural effects of low-level lead exposure: (1) use of weak markers of exposure; (2) use of insensitive measures of outcome; (3) inadequate attention to confounders; and (4) ascertainment bias. Two of these factors, weak exposure markers and insensitive measures of outcome, tend to bias conclusions towards the null; ascertainment bias and inadequate attention to confounders, on the other hand, may bias conclusions in either direction — towards or away from the null.

FACTORS INCREASING THE RISK OF TYPE II ERRORS

We now focus on 7 previously undiscussed tactics in design or interpretation which increase the risk of Type II errors.

The sacrament of $p < 0.05$

In evaluating whether a given set of observed differences in IQ scores between lead-exposed and non-exposed children should be taken as causally related, some investigators dismiss any studies in which the p value is greater than 0.05. Differences of $p = 0.07$ or 0.10 are said to be due to chance and, even further, are taken as evidence that no relationship between lead and a given type of deficit exists in nature (Smith, 1985; Ernhart *et al.*, 1981).

This use of a significance level as a dichotomous classifier to sort out causal from chance associations ignores the genesis of the test of statistical significance. Most writers acknowledge Sir Ronald Fisher as the source of the now sacramental criterion value, $p = 0.05$. Fisher's own position on the matter is interesting. In his 1925 edition of *Statistical Methods for Research Workers*, he stated:

It is convenient to take this point [$p = 0.05$] as a limit in judging whether a deviation is to be considered significant or not. Deviations exceeding twice the standard deviation are thus formally regarded as significant.

In 1926 Fisher went on to assert:

If one in twenty does not *seem* high enough odds, we may *if we prefer*, draw the line at one in fifty, or one in a hundred.

The terms 'convenient' or 'If we prefer' are italicized here to emphasize their intended use. These words were obviously not chosen to establish a fixed boundary; rather, they state a preference. It is simply time and unexamined practice that has served to harden this preference into an icon.

The convention of using 1 in 20 odds to choose between randomness and causality or as a discriminator between null and causal hypotheses actually preceded Fisher. Pearson, who promulgated the concept of standard deviation, commenting on a goodness of fit analysis, stated that at $p = 0.5586$ 'we may consider the fit remarkably good'; that $p = 0.10$ was *'not very improbable'* that the observed frequencies are compatible with a 'random sampling'; and that $p = 0.01$ was taken as 'this very improbable result' (Cowles and Davis, 1982). The subjective nature of this psychophysical trichotomy is once more worthy of note. It is quite clear that people begin to define 'unlikely' as occurring at a frequency of 1/10, and are convinced at 1/100. The value 0.05 is placed at the midpoint of this clearly subjective psychophysical function. Jerome Cornfield's comments (1976) on this point are pertinent:

[T]he prespecification of a significance level, e.g., .05 or .01 has no sound logical basis and remains unjustified.

Reliance on phantom covariates

Because cognitive function is determined by multiple factors, careful investigators of lead's effects try to identify and evaluate those non-lead covariates which could confound. This partitioning of the variance usually, but not always, has the effect of reducing the size of the lead effect (for an exception, see Bellinger *et al.*, this volume). Some investigators (for example Smith *et al.*, 1983) extrapolate from this reduction of effect size after covariate adjustment to argue that since controlling for non-lead variates reduced the variance due to lead, if the proper unnamed variate should be found, controlling for it would set the lead coefficient at zero. In the paper cited, Smith states:

The findings in this study show that if outcome measures are controlled, differences between lead groups on all tests *become non-significant* and the *null hypothesis* that the differences are not statistically different from zero *must be accepted*. In other words, social factors explain the differences in test performance to such a considerable degree that it is likely that the *very small* differences that remain once social factors have been taken into account are due to chance or to other social factors not measured.

295

This is, of course, formally incorrect: One is not forced to accept the null hypothesis; one cannot reject it at the odds given by the p value. More importantly, studies of child development have established a body of prior information which specifies to a considerable extent those social factors which enhance or interfere with cognitive development. It does not seem likely that some new variate (which to be a confounder is required to be both correlated with lead exposure and deleterious to psychological performance) remains undiscovered. Given that lead's neurotoxic properties have been repeatedly and unequivocally demonstrated, both in humans at high dose and in experimental animals under carefully controlled conditions resembling low-level exposure (see papers by Rice and Cory-Schlecta, this volume), it is neither necessary nor scientifically rigorous to invoke unnamed ghosts ('other social factors not measured') in the epidemiological machinery to explain away neurotoxic effects that remain after control of covariates.

Building non-veridical causal models

Variates which are measured in a study may be independent variables that affect the outcome under examination, or they may themselves be affected by lead. They may in fact occupy both positions in the causal chain. The question of simultaneity, which is just beginning to gain attention in the area of lead toxicity, will not be addressed here. To control for such outcome measures as school placement (Winneke et al., 1983), hyperactive behaviour (Harvey et al., 1984), or developmental delay (Smith et al., 1983) may be to subtract out variance which properly belongs to the main effect, lead. Since it has been shown that lead exposure during pregnancy can affect later development (Bellinger et al., this volume), control of early development or temperament may result in overcontrolling for lead. It would be important for investigators at the least to report the results with and without controlling for these variates.

In the study of prenatal exposure, the transgenerational influence of lead has received little attention. Since most economically disadvantaged parents have little economic mobility, they tend to reside in the same or similar neighbourhoods from childhood through their adult years. It is reasonable then to expect that mothers (and fathers) share lead exposures and burdens similar to those of their offspring. It has been suggested (Dietrich et al., 1985; Milar et al., 1980) that higher lead burdens in infants and children are associated with poor maternal rearing, as measured by scaled scores such as the Caldwell Home Observation for Measurement of the Environment (HOME). What has not been widely appreciated is that some of the poorer rearing scores in mothers of children with higher lead levels may derive from deficits in the mother's behaviour, and that this might be a result of the mother's exposure to lead when she was a child. This effect of lead exposure on rearing patterns has been experimentally demonstrated in the rodent (Barrett and Livesey, 1983).

Accepting the null hypothesis from studies with inadequate power

Focusing attention on the alpha (Type I error) risk in a study can lead the investigator away from attention to the beta (Type II error) risk. Most published studies cite the alpha risk, but infrequent attention is given to the accompanying beta risk. Inescapably, value choices are expressed in this regard. Scientific rigour is thought to be defended by lowering alpha levels, preventing or minimizing the number of spurious facts inserted into the literature, and reducing the number of unnecessary replications. But exclusive concern for minimizing alpha risks narrows the gate for new observations and hypotheses. This can have unfortunate implications, particularly in the arena of preventive medicine where putative health effects are frequently difficult to measure.

The relative value placed upon avoiding Type I and Type II errors can be appreciated by examining the ratio of beta level to alpha level at sample sizes generally seen in the lead literature. Table 1, taken from a recent communication by Rosenthal and Rubin (1985), is informative. It shows that for a sample size between 80 and 200, at an r of 0.10, the ratio of accepted beta to alpha error can be as high as 17 to 1.

In the 14 studies reviewed later in this paper, none presented a formal power analysis. We calculated the power to find a 'medium effect' for all studies and found the range to be 0.30 to 0.99. For a 'small' effect the power ranged from zero to 0.70. One study that reported no relationship between lead and IQ used multiple-regression analysis with 17 covariates. The sample size was 48. This study had a power of between zero and 0.30 to reject the null hypothesis (Harvey et al., 1984). In the univariate analysis, before control of covariates and stratification of subjects by social class, the sample size was 133. The power for this n was 0.10. It is of interest that this analysis did show a relationship between lead level and outcome that was significant at the $p = 0.05$ level. In another study, not included here, Ernhart et al., reanalysed an earlier data set that had shown an association between lead and IQ. The reanalysis eliminated a number of subjects and reduced the sample size from 80 to 45. These authors reported no significant effect. The power in that study to find a small effect was 0.32 (Ernhart et al., 1985). The authors concluded that lead effects, if present, were small and outweighed by social factors. These authors then proceeded to generalize from these no-effect studies to more global conclusions about the relationship between lead and neurocognitive function.

Table 1 Ratio of beta to alpha risks for certain effect sizes

	$r = 0.10$		$r = 0.30$	
N subjects	alpha = 0.05	alpha = 0.01	alpha = 0.05	alpha = 0.02
50	18	97	9.0	67
80	17	96	4.0	44
100	17	94	3.0	31
200	16	88	0.2	31

After Rosenthal and Rubin, 1985

Underestimating the biological significance of a demonstrated effect size

Studies of lead have shown effect sizes of approximately 4–6 points. Differences of this magnitude have effect sizes of 0.30 to 0.45 standard deviations. A number of commentators have defined these differences as 'minimal' or unlikely to be of clinical significance (Smith *et al.*, 1983; Ernhart *et al.*, 1981). We have pointed out that a difference between median IQ scores of 6 points predicts a four-fold increase in the proportion of significantly impaired children (Needleman *et al.*, 1982) (Figure 1).

Ernhart and colleagues (1985), in a reanalysis of their first study, report a partial r^2 of 0.028 for lead level and cognitive IQ, and describe this as minimal. An r^2 of this magnitude can be expressed as the binomial effect size, that is, the proportion of subjects whose IQ scores would be reduced below the

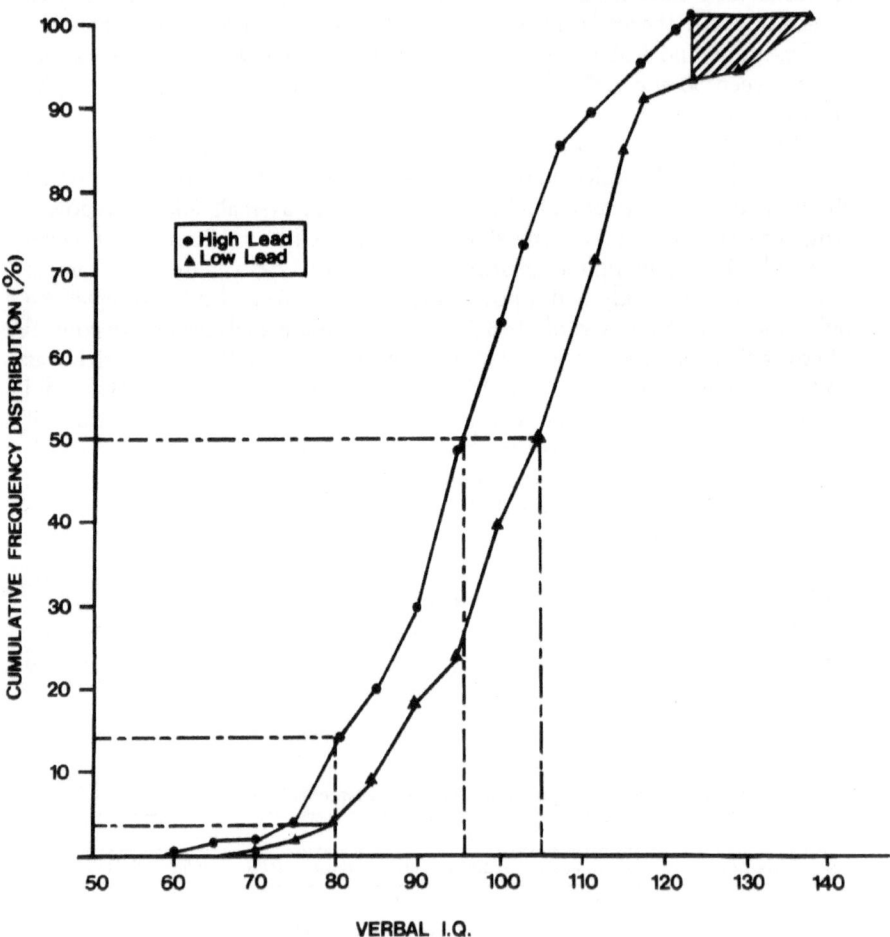

Figure 1 Cumulative frequency distribution of verbal IQ scores in high and low lead subjects. A shift in the median score of 6 points is associated with a four-fold increase in the risk of IQ below 80

median by their lead exposure. The difference in binomial effect attributable to lead in that study was 0.16. This means that the proportion of children with reduced cognitive scores was increased from 0.42 to 0.58 by their lead exposure. This can in no way be described as a minimal effect.

The mean effect size in the 14 studies we reviewed was 0.37 standard deviations, and the range was 0.07 to 0.64 standard deviations. At an effect size of 0.4, the area of non-overlap of the two samples is 27.4%. The upper 50% of the unexposed group exceeds in IQ 65.5% of the exposed group. While an effect size of this magnitude may be difficult to detect, it is of major biological consequence.

Expecting proof of causality

Numerous critics of studies which assert that an association between lead and outcome has been demonstrated reject the studies because the causal relationship has not been proven. This criticism usually depends on three arguments: (1) flaws in design or execution of the paper under examination; (2) the possibility that some covariate may not have been recognized and controlled; or (3) the failure of the difference found to reach the 0.05 significance level. We have earlier discussed the misuse of the 0.05 level. It should also be noted that the 0.05 significance level is not the only, or even the most important, criterion for causality. Relationships with p values smaller than 0.05 may not be causal, and relationships at higher values may be causal.

No real-world epidemiological study is without flaw. As a consequence all studies are vulnerable. Since multivariate space has infinite dimensions (for example, has the study controlled for birth weight, haemoglobin, degree of neonatal icterus, serum iron level, school quality, hair colour, handedness, marital adjustment, early temperament, etc.?) and the supply of subjects is finite, the investigator will necessarily be confronted with an unsaturated structural model. Any clever biostatistician with access to a rather dull computer can fit an infinite number of regression equations to the data in that circumstance (Leamer, 1983). In addition, the variates measured only imperfectly capture the factors of real interest to the study. Family size, socioeconomic status and mother's IQ do not, after all, directly influence the child's intellectual function. They are surrogates for other variables more proximate to those mechanisms that affect the outcomes of interest. These variables, specified imperfectly, are also unavoidably measured with some error. These inescapable design hurdles, taken in sum, provide the investigator with fixed constraints upon the demonstration of causal relationships.

But even if these design difficulties were surmounted, the demonstration of causal proof could not be accomplished. David Hume, 200 years ago, stated that causality is a concept not susceptible to empirical demonstration. Epidemiologists, and bench scientists as well, are generally modest folk who accept more limited goals for themselves. They are in most cases content to contribute to the incremental and somewhat painful accretion of bits of data which one hopes can be assembled into a coherent picture, from which lawfulness can be inferred.

Evaluating studies in isolation

Most narrative reviews (Bornschein et al., 1980, Pocock and Ashby, 1985; Smith, 1985; Needleman and Landrigan, 1981; Bellinger and Needleman, 1982; Yule and Rutter, 1985), examine each study's methodology, detail their strengths and weaknesses, and then attempt a narrative summary of the combined importance of the studies. Often a simple tally of those studies that showed an effect and those that showed no effect is presented in the conclusion. This balloting approach to seeking a consensual summary of the studies seriously degrades the data. Some authors, for example, still persist in reporting p-values > 0.05 as 'N.S'. If four investigators were to report differences between lead-exposed groups at the $p = 0.10$ level, this method would count them as no-effect studies. In fact the joint probability of this outcome is 0.02 (see Table 2).

Discarding individual studies on the basis of flawed design or execution can be seen as another form of requiring causal proof. Inferences do not grow from single studies. They are a product of the interaction of many scientists whose studies build upon earlier work; and, while imperfect themselves, the collective nonlinear sum of their conclusions permits the making of causal inferences.

The method of narrative reviewing has inherent limitations; the method of selection is often subjective, and the evaluation of the merits of each study is not separated from the bias of the reviewer. One response to this dilemma is the quantitative integrative review, or meta-analysis (Light and Pillemer, 1984; Rosenthal and Rosnow, 1984; Glass et al., 1981). In meta-analysis each study is treated as a subject in a study of studies, and the combined, integrated effects of the agent under question are evaluated. While this method does not completely insulate the study from bias in selection or interpretation, the criteria for selection (which should be determined a priori) can be made explicit and inclusive.

A META-ANALYSIS OF RECENT STUDIES OF LEAD AND IQ

We reviewed all studies published since 1974 in refereed journals, meeting proceedings, or PhD dissertations, using computer search. The only other meta-analysis for studies in this area of which we are aware was done by Schwartz et al. (1985) on six studies. Two studies presented in this volume (Hatzakis et al., Raab et al.) were added to the present analysis. In order to

Table 2 A simulated meta-analysis of four studies

	p-value	$-2 \log_e p$
Study 1 $p[\text{IT}] = 0.1$		4.6
2	0.1	4.6
3	0.1	4.6
4	0.1	4.6
		18.4, d.f. $= 8$
		$p = 0.02$

be included in the meta-analysis the studies had to meet the following criteria:

1. The methodology section of the study must have been informative enough to permit calculation of effect size and p values. That is, the author must have presented differences between groups and standard deviations, or r-values. In those cases where multiple regression was used, the effect size of IQ differences at blood levels of 10 μg/dl and 20 μg/dl was calculated from the regression equation. The standard deviation of the control group was the denominator.
2. The subjects must have been children under 12; the exposed group must have been exposed to doses considered to be 'low-level', e.g., 40 μg/dl in the blood or below.
3. The section on data analysis must have been informative enough to permit understanding of the methods employed. Where regression was used, the actual n, the regression coefficients, and the analysis of variance must have been available.
4. Only one version of each study was analysed. In some circumstances authors have submitted their study to reanalysis (Ernhart, et al., 1981; Needleman et al., 1985). Since both the original and the reanalyses cannot be considered independent measures, only the original of each was included in the present analysis.

Each study was reviewed for specific design and substantive features (Table 3). Power for each study was calculated by algorithms appropriate for the type of analysis used. Jacob Cohen's book was the source text (Cohen, 1977). Effect size for each study was calculated by the following formula:

$$ES = \frac{M1 - M2}{SDc}$$

where: M1 = mean IQ score for the unexposed group,
M2 = mean IQ score for the exposed group,
SDc = standard deviation of the unexposed group

One-tailed p values for the lead effect on verbal IQ were calculated, and the value transformed by taking $-2 \log_e p$. The transformed values were then summed. This sum has a chi-square distribution with $2N$ degrees of freedom. The sum was 109.13 for 26 degrees of freedom ($p = 2.97 \times 10^{-12}$).

We then addressed the 'file drawer question' and calculated the number of unpublished studies at $p = 0.5$ which would be required to bring the combined p-value to 0.05. The formula for the number of cases was:

Chi square for $[p(0.05)]$ $(2N + 26)$ $= 110 + 1.38 \times N$
Chi square for $[p(0.05)]$ (190) $= 110 + 1.38 \times 82$

Eighty-two cases with significance values of 0.5 would be required to raise the collective p-value to > 0.05. We do not believe that there are that number (82) of unpublished papers with this result lying fallow and anonymous in the files of investigators around the world.

Table 3 Meta-analysis, studies of the lead–IQ relationship

Authors	Year	n	Effect size	Power small effect	p val [IT]	$-2 \log_e p$
Ernhart et al.	1974	80	0.6	0.2	0.025	7.38
Needleman et al.	1979	73	0.35	0.47	0.015	8.4
Yule et al.	1981	82	0.573	0.42	0.021	7.73
Winneke et al.	1982	26	0.26	0.18	0.15	3.7
Smith et al.	1983	185	0.17	0.7	0.12	4.24
Winneke et al.	1983	115	0.351	0.25	0.4	1.83
Harvey et al.	1984	47		0		
Shapiro and Maracek	1984	193	0.46	0.48	0.025	7.38
Lansdown et al.	1986	162	0.07	0.48	0.66	0.83
Hansen et al.	1985	82	0.5	0.34	0.0005	15.2
Hawk et al.	1985	75	0.64	0.25	0.0004	15.64
Schroeder et al.	1985	104	0.5	0.33	0.005	10.6
Fulton et al. (this volume)	1986	501	0.4	0.52	0.003	11.6
Hatzakis et al. (this volume)	1986	509	0.4	0.52	0.00065	14.6

$$\Sigma \bar{x} = 109.13$$
$$p = 2.97 \times 10^{-12}$$

CONCLUSION

Making causal connections in the real world is not a pure, value-free enterprise. The present paper has attempted to show how causal interpretation is influenced by perceptions of the relative adversiveness of Type I and Type II errors. It seems clear that differences in style exist among investigators and interpreters of the same data base. These stylistic, value-laden differences in interpreting the data seem to be rather stable traits. It would be of considerable interest to determine whether they segregate with differences in training, discipline, or other variables.

In this paper we have catalogued seven methodological solecisms that cloud the valid interpretation of an ever-growing and converging data base on lead and neurocognitive function. Examining arguments raised against the toxicity of lead, tobacco, formaldehyde, and asbestos persuades us that these errors have also been made many times in other domains, with other toxicants. Cautious investigators will want to keep these errors in mind when making future causal judgements about lead and other substances that may produce small (by this we mean unobservable to the naked eye) but important changes in a complex chemical, economic and social surrounding.

REFERENCES

Barrett, J. and Livesey, P.J. (1983) Lead induced alterations in maternal behavior and offspring development in the rat. *Neurobehav. Toxicol. Teratol.*, **5**, 557–563

Bellinger, D. and Needleman, H.L. (1982) Low level exposure and psychological deficit in children. In Wolraich, M. and Routh, D.K. (eds) *Advances in Developmental and Behavioral Pediatrics*, Vol. 3 (Greenwich, Conn.: JAI Press)

Bornschein, R., Pearson, D. and Reiter, L. (1980) Behavioral effects of moderate lead exposure in children and animal models. Part 2: animal studies. *CRC Crit. Rev. Toxicol.*, **8**, 101–152

Cohen, J. (1977) *Statistical Power Analysis for the Behavioral Sciences*, rev. edn (London: Academic Press)

Cohen, J. and Cohen, P. (1975) *Applied Multiple Regressional/Correlation Analysis for the Behavioral Sciences*, (Hillsdale, NJ: Lawrence Erlbaum), pp. 123–167

Cornfield, J. (1974) Recent methodological contributions to clinical trials. *Am. J. Epidemiol.*, **104**, 408–421

Cowles, M. and Davis, C. (1982) On the origins of the .05 level of significance. *Am. Psychol.*, **37**, 553–558

Dietrich, K.N., Krafft, K.M., Pearson, D.T., Harris, L.C., Bornschein, R. L. Hammond, P.B. and Succop, P.A. (1985) Contribution of social and developmental factors to lead exposure during the first year of life. *Pediatrics*, **75**, 1114–1119

Ernhart, C., Landa, B. and Schell, N. (1981) Subclinical levels of lead and developmental deficit – a multivariate follow-up reassessment. *Pediatrics*, **67**, 911–919

Ernhart, C., Landa, B. and Wolf, A.W. (1985) Subclinical lead level and developmental deficit: re-analyses of data. *J. Learning Disabil.*, **18**(8), 475–479

Fisher, R.A. (1925) *Statistical Methods for Research Workers*, (Edinburgh: Oliver & Boyd)

Fisher, R.A. (1926) *Statistical Methods for Research Workers*, 2nd edn (Edinburgh: Oliver & Boyd)

Glass, G.V., McGaw, B. and Smith, M.L. (1981) *Meta-analysis in Social Research* (Beverly Hills: Sage)

Hansen, O.N., Lyngbye, T., Trilingsgaard, A., Beese, I. and Grandjean, P. (1985) A neuropsychological and behavioral assessment of children with low level lead exposure. (T.D. Lekkas (ed.) *International Conference on Heavy Metals in the Environment*, Athens

Harvey, P.G., Hamlin, M.W., Kumar, R. and Delves, H.T. (1984) Blood lead, behaviour and intelligence test performance in preschool children. *Sci. Total Environ.*, **40**, 45–60

Hawk, B.A., Schroeder, S.R., Robinson, G., Otto, D.A., Mushak, P. and Barton, C. (1985) Relation of lead to cognitive function of children at risk for sociocultural mental retardation. T. D. Lekkas (ed.) *International Conference on Heavy Metals in the Environment.* Athens

Lansdown, R., Yule, W., Urbanowicz, M.A. and Hunter, J. (1986) The relationship between blood-lead concentrations, intelligence, attainment, and behavior in a school population: the second London Study. *Int. Arch. Occup. Environ. Health,* **57**, 225–235

Leamer, E.E. (1983) Let's take the con out of economics. *Am. Econ. Rev.,* **73**, 31–43

Light, R. and Pillemer, D.B. (1984) *Summing Up* (Cambridge, Mass.: Harvard University Press)

Milar, C.R., Schroeder, S.R., Mushak, P., Dolcourt, J.L. and Grant, L.D. (1980) Contributions of the care giving environment to increased lead burden of children. *Am. J. Ment. Defic.,* **84**, 339–344

Needleman, H.L., Geiger, S.K. and Frank, R. (1985) Lead and IQ scores: a reanalysis [letter]. *Science (Washington, DC),* **227**, 701–704

Needleman, H., Gunnoe, C., Leviton, A., Reed, R.R., Peresie, H., Maher, C. and Barrett, P. (1979) Deficits in psychologic and classroom performance in children with elevated dentine lead levels. *N. Engl. J. Med.,* **300**, 584–695

Needleman, H.L. and Landrigan, P.J. (1981) The health effects of low level exposure to lead. *Ann. Rev. Public Health,* **2**, 277–298

Needleman, H., Leviton, A. and Bellinger, D. (1982) Lead-associated intellectual deficit. *N. Engl. J. Med.,* **306**, 367

Pocock, S.J. and Ashby, D. (1985) Environmental lead and children's intelligence: a review of recent epidemiological studies. *Statistician,* **34**, 31–44

Rosenthal, R. and Rosnow, R. (1984) *Essentials of Behavioral Research* (New York: McGraw Hill)

Rosenthal, R. and Rubin, D.B. (1985) Statistical analysis: summarizing evidence versus establishing facts. *Psychol. Bull.,* **97**, 527–529

Schroeder, S.R., Hawk, B., Ottot, D., Mushak, P. and Hicks, R.E. (1985) Separating the effects of lead and social factors on IQ. *Environ. Res.,* **38**, 144–154

Schwartz, J., Pitcher, H., Levin, R., Ostrow, B. and Nichols, A. (1985) Cost and benefits of reducing lead in gasoline: final regulatory impact analysis. USEPA: EPA 230-05-85-006

Smith, M. (1985) Recent work on low level lead exposure and its impact on behavior, intelligence and learning: a review. *J. Am. Acad. Child Psychiatry,* **24**, 24–32

Smith, M., Delves, T., Lansdown, R., Clayton, B. and Graham, P. (1983) The effects of lead exposure on urban children: the Institute of Child Health/Southampton Study. *Dev. Med. Child Neurol.,* **25**, 47

Winneke, G., Hrdina, K. and Brockhaus, A. (1982) Neuropsychological studies in children with elevated tooth lead concentrations. Part I: Pilot study using a matched pair approach. *Int. Arch. Occup. Environ. Health,* **51**, 169

Winneke, G., Kramer, G., Brockhaus, A., Ewers, U., Kujanaek, G., Lechner, H. and Janke, W. (1983) Neuropsychological studies in children with elevated tooth lead concentration. *Int. Arch. Occup. Environ. Health,* **51**, 231

Yule, W. and Rutter, M. (1985) Effect of lead on children's behavior and cognitive performance: a critical review. In *Dietary and Environmental Lead: Human Health Effects* (Amsterdam: Elsevier)

Section 4

PREGNANCY OUTCOME, NEONATAL AND PROSPECTIVE STUDIES

Introduction

The prospective studies have investigated groups of children followed over periods of several years. They were set up for a number of reasons: to allow examination of body lead burden over time, and at different developmental stages, and to allow examination of the relationship of exposure variables to indices of body lead; to allow examination of the association of measures of body lead obtained at different ages and outcome measures, and therefore an examination of critical periods of exposure; and to allow the examination of the impact of social and environmental variables on lead uptake, and on development. Unlike the cross-sectional studies where there is much reliance on retrospective data for information on past exposure, and on social and environmental variables, in prospective studies measures can be made or information collected at one stage, for use at a later stage of the study. The prospective studies, starting at or before birth, have also enabled investigation of the effects of low levels of lead on pregnancy outcome, and on neonatal measures.

Compared with the cross-sectional studies, many of the prospective studies reported in this section are situated in areas of relatively high lead exposure. The design of many is similar as they are, to some extent, following a common protocol. The papers describe research being carried out in an industrially polluted area in Australia (Vimpani *et al.*), and a similarly polluted area in Yugoslavia (Graziano *et al.*); in areas of high urban pollution in USA (Bornschein *et al.* and Dietrich *et al.*) and in Mexico (Rothenberg *et al.*), in a high water-lead urban area in UK (Moore *et al.*); and in an urban area in USA with relatively low exposure (Bellinger *et al.*). As in the cross-sectional studies, most of the populations studied have been socially disadvantaged, but that studied in Boston by Bellinger *et al.* was unusual in that it was relatively advantaged. The studies reported are at different stages of progress: those in Yugoslavia and Mexico are in the early stages with few results, while others report the results from several years of investigation. The paper by Ernhart and colleagues is a review of results on pregnancy outcome and birth defects in relation to some of the methodological isues involved.

4.1

Effects of Prenatal Lead Exposure on Infant Size at Birth

R. L. BORNSCHEIN, J. GROTE, T. MITCHELL, P. A. SUCCOP,
K. N. DIETRICH, K. M. KRAFFT and P. B. HAMMOND

SUMMARY

It is well established that high levels of maternal lead exposure during pregnancy can result in a spectrum of adverse outcomes for the foetus, including spontaneous abortion, stillbirth, preterm delivery, and small-for-gestational-age deliveries. Less is known about lead-related intrauterine growth retardation at levels of lead exposure encountered by the general population. In an interim analysis of data from 202 inner-city infants, prenatal lead exposure was inversely related to birth weight and birth length. Maternal blood lead (PbB) concentrations ranged from 1 to 26 μg dl^{-1} ($\bar{x} = 7.6$). The lead effect varied from a negative 58 g per natural log unit increment in PbB for 18-year-old mothers to a negative 601 g per natural log unit increment in 30-year-old mothers.

The reproductive toxicity of high-level lead exposure is well known and supported by an extensive literature (Rom, 1976). Much of this literature focuses on an increased incidence of spontaneous abortions and stillbirths associated with lead exposures in the workplace (Oliver, 1911; Lane, 1949). Based on a renewed awareness of these earlier findings, women have been largely excluded from occupational lead exposure. Therefore, exposures have declined and the attention of researchers and regulatory agencies has shifted to more subtle manifestations of lead-related reproductive toxicity in the general population.

Recently, several large epidemiological studies have reported an association between low-level maternal blood lead (PbB) concentrations and various indices of adverse reproductive outcome, including preterm delivery (McMichael et al., 1986), low birth weight (Dietrich et al., in press), an increased incidence of minor anomalies (Needleman et al., 1984), and indices of neurological involvement (Ernhart *et al.*, 1986; Dietrich *et al.*, 1987; and Bellinger *et al.*, 1984). The purpose of the present report is to provide an update on interim analyses of the relationship between *in utero* lead exposure and foetal development as indexed by physical size at birth. The data were derived from a cohort of pregnant women recruited to participate in the Cincinnati Lead Study.

METHODS

Sample

Expectant mothers residing in previously defined high-risk-for-lead-exposure neighbourhoods were contacted at the time of their first prenatal clinic visit. Women were eligible to participate if they resided in the designated study area, were not more than 28 weeks pregnant, and had no documented history of diabetes, current treatment for drug or alcohol abuse or recent treatment for psychiatric disorders. They also had to grant informed consent and indicate an intention to remain in Cincinnati following delivery. At delivery, the mother was asked to consent to the long-term study of her infant if the infant weighed more than 1500 g; was equal to or greater than 35 weeks gestational age at delivery; was free from serious medical conditions, such as Down's syndrome, phenylketonuria, and significant congenital anomalies; and had an Apgar score of 6 or greater at 5 minutes postparturition. The initial recruitment of expectant mothers took place between January 1980 and May 1985 and yielded over 700 women for whom lead exposure data and relevant covariate and outcome data were available. The recruitment of infants at delivery yielded over 400 subjects. This analysis is limited to the 202 mother–infant pairs for whom complete data are currently available. Six sets of twins were excluded from this analysis. A brief summary of key descriptive statistics for the sample is provided in Table 1.

Blood collection and analysis

Maternal blood samples were collected by venipuncture at the first prenatal visit, which occurred between the sixth and twenty-eighth week of gestation ($x = 16$ weeks). Lead-free Vacutainer® tubes were used. Prenatal PbB analyses were carried out by anodic stripping voltammetry on an ESA Model 2014. All samples were analysed in duplicate by Environmental Sciences Associates, Inc. and approximately 20% of the samples were also analysed in duplicate in our laboratory, using an ESA Model 3010A, as a means of establishing interlaboratory confirmation of accuracy and precision. All PbB values, expressed as μg Pb dl^{-1} whole blood, were subsequently adjusted to a standard haematocrit (packed cell volume) of 35% and transformed to their natural logarithm equivalent for data analysis.

Table 1 Descriptive statistics for sample ($n = 202$)

	x̄	SD	Range
Gestational age (wk)	39.6	1.6	35–43
Prenatal PbB (μg dl^{-1})*	7.5	1.6	1–27
Maternal age (y)	22.6	4.4	15–39
Prenatal care (clinic visits)	8.9	3.8	1–22
Maternal height (cm)	162.5	6.5	148–181
SES score	17.1	5.6	8–50
Race (% black)	83.2%		
CITAC (% users)	57.8%		
Marital status (% single)	82.4%		
Birth weight (g)	3160	449	2010–4400
Birth length (cm)	49.4	2.4	42–56
Birth head circumference (cm)	33.8	1.3	30–39

*Geometric mean and standard deviation (SD)

Obstetric history and perinatal data

A comprehensive set of standardized definitions and scoring criteria was developed to encode information on 342 items. These items, which were extracted from hospital charts of the mothers and infants, pertained to obstetric history, the course of the pregnancy, and neonatal status. An experienced neonatologist assisted in the formulation of these definitions and resolved any ambiguities in the interpretation of items in the charts. The same team of two experienced research staff independently reviewed and encoded each chart. The intercoder reliability was very high. In a sample audit of 20 records, 10 of 6840 items were disparate, none of which was of a substantive nature. This data base was subsequently used to complete the Littman–Parmelee Obstetrical and Postnatal Complications Scales (Littman and Parmelee, 1978) and the Problem Oriented Perinatal Risk Assessment System (POPRAS) developed by Hobel et al. (1979). The POPRAS is divided into an Initial Risk Assessment Scale, a Developing Problems Scale, and a Newborn Risk Assessment Scale. The Composite Index of Tobacco and Alcohol Consumption (CITAC), taken from the POPRAS, was scored dichotomously, with a value of 0 indicating abstention from use of cigarettes and alcohol during pregnancy. Fifty-eight percent of this sample of mothers reported use of these substances at the time of their initial prenatal interview.

Socioeconomic status (SES)

During the first year postpartum, each infant's family was assessed and a determination of SES made with the use of the Hollingshead Four-Factor Index of Social Status (Hollingshead, 1975). The mean SES for the sample was 17.1 ± 5.6, which reflects the large number of single parent, low-income households in this sample.

Gestational age

Study infants were examined during the first 72 h postparturition to assess the gestational age of the infant. The Ballard Assessment of Gestational Age (Ballard *et al.*, 1979) was used for this purpose.

Statistical methods

Variables that might serve as confounders of the prenatal PbB:birth weight relationship were chosen, *a priori*, on the basis of their theoretical and/or known empirical relationship with blood lead and/or birth weight (see Table 2).

Each of the 21 variables so chosen was interacted with the prenatal PbB variable, so that PbB effects which might be specific to subpopulations could also be detected. Beginning with this model, which included 21 potential confounders and covariates, PbB, and 21 first-order interaction terms, a backward-elimination stepwise procedure was executed. Interaction terms were inspected and dropped from the model before the potential confounder, from which it was formed, was inspected for significance. A single interaction

Table 2 Candidate covariables in regression models examining the effect of maternal prenatal blood Pb on birth weight*, birth length, and head circumference

---

** Gestational age by physical examination†

** (Gestational age)^2

** Use of alcohol or tobacco products during pregnancy†† (CITAC)

** Maternal age
(Maternal age)^2
Gravidity

** Number of prenatal visits
(Number of prenatal visits)^2
Persistent prenatal anaemia
Maternal prenatal infections
Race
Initial Risk Assessment Score††
Socioeconomic status†††
Obstetrical Complications Scale††††
Marital status

** Maternal height
Current hypertension
History of hypertension
1-minute Apgar score
5-minute Apgar score
Date of infant birth (to assess potential cohort effects)

---

† Ballard *et al.* (1979)
†† Hobel (1979)
††† Hollingshead (1975)
†††† Littman and Parmelee (1978)
* All first-order interactions with prenatal PbB were tested.
** Significant covariates ($p = 0.05$) in final model. The prenatal PbB × maternal age interaction was also statistically significant

or confounder was eliminated at each step of this procedure. When all confounders and interactions remaining in the model were significant at $p < 0.05$, eliminated variables were tested for possible reentry into the model. If the partial bivariate relationship between any eliminated variable and birth weight residualized from this tentative model was found to be significant at $p < 0.05$, the variable was once again included in the model for birth weight. This process was repeated until all confounders and interaction terms in the final model were significant at $p < 0.05$, and each of the partial relationships between residualized birth weight and the excluded variables was not significant at $p > 0.05$. In the absence of any significant interaction variables, the significance of the PbB:birth weight effect was tested in this final model. A similar procedure was used to derive models for birth length, head circumference, ponderal index (PI) and duration of gestation.

RESULTS

Table 3 summarizes the intercorrelation among target-dependent variables birth weight, birth length, head circumference, ponderal index (birth weight in grams ÷ [birth length in cm]³) and duration of gestation; the main independent variable (maternal–prenatal PbB) and covariate and confounder variables which remained in the final models. Of particular interest are the statistically significant negative bivariate correlations between PbB and birth weight ($r = -0.18, p < 0.001$) and between PbB and birth length ($r = -0.13$, $p < 0.05$). These two relationships are shown in Figures 1 and 2.

The results of three multiple regression analyses, which relate maternal PbB to infant size at birth, are summarized in Table 4. The final model for birth weight accounted for 29% of the observed variance. Maternal PbB interacted with maternal age to produce a statistically significant ($p < 0.007$) depression in covariate-adjusted birth weight. This interaction is depicted in Figure 3. The lead effect varies from -58.1 g per natural log unit increment in PbB for 18-year-old mothers to -600.9 g per natural log unit increment in PbB for 30-year-old mothers.

The final model for birth weight accounted for 24% of the observed variance in birth length. Maternal PbB interacted with race to produce a significant ($p < 0.025$) depression in birth length. This effect was contained entirely within the white infants. The birth length of white infants decreased approximately 2.5 cm per natural log unit increment in maternal PbB. This interaction is shown in Figure 4.

A significant maternal lead × race interaction ($p < 0.01$) was found in the model describing lead's effect on ponderal index (weight in grams/[length in cm]³). This interaction was due to the significant effect of maternal PbB on infant length within white infants.

No significant covariate-adjusted effect of maternal PbB on head circumference or duration of gestation (estimated by Ballard exam) was observed.

DISCUSSION

This interim report has examined the potential impact of elevated maternal blood lead concentrations during pregnancy on indices of physical size at

Table 3 Correlation among potential covariates and confounders

	Birth weight	Birth length	Head circumference	Ponderal index	Race	Gestation	CITAC	Visits	Maternal age	Maternal height	SES
Length	0.72										
Head circumference	0.63	0.52									
PI	0.35	-0.40	0.12								
Race	-0.07	-0.12	-0.09	0.05							
Gestation	0.32	0.27	0.33	0.05	0.05						
CITAC	-0.29	-0.26	-0.16	-0.02	-0.12	-0.02					
Visits	0.20	0.09	0.12	0.11	0.10	0.06	-0.11				
Maternal age	0.03	0.04	-0.02	0.09	0.02	0.03	0.04	0.12			
Maternal height	0.28	0.30	0.11	-0.03	-0.05	0.05	0.04	0.01	0.02		
SES	0.07	0.09	0.01	-0.01	0.07	0.13	-0.03	0.15	0.09	-0.00	
Ln PbB	-0.18	-0.13	-0.04	-0.06	-0.11	-0.07	0.15	-0.03	0.04	-0.09	-0.11

r must be > 0.11 to be statistically significant at $p < 0.05$
r must be > 0.16 to be statistically significant at $p < 0.001$

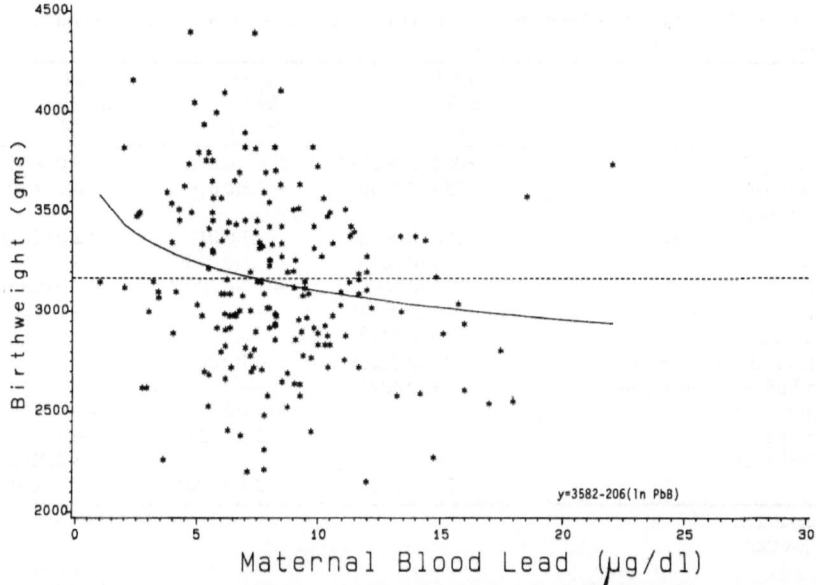

Figure 1 The unadjusted relationship between maternal blood lead concentration and infant weight at birth; $n = 202$; $r = -0.18$; $p = <0.001$

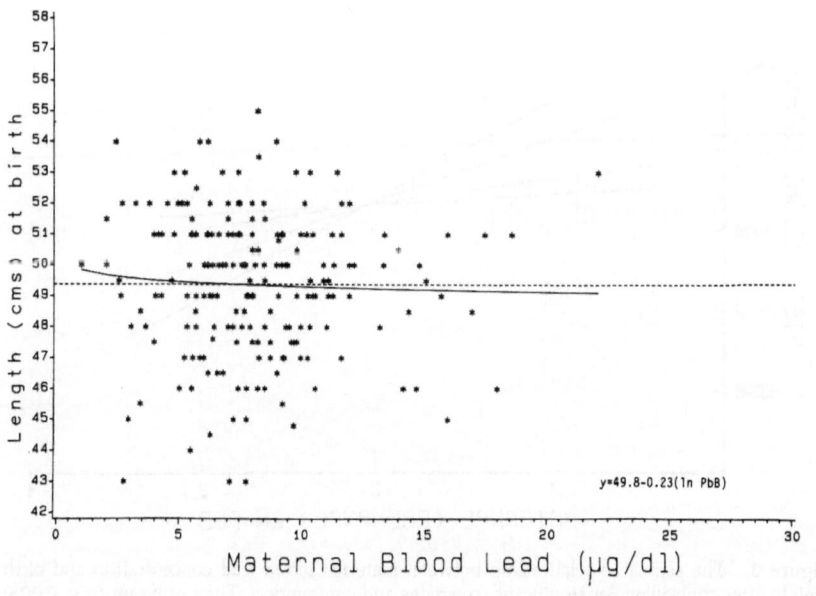

Figure 2 The unadjusted relationship between maternal blood lead concentration during pregnancy and infant length at birth; $n = 202$; $r = -0.13$; $p < 0.05$.

313

Table 4 Multiple regression models for association between maternal blood lead and foetal size at birth ($n = 202$)

	Birth weight model	Birth length model	Head circumference model
Intercept	−43082*(0.0007)**	−128.8(0.058)	25.9(0.0001)
Maternal (prenatal) Ln PbB	756 (0.0340)	−2.5(0.019)	−0.0(0.9670)
Gestational age (wk)	2079 (0.0012)	8.3(0.017)	0.2(0.0001)
(Gestational age)^2	−26 (0.0016)	−0.1(0.020)	—
CITAC (0,1)	−182 (0.0009)	−1.3(0.0001)	−0.3(0.0436)
Maternal age (y)	92 (0.0074)	—	—
Prenatal visits	19 (0.0174)	—	—
Maternal height (cm)	16 (0.0002)	0.1(0.0001)	—
Ln PbB × maternal age	−45 (0.0073)	—	—
Race	—	−5.9(0.013)	—
Ln PbB × race	—	2.5(0.025)	—
Child's sex	—	—	−0.3(0.0263)
r^2	0.29 (0.0001)	0.24(0.0001)	0.11(0.0001)

* parameter estimate
** p-value

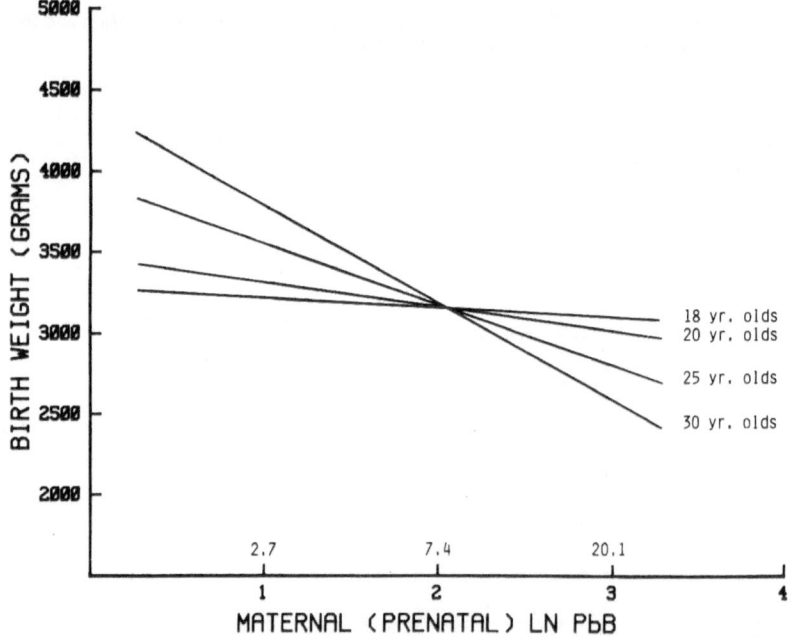

Figure 3 The estimated relationship between maternal blood lead concentration and birth weight after controlling for significant covariates and confounders. The significant ($p < 0.008$) blood lead by maternal age interaction is show; $n = 202$

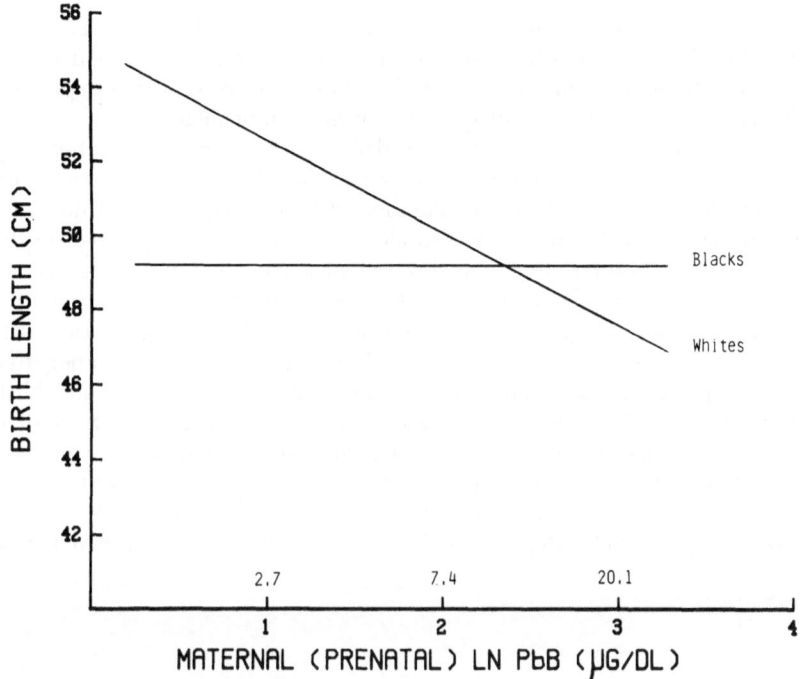

Figure 4 The estimated relationship between maternal blood lead concentration and birth length after controlling for significant covariates and confounders. The significant blood lead by race interaction is show; $n = 202$

birth and preterm deliveries. Contrary to the recent report by McMichael *et al.* (1986), we did not find an association between maternal blood lead and preterm deliveries. This could be due to the fact that the present analysis was restricted to infants carried to at least 35 weeks of gestation. An alternative explanation might be that the majority of the Cincinnati cohort had PbB concentrations below the threshold for causing preterm delivery. The PbB distribution for the Cincinnati cohort was as follows ($\bar{x} = 7.5$; SD = 1.6; range = 1 to 27), whereas the Port Pirie cohort distribution was ($\bar{x} = 10.6$; SD = 4.1; range = 1 to 32). Other yet-to-be-identified differences in key risk factors could also account for this discrepancy.

Indices of physical size at birth were significantly associated with maternal PbB. Of particular interest is the apparent impact of maternal PbB on infant birth weight. This lead effect interacts strongly with maternal age, itself a risk factor for adverse pregnancy outcome. The lead × maternal age interaction may indicate that older women are more sensitive to the additional insult of lead exposure, or that older women have higher total lead burden resulting from the greater number of years of exposure and exposure to higher ambient lead levels when they were children. Again, in contrast to the Port Pirie cohort, the Cincinnati cohort was generally younger and had slightly lower mean PbB concentrations. Perhaps the most lead sensitive of the older, more highly exposed pregnant women in the Port Pirie cohort delivered preterm

315

infants, whereas the remaining, less sensitive women in Port Pirie had term deliveries of normal-weight infants. Conversely, since the Cincinnati cohort was younger and had slightly lower PbB values, lead did not result in preterm delivery, but rather term delivery of low-birth-weight infants.

In a separate but related analysis of data from the Cincinnati cohort, the PbB:birth weight relationship was examined in a cohort of 861 women with pregnancies of at least 20 weeks duration. This cohort contained not only the 202 cases reported here, but also all women and infants rejected on the basis of the exclusion criteria and those women who declined to participate in the subsequent study of their infants. This analysis, which controlled for duration of gestation, gravidity, marital status, marital age, prenatal care, race and child's sex, indicated that a statistically significant ($p < 0.0006$) negative relationship existed between maternal blood lead concentration and birth weight after controlling for the statistically significant covariate and/or confounder variables (see Figure 5). The maternal blood lead range was $1-27\,\mu g\,dl^{-1}$ ($\bar{x} = 7.6$), and the birth weight range was $540-4649\,g$ ($\bar{x} = 3091$). The observed decrement in birth weight attributable to lead exposure was approximately 114 g per natural log unit increment in maternal

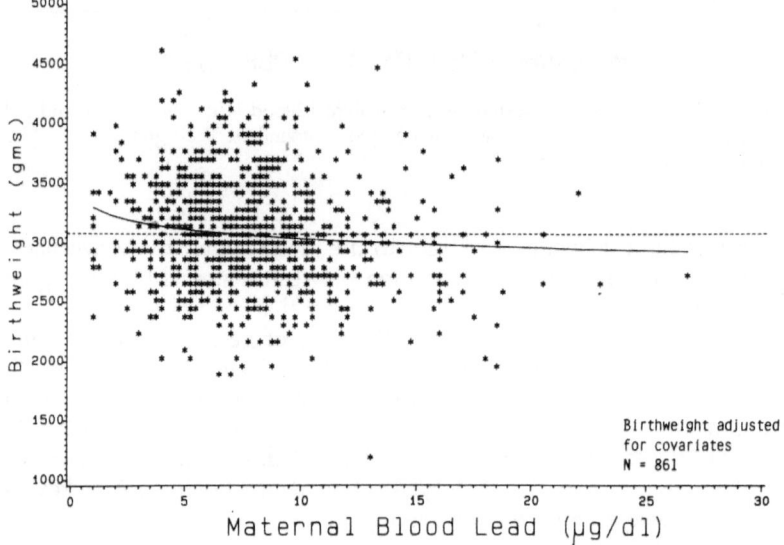

Figure 5   The dose–effect relationship between maternal blood lead concentration and infant birth weight after controlling for significant covariates and confounders.

Birth weight (g) $= -8050 - 114$ (1n PbB) $+ 472$ (gestation age)
$\qquad\qquad\qquad + 4$ (gestational age)^2 $+ 18$ (gravidity)
$\qquad\qquad\qquad - 139$ (child's sex) $- 190$ (race)
$\qquad\qquad\qquad + 67$ (married).

where: gestational age in wk
$\qquad$ child's sex: male $= 1$; female $= 2$
$\qquad$ maternal race: white $= 1$; black $= 2$
$\qquad$ married: yes $= 1$; no $= 0$
$r^2 = 0.45$; $p < 0.0001$; $n = 861$

316

blood lead concentration. This was equivalent to a 376-g decrement over the observed range for maternal PbB. An analysis was also performed using the infant's blood lead concentration at 10 days of age instead of the maternal blood lead as an indicator of foetal lead exposure. Lead remained a significant determinant of birth weight, further validating the PbB:birth weight relationship. A preliminary dose-response analysis was also undertaken. A response was defined as a covariate-adjusted birth weight less than 2750 g (controlling for all covariates found to be statistically associated with birth weight). The PbB exposure scale was divided into five $6 \mu g \, dl^{-1}$ intervals as follows: 1–6, 7–12, 13–18, 19–24, and 25–30. Since the last two intervals contained only six cases, these cases were combined with those having PbBs between 13 and $18 \mu g \, dl^{-1}$. The percentages of women delivering infants weighing less than 2750 g were 19, 21 and 33% for the intervals 1–6, 7–12, and $> 12 \mu g \, dl^{-1}$, respectively (see Figure 6). Employing a more severe criterion of this response, i.e. a birth weight less than 2500 g, resulted in incidences of 6.1, 9.3, and 12.2%, respectively, for these three PbB intervals.

It has been suggested that distressed foetuses may absorb more lead than healthy infants, thereby resulting in a spurious association between elevated PbB and low birth weight (Wibberly et al., 1977; Khera et al., 1980; Ernhart et al., in press). Data from the present study do not support this hypothesis. If Apgar scores at 5 minutes postparturition or Littmann–Parmelee Obstetrical and Postnatal Complications Scores are used as an indicator of infant distress, the aforementioned hypothesis would predict that low Apgar scores or low Littman–Parmelee scores would be associated with low birth weight and high PbB (either maternal or infant). No such pattern was found in this data set. In fact the PbB:birth weight relationship is most apparent in mother–infant

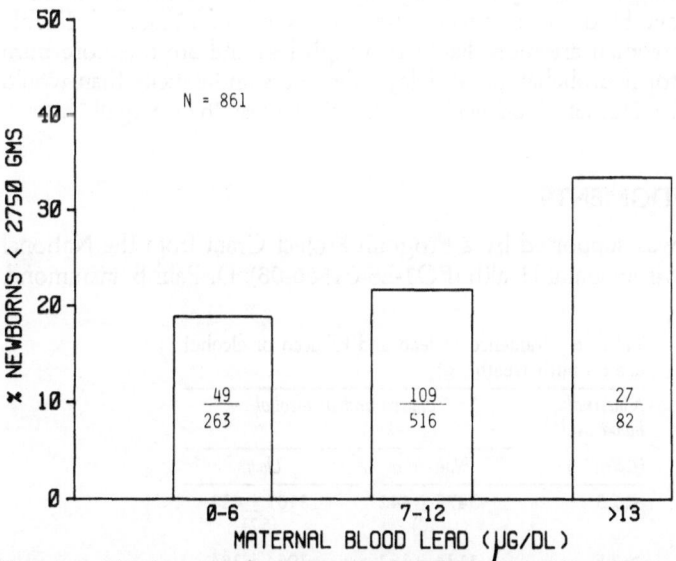

Figure 6 The dose–response relationship between maternal blood lead concentration and the percent of newborns weighing less than 2750 g at birth; $n = 861$

pairs *not* subjected to other risk factors. For example, it is well established that cigarette and/or alcohol use during pregnancy is associated with an increased incidence of low-birth-weight infants. If the sample discussed in this report is dichotomized on the basis of 'users' or 'abstainers' from alcohol or cigarettes, we can then examine the impact of maternal blood lead on birth weight within each of these subsamples. The results are presented in Table 5. The maternal prenatal PbB distribution was split at $7.5\,\mu g\,dl^{-1}$. Among non-users of alcohol and/or cigarettes, the mean birth weight difference between the high and low lead groups was 341 g. Among users, the difference was only 53 g. These data suggest that, if a study sample is composed of a high percentage of users of alcohol and/or cigarettes, it might be very difficult to detect an effect of PbB on birth weight. This might explain the non-significant PbB:birth weight findings reported in the Cleveland study (Ernhart *et al.*, in press).

Numerous risk factors have been shown to depress birth weight. However, these data suggest that they are not simply additive. There probably exists some lower limit beyond which birth weight cannot be depressed and still result in a term or near-term delivery. If multiple high-risk factors occur in the same pregnancy, the occurrence of preterm delivery, stillbirth, or spontaneous abortion is more likely to increase.

The findings of this report are of potentially great significance. Low birth weight is associated with numerous adverse neurobehavioural sequelae, including developmental delays, disorders and deficits. Any factor that contributes to the likelihood of low birth weight also increases the likelihood of poor developmental outcome.

The findings are also significant when one considers the level of lead exposure associated with this effect. Based on the recent National Health and Nutrition Examination Survey (Annest *et al.*, 1982), 500 000 women of child-bearing age have blood lead concentrations in excess of $12\,\mu g\,dl^{-1}$. Infants born to these women are more likely to weigh less and are therefore born at higher risk for neurobehavioural delays, disorders and deficits than would be expected at maternal blood lead concentrations less than $6\,\mu g\,dl^{-1}$.

ACKNOWLEDGMENTS

This research was supported by a Program Project Grant from the National Institute of Environmental Health (PO1-ES-01566-08), Dr Paul B. Hammond,

Table 5 Influence of lead and tobacco or alcohol use on birth weight (g)

Maternal blood lead	Tobacco and/or alcohol	
$(\mu g\,dl^{-1})$	Non-users	Users
<7.5	3475 ± 442 (40)	3107 ± 428 (52)
>7.5	3134 ± 382 (44)	3054 ± 384 (66)

Principal Investigator.

We are grateful to the many staff members who made significant contributions to this research, including Sandy Roda, Robert Greenland and Veronica Ratliff. We would also like to thank the Cincinnati Health Department, the Babies Milk Fund Association and the University Hospital for their co-operation and assistance during the recruitment phase of this study. Thanks also to Nancy Knapp who typed this manuscript.

REFERENCES

Annest, J.L., Mahaffey, K.R., Cox, D.H. and Roberts, J. (1982). Blood lead levels for persons 6 months–74 years of age: United States, 1976–1980. Hyattsville, MD: U. S. Department of Health and Human Services; DHHS pub no. (PHS) 82–1250. (Advance data from vital and health statistics of the National Center for Health Statistics: no. 79)

Ballard, J.L., Novak, K.K. and Driver, M. (1979). A simplified score for assessment of fetal maturation of newly born infants. *J. Pediatr.*, **95**, 766–774

Bellinger, D.C., Needleman, H.L., Leviton, A., Waternaux, C., Rabinowitz, M.B. and Nichols, M. (1984). Early sensory–motor development and prenatal exposure to lead. *Neurobehav. Toxicol. Teratol.*, **6**, 387–402

Dietrich, K.N., Krafft, K.M., Shukla, R., Bornschein, R.L. and Succop, P.S. (1987). The neurobehavioral effects of prenatal and early postnatal lead exposure. AAMD Monograph: Mental Retardation, Neurobehavioral Toxicology and Teratology, **8**, 71–95

Ernhart, C.B., Wolf, A.W., Kennard, M.J., Erhard, P., Filipovich, H.F. and Sokol, R.J. (1986). Intrauterine exposure to low levels of lead: the status of the neonate. *Arch. Environ. Health*, **41**, 287–291

Hobel, C.J., Youkeles, L. and Forsythe, A. (1979). Prenatal and intrapartum high-risk screening: II. Risk factors reassessed. *Am. J. Obstet. Gynecol.*, **135**, 1051–1056

Hollingshead, A.B. (1975). *Four Factor Index of Social Status.* Unpublished manual. (New Haven, Connecticut)

Khera, A.K., Wibberly, D.G. and Dathan, J.G. (1980). Placental and stillbirth tissue lead concentrations in occupational exposed women. *Br. J. Ind. Med.*, **37**, 394–396

Lane, R.E. (1949). The care of the lead worker. *Br. J. Ind. Med.*, **6**, 125–143

Littman, B. and Parmelee, A.H. (1978). Medical correlates of infant development. *Pediatrics*, **61**, 470–474

McMichael, A.J., Vimpani, G.V., Robertson, E.F., Baghurst, P.A. and Clark, P.D. (1986). The Port Pirie cohort study: maternal blood lead and pregnancy outcome *J. Epidemiol. Community Health*, **40**, 18–25

Needleman, H.L., Rabinowitz, M., Leviton, A., Linn, S. and Schoenbaum, S. (1984). The relationship between prenatal exposure to lead and congenital anomalies. *J. Am. Med. Assoc.*, **251**, 2956–2959

Oliver, T. (1911). Lead poisoning and the race. *Br. Med. J.*, **1(2628)**, 1096–1098

Rom, W.N. (1976). Effects of lead on the female and reproduction: a review. *Mount Sinai J. Med.*, **43**, 542–552

Wibberly, D.G., Khera, A.K., Edwards, J.H. and Rushton, D.I. (1977). Lead levels in human placenta from normal and malformed births. *J. Med. Genet.*, **14**, 339–345

4.2

Neurobehavioural Effects of Foetal Lead Exposure: The First Year of Life

K. N. DIETRICH, K. M. KRAFFT, M. BIER, O. BERGER,
P. A. SUCCOP and R. L. BORNSCHEIN

SUMMARY

Evidence from several recent prospective and retrospective studies indicates that lead may be psychoteratogenic at relatively low levels of foetal exposure. In the present interim study, lead measured in whole blood during the prenatal (maternal blood lead) and neonatal periods was found to be inversely related to a complex of sensorimotor developmental indices at 6 and 12 months. Prenatal blood lead was also related to lower birth weight, which in turn was related to poorer sensorimotor performance in infants during the first year. These adverse effects were observed at levels of lead exposure common in pregnant women in the United States, Europe, and other developed areas.

Mounting evidence suggests that lead is both a behavioural and physiological teratogen at typical levels of community exposure in the United States and other countries. This paper briefly reviews reports of some recent prospective studies and presents some additional work of the present authors in this area.

In a study of 185 infants in Boston, Massachusetts, Bellinger and his associates demonstrated a consistently negative relationship between umbilical cord blood lead (PbB) level and Bayley Mental Development Index (MDI) at 6 and 12 months (Bellinger et al., 1986). At each age, the difference between the low and high cord blood lead groups was equal to about one-third of a standard deviation (6–7 points). These adverse effects were found after statistical adjustments for developmentally relevant social and biological covariables. The findings of Bellinger et al. are particularly noteworthy because of their consistency across development and because cord PbB levels were relatively low (M = 6.6 μg dl^{-1}, SD = 3.2).

In another prospective study, 600 infants living near a primary lead smelter in Australia were given the Bayley Scales at 24 months (Vimpani *et al.*, 1987). Data analyses showed that the Bayley MDI was inversely related to early postnatal PbB levels measured at 6 months and to an integrated index of postnatal lead exposure that included repeat PbB assessments to 24 months. These effects were observed after statistical control for relevant developmental covariables, including maternal IQ. The Australian infants had, on average, higher postnatal PbB levels than typically found among US infants living in good housing (e.g. mean PbB at 24 months was $21 \mu g \, dl^{-1}$). However, this level of intoxication is commonly found among urban, innercity infants in the United States who reside in old deteriorating residences where lead is found in dusts, soils and flaking paint (Clark *et al.*, 1985).

In an interim study of 185 innercity infants in Cincinnati, Ohio, we previously reported (Dietrich *et al.*, 1986) an 'indirect' adverse effect of prenatal lead exposure on the 6-month Bayley MDI and Psychomotor Development Index (PDI). The effect was mediated by lead-related deficits in foetal growth (birth weight) and maturation (gestational age by physical examination). These relationships are illustrated by the structural equation model shown in Figure 1.

The variables in this structural equation model represent the final trimmed multivariate regression equation obtained after backward elimination of non-significant developmental covariates and confounders. As the figure shows, log maternal prenatal PbB (PbBPre) and the Composite Index of Tobacco and Alcohol Consumption (CITAC) were both inversely related to infant birth weight (in grams). PbBPre was also inversely related to gestational age (in weeks). As one would predict, both birth weight and gestational age were positively associated with Bayley MDI and PDI. Thus, the structural equation model suggests that sensorimotor deficits were apparently mediated by lead-related deficits in foetal growth and maturation. As in the study by Bellinger

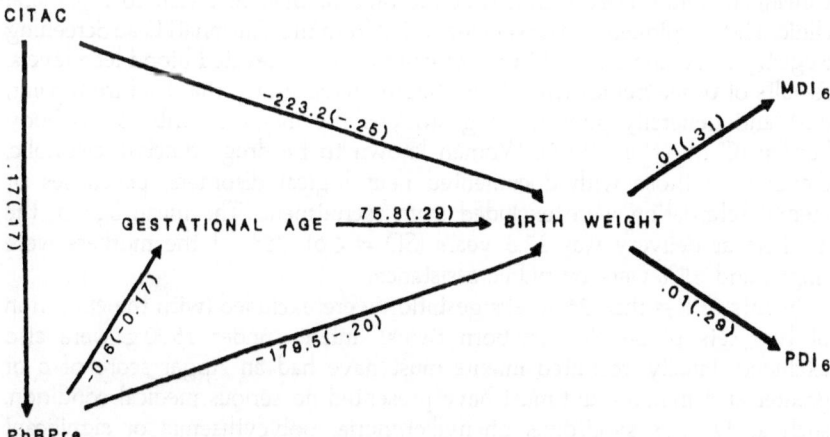

Figure 1 Relationships among variables affecting 6-month MDI/PDI, as revealed through structural equation analyses. Covariate-adjusted parameter estimates (and standardized regression coefficients) are indicated. All relationships significant at $p = 0.05$ or less, one-tailed tests. After Dietrich *et al.* (1986)

et al. (1986), adverse effects were observed at relatively low levels of exposure (mean PbBPre = 8.3, SD = 3.8).

In addition to the alleged psychoteratogenic properties of low-level foetal lead exposure, low birth weight (Bornschein *et al.*, 1988) and shortened gestation (McMichael *et al.*, 1986) have been found as well. Bellinger *et al.* (1984) did not find a relationship between cord PbB and birth weight. However, the percentage of intrauterine growth retardation was 1.2, 2.4 and 8.1 in the low, medium and high cord PbB groups, respectively. This same group of investigators examined the relationship between prenatal exposure to lead and minor congenital anomalies in 4354 births in Boston, Massachusetts (Needleman *et al.*, 1984). Umbilical cord PbB level was found to be associated, in a dose-related manner, with an increased risk for minor anomalies. While minor anomalies carry little health significance in themselves, they may be clues to more serious malformations which could potentially contribute to later functional deficits (Waldrop *et al.*, 1978).

Bellinger *et al.* (1986) have correctly noted that the implications of these adverse low-level lead effects for regulatory policy depend on the magnitude of the inverse relationships and their stability over time. The central questions for the present study are:

(1)   Do lead-related sensorimotor deficits persist beyond 6 months of age;
(2)   Do lead-related neurobehavioural deficits, if any, observed at 12 months differ from those previously observed at 6 months; and
(3)   Are the developmental deficits associated with prenatal lead exposure still mediated through foetal growth and maturational factors?

SUBJECTS

A total of 192 mothers, residing in predesignated lead-hazardous areas of Cincinnati, Ohio, were recruited at the time of their first visit to a prenatal clinic. The recruitment areas were identified from the Cincinnati Lead Screening Registry as having a long history of children with elevated blood lead levels. Results of other studies with these children have shown that lead from paint, dust and generally poor housing stock is the major contributor to body burden (Clark *et al.*, 1985). Women known to be drug addicted, alcoholic, diabetic, or those with documented neurological disorders, psychoses or mental retardation were excluded from recruitment. The mean age of the mothers at delivery was 22.8 years (SD = 4.6); 88% of the mothers were single, and 85% were on public assistance.

Infants of less than 36 weeks gestation were excluded (with the exception of two sets of healthy newborn twins). Infants under 1500 g were also excluded. Finally, recruited infants must have had an Apgar score of 6 or greater at 5 minutes and must have presented no serious medical condition, such as Down's syndrome, phenylketonuria, polycythaemia or significant congenital anomaly. With a few exceptions, the infants in this sample were the same as those in the aforementioned 6-month Bayley Scale analyses (Dietrich *et al.*, 1986). Study infants had a mean birth weight of 3153.3 g (SD = 443.8) and a mean gestational age by physical examination of 39.6

weeks (SD = 1.5). Table 1 presents these and other descriptive statistics on selected study variables.

MATERIALS AND PROCEDURES

Assessment of potential confounders and covariates

Undue lead exposure is known to covary with a number of social and biological risks which may mimic or otherwise interact with the effects of toxic exposure on neurobehavioural development (Dietrich *et al.*, 1985; Hunt, Hepner and Seaton, 1982; Milar *et al.*, 1980; Stark *et al.*, 1982). Therefore, substantial medical and social background data were collected on all subjects. Table 2 lists the candidate confounders and covariates which were chosen *a priori*, based upon their theoretical and/or known empirical association with both the target independent variable (lead exposure) and/or target-dependent variable (Bayley Scale performance).

Obstetric history and pertinent perinatal data were recorded from the mothers' and neonates' charts. These data were coded using the Littman–Parmelee Obstetrical and Postnatal Complications Scales (Littman and Parmelee, 1978). The Composite Index of Tobacco and Alcohol Consumption (CITAC), taken from the Problem Oriented Perinatal Risk Assessment System (POPRAS) by Hobel (1982), was also used. The CITAC variable was dichotomously scored, with a value of '1' indicating use of tobacco and/or consumption of alcohol during pregnancy. Of the mothers in the sample, 59% reported use of these substances during the prenatal period. There was

Table 1 Descriptive statistics on selected study variables ($n = 192$)

Variable	M	SD	Low	High	Percentage
12-month Bayley MDI	113.3	13.2	50	134	
12-month Bayley PDI	104.8	12.9	50	143	
Prenatal (maternal) PbB[a]	8.2	3.6	1	27	
10-day (neonatal) PbB	4.8	3.1	1	23	
3-month PbB	6.0	3.5	1	20	
6-month PbB	7.9	4.8	1	35	
9-month PbB	11.5	6.9	2	57	
12-month PbB	14.2	7.3	4	47	
3 to 12-month maximum PbB	15.1	7.8	5	57	
Birth weight (g)	3153.5	443.8	1814	4400	
Gestational age (weeks)[b]	39.6	1.5	35	43	
Percentage black					86
Percentage female					51
Maternal age (years)	22.8	4.6	15	37	
Number of children in home	2.5	1.3	0	6	
Total HOME score[c]	31.2	4.5	19	41	
Social class[d]	17.1	5.4	8	50	
Percentage married					12

[a] All in $\mu g\,dl^{-1}$ whole blood lead, arithmetic mean (M) and standard deviation (SD)
[b] By physical examination (Ballard, Novak and Driver, 1979)
[c] Caldwell and Bradley, 1978
[d] Hollingshead, 1975

Table 2 Candidate confounders and covariates in the disease-primary trait covariance matrix

Perinatal variables	Child health variables	Socio-hereditary variables
Birth weight	Number of infections during	Socioeconomic status
Gestational age by physical	the last year	Developmental stimulation
examination	Current illness	(HOME)
Child race	Iron status	Maternal IQ[a]
Child sex	Haemoglobin	Number of children in home
Obstetrical complications	Serum iron	
scale	Total iron binding	
Postnatal complications scale	capacity	
Tobacco and/or alcohol	Haematocrit	
consumption (CITAC)		
Maternal age		
Gravidity		
Parity		
Maternal total iron binding		
capacity		

[a] Wechsler Adult Intelligence Scale – Revised (Wechsler, 1981), short form

no evidence of alcoholism during any of the sample pregnancies.

The socioeconomic status (SES) of the infant's family was assessed at three months postpartum with the Hollingshead Four-Factor Index of Social Status (Hollingshead, 1975). The mean SES for families in this sample was 17.1 (SD = 5.4), reflecting the preponderance of single-parent low-income households. At 6 and 12 months, the quality of the infant's domestic environment was assessed with Caldwell and Bradley's Home Observation for Measurement of the Environment (HOME) (Caldwell and Bradley, 1978). The HOME combines interviewers' questions with direct observations to yield subscale and total HOME scores. In general, the HOME measures both the parent's responsivity and personal involvement with her infant and the extent to which the physical and temporal environment is stimulating and safe. The mean of the 6- and 12-month HOME scores was calculated for each subject and tested as a potential developmental covariate or confounder in regression analyses.

Assessment of lead exposure and behavioural development

Maternal blood samples were collected by venipuncture at the first prenatal visit. Of these samples, 43% were collected during the first trimester, and 51% and 6% during the second and third trimesters, respectively. Infant blood samples were collected at 10 days postparturition (corrected for gestational age) and at 3, 6, 9 and 12 months thereafter. Blood was drawn by either heel stick, finger stick or venipuncture, depending upon the physical characteristics of the infant. The percentage of blood samples drawn by a method other than venipuncture was very low after 3 months of age. The arithmetic means and standard deviations for prenatal and postnatal PbB values are presented in Table 1. The mean maximum PbB value between 3 months and 12 months was 15.1 μg dl^{-1}. Approximately 10% of the sample had at least one postnatal

PbB determination in excess of 25 μg dl^{-1} during the first year of life. Prenatal PbB measurements were conducted by Environmental Sciences Associates using a Model 2014 anodic stripping voltammeter (ASV) strip chart recording. All postnatal blood samples were analysed in the authors' laboratory using a Model 3010 ASV instrument. To increase precision of measurement, instrument digital readout was abandoned in favour of peak height determination using a strip chart recorder. All prenatal and postnatal PbB values were corrected for haematocrit and transformed to their natural logarithm. The analytical laboratory used in this study participates in several quality assurance programmes (see Bornschein *et al.*, 1985).

These analyses focused on four lead exposure variables: prenatal (maternal) blood lead (PbBPre) as an index of prenatal exposure; 10-day neonatal blood lead (PbB1) as another index of prenatal exposure; and maximum first-year blood lead (MaxPbB) and cumulative 12-month blood lead (CumPbB) as indices of postnatal exposure. MaxPbB was the highest postnatal PbB value recorded for each infant at any assessment between 3 and 12 months of age. CumPbB was derived from calculation of the area under the curve of each child's PbB profile from 10 days to 12 months. This integrated index was used to characterize historical postnatal lead exposure in assessing developmental effects.

Behavioural development was assessed at 12 months with the Mental Development Index (MDI), Psychomotor Development Index (PDI) and Infant Behavior Record (IBR) of the Bayley Scales of Infant Development (Bayley, 1969). The Bayley Scales were administered in the morning at an innercity clinic by one of three psychometricians trained by the same developmental psychologist (KND). Behavioural assessments were completed prior to the medical examination and phlebotomy. Care was taken to ensure that the infant was not noticeably ill, fatigued, hungry or under medication when examined. Intertester reliability was assessed at regular intervals and averaged 0.96 (Pearson *r*) for the Bayley MDI and PDI. In addition, at least 85% agreement was maintained for each rating scale item from the Bayley IBR.

A principal axis factor analysis (Statistical Analysis System, 1985) of the 12-month IBR data set was executed to reduce the 30 rating scale variables to a few meaningful behavioural factors. A predetermined eigenvalue of 1.0 was used as the cut off for factor extraction. Table 3 shows that three factors emerged from the analysis: activity level, attention and social–emotional tone.

Data analyses

The data analytical strategy used, which has been outlined in detail in a previous methodological publication (Dietrich *et al.*, 1986), is basically designed to achieve the best compromise possible between the conflicting goals of reducing the probability of Type I (false positives), Type II (false negatives) and Type III (model misspecification) errors. The analytical strategy involves *a priori* specification of potential developmental confounders and covariates; pretesting variables for confounding potential ($p = 0.10$ or less); backward elimination by multiple regression analyses to a trimmed regression model;

Table 3 Factor analysis of the Bayley Infant Behavior Record at 12 months*

IBR items	Factor 1 (Activity level)	Factor 2 (Attention)	Factor 3 (Social → emotional tone)
Activity level	0.89		
Body motion	0.82		
Fearfulness	−0.44		−0.51
Banging toys	0.37		
Reactivity	0.32	0.55	
Tension	0.30		
Vocalizations	0.30		
Attention span		0.71	
Object orientation		0.63	
Goal direction		0.58	0.31
Co-operativeness		0.41	0.52
Interest in sights		0.37	
Fine motor co-ordination		0.35	
Social orientation: persons		0.33	
Emotional tone			0.76
Social orientation: examiner			0.68
Endurance			0.52

*Only variables with a loading of ±0.30 or greater are shown. Exact factor scores were calculated for each subject in the study from the factor scoring coefficients

and, finally, the testing of potential dynamic interactions among lead exposures, biological outcomes, and behavioural performance through structural equation analysis.

RESULTS

No adverse effects of postnatal lead exposure (CumPbB, MaxPbB) on Bayley developmental outcomes were found. However, Table 4 shows that a number of effects were found for the foetal lead exposure variables (PbBPre, PbB1) PbBPre was negatively associated with 12-month PDI. The significant PbBPre-by-race interaction indicates that this effect was most pronounced among white infants. Foetal exposure variables were directly related to two IBR

Table 4 Results of multiple regression analyses of the effects of foetal lead exposure on Bayley developmental variables

Dependent variable	Independent variable	Beta	SE	t	p*
Psychomotor development index (PDI)	Log PbBPre	−14.09	7.26	−1.94	0.054
	Gestation	1.64	0.73	2.26	0.025
	Race	−28.68	16.32	−1.76	0.081
	Log PbBPre x race	16.51	7.62	2.16	0.032
Activity level (IBR)	Log PbBPre	0.31	0.14	2.10	0.037
	Number of children in home	−0.13	0.05	−2.45	0.016
Social−emotional tone (IBR)	Log PbB1	−0.20	0.10	−1.97	0.050
	Number of children in home	−0.12	0.05	−2.50	0.013

* two-tailed test

factors. Foetal exposure variables were directly related to two IBR factors. PbBPre was associated with higher levels of motor activity during testing. PbB1 was associated with more negative social–emotional response.

The hypothesis that lead-related deficits in foetal growth lead to lower MDI and PDI at 12 months was tested in a structural equation analysis (SYSREG PROCEDURE, Statistical Analysis System, 1984). Figure 2 presents the results of this work. The variables in this structural model are those potential confounders (or mediators) of lead effects selected *a priori* and tested for their confounding potential. As in the multiple regression analyses, all variables originally considered were bivariately associated with PbB and Bayley MDI/PDI at $p = 0.10$ or lower. All pathways in Figure 2 were statistically significant at $p = 0.05$ or lower, one-tailed tests.

As in the 6-month Bayley analysis, PbBPre was indirectly related to Bayley MDI through birth weight. However, PbBPre was not related to gestational age in this model as it was at 6 months, and there was no evidence of an indirect effect of PbBPre on PDI. As in the earlier analysis, use of tobacco and/or alcohol products was related to shortened gestation. Finally, as in the

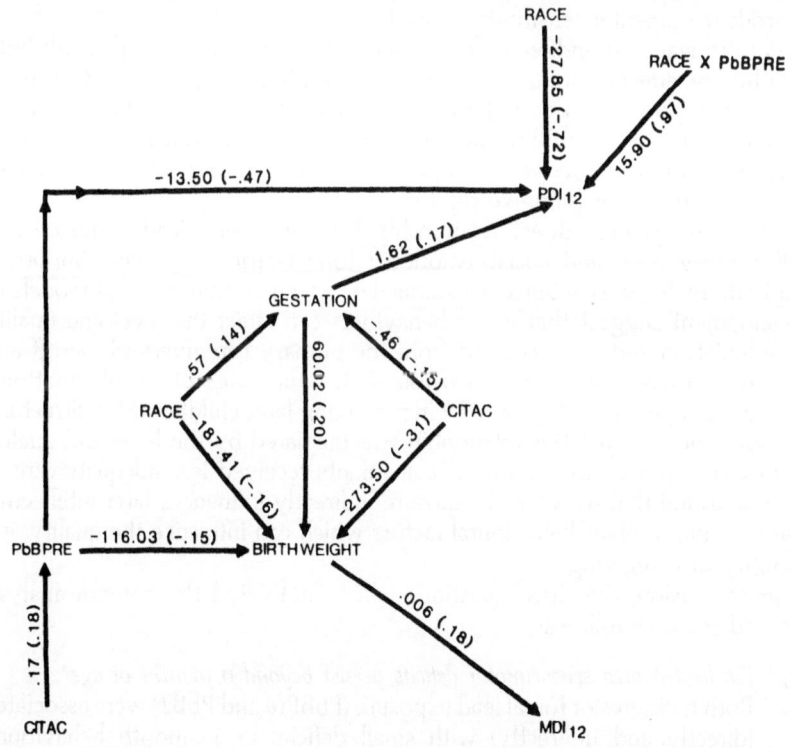

Figure 2 Relationships among variables affecting 12-month MDI/PDI, as revealed through structural equation analyses. Covariate-adjusted parameter estimates (and standardized regression coefficients) are indicated. All relationships significant at $p = 0.05$ or less, one-tailed tests

standard multiple regression analyses reported above, the PbBPre-by-race interaction on PDI was statistically significant in the structural model.

SUMMARY AND DISCUSSION

Early postnatal PbB levels were not found to be inversely associated with 12-month infant mental, motor or behavioural development. This finding is consistent with previously published reports (e.g. Bellinger et al., 1986). Foetal exposure variables, however, were associated with a complex of neurobehavioural indices at 12 months. PbBPre was inversely associated with 12-month motor performance as assessed by the Bayley PDI. This association was most pronounced among white infants, as evidenced by a statistically significant PbBPre-by-race interaction. In fact, the main effect of PbBPre on PDI in this analysis was entirely dependent upon presence of the interaction term in the regression equation. This result is interesting in light of our previously reported analysis which found a significant 3-month PbB-by-race interaction and cumulative 6-month PbB-by-race interaction on 6-month Bayley MDI, PDI, and Attention/Motor Maturity Factor from the Bayley IBR (Dietrich et al., 1986). Our evidence at both 6 and 12 months is consistent with the hypothesis that there may be racial differences in the early neurodevelopmental sensitivity to lead.

PbBPre was also 'indirectly' associated with deficits in MDI through birth weight. The effect of prenatal (maternal) PbB on birth weight in the Cincinnati cohort is reported in this volume (Bornschein et al., 1988). The continuing indirect influence of PbBPre on MDI reflects the expected persistence of a positive relationship between weight at birth and neurodevelopmental status during the first year (Illingworth, 1983).

The findings of a direct relationship between foetal lead exposure and IBR activity level and social–emotional tone factors may have important implications for later intellectual status. For example, transactional models of development suggest that infant behaviours can affect the level and quality of stimulation and care received from the primary caregivers (Sameroff and Chandler, 1975). Sameroff (1978) found that measures of infant emotional tone were superior to Bayley MDI in predicting later childhood IQ. Structural analyses showed that this relationhip was mediated by the level and quality of maternal stimulation; more difficult infants received less adequate care. It may be found that foetal lead exposure indirectly influences later intellectual status through infant behavioural factors which can influence the quality and quantity of caregiving.

In conclusion, the three questions which motivated this interim analysis are addressed as follows:

(1) *Do lead-related sensorimotor deficits persist beyond 6 months of age?*
    Both measures of foetal lead exposure (PbBPre and PbB1) were associated (directly and indirectly) with small deficits in 12-month behavioural performance.

(2) *Do lead-related neurobehavioural deficits observed at 12 months differ from those previously observed?*

In addressing this question, complications arise because the types of behaviours assessed by instruments such as the Bayley Scales change as the infant matures. While 6-month MDI reflects more purely sensorimotor skill assessment, 12-month Bayley items also tap rudimentary problem-solving skills and the precursors of language behaviour. Nevertheless, some differences between the 6- and 12-month Bayley results are notable. Direct effects of foetal exposure on behavioural performance as measured by the Bayley IBR were not previously observed at 6 months, despite a very similar factor structure at both ages. Perhaps such observations are more reliable in the older infant. The indirect effect of PbBPre on PDI through foetal growth variables was no longer present at 12 months. However, PbBPre was still indirectly associated with 12-month MDI through birth weight.

(3) *Are the developmental deficits associated with prenatal lead exposure still mediated through foetal growth and maturational factors?*
This question has already been addressed under the previous heading. Higher prenatal (maternal) blood lead levels were associated with lower birth weight. As expected, birth weight continued to be positively related to Bayley MDI at 12 months.

From these findings, it may be concluded that the adverse effects of foetal lead exposure on neurobehavioural development are relatively stable over the first year of life, and, indeed, may even expand to include 'non-cognitive' behavioural characteristics of the infant. The magnitude of these effects, however, is another matter. The magnitude and 'health-significance' of lead–behaviour relationships has been a topic of considerable, sometimes rancorous, debate. Our own structural analyses of the 6-month Bayley data have shown that each log increment in prenatal PbB was associated with a decrement in Bayley MDI of 2.25 points (through lead effects on birth weight and gestational age). This translates into a net loss of about 7.5 MDI points over the entire range of foetal exposures observed in the sample. The decrement in MDI-associated prenatal exposure at 12 months was somewhat reduced due to the decreased association between birth weight and mental developmental status.

It is always difficult to evaluate the health significance of parameter estimates obtained from regression analyses because they reflect only 'average' effects. There may be sensitive individuals or defined groups within the population for whom the effects of exposure are far more serious. For example, our analyses of the 6- and 12-month Bayley data show consistent evidence of racial differences in the PbB–behaviour dose–effect relationship; in this instance, each log increment in prenatal PbB was associated with an average decrement of 14 points in 12-month Bayley PDI among white infants (0.87 SD).

While current or longer-term health significance of these effects for all individuals cannot be precisely determined, results of studies of the early neurobehavioural effects of low-level foetal lead exposure should be seriously considered by public health officials when setting standards for human exposure.

ACKNOWLEDGMENTS

This research was supported by a grant from the National Institute of Environmental Health Sciences, Dr Paul B. Hammond, Principal Investigator. We wish to thank the many technicians and support personnel at the University of Cincinnati College of Medicine and Babies Milk Fund Clinic who helped to make this research possible.

REFERENCES

Ballard, J.L., Novak, K.K. and Driver, M. (1979). A simplified score for assessment of fetal maturation of newly born infants. *J. Pediatr.*, **95**, 766–774

Bayley, N. (1969). *Bayley Scales of Infant Development*. (New York: Psychological Corporation)

Bellinger, D.C., Needleman, H.L., Leviton, A.L., Waternaux, C., Rabinowitz, M.B. and Nichols, M.L. (1984). Early sensory-motor development and prenatal exposure to lead. *Neurobehav. Toxicol. Teratol.*, **6**, 387–402

Bellinger, D.C., Leviton, A., Needleman, H., Waternaux, C. and Rabinowitz, M. (1986). Low-level lead exposure and infant development in the first year. *Neurobehav. Toxicol. Teratol.*, **8**, 151–161

Bornschein, R.L., Hammond P.B., Dietrich, K.N., Succop, P., Krafft, K.M., Clark, S., Berger, O. and Que Hee, S.S. (1985). The Cincinnati Prospective Study of low level lead exposure and its effects on child development. *Environ. Res.*, **38**, 4–18

Bornschein, R.L., Grote, J., Mitchell, T., Succop, P.A., Dietrich, K.N., Krafft, K.M. and Hammond, P.B. (1988). Effects of prenatal lead exposure on infant size at birth. (this volume)

Caldwell, B.M. and Bradley, R.H. (1978). *Administration Manual for the Home Observation for Measurement of the Environment*. (Little Rock: University of Arkansas at Little Rock) (manual available from the authors)

Clark, C.S., Bornschein, R.L., Succop, P., Que Hee, S., Hammond, P.B. and Peace, B. (1985). Condition and type of housing as an indicator of potential environmental lead exposure and pediatric blood lead levels. *Environ. Res.*, **38**, 46–53

Dietrich, K.N., Krafft, K.M., Pearson, D.T., Harris, L.C., Bornschein, R.L., Hammond, P.B. and Succop, P.A. (1985). Contribution of social and developmental factors to lead exposure during the first year of life. *Pediatrics*, **75**, 1114–1119

Dietrich, K.N., Krafft, K.M., Shukla, R., Bornschein, R.L. and Succop, P.A. (1986). The neurobehavioral effects of prenatal and early postnatal lead exposure. In Schroeder, S. (ed.) *Toxic Substances and Mental Retardation: Neurobehavioral Toxicology and Teratology*. (Washington, DC: American Association on Mental Deficiency)

Hobel, C.J. (1982). Development of POPRAS-problem oriented perinatal risk assessment system. In Harris, T.R. (ed.). *The Use of Computers in Perinatal Medicine*. (New York: Praeger)

Hollingshead, A.B. (1975). *Four Factor Index of Social Status*. (New Haven, Connecticut: Yale) (manual available from the author)

Hunt, T.J., Hepner, R. and Seaton, K.W. (1982). Childhood lead poisoning and inadequate child care. *Am. J. Dis. Child.*, **136**, 538–542

Illingworth, R.S. (1983). *The Development of the Infant and Young Child*. (Edinburgh: Churchill-Livingstone)

Littman, B. and Parmelee, A.H. (1978). Medical correlates of infant development. *Pediatrics*, **61**, 470–474

McMichael, A.J., Vimpani, G.V., Robertson, E.F., Baghurst, P.A. and Clark, P.D. (1986). The Port Pirie cohort study: Maternal blood lead and pregnancy outcome. *J. Epidemiol. Commun. Health*, **40**, 18–25

Milar, C.R., Schroeder, S.R., Mushak, P., Dolcourt, J.L. and Grant, L.D. (1980). Contributions of the caregiving environment to increased lead burden of children. *Am. J. Ment. Defic.*, **84**, 339–344

Needleman, H.L., Rabinowitz, M., Leviton, A., Linn, S. and Schoenbaum, S. (1984). The relationship between prenatal exposure to lead and congenital anomalies. *J. Am. Med. Assoc.*, **251**, 2956–2959

Sameroff, A.J. (1978). Caretaking or reproductive casualty? Determinants of developmental deviancy. In Horowitz, F.D. (ed.) *Early Developmental Hazards: Predictors and Precautions.* (Boulder Colorado: Westview Press)

Sameroff, A.J. and Chandler, M.J. (1975). Reproductive risk and the continuum of caretaking casualty. In Horowitz, F.D., Hetherington, M., Scarr-Salopatek, S. and Siegel, G. (eds.) *Review of Child Development Research,* Vol. 4. (Chicago: University of Chicago Press)

Stark, A.D., Quah, R.F., Meigs, J.W. and DeLouise, R.R. (1982). Relationship of sociodemographic factors to blood lead concentrations in New Haven children. *J. Epidemiol. Commun. Health,* **36,** 133–139

SAS Institute Inc. (1984). *SAS/ETS User's Guide, Version 5 Edition.* (Cary, North Carolina: SAS Institute Inc.)

SAS Institute Inc. (1985). *SAS User's Guide: Stastics, Version 5 Edition.* (Cary, North Carolina: SAS Institute Inc.)

Vimpani, G.V., Wigg, N.R., Robertson, E.F., McMichael, A.J., Baghurst, P.A. and Roberts, R.J. (1987). The Port Pirie cohort study: Blood lead concentration and childhood developmental assessment. In Goldwater, L.J., Wysocki, L.M. and Volpe, R.A. (eds.) *Proceedings of Lead Environmental Health: The Current Issues.* (Durham NC.: Duke University Press)

Waldrop, M.F., Bell R.Q., McLaughlin, B. and Halverson, C.F. (1978). Newborn minor physical anomalies predict shorter attention span, peer aggression and impulsivity at age 3. *Science,* **179,** 563–564

Wechsler, D. (1981). *Wechsler Adult Intelligence Scale – Revised.* (New York: Psychological Corporation)

4.3

The Port Pirie Cohort Study – Cumulative Lead Exposure and Neurodevelopmental Status at Age 2 Years: Do HOME Scores and Maternal IQ Reduce Apparent Effects of Lead on Bayley Mental Scores?

G. V. VIMPANI, P. A. BAGHURST, N. R. WIGG,
E. F. ROBERTSON, A. J. McMICHAEL and R. R. ROBERTS

SUMMARY

As part of a longitudinal study examining the effects of cumulative lead exposure on pregnancy outcome and childhood growth and development in the first seven years of life, 595 children living in the lead smelter town of Port Pirie and several surrounding rural communities in South Australia have now been followed up from 14–20 weeks gestation until aged three years.

Initial analysis of the relationship between cumulative lead exposure (as measured by blood lead levels) and scores on the Bayley Mental Development Scales (MDI) showed a significant negative correlation between blood lead levels at ages 6, 15 and 24 months and integrated postnatal blood lead (PbB) levels and Bayley scores. Some 13 other biological and sociodemographic variables were also found to be statistically significantly related to Bayley scores. When multiple regression analysis of the relationship between blood lead and Bayley scores was undertaken with these covariates entered into the model, lead levels at all postnatal ages except 24 months were found to have an independent effect on Bayley scores. This relationship was not eliminated by entering maternal IQ scores (for the 246 mothers for which these had been obtained) into the model. HOME scores were also significantly positively correlated with Bayley MDI scores. Inclusion of HOME scores in the multiple regression model reduced but did not eliminate the independent association of PbB with MDI. The strongest independent association was between 6-month PbB and Bayley MDI. The significance of these findings is discussed.

Port Pirie is an industrial city of 15 000 people of European descent located about 250 km north of Adelaide on the south-central coast of Australia, with a large lead–zinc smelter as its major industry. In 1979, a study (the Port Pirie Cohort Study) was begun to investigate further the relatively high and unexplained late foetal death rate which had been observed during the period 1968 to 1976.

The initial aim of this study was to examine the relationship between cumulative lead exposure during pregnancy and its subsequent outcome. A total of 831 pregnancies was registered during a three-year period (1979 to 1982), 749 of which were followed to birth. Three-quarters of the enrolled women were resident in Port Pirie; the remainder lived in the surrounding grain-farming districts. During this phase of the study a statistically significant, dose–response-related, association between maternal blood lead at delivery and preterm birth was found (McMichael et al., 1986). This association remained significant when a variety of other potentially confounding variables was taken into account.

This birth cohort is being followed until all children are aged seven years in order: (1) to examine prospectively the relationship between cumulative lead burdens and other possible genetic and sociodemographic influences on developmental outcome at ages 2, 4 and 7 years; and (2) to examine longitudinal trends in mother–child lead parameters, and the relationship between antenatal and postnatal blood lead levels and tooth lead.

METHODS

Approximately 595 children at 2 years of age and about 560 children at 3 years remained in the study. Most of the withdrawals from the original cohort occurred during the first 6 months after birth (Figure 1). Children remaining in the study were aged between 4 and 7 years at the beginning of 1987.

Umbilical cord blood and capillary blood samples, collected using standardized techniques (Australian Standards Association, 1983) at age 6 months, 15 months, 2 years, and annually thereafter, were assayed for blood lead (PbB). Blood lead assays were made using electrothermal atomic absorption spectrophotometry, after standard complexing and extraction of lead (Australian Standards Association, 1984). The laboratory undertaking the analyses participates in several national and international quality control programmes. Crude blood lead levels were standardized to a packed cell volume (PCV) of 35% before being included in subsequent data analysis (except in cord blood where standardization was to a PCV of 50%). A capillary–venous correlation coefficient of +0.97 has been achieved in a sample of children of this age using these techniques (ACH, unpublished data).

Structured interviews were undertaken, at the time of each blood sampling,

333

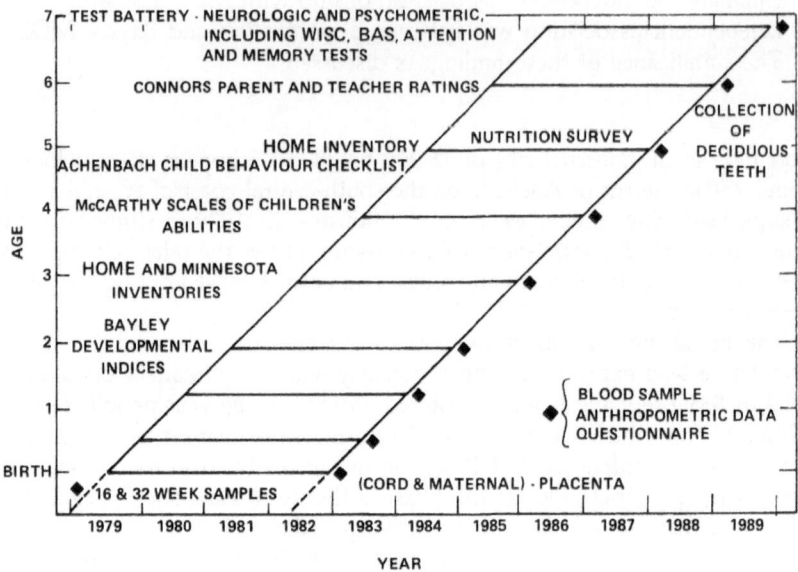

Figure 1   The Port Pirie cohort data collection schedule

by the nurse to obtain data on a comprehensive range of demographic, psychosocial, medical and developmental factors.

At age 24 months, the developmental status of each child was formally measured using the mental (MDI) and psychomotor (PDI) subscales of the Bayley Scales of Infant Development (Bayley, 1969). These scales were administered to all children by one clinical psychologist who has remained blind to blood lead results throughout the study. Testing was undertaken on a different day from that on which other interviewing and blood collection took place.

Maternal IQ was assessed using the Wechsler Adult Intelligence Scale (WAIS) (Wechsler, 1981).

The HOME inventory (Caldwell and Bradley, 1979) (preschool version) was administered at age 3 years by a nurse trained in its use by a psychologist. This instrument, developed by Bradley and Caldwell (1977), has revealed a substantial relationship between aspects of the home environment and children's intellectual and language development during early childhood. The decision to include this measure, rather than the Parent Attitude Research Inventory, was made after the study group participated in the First International Lead Workshop in Cincinnati in 1981 (Bornshein, 1962). At that time, its administration at 2 years of age was precluded, as some of the cohort had already passed their second birthday. Because the HOME inventory will be administered again at age five years, a measure of its stability over time will be possible.

In addition, a range of neurodevelopmental, behavioural and cognitive tests will be undertaken at ages 4, 5, 6 and 7 years as shown in Table 1.

334

RESULTS

At a May, 1985 international meeting in Durham, NC (USA) (Vimpani *et al.*, 1987), the following results were reported and discussed.

The distribution of blood lead levels in our sample by age and sex

The mean PbB concentration rose sharply between 6 and 15 months of age, reaching a peak at 24 months and declining steadily from 2 to 5 years (Figure 2). Strongest correlates of blood lead concentration were area of residence and having a father involved in manual work at the smelter. Children who spent more time playing outdoors and who were classified as engaging in frequent mouthing of objects, sucking fingers and eating dirt had consistently elevated PbB concentrations (Baghurst *et al.*, 1985).

The relationship between Bayley scores and PbB levels

There was a statistically significant correlation between Bayley MDI scores at 2 years and PbB levels at all ages except for samples collected at the time of delivery. There was no correlation between Bayley PDI scores and PbB levels (Table 2).

When children were classified into three groups on the basis of their cumulative postnatal lead exposure, a strong crude association between MDI and PbB was evident (Table 3).

An association was observed between a number of sociodemographic and biological covariates, including maternal WAIS and Bayley MDI scores. These conditions, either directly or indirectly, could have accounted for some or all

Table 1 Tests proposed at 4, 5, 6 and 7 years of age

Age 4 years
    McCarthy Scales of Children's Abilities
    Achenbach Child Behaviour Checklist

Age 5 years
    Achenbach Child Behaviour Checklist

Age 6 years
    Conner's parent and teacher rating questionnaires

Age 7 years
    Wechsler Intelligence Scale for Children – Revised
    British Ability Scales – Word Reading
                   – Mathematics
    Conner' Scales – parents
               – teachers
    Auditory Verbal Learning Test (Rey)
    Continuous performance test
    Reaction time test
    Selective attention (Geffen)
    Beery visual–motor integration test
    Finger localization
    Neurological assessment

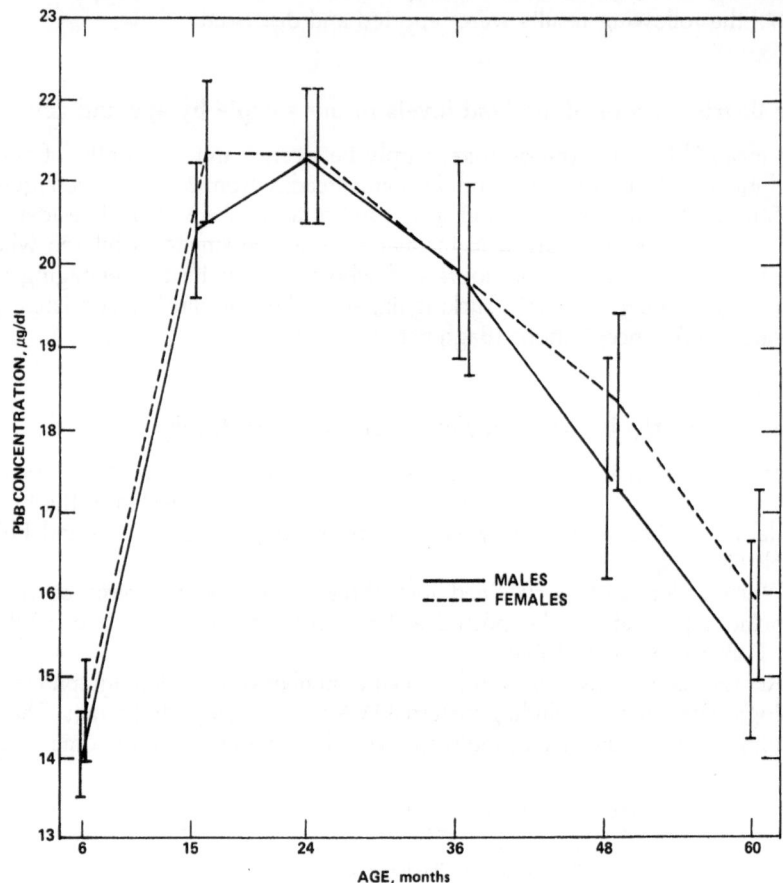

Figure 2 Early childhood geometric mean blood concentration (μg dl^{-1}) and 95% confidence intervals, by age and sex

Table 2 Correlations between Bayley MDI at 24 months and blood lead measurements

Blood sample		Pearson Correlation Coefficient*	
Maternal:	14–20 weeks gestation	−0.089	(509)
	after 20 weeks gestation	−0.094	(560)
	average prepartum	−0.125	(586)
	at delivery	−0.043	(524)
Infant:	cord blood	−0.041	(520)
	6 months	−0.135	(575)
	15 months	−0.140	(579)
	24 months	−0.185	(586)

Number of children/blood samples shown in parentheses
*Coefficients with absolute values exceeding approximately 0.08 are significant at $p = 0.05$ or less

Table 3   Association of Bayley MDI at 24 months of age with blood lead history

Blood lead concentration	Mean MDI	No. children	SE
Persistently high[1]	102.2	51	1.6
Intermediate[2]	109.7	451	0.6
Persistently low[3]	112.2	62	1.6

[1]PbB concentrations in highest quartile of PbB distribution on all three postnatal samplings (6, 15 and 24 months)
[2]All except high and low group
[3]Lead levels in lowest quartile on all three occasions

of the observed reduction in Bayley MDI scores with elevated PbB concentrations. The mean Bayley MDI was found to be depressed in children of women aged less than 21 years, women who were unable to recall the extent of the father's secondary education, parents who were living apart, and women whose antenatal marital status was single, widowed or divorced. Higher than average scores were found among children for whom either parent had more than 3 years secondary education or whose fathers were engaged in office work. Children who had less than optimum perinatal histories (oxygen required at birth, Apgar < 8 after 5 minutes, small for gestational age) also had lower mean MDI scores, but there was no obvious relationship between MDI and either birth rank or the occurrence of neonatal jaundice.

Maternal intelligence is known to be a determinant of a child's mental development, and the results of this study are not inconsistent with this observation. At present, only 246 maternal IQ scores have been determined and the data are thus incomplete. The strength of the association is evident in Table 4.

A multiple regression analysis was then undertaken with and without maternal IQ entered in the model. Blood lead measures were entered as explanatory variables *after* all the other perinatal and sociodemographic variables had been entered (Table 5). A statistically significant association was found between various PbB measures and Bayley MDI scores, which was not attenuated by including maternal WAIS in the model. At that stage, the implication of these preliminary findings was that "when the influence of a range of possible confounders was accounted for, there was still an independent effect of PbB on MDI to the extent that for a rise in PbB of $10 \mu g \, dl^{-1}$ at 6 months one would expect a fall of 4 units in the MDI" (Vimpani *et al.*, 1987).

Table 4   Bayley MDI at 24 months tabulated by maternal WAIS

Maternal WAIS	Bayley MDI	n	SE
< 80	100.0	27	3.4
81–90	108.2	65	1.7
91–100	110.1	88	1.6
> 100	113.9	66	1.9
Not yet completed	109.1	280	0.8
Refused	105.1	12	6.3
All mothers	109.2	538	0.6

Table 5 Partial linear regression coefficients for each blood lead measure with and without maternal IQ included in the model

	Regression coefficient (MDI μg dl^{-1})	
Blood lead measure	Ignoring maternal IQ	Controlling for maternal IQ
Average antenatal	−0.250	−0.064
Delivery	0.181	0.001
Cord	0.053	0.026
6 months	−0.231*	−0.396*
15 months	−0.084	−0.103
24 months	−0.152*	−0.061
Integrated postnatal	−0.240*	−0.310*

*Statistically significantly different from zero at $p < 0.05$ (one-tailed test)

These preliminary results were qualified by recognizing the need to examine the impact of a measure of the child's caretaking environment (HOME) on Bayley MDI, as well as maternal intelligence assessments, from the whole cohort when these analyses were available.

Since our May, 1985 report, further results have been obtained by means of additional analyses, as described below.

The interrelationship between caretaking environment (HOME), PbB measures and Bayley scores

The total HOME score modal value was 44, which is somewhat higher (more favourable) than the mean score in the standardizing sample of Bradley and Caldwell (37.54 with a SD of 10.4). The distribution was significantly skewed to the left.

There was a strong positive correlation between the HOME score and the Bayley MDI. These two measures were negatively correlated with postnatal PbB concentrations (expressed as 'integrated PbB' which is derived by trapezoidal integration of each individual's blood lead curve derived from PbB estimates of cord, 6-, 15- and 24-month samples) (Table 6). A very low HOME score also appeared to be associated with a low Bayley PDI, but no significant relationship was found between these two measures across the rest of the HOME score range.

Table 6 Mean Bayley MDI at 2 years and geometric mean of integrated PbB according to total HOME score at 3 years

HOME scare	MDI (n)	95% CI*	PDI	95% CI*	Int. PbB (n)
<39	99.5 (108)	96.8−102.2	99.4	96.6−102.2	20.95 (88)
39−41	105.3 (115)	102.7−107.9	106.1	103.2−108.9	19.55 (94)
42−44	113.0 (147)	110.8−115.2	106.9	104.7−109.2	18.04 (128)
45−47	111.7 (110)	109.0−114.4	107.6	104.9−110.3	15.72 (90)
>47	118.7 (83)	115.3−122.1	105.8	102.5−109.1	16.20 (71)
Total	109.4 (563)	108.1−110.7	105.3	104.1−106.5	18.07 (471)

*95% CI = 95% confidence interval

The association of a number of maternal, sociodemographic and perinatal variables with total HOME score was evaluated before assessing the effect of including the child's HOME score at age 3 years along with these variables in a multivariate analysis examining the explanatory power of the various PbB measures.

A clearly positive association between mother's age, years of secondary education of both parents, mother's and father's workplace, parental relationship, marital status and maternal WAIS and the total HOME score was observed. Perinatal variables – with the exception of oxygen use which was of borderline significance – had no statistically significant relationship to HOME score (Table 7).

A second multiple regression analysis was undertaken in which PbB measures were entered as explanatory variables before and after HOME scores and maternal WAIS had been entered in the model. This analysis strategy is conservative in that it assumes that the effects of all the 'non-lead' variables are associated with MDI via independent (i.e. direct) mechanisms that do not involve lead exposure (i.e. they are pure confounders as shown in Model 1, Figure 3). In reality, it is plausible – even likely – that part of the effect of some non-lead variables is mediated via altered exposure to lead.

The inclusion of the HOME score in the regression model has the effect of markedly attenuating the independent effect of PbB on Bayley MDI. Nevertheless, it should be noted that the relationship between PbB at 6 months and Bayley MDI at 2 years remains statistically significant at the 5% level using a one-tailed test. Furthermore, the estimated partial regression coefficients for all PbB measures (excluding those measured at birth) are negative (Table 8). Briefly interpreted, these results suggest that, conservatively, other factors remaining constant, a child's MDI at 24 months will decrease by 1.9 points for every 10 μg dl^{-1} rise in PbB at six months of age.

There are two other possible explanations for the observed relationships between PbB, HOME scores, other explanatory sociodemographic and perinatal variables, and Bayley MDI scores (Figure 3).

First, it is possible that the observed effect on Bayley MDI of some of the explanatory variables, including the caretaking environment (as reflected by the HOME score), is mediated by the amount of lead in the home environment which becomes ingested or inhaled and leads to elevated PbB concentrations (Model 2, Figure 3). It is plausible that, in homes in which parents are less well educated and in which less attention is given to providing a developmentally enriching milieu, that less attention is also paid to other aspects of child and family care, such as domestic cleaning and maintenance. Although there is a well-documented association in other studies of a significant positive association between HOME scores and developmental outcome measures, such as the Bayley MDI, in few of these studies has a possible mediating effect of the absorption of lead from the domestic environment been considered. Most studies, although urban-based, have not included PbB as a possible confounder.

The possibility of this explanation was investigated by examining the relationship between HOME scores and Bayley MDI in children with high, intermediate and low integrated PbB levels to see whether the association between HOME and MDI was consistent across the whole spectrum of lead

Table 7 Mean HOME score tabulated by sociodemographic factors, maternal IQ and perinatal factors

Sociodemographic factor	n	Mean HOME	95% CI*
Maternal age (years)			
≤21	95	39.9	38.9−41.0
22−29	363	42.4	41.9−43.0
≥30	101	43.9	43.0−44.7
Father's secondary education			
unknown	65	38.2	37.0−39.5
<3 years	242	42.0	41.4−42.6
≥3 years	257	43.6	43.0−44.2
Mother's secondary education			
<3 years	271	41.2	40.6−41.9
≥3 years	274	43.5	42.9−44.0
Father's workplace			
office	135	43.6	42.6−44.6
non-office	420	41.9	41.4−42.4
Mother's workplace			
home	227	43.0	42.4−43.7
outside home	329	41.8	41.2−42.4
Parental relationship			
living together	516	42.7	42.3−43.1
living apart	44	37.2	35.6−38.8
Mother's antenatal marital status			
single, widowed, divorced	53	38.5	37.1−39.8
married or defacto	506	42.7	42.2−43.1
Child's birth rank			
first born	255	42.1	41.5−42.7
second born	194	42.3	41.6−43.0
subsequent born	115	42.6	41.6−43.6
Maternal IQ			
<81	26	39.7	37.7−41.7
81−90	64	42.7	41.8−43.7
91−100	87	43.5	42.7−44.3
>100	65	45.6	44.6−46.5
lost	3	38.7	35.0−42.3
not yet completed	265	41.6	41.0−42.2
Oxygen use at birth			
required	166	41.3	40.5−42.2
not required	388	42.6	42.1−43.1
Apgar score at 5 minutes			
<8	124	41.2	40.3−42.2
8−10	426	42.5	42.0−43.0
Neonatal jaundice			
present	206	42.1	41.4−42.8
not present	349	42.4	41.8−42.9
Size for gestational age			
small	29	40.4	38.0−42.9
appropriate	467	42.5	42.0−42.9
large	52	41.5	40.0−43.9

* 95% = 95% confidence interval

MODEL 1

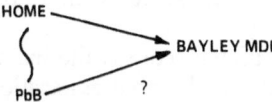

ASSUMPTION:

THE EFFECT OF PbB ON MDI IS REAL BUT THE MAGNITUDE OF EFFECT IS OVER-ESTIMATED IF HOME (OR ANY OTHER COVARIATE WHICH HAS AN INDEPENDENT EFFECT ON MDI, AND THUS ACTS AS A PURE CONFOUNDER) IS NOT CONTROLLED FOR BY MULTIPLE REGRESSION ANALYSIS.

MODEL 2

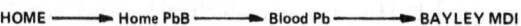

HOME ⟶ Home PbB ⟶ Blood Pb ⟶ BAYLEY MDI

ASSUMPTION:

THE COVARIATE HAS A REAL EFFECT BUT IT IS ENTIRELY MEDIATED BY ITS EFFECT ON PbB. THUS THERE IS NO DIRECT EFFECT OF THE COVARIATE (HOME) UPON MDI. MULTIPLE REGRESSION ANALYSIS IS INAPPROPRIATE.

MODEL 3

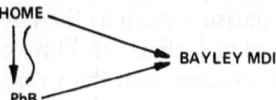

ASSUMPTION:

THE COVARIATE HAS AN INDEPENDENT EFFECT, ACTING AS A CONFOUNDER, BUT ALSO HAS A REAL EFFECT WHICH IS MEDIATED THROUGH PbB. THERE IS NO DIRECT REAL EFFECT OF PbB ON MDI AND THUS MULTIVARIATE CONTROL IS A CONSERVATIVE STRATEGY.

Figure 3 Three alternative explanations for the relationship between PbB, HOME and MDI

Table 8 Partial linear regression coefficients of MDI with each blood lead measure – with and without maternal IQ and HOME score in the model[1]

	Regression coefficient (MDI μg dl^{-1})		
Blood lead measure	Ignoring maternal IQ and HOME	Controlling for maternal IQ only	Controlling for maternal IQ and HOME
Average antenatal	−0.250	−0.150	−0.007
Delivery	0.181	0.206	0.166
Cord	0.053	0.097	0.120
6 months	−0.231*	−0.258*	−0.191†
15 months	−0.084	−0.065	−0.012
24 months	−0.151	−0.082	−0.006
Integrated postnatal	−0.240†	−0.222†	−0.111

[1]The model contains the 13 socioeconomic, demographic and behavioural factors, with each lead measure being tested singly (i.e. in the absence of other lead measures)
*$p < 0.05$
†$p < 0.01$

exposure (Table 9). Although there is no significant difference in the distribution of MDI scores within the study population at the extremes of the lead exposure distribution, the more pertinent observation would be whether the range and distribution of MDI scores within PbB categories is less than that observed for all children.

A second explanation is that the HOME score is the main predictor (i.e. effector variable) of Bayley MDI, and the observed association of PbB with MDI is found because of the high correlation between PbB and HOME (Model 3, Figure 3). In these circumstances, PbB could be considered as a surrogate for HOME. If, indeed, total HOME score is highly correlated with PbB it would be difficult to demonstrate much additional effect of PbB on Bayley MDI in the regression analysis (after allowing for HOME score), even if it did have some independent effect. It is clear from preliminary analyses that these variables are correlated to an extent which makes such considerations important.

CONCLUSIONS

These results show that even after a range of variables with independent effects on a developmental outcome measure (such as the Bayley MDI) have been taken into account, a small residual effect of PbB on MDI can be demonstrated. Interestingly, the PbB measure with the strongest association with MDI appears to be that obtained at six months of age. Unlike other studies (Bellinger et al., 1988), no significant relationship between PbB measures obtained at, or prior to, birth and MDIs at age 2 years has been observed, nor has a relationship between lead exposure and PDI been demonstrated (Dietrich et al., this volume). As MDI is the component of the Bayley scores which correlates most closely with measures of intelligence in older children, whereas PDI is a measure of a child's motor abilities, the differences in association between PbB and MDI and PDI might have been expected in the light of evidence in older children showing a small, but significant relationship between lead exposure and measures of intelligence (such as those reported by Fulton et al., 1988).

The relative crudity of the outcome instruments at this age indicates the need for continuing caution about reaching final conclusions at this stage of the study. Clearly, the results at older ages, at 4 and particularly 7 years,

Table 9 Relationship between HOME score and Bayley MDI according to integrated PbB (n in brackets)

HOME score	Bottom quartile (PbB $< 14 \mu g\,dl^{-1}$)		Middle 50 percentile (PbB $14–23 \mu g\,dl^{-1}$)		Top quartile (PbB $> 23 \mu g\,dl^{-1}$)	
	Mean MDI (n)	SE	Mean MDI (n)	SE	Mean MDI (n)	SE
<39	101.8 (8)	6.8	102.3 (42)	1.7	98.1 (38)	2.5
39–41	106.4 (14)	5.7	105.0 (54)	2.0	103.1 (26)	2.0
42–44	111.6 (29)	2.6	114.7 (66)	1.6	109.8 (33)	2.2
45–47	110.1 (31)	2.8	112.8 (47)	1.8	110.3 (12)	4.4
>47	122.7 (26)	2.7	117.5 (36)	2.8	120.2 (9)	5.7

when more extensive neurodevelopmental testing will be undertaken, are needed before final conclusions can be reached. Preliminary analyses, to be reported at a later date, indicate a stronger inverse association between lead exposure and scores on the McCarthy Scales of Children's Abilities, which were administered at age four years.

ACKNOWLEDGMENTS

The authors acknowledge the excellent co-operation of families in Port Pirie and the surrounding towns who were involved in this study, their doctors and the staff of local hospitals. The study would have been impossible without the skilled participation of Barbara Hobson RN, Chris Mavromatis RN, Mary-Anne Lange RN, Bronwen Morgan RN and Louise Thomson RN. We also thank members of the Adelaide Children's Hospital Chemical Pathology Department (Ms B. King, Mr R. Oldfield, Dr A. Pollard) who undertook the lead assays, staff of the CSIRO Division of Human Nutrition who assisted with the data analysis (Ms M. Padhye, Ms J. Rogers, Ms J. Syrette) and Mr C. Greeneklee, Manager of the Commonwealth Health Department Laboratory in Port Pirie who was responsible for the determination of packed cell volumes. The study was supported by grants from the Australian National Health and Medical Research Council and the South Australian Health Commission. We are grateful to the United States Environmental Protection Agency for travel assistance, enabling Dr Vimpani and Dr Baghurst to participate in this Edinburgh workshop.

REFERENCES

ACH. Department of Chemical Pathology, Adelaide Children's Hospital (unpublished data)

Australian Standards Association (1984). Australian Standard Project No. CH/006-0030. Method for the determination of lead in whole blood (Electrothermal atomisation Atomic Absorption Spectrophotometric Method). (Melbourne: Australian Standards Association)

Australian Standards Association (1983). Australian Standard 2636: Sampling of venous and capillary blood for the determination of lead content. (Melbourne: Australian Standards Association)

Baghurst, P.A., Oldfield, R.A., Wigg, N.R., McMichael, A.J., Robertson, E.F. and Vimpani, G.V. (1985). Some characteristics and correlates of blood lead in early childhood: preliminary results from the Port Pirie Study. Environ. Res., 38, 24–30

Bayley, N. (1969). Manual for the Bayley Scales of Infant Development. (New York: Psychological Corporation)

Bellinger, D., Leviton, A., Waternaux, C., Needleman, H. and Rabinowitz, M. (1988). Low-level lead exposure and early development in socioeconomically advantaged urban infants. (this volume)

Bornshein, R.L. (ed.) (1982). Proceedings of the First International Workshop on the effects of lead on child development, September 1981, Cincinnati, OH., University of Cincinnati

Bradley, R. and Caldwell, B. (1977). Home observation for measurement of the environment: a validation study of screening efficiency. Am. J. Ment. Defic., 81, 417–420

Caldwell, B.M. and Bradley, R.H. (1979). Home Observation for Measurement of the Environment. (Little Rock. University of Arkansas)

Fulton, M., Raab, G., Thomson, G., Laxen, D., Hunter, R. and Hepburn, W. (1988). Abilities of children and exposure to lead in Edinburgh. (this volume)

McMichael, A.J., Vimpani, G.V., Robertson, E.F., Baghurst, P.A. and Clark, P.D. (1986). The

Port Pirie cohort study: maternal blood lead and pregnancy outcome. *J. Epidemiol. Commun. Health*, **40**, 18–25

Vimpani, G.V., Wigg, N.R., Robertson, E.F., McMichael, A.J., Baghurst, P.A. and Roberts, R.J. (1987). The Port Pirie cohort study: Blood lead concentration and childhood developmental assessment. In: Goldwater, L.J., Wysocki, L.M. and Volpe, R.A. (eds.) *Lead Environmental Health: The Current Issues*. (Durham, NC: Duke University Press).

Wechsler, D. (1981). Wechsler Adult Intelligence Scale – Revised. (New York: Psychological Corporation)

4.4

Low-level Lead Exposure and Early Development in Socioeconomically Advantaged Urban Infants

D. BELLINGER, A. LEVITON, C. WATERNAUX, H. NEEDLEMAN and M. RABINOWITZ

SUMMARY

To assess the association between prenatal/early postnatal lead exposure and development, we followed a group of urban US infants from birth to 2 years of age. Estimates of the association between lead and Bayley Mental Development Index (MDI) scores at ages 6, 12, 18, and 24 months were obtained using several regression options. In all multivariate models examined, MDI scores were associated with umbilical cord blood lead levels, but not with postnatal blood lead levels. Infants with high cord blood lead levels (10–25 μg/dl) consistently scored 4 to 8 points lower than infants with low cord blood lead levels (< 3 μg/dl). Infants' vulnerability to lead's developmental toxicity appears to be greatest during the fetal period.

In previous reports we discussed various aspects of our ongoing prospective cohort study of infants who experienced low-level lead exposure in the late prenatal and early postnatal periods: performance on tests of development within the first 2 years of life (Bellinger et al., 1984, 1985a, 1986a); sources and correlates of exposure (Bellinger et al., 1985b, 1986b; Rabinowitz et al., 1985); implications for developmental models (Bellinger and Needleman, 1985); and statistical approaches (Bellinger et al., 1985b; Waternaux et al., 1989). Assessments of the infants at age 5 were completed in the spring of 1986, and will be reported in later publications.

Descriptions of the study design and methods (e.g. sample recruitment, attrition and characteristics, data collection, and analytical methods) are available elsewhere (Bellinger et al., 1984; Rabinowitz et al., 1985; Needleman et al., 1981). Briefly, infants were recruited on the basis of umbilical cord blood lead levels: low ($<3\,\mu g/dl$, $\bar{X} = 1.8$, SD $= 0.6$, $n = 85$), mid (6–7 $\mu g/dl$, $\bar{X} = 6.5$, SD $= 0.3$, $n = 88$), and high ($\geq 10\,\mu g/dl$, $\bar{X} = 14.6$, SD $= 3.0$, range $= 10.0$–24.9, $n = 76$).

After birth the sharp distinctions among groups in terms of blood lead levels were lost. In the sample as a whole, mean postnatal blood lead level did not exceed 8 $\mu g/dl$ at any age and, on most occasions, postnatal levels were not associated with infants' cord blood lead classifications. In contrast to the trimodal distribution of cord blood lead levels created by our sampling strategy, the distribution of postnatal blood lead levels more closely approached normality (Rabinowitz et al., 1984). Because extreme postnatal values are much less frequent in our sample than are extreme cord blood values, we can evaluate the hypothesis of an association between infant development and prenatal lead exposure more efficiently than the hypothesis of an association between infant development and postnatal exposure. Moreover, the weak correlations between infants' cord blood lead levels and their postnatal lead levels (Rabinowitz et al., 1984) mean that any cord blood lead level–outcome relationship is not likely to be confounded by infants' postnatal lead exposures.

Most of our subjects are middle to upper-middle class white infants, for whom socioeconomic status and quality of caregiving are at most only weakly associated with prenatal or postnatal blood lead levels (Bellinger et al., 1985b, 1986b). They do not display the typical association between demographic/economic risk factors and increased lead exposure seen in most samples. As a consequence, the likelihood of observing a spurious association between elevated lead exposure and poor outcome is lower in this sample than it is in most samples recruited to study the developmental impact of lead.

In this paper we examine two aspects of the association between lead exposure and infants' scores on the Mental Development Index (MDI) of the Bayley Scales of Infant Development at 6, 12, 18 and 24 months of age: (1) the stability of the estimate when different approaches to data analysis are taken; and (2) inter- and intra-individual stability of the estimate of the association over time.

ROBUSTNESS OF THE CORD BLOOD LEAD–MDI ASSOCIATION

Much of the controversy in this literature concerns the methods used to account for the fact that naturally constituted exposure groups inevitably differ in terms of many factors associated with infant development. To explore the robustness of the cord blood lead–MDI association, we applied a sequence of different analytical approaches to see whether the results are sensitive to the particular assumptions that underlie the alternative modelling strategies. The strategies are defined in terms of two key aspects of the process of adjusting for confounders: (1) the choice of potential confounders; and (2) the method used to construct (and modify) models from these factors (Robins and Greenland, 1986). The hierarchical relationships among the data analysis methods we compared are depicted in Figure 1.

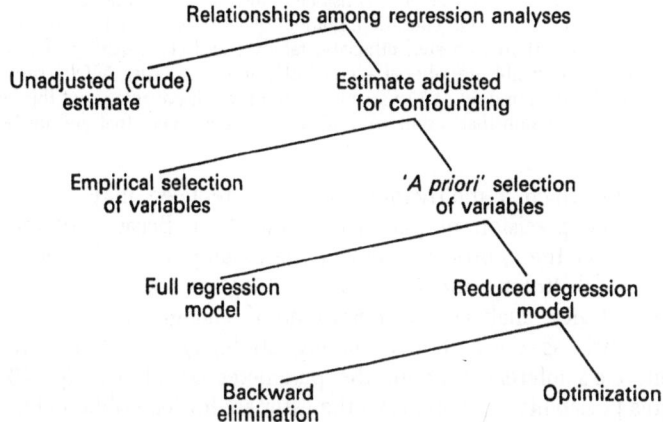

Figure 1 Hierarchical relationships among the regression strategies used to evaluate the association between infants' cord blood lead category and MDI scores

Methods

We compared two methods, empirical and *a priori*, for selecting the factors to consider in modelling the cord blood lead association:

(1) *Empirical*. Selection was based on evidence that, in our sample, adjusting for a variable altered the estimate of lead's association with development. In some previous analyses (Bellinger *et al.*, 1984, 1985a,b, 1986a) potential confounders were selected (from a list of more than 100 candidates) by identifying the set of variables most strongly associated with MDI scores and reducing it to only those whose presence in the regression model affected the estimate of the lead variable being evaluated. Preserving the validity of this estimate was the primary goal. Maximizing its precision was a secondary goal. A step-by-step description of this strategy is presented elsewhere (Bellinger *et al.*, 1985b).

Using this strategy the following variables were identified as potential confounders at the four ages:

6 months:	length of gestation
	HOME total score at 6 months
12 months:	length of gestation
	HOME scale 1 score at 6 months
18 months:	length of gestation
	HOME scale 1 score at 18 months
	ethnicity (white/nonwhite)
	maternal teaching style (Barnard, 1978)
24 months:	length of gestation
	HOME scale 1 score at 18 months
	HOME total score at 24 months
	ethnicity (white/nonwhite)
	paternal social class

Note that a different model of MDI was constructed at each age. This strategy permits recognition of the fact that some covariates may be time-varying (e.g. paternal social class), while others are fixed but vary over time in their relationship with infant's performance (e.g. ethnicity).

(2) *A priori*. Selection of confounders was based on prior knowledge of important correlates/determinants of infants' performance rather than on the statistical significance of patterns noted in the data collected (Kleinbaum *et al.*, 1982). Biological or psychological

347

plausibility is the paramount criterion. We considered such 'a priori' confounders to include maternal age, IQ (Dunn, 1965), and education, number of years of cigarette smoking, alcohol consumption during the third trimester, ethnicity, family social class, quality of care-giving (HOME), gender, birth weight, gestational age at birth, and birth order. MDI scores at each age were adjusted for the same set of 12 variables. One of the disadvantages of this approach is a possible loss of precision that results from adjusting for variables that are not bona-fide confounders.

The way in which a multivariate model is reduced may affect model validity and the precision of parameter estimation. Because of inevitable uncertainty about the appropriateness of the assumptions that underlie any regression model, Robins and Greenland (1986) suggest that investigators conduct 'sensitivity analyses' to determine if changes in 'one's analytic procedures (such as one's model-building strategy) would lead to large changes in one's inferences about the parameter of interest' (p. 402). To evaluate this possibility we compared the estimate for lead obtained from the full regression model (i.e. all 12 *a priori* confounders) to the estimates obtained from 'reduced' models derived by backward elimination (Kleinbaum *et al.*, 1982) and by optimization (Pocock and Ashby, 1985). In the backward stepwise procedure the p value required for retention in the model was $p < 0.10$. In the optimization method the computer is allowed to select the combination of candidate variables that is the best compromise in terms of complexity and fit. Operationally, this is the model that minimizes Mallows' C_p, where $C_p = (SSEp/s^2)-(N-2p)$. (SSEp is the error sum of squares for a model with a subset of p variables, and s^2 is the error mean squares for the full model of p variables.) In using this method to re-analyse the data of Smith *et al.* (1983), Pocock and Ashby (1985) forced tooth lead into all models. In our analyses cord blood lead category competed with other variables for inclusion in the 'best' model. All analyses were carried out using the BACKWARD (backward elimination) or the RSQUARE and GLM (optimization) procedures in the Statistical Analysis System (SAS, 1982).

Results

Method of confounder selection

Table 1 contrasts the results of three methods of estimating the association between cord blood lead category and infants' MDI scores: unadjusted for confounders, adjusted for confounders selected empirically, and adjusted for confounders selected *a priori*. In these analyses cord blood lead category was coded ordinally (1 = low, 2 = mid, 3 = high). This assumes linearity in the dose–response relationship between MDI and exposure category. The parameter estimate corresponds to the estimated difference in the mean adjusted MDI scores of infants in adjacent exposure groups (e.g. low versus mid, or mid versus high). In additional analyses the three exposure groups were represented by two indicator variables, permitting the estimation of nonlinear relationships. In general, both coding strategies suggested a significant association between cord blood lead and MDI scores.

At the later ages the use of indicator variables provided a somewhat better fit to the data. The reason is apparent from a plot of the least-squares mean

348

Table 1 Crude and adjusted parameter estimates for cord blood lead category

| Age (months) | Crude[a] | Adjusted[b] | |
		Empirical confounders	A priori confounders
6	-1.5 ± 1.0[c]	-2.9 ± 0.9	-2.1 ± 1.0
	$(0.5, -3.5)$[d]	$(-1.1, -4.7)$	$(-0.2, -4.1)$
12	-2.0 ± 1.1	-3.6 ± 1.1	-2.9 ± 1.2
	$(0.2, -4.2)$	$(-1.4, -5.8)$	$(-0.6, -5.2)$
18	-1.8 ± 1.5	-2.0 ± 1.4	-3.4 ± 1.4
	$(1.1, -4.7)$	$(0.7, -4.6)$	$(-0.5, -6.2)$
24	-2.5 ± 1.5	-2.7 ± 1.3	-4.0 ± 1.3
	$(0.4, -5.4)$	$(-0.2, -5.2)$	$(-1.3, -6.6)$

[a]Crude estimates were obtained by regressing MDI scores on cord blood lead category coded as an ordinal scale ($1 =$ low, $2 =$ mid, $3 =$ high)
[b]Descriptions of the methods used to choose the variables included in the empirical and a priori sets of confounders are given in the text
[c]Parameter estimate $\pm$ standard error; parameter estimate corresponds to the estimated difference in the mean adjusted MDI scores of infants in adjacent exposure groups (i.e. low versus mid or mid versus high); the sign indicates whether the group with higher exposure has a higher ($+$) or lower ($-$) mean adjusted score
[d]95% (two-sided) confidence interval for the parameter estimate

scores for the three exposure groups (Figure 2). Infants in the low and midrange lead groups tended to perform at roughly the same level, with both considerably higher than infants in the high lead group.

Two features of the results stand out. First, although the unadjusted estimate is negative at all four ages (indicating an inverse association between cord blood lead level and MDI), it is always smaller than the two adjusted estimates. In fact, the unadjusted estimate did not achieve nominal statistical significance ($p < 0.05$) at any age. This enhancement of the lead estimate by adjustment is unique among lead studies and probably reflects the fact that children from the most advantaged families tended to have slightly higher lead levels (Bellinger et al., 1985b).

Second, the 95% confidence intervals produced by the two adjustment strategies were generally quite similar. In the empirical method the lower bound for the interval associated with the difference between the low and high exposure groups (twice the parameter estimate) varies from $+1.4$ to -2.8 points, and the upper bound varies from -9.2 to -11.6. In the a priori method the ranges for the lower and upper bounds are -0.4 to -2.6 and -8.2 to -13.2 points, respectively. During the second year, when sociodemographic factors typically become potent predictors of infant development, the more potential confounders considered, the greater the estimate of the association of cord blood lead with MDI scores. This provides another illustration of the unusual manner in which cord blood lead level relates to other significant predictors of performance in this sample of infants.

To demonstrate that infants with high cord blood lead levels are not at risk for poor development based on other aspects of their rearing context, we calculated least-squares mean MDI scores for infants in the three lead groups, using a regression equation that included the 12 a priori variables but not cord blood lead category (Figure 3). These are the scores that would be

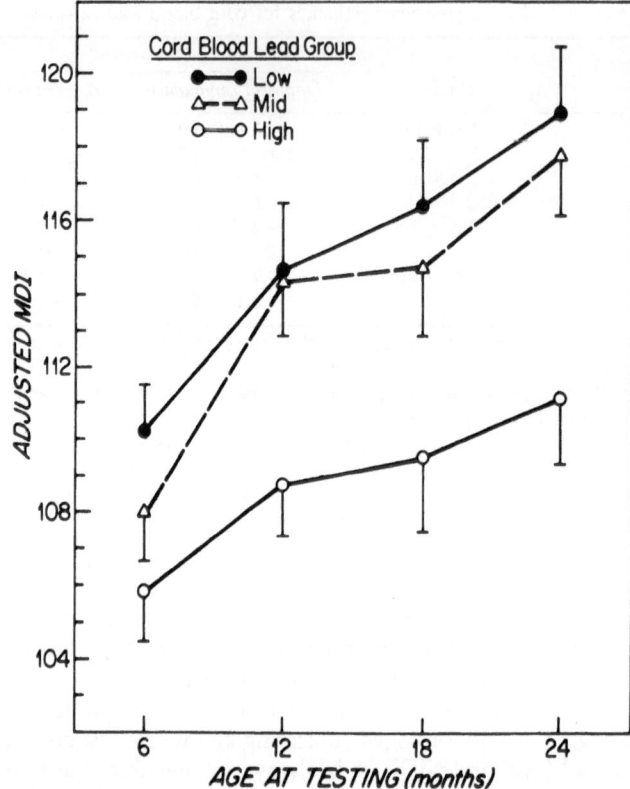

Figure 2   Mean mental development index (MDI) scores at four ages for infants in the three umbilical cord blood lead categories. Scores are least-squares means, derived from a regression equation that included the 12 'a priori' confounders and the cord blood lead category (represented by two indicator variables). Error bars represent one standard error

expected under the null hypothesis of no association between cord blood lead category and MDI scores. Expected performance did not relate to infants' lead levels in the way that would be anticipated based on the assumption that it is children who are at higher risk of poor outcome for other reasons who tend to suffer greater exposure to lead. In this sample, infants with midrange lead levels had covariate values that are associated with the best performance. Low lead infants, not high lead infants, had the least optimal covariate values.

Partly as a result of this, infants' MDI scores tended to be more strongly associated with cord blood lead grouping when it was coded by indicator variables rather than by a single ordinal scale. For instance, in crude analyses the p values associated with lead coded as indicator variables were 0.29, 0.011, 0.063, and 0.007 at 6, 12, 18, and 24 months of age, respectively. They are considerably more extreme than the corresponding p values associated with the crude parameter estimates presented in Table 1. Because the infants in the midrange lead group possessed covariate values associated

350

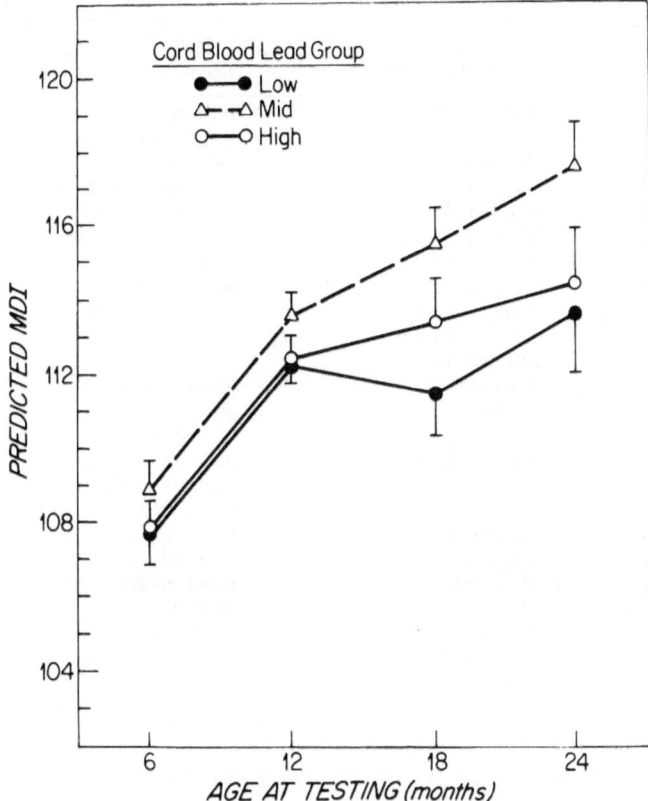

Figure 3 Mean 'predicted' mental development index scores at four ages for infants in the three umbilical cord blood lead categories. Scores are least-squares means, derived from a regression equation that included only the 12 'a priori' confounders. These are the scores that infants in the three exposure groups would be expected to achieve based solely on the confounders. Error bars represent one standard error

with the highest MDI scores, fitting a straight line to the unadjusted scores of the three exposure groups (the assumption that underlies ordinal coding), resulted in large standard errors for the parameter estimates and, hence, distorted p values.

Method of refining the multivariate model
Table 2 presents the models produced by applying backward elimination and optimal regression methods to the full set of 12 variables selected *a priori*. At all four ages, cord blood lead category was selected for inclusion in the 'best' model regardless of method. At 6, 12, and 24 months the models produced by the two methods are identical.

Table 3 presents the parameter estimates for cord blood lead category in the full regression model (i.e. all 12 *a priori* variables) and the final models produced by the two reduction methods. At all ages but one (6 months), the

Table 2 'Best' regression models produced by backward elimination and optimization

Age (months)	Method for reducing full model	
	Backward elimination	Optimization
6	Birth weight	birth weight
	length of gestation	length of gestation
	HOME score[a]	HOME score
	maternal education	maternal education
	cord blood lead	cord blood lead
12	length of gestation	length of gestation
	maternal IQ[b]	maternal IQ
	infant gender	infant gender
	maternal alcohol[c]	maternal alcohol
	cord blood lead	cord blood lead
18	birth weight	birth weight
	infant gender	infant gender
	ethnicity[d]	ethnicity
	HOME score	HOME score
	cord blood lead	maternal smoking[e]
		maternal alcohol
		cord blood lead
24	birth weight	birth weight
	maternal age	maternal age
	infant gender	infant gender
	ethnicity	ethnicity
	HOME score	HOME score
	maternal education	maternal education
	cord blood lead	cord blood lead

[a]Mean of the total scores assigned at the 6 and 24 month administrations of the Home Observation for Measurement of the Environment (HOME)
[b]Peabody Picture Vocabulary Test, administered to mothers when infants were 12 months of age
[c]Mean number of drinks (beer, wine, spirits) consumed per week in the third trimester of pregnancy
[d]White versus nonwhite
[e]Number of years of maternal smoking

parameter estimate assigned to lead in the full model slightly exceeded the estimate in either reduced model. On the other hand, at each age the 95% confidence intervals for the estimates are slightly narrower in the reduced models than in the full models. This may be an example of the loss of precision that results when adjustment is made for variables that are not true confounders.

The parameter estimates for cord blood lead group obtained using the different adjustment methods define the range within which the true value is likely to lie for this sample (assuming that appropriate adjustment has been made for all true confounders). The minimum and maximum estimates range from -2.0 to -4.0 at the various ages (Table 4). (This is the range for the estimated mean differences between adjacent exposure groups. The 95% confidence intervals around these bounds are considerably wider and can be calculated using the standard errors given in Tables 1 and 3.) The consistency of the estimate among analytic methods and ages is evidence that the prenatal exposure–development association is indeed robust.

Table 3 Adjusted parameter estimates for cord blood lead category: comparison of full and reduced regression models

Age (months)	Full model	Reduced models	
		Backward elimination	Optimization
6	−2.1 ± 1.0[a]	−2.4 ± 0.9	−2.5 ± 0.9
	(−0.2, −4.1)[b]	(−0.7, −4.2)	(−0.7, −4.2)
12	−2.9 ± 1.2	−2.6 ± 1.1	−2.4 ± 1.1
	(−0.6, −5.2)	(−0.4, −4.7)	(−0.2, −4.5)
18	−3.4 ± 1.4	−3.1 ± 1.3	−3.3 ± 1.4
	(−0.5, −6.2)	(−0.5, −5.8)	(−0.5, −6.0)
24	−4.0 ± 1.3	−3.4 ± 1.2	−3.4 ± 1.2
	(−1.3, −6.6)	(−1.0, −5.8)	(−1.0, −5.7)

[a]Parameter estimate ± standard error
[b]95% (two-sided) confidence interval for the parameter estimate
Note: As described in the text, the backward elimination and optimization methods selected the same sets of variables for the 'best' models at 6, 12, and 24 months. Differences between the parameter estimates and standard errors presented for the two methods are due to the fact that slightly different numbers of cases were used in the two sets of analyses. Cases with missing values for any of the 12 variables were eliminated from the backward elimination analyses. In the optimizing regressions, only cases with missing values for variables selected for the 'best' model were eliminated

Table 4 Summary of results obtained using several regression models

Age (months)	Range of adjusted parameter estimates (± SE) for cord blood lead category)	Estimated MDI advantage of infants in low v. high cord blood lead category
6	−2.1 ± 1.0 to −2.9 ± 0.9	4.2 to 5.8 points
12	−2.4 ± 1.1 to −3.6 ± 1.1	4.8 to 7.2 points
18	−2.0 ± 1.4 to −3.4 ± 1.4	4.0 to 6.8 points
24	−2.7 ± 1.3 to −4.0 ± 1.3	5.4 to 8.0 points

INTER- AND INTRA-INFANT STABILITY

Conventional statistical tests, involving comparisons of group means, may contribute little information about the distribution of susceptibility to a toxin within a sample. The magnitude and variance of the average response is highly influenced by the ratio of responders to non-responders. As a result, these methods may not adequately address issues of prime interest in toxicological studies (Good, 1979; Weiss, 1980). For example, we evaluated whether the differences in mean MDI scores of infants in the different cord blood lead categories were due to small deficits in the performance of most infants with the highest exposures, or to large deficits in the performance of only a few infants with such exposures. We also investigated whether the same group of high lead infants tended to perform relatively poorly at each age.

Methods

We calculated a 'residual' score at each age for each infant. The MDI score 'expected' for an infant, calculated from the regression equation consisting of the 12 *a priori* confounders, was subtracted from the score the infant actually achieved. Infants were assigned a summary score of 0 to 4, depending on the number of ages at which the residual was greater than zero (i.e. observed score exceeded expected score). A plot of the percentage of infants in the three cord blood lead groups who achieved each summary score (Figure 4) shows that 3 to 4 times as many infants in the high lead group as in the low or midrange lead groups did not score higher than expected on any occasion (23.6% versus 8.5% and 6.5%, respectively). Fewer than half of the high lead infants scored higher than expected on more than one of the four occasions

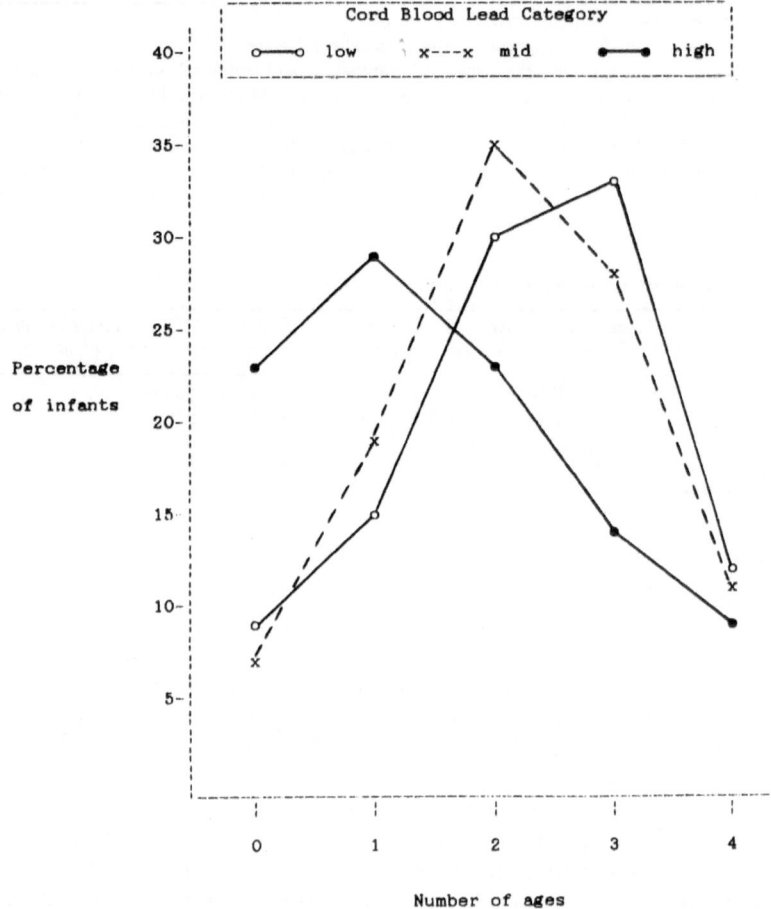

Figure 4 Percentage of infants in the three cord blood lead categories displaying various performance profiles. 'Profile' is defined as the number of ages (maximum of four) at which an infant's observed mental development index (MDI) score exceeded the expected score. Expected score at each age was defined as the least-squares mean based on a regression model of MDI consisting of the 12 'a priori' confounders

they were tested. Thus, it appears that a substantial percentage of infants in the high lead group consistently performed worse than expected.

CONCLUSION

The inverse association in this sample between MDI scores and umbilical cord blood lead levels in the 0 to 25 μg/dl range appears to be robust. Estimates of its magnitude and precision are relatively independent of analytic approach. Furthermore, the association does not appear to be attributable to the inordinate influence of outliers. Most infants with high lead levels contribute to the overall poorer performance of this group relative to infants with lower levels of prenatal exposure.

The generalizability of this association to infants of lower socioeconomic standing is uncertain. The correlation between lead exposure and other developmental risk factors may vary substantially across samples. This has important conceptual and statistical implications. Social class may be an effect modifier, with the adverse effects of lead, like those of some other biological insults, greater among infants already stressed by socioeconomic disadvantage. Support for this hypothesis has been obtained in studies of older children (Winneke and Kraemer, 1984; Harvey et al., 1984) and it appears to be supported in our own sample of infants despite the relatively limited representation of lower class families (Bellinger et al., 1989a).

Social class may be both a confounder and an effect-modifier, however. The statistical methods generally used to adjust for social class may not be equally effective across variations in the strength of the association between lead exposure and social class. In exploratory simulations we have found that semipartial correlations (and, by extension, regression coefficients) increasingly underestimate the association between lead and development as the link between increased lead exposure and social disadvantage becomes stronger (Bellinger et al., 1989b).

Because the association between lead exposure and social class is not uniform among studies, adjustments for the resulting confounding vary in their efficiency. This may help to account for some of the inconsistency among different studies in the statistical significance of the 'adjusted' association between lead and development.

ACKNOWLEDGMENTS

This work was supported by grants HD-08945 and HD-17407 from the National Institute of Child Health and Human Development. D.B. is supported by a Research Career Development Award (ES-00138) from the National Institute of Environmental Health Sciences.

REFERENCES

Barnard, K. (1978) *The Nursing Child Assessment Teaching Scales*, (Seattle: University of Washington)

Bellinger, D. and Needleman, H (1985). Prenatal and early postnatal exposure to lead: developmental effects, correlates and implications. *Int. J. Ment. Health*, **14**, 78–111

Bellinger, D., Needleman, H., Leviton, A., Waternaux, C., Rabinowitz, M. and Nichols, M. (1984). Early sensory-motor development and prenatal exposure to lead. *Neurobehav. Toxicol. Teratol.*, **6**, 387–402

Bellinger, D., Leviton, A., Waternaux, C., Needleman, H. and Rabinowitz, M. (1985a) A longitudinal study of the developmental toxicity of low-level lead exposure in the prenatal and early postnatal periods. In Lekkas, T. (ed.) *Proceedings of the International Conference Heavy Metals in the Environment*, (Edinburgh: CEP Consultants), pp. 32–34

Bellinger, D., Leviton, A., Waternaux, C. and Allred, E. (1985b) Methodological issues in modeling the relationship between low-level lead exposure and infant development: Examples from the Boston Lead Study. *Env. Res.*, **38**, 119–129

Bellinger, D., Leviton, A., Needleman, H., Waternaux, C. and Rabinowitz, M. (1986a) Low-level lead exposure and infant development in the first year. *Neurobehav. Toxicol. Teratol.*, **8**, 151–161

Bellinger, D., Leviton, A., Rabinowitz, M., Needleman, H. and Waternaux, C. (1986b) Correlates of low-level lead exposure in urban children at 2 years of age. *Pediatrics*, **77**, 826–833

Bellinger, D., Leviton, A., Waternaux, C., Needleman, H. and Rabinowitz, M. (1989a) Low-level lead exposure, social class, and infant development. *Neurotoxicol. Teratol.* (in press)

Bellinger, D., Leviton, A. and Waternaux, C. (1989b) Lead, IQ, and social class. *Int. J. Epidemiol.* (in press)

Dunn, L. (1965) *Peabody Picture Vocabulary Test* (Circle Pines, MN: American Guidance Service)

Good, P. (1979) Detection of a treatment effect when not all experimental subjects will respond to treatment. *Biometrics*, **35**, 483–489

Harvey, P., Hamlin, M. and Kumar, R. (1984). Blood lead, behavior and intelligence test performance in pre-school children. *Sci. Total Env.*, **40**, 45–60

Kleinbaum, D., Kupper, L. and Morgenstern, H. (1982) *Epidemiologic Research: Principles and Quantitative Methods* (Belmont, CA: Lifetime Learning Publications)

Needleman, H., Leviton, A., Rabinowitz, M. and Bellinger, D. (1981) The perinatal lead exposure study. In Bornschein, R. (ed.), *Proceedings of the First International Conference of Lead Exposure in Children, Cincinnati*, pp. 15–18

Pocock, S. and Ashby, D. (1985) Environmental lead and children's intelligence: A review of recent epidemiological studies. *Statistician*, **34**, 31–44

Rabinowitz, M., Leviton, A. and Needleman, H. (1984) Variability of blood lead concentrations during infancy. *Arch. Env. Health*, **39**, 74–77

Rabinowitz, M., Leviton, A., Needleman, H., Bellinger, D. and Waternaux, C. (1985) Environmental correlates of infant blood lead levels. *Env. Res.*, **38**, 96–107

Robins, J. and Greenland, S. (1986) The role of model selection in causal inference from nonexperimental data. *Am. J. Epidemiol.*, **123**, 392–402

SAS User's Guide (1982) (Cary, NC: SAS Institute)

Smith, M., Delves, T., Lansdown, R., Clayton, B. and Graham, P. (1983) The effects of lead exposure on urban children: the Institute of Child Health/Southampton Study. *Dev. Med. Child Neurol.*, **25**, Suppl. 47

Waternaux, C., Laird, N. and Ware, J. (1989) Methods for analysis of longitudinal data: Blood lead concentrations and cognitive development. *J. Am. Stat. Assoc.* (in press)

Weiss, B. (1980) Conceptual issues in the assessment of lead toxicity. In Needleman, H. (ed.), *Low Level Lead Exposure: Clinical Implications of Current Research* (New York: Raven Press)

Winneke, G. and Kraemer, U. (1984) Neuropsychological effects of lead in children: interactions with social background variables. *Neuropsychobiologica*, **11**, 195–204

4.5

Lead-related Birth Defects: Some Methodological Issues

C. B. ERNHART, G. BRITTENHAM, M. R. MARLER and
R. J. SOKOL

SUMMARY

In the course of reviewing our findings on the topic of foetal lead effects, several methodological problems are noted. The first is the effective measurement and control of important confounding variables. In our studies, we demonstrated that failure to consider the effect of foetal lead exposure with the effects of maternal use of alcohol and cigarettes during pregnancy can lead to discrepant findings in the association of lead exposure and the gestational age, birth weight, length and head circumference of the neonate. We also demonstrated that similar discrepancies in findings for the size measurements might follow from failure to consider parental size. Similarly, the association of lead level and neonatal anomalies might be a function of failure to obtain adequate measurements of maternal alcohol use and to control for this confounding condition in statistical models. The second concern is the effect of adjusting cord blood lead (PbB) data for haematocrits. We demonstrated that effect sizes tend to be reduced when PbB corrected for haematocrits is used in place of uncorrected values. Although the haematocrit measure in our data was correlated with cord PbB, it did not appreciably alter a previously reported association of foetal lead exposure and neonatal status.

Various investigators have reported an association of low-level lead exposure in the foetal period and neonatal outcome measures. These studies differ, of course, with respect to the populations sampled and other procedural features. What is striking, however, in reviewing these is the lack of consistency between studies in the specific outcome measures related to foetal lead exposure. Several features of the research designs that could account for some

357

of these discrepancies are noted. This review was initiated in the hope that exploration of the ways in which the studies differ might clarify these discrepant results.

First, the possibility will be considered that some unmeasured or undermeasured confounding conditions may be particularly crucial to gestational lead exposure and to neonatal outcome measures. The second possibility to be considered is whether discrepancies between studies with respect to correction of blood lead level (PbB) for haematocrit percent (Hct%) may be related to discrepant results. Data from our Cleveland study will be used to illustrate some of these issues. While this commentary is limited to neonatal outcome measures, the issues raised are also relevant to prospective analyses relating foetal lead exposure to later development.

UNMEASURED OR UNDERMEASURED CONFOUNDING CONDITIONS

Table 1 includes neonatal outcome variables reported to be significantly related to low-level maternal, placental, cord, or very early infancy PbB in one or more studies. Case reports and some older studies that include additional adverse outcomes, usually as a result of high-level exposure (Rom, 1976), have been excluded. To save space, Table 1 excludes reports of assessed outcome measures not significantly related to PbB in any study in the review. These variables are pre-eclampsia, spontaneous abortion, foetal distress, ponderal index, intrauterine growth retardation, meconium staining, Apgar scores, jaundice, blood type, sex of infant and most scales of the Brazelton Newborn Assessment Scale.

Birth weight and gestational age are inherently important outcome measures. Furthermore, they are of particular methodological interest in that they may be controlled as confounders in prospective analyses of later outcome measures. Thus, statistical control of gestational age was crucial to the Bellinger *et al.* (1986) finding of a relationship between cord PbB and Bayley Mental Development Index (MDI) at later ages in the data of the Boston study. Dietrich *et al.* (1986) controlled both birth weight and gestational age in their analyses of six month MDI.

It has been suggested that stunting of growth results from lead exposure and that such stunting might be observed in the newborn. Of the sixteen studies reviewed, four reported decreased birth weight associated with lead level. In one (Bogden *et al.*, 1978), the effect was not statistically significant; in another (Nordstrom *et al.*, 1979), the lead effect may be confounded by other toxic exposures; and a third study (Bryce-Smith, 1986) is a preliminary report with little information. The most clearly documented finding is that from the Cincinnati study, as reported by Dietrich *et al.* (1986).

The Cincinnati study measured alcohol and tobacco exposure by a dichotomous score that was positive if the mother reported use of alcohol, tobacco, or both. The relationship of birth weight to use of tobacco has been fairly well established, and reduced birth weight has been related to foetal alcohol exposure (Abel, 1983). We considered the possibility that this simple

Table 1 Neonatal outcome measures related to one or more indicators of foetal lead exposure in one or more studies

Study	Lead indicator	Neonatal size			Adverse obstetrical outcomes					Abnormalities		Neurological findings		
		Birth weight	Length	Head circumference	Death	GA	PROM	Premature labour	Respiratory distress	Major	Minor	Abnormal reflexes	Neuro SS	Muscle tonus
Rajegowda et al. (1972)	C	0			0									
Gershanik et al. (1974)	C	0				0								
Fahim et al. (1976)	M,C,L					+*	+*							
Clark (1977)	M,C,L	0				0				0				
Wibberly et al. (1977)	P	0			+*									
Bodgen et al. (1978)	M,C	+												
Roels et al. (1978)	P,M,C	0												
Nordstrom et al. (1979)	L	+								+				
Alexander and Delves (1981)	M,6-DL				0					−				
Angell and Lavery (1982)	C					0	0							
Moore et al. (1982, 1984)	M,C	0	0[a]	0[a]		+*								
Boston (Needleman et al., 1984; Bellinger et al., 1985)	C	0				−*	0	−*	−*	0	+*			
Pt. Pirie (McMichael et al., 1986)	M[b],C[c],L	−	0	+*[c]	+,−*	+*	0				0			
Bryce-Smith (1986)	P	+*	0	+*		+*								
Cincinnati (Dietrich et al., 1986)	M[b],10-D[b]	+*				+*								
Cleveland (Ernhart et al., 1986)	M,C	0	0	0		0[d]				0		+*	+*	+*

Symbols: 0 no evident relationship; + results consistent with adverse lead effect; − results contrary to adverse lead effect; * statistically significant at p < 0.05. If any lead indicator in the study was reported as + or − for the outcome, this was coded, even if other lead indicators were unrelated.

Abbreviations, Obstetrical Outcomes: Death: late foetal, stillborn, or neonatal. GA: Preterm delivery or gestational age; PROM: premature rupture of membranes.

Abbreviations, Neurological findings: Abnormal reflexes: the Abrormal Reflexes Scale of the Brazelton Scales; Neuro SS: The Neurological Soft Signs Scale of the Graham/Rosenblith Examination; Muscle tonus: the Muscle Tonus Scale of the Graham/Rosenblith Examination.

Code for lead indicator: M maternal (pregnancy or delivery): C cord: 6-D age 6 days; 10-D age 10 days; P placenta; L contrast in locations.

[a] From notes made at meeting
[b] Corrected for Hct%
[c] May be due to hospital differences
[d] Not previously published

index, based on routine antenatal obstetric information, undercorrects for these exposures. We also considered the contribution of parental size to infant size.

The data of the Cleveland study are used here to evaluate the way in which these factors, as well as gestational age, can affect the relationship of cord lead level and three measures of neonatal size. As shown in Table 2, the Pearson correlations (r) for length and head circumference were statistically significant; the correlation for birth weight might be called marginal. Although gestational age of less than 37 weeks was an exclusion criterion, the range was related, reasonably enough, to each size measure. Gestational age was correlated -0.17 ($n = 162$, $p < 0.05$) with cord PbB. Clearly, the effect of gestational age should be controlled; when it is, the effect size for PbB is reduced for each size measure.

Although the inference might be drawn at this point that there exist marginal, but statistically significant, effects for length and head circumference, this analysis was continued to assess the influence of additional factors. We had hypothesized, a priori, that specified other variables were particularly crucial to the assessment of infant size. These were maternal height, paternal height, maternal head circumference, number of cigarettes smoked per day, and an index (AA/day) of maternal alcohol consumption throughout pregnancy. The analysis was continued to assess the contribution of these to lead-related variance in the outcome measures. To simplify matters, these were grouped into a size set and a substance set for model entry. With the addition of either set, the lead-related variance decreased; with the inclusion of both, the effect sizes became quite small and none were statistically significant.

The point made is that both the inclusion of more comprehensive measures of the confounding effects of alcohol and smoking and also the control of parent size, an obvious correlate of infant size, might modify the results. The inclusion of parent size measures in analyses relating lead level and size might also be pertinent to analyses of childhood size. The possibility of confounding due to this source was not considered in the Schwartz, Angle, and Pitcher (1986) analyses of the NHANES II data. We will be including parent size measures in the analyses we will make of our preschool-age size data. Even if parent size is not a confounder in studies of child size, its inclusion in analytic models should increase the statistical power of the analyses by reducing error variance in the linear models.

In addition to our published analyses of size measures and those provided in Table 2, we conducted a series of additional analyses involving different alcohol exposure variables, substitution of serum thiocyanate data for the cigarettes per day measure, transformations of several measures, and the use of missing data techniques to avoid reductions in sample size. This deliberate analytical dredging of the data yielded results consistent with the findings provided in Table 2. These analyses increased our confidence in the analytical plan and in the robustness of the findings regarding these outcome measures.

The present study now considers whether gestational age (or the dichotomous variable, preterm delivery) is related to lead level. This, too, is an important outcome measure and is a covariate in some studies of later

Table 2 The relationship of cord PbB and size measures with and without control of relevant variables, $n = 162$

Measure	r	Shared variance, % (r^2)	Variance (%) after control of				
			Gestational age (GA)	GA and parent size	GA and substance use	GA, parent size, and substance use	Substance use
Birth weight	0.15 (0.06)	2.3 (0.06)	1.4 (0.13)	0.9 (0.20)	0.5 (0.34)	0.3 (0.50)	
Length	0.20 (0.01)	4.2 (0.01)	2.9 (0.03)	2.3 (0.05)	2.4 (0.05)	1.8 (0.08)	
Head circumference	0.20 (0.01)	4.1 (0.01)	2.6 (0.04)	1.3 (0.11)	1.9 (0.07)	0.9 (0.20)	
Gestational age	0.17 (0.03)	2.8 (0.03)					1.8 (0.08)

Note: p values are indicated in parentheses

361

development. Once again, we have tried to integrate inconsistent findings. Some studies found no significant lead effects. Fahim, Fahim, and Hall (1976) reported a higher incidence of preterm delivery, as well as premature rupture of membranes, in a lead belt area in Missouri, but maternal lead levels did not differ with locale. Moore *et al.* (1982) reported significant associations of gestational age with both maternal and cord PbB. An increase in the incidence of preterm delivery was the only consistently significant effect reported by the Port Pirie group (McMichael *et al.*, 1986).

In an interim report (Dietrich *et al.*, 1986) on the Cincinnati study, maternal PbB, but not PbB at age 10 days, was related at a minimal level (-0.17) to gestational age. The dichotomous indicator of alcohol and tobacco exposure did not alter this relationship, and no other confounding variables were found to modify the effect. The Boston study (Bellinger *et al.*, 1985) is most discrepant, since the direction of effect was reversed, with a significantly larger number of preterm infants found in the low-lead group. The positive relationship between gestational age and PbB did not reach statistical significance, but it was large enough to be identified as a *bona fide* covariate in analyses of later outcome measures (Bellinger *et al.*, 1986).

The Cleveland study was limited by exclusion of infants with gestational age < 37 weeks; thus the relationship of lead level to preterm delivery cannot be tested. The correlation of gestational age and maternal PbB was -0.11 (non-significant) and, as noted above, for cord PbB was -0.17 ($p < 0.05$). Covariate control of substance measures (average ounces of alcohol per day and cigarettes per day) attenuated the relationships. As shown in Table 2, the variance accounted for by cord PbB was reduced from 2.8% to 1.8%. This was not statistically significant.

Malformations or anomalies are next considered. Major malformations were not found to be related to lead in the Boston study (Needleman *et al.*, 1984), possibly because they were infrequent. Malformations of unspecified seriousness were related to residence in a low, as opposed to a high, lead area in the Alexander and Delves (1981) study. Although Wibberley *et al.* (1977) reported higher placental lead levels among stillborn and neonatal death infants, there was no significant difference in lead levels for malformed deceased infants, as opposed to non-malformed deceased infants. Wibberley suggested that one explanation of their results is that infants under stress might tend to accumulate lead, an interpretation that could be tested by analyses of maternal tissues that were not available to him.

Minor anomalies were related to lead level in the Boston study (Needleman *et al.*, 1984) but not in the Port Pirie (McMichael *et al.*, 1986) or the Cleveland (Ernhart *et al.*, 1986) studies. While there were a number of methodological differences between the Boston and the Cleveland studies, one discrepancy in findings that may be meaningful is that the Boston group failed to find an association between their alcohol-use measure and neonatal anomalies. This is notable, since it has been estimated that 5% of anatomic congenital defects may be attributable to prenatal alcohol exposure (Sokol, 1981).

In the Cleveland study, we followed a very detailed gestational period protocol (Sokol, Martier and Ernhart, 1985) for assessing foetal alcohol exposure and for obtaining a history of maternal alcohol abuse. Furthermore, since the anomalies were identified through a careful examination under a research protocol, the likelihood of underascertainment was much less than is the case for chart review ascertainment. We have reported (Ernhart et al., 1987) dose–response relationships illustrating the relationship of alcohol use and two tallies of neonatal anomalies. The craniofacial anomalies, which are relatively specific to fetal alcohol effects, were related in a positively accelerated manner to ounces of alcohol consumed per day during the embryonic period. The other anomalies, including cardiac murmur, haemangiomas, hydrocoele, etc. were also increased for the offspring of heavy drinkers, but the effect was not as dramatic as was the case for craniofacial anomalies.

Since (a) maternal alcohol consumption during early pregnancy is related to neonatal anomalies in this and other studies (Abel, 1982), and (b) alcohol consumption is related to lead level in this and other studies of pregnant and non-pregnant adults (Grandjean, Olsen, and Hollnagel, 1981; Pocock et al., 1983; Ernhart et al., 1985), we believe that foetal alcohol exposure cannot be considered irrelevant. (A new study of alcohol-related birth defects, now beginning at Wayne State University, will incorporate cord PbB measures so that a replication of the tests of a possible lead effect with adequate control of alcohol exposure confounding will be available.)

This discussion has demonstrated that the introduction of covariates which were not previously included (parental size in the case of child size) or which may not have been measured in detail (such as maternal alcohol and cigarette consumption) can influence the association of lead level and neonatal outcome. As usual, the possibility must be considered that statistical control might be diminishing a true lead effect. It is hard to believe that lead exposure caused, or was caused by, variation in parent size. It could be argued, perhaps, that control of alcohol and tobacco exposure in a lead-effects model is improper, since it appears that these factors influence lead level. Here we can only ask whether the portion of the lead variance that is not dependent on alcohol and smoking contributes significantly to the variance of the outcome measures. For the variables reviewed, the answer appears to be no. Perhaps the joint or common effects of the respective risk factors cannot be wholly untangled, but the evidence regarding alcohol-related birth defects and smoking-related intrauterine growth retardation cautions against taking a minimal approach to the measurement of these variables.

CORRECTION FOR HAEMATOCRIT LEVELS

As we attempted to resolve some discrepancies between studies, we noted that two groups of investigators, those from Port Pirie (McMichael et al., 1986) and those from Cincinnati (Dietrich et al., 1986), corrected for haematocrit levels. This correction presumably increases the accuracy of the estimate of the lead available to the soft tissues perfused by the blood (Kochen and Greener, 1973). Although some investigators assert that haematocrit correction is not necessary (Rosen, Zarate-Salvador, and Trinidad, 1974; Chisolm, 1974), the issue is not settled (DeSilva, 1984). The usual use is to correct for anaemia, and this may be appropriate for maternal PbB. In the case of the foetus or neonate, it may also be correct, in the opposite direction, for excessive erythrocyte concentration, or polycythaemia. Since haematocrit (Hct%) in the foetus and neonate may be affected by conditions unique to the age (gestational hypoxaemia, for example, and, under some circumstances, placental transfusion), the possibility is considered here that Hct% correction may alter the results or the inferences drawn in studies of foetal lead exposure. This possibility does not appear to have been explored in studies of lead exposure in the perinatal period. This issue is examined from two perspectives. First, it is considered whether effect sizes are influenced by Hct% adjustment. Second, it is considered whether the variance of Hct% is itself a confounding factor in the aetiology of the conditions attributed to lead exposure.

Data from our Cleveland study were used to demonstrate the effect of Hct% correction. The correlation of cord PbB and Hct% was 0.26, $p = 0.001$. Most investigators have not reported the relationship between cord PbB and Hct% in their data; some (Rajegowda, Glass, and Evans, 1972; Clark, 1977; Needleman et al., 1984) have stated that no significant relationship was found. (Although the Kochen and Greener (1973) argument against Hct% correction states that they found no correlation of PbB and Hct%, the report includes a series of correlations ranging from 0.20 to 0.66; none were significant with the small substudy sample sizes.) The correlation between maternal PbB and Hct% in our data was 0.10 (non-significant).

Since lead level in sera is minimal (Rosen, Zarate-Salvador, and Trinidad, 1974), the Hct%-adjusted values for each person in the present study were estimated by dividing the obtained PbB by the Hct% and multiplying by a constant. For cord blood, the adjustment was to $50 \, \mu g \, dl^{-1}$; for maternal blood, it was to $35 \, \mu g \, dl^{-1}$. In addition to this form of adjustment, demonstration analyses were also made with Hct% entered as a covariate. In this way, we could determine whether this form of correction would have a different effect on the basic analyses as contrasted with the simple Hct% correction. Furthermore, with Hct% entered with PbB in the statistical model, the possibility that the particular outcome measure was directly dependent on Hct% could be assessed.

The illustrative data are those for cord PbB as it relates to gestational age, birth weight, length, and head circumference. As shown in Table 3, the adjustment for Hct% attenuated the effect size for each measure in models without control of confounding variables. In models with covariate control, Hct% correction made little difference, probably because there was little variance that could be attenuated. In the absence of a definitive basis of choice for the perinatal period, these analyses are reported as empirical findings that may be related to the methodology employed in these studies.

The present study also considered whether neonatal polycythaemia (elevated Hct%) might be a confounding condition for research on lead effects. Neonatal polycythaemia is not uncommon; the incidence estimates range from 2.5% (Wirth, Goldberg and Lubchenco, 1979) to 20% (Shohat, Merlob and Reisner, 1984) of all newborns. It can result from such risk conditions as foetal hypoxaemia, which apparently stimulates the production of erythrocytes, maternal hypertension, maternal diabetes, and some other relatively rare conditions (Shohat, Merlob and Reisner, 1984; Gross, Hathaway and

Table 3 The relationship of cord PbB with size measures and gestational age with and without Hct% correction

Measure	Shared variance (%) without covariate[a] control		Shared variance (%) with covariate[a] control	
	No Hct% adjustment[b]	Hct% adjusted[c]	No Hct% adjustment[b]	Hct% adjusted[c]
Birth weight	2.3 (0.06)	0.8 (0.22)	0.3 (0.50)	0.2 (0.60)
Length	4.2 (0.01)	2.1 (0.07)	1.8 (0.08)	1.1 (0.17)
Head circumference	4.1 (0.01)	1.9 (0.09)	0.9 (0.20)	0.5 (0.34)
Gestational age	2.8 (0.03)	0.8 (0.29)	1.8 (0.08)	0.6 (0.30)

Note: p values are indicated in parentheses.
[a] Covariates included gestational age, parent size measures and substance use measures for birth weight, length and head circumference.
[b] These columns were reproduced from Table 2 for reference purposes.
[c] A missing data variable was used for 13 cases lacking Hct%. Missing data were related significantly to length such that smaller infants were more likely to lack Hct%.

McGaughey, 1973; Wesenberg, 1978). It may also result from placental transfusion, the extent of which may vary with time of cord clamping and positioning of the neonate if clamping is delayed. Polycythaemia and hyperviscosity have been related to later motor and neurological abnormalities (Allen and Chilcote, 1979; Black et al., 1982).

Although the criteria for screening vary somewhat, a diagnosis of neonatal polycythaemia may be considered when a central venous haematocrit of 65% or more is obtained (Wirth, Goldberg and Lubchenco, 1979). Assessment is complicated by rapid changes in Hct% during the first hours of life, which reach a peak at about two hours (Shohat, Merlob and Reisner, 1984), and by marked discrepancies between capillary and venous sampling (Oski and Naiman, 1972). Although the mean Hct% increases from cord blood sampling to that obtained at two hours, the two measures have been described as being correlated, and it has been suggested that cord blood Hct% < 56 can predict polycythaemia at two hours.

In an initial test of the possibility that this problem might confound results, we selected the 26 cases with Hct% < 56 and contrasted their mean cord cord PbB with the mean for the 123 cases with lower Hct%. The t-test revealed a higher mean for the high Hct% group (6.89 and 5.64 μg dl^{-1}, respectively) and a significant difference in variances (SDs equalled 2.56 and 1.86, respectively). Given the differences in variances and sample sizes, the significance of the differences between the means cannot be specified exactly. The differences obtained between groups, combined with the overall significant correlation of Hct% and cord PbB, suggest a possible confound of PbB and Hct%.

For the first set of analyses of the confounding of PbB and Hct%, size and gestational age measures were considered. As shown in Table 4, the size of the lead effect is changed little by the inclusion of Hct% in the models. Furthermore, Hct% was not related significantly to the size and gestational age variables.

The issue of possible confounding was further considered in analyses of

Table 4 The relationship of cord PbB and Hct% with size measures and gestational age, $n = 162$

Measure	Shared variance (%) without other[a] covariate control			Shared variance (%) with control of other covariates		
	PbB without Hct% as covariates	PbB with Hct%[b] covaried	Hct% with PbB[b] covaried	PbB without Hct% as covariates	PbB with Hct%[b] covaried	Hct% with PbB[b] covaried
Birth weight	2.3 (0.06)	2.4 (0.05)	0.1 (0.24)	0.3 (0.50)	0.4 (0.42)	1.8 (0.12)
Length	4.2 (0.01)	3.4 (0.02)	0.4 (0.37)	1.8 (0.08)	1.5 (0.10)	0.9 (0.19)
Head circumference	4.1 (0.01)	4.4 (0.01)	0.5 (0.35)	0.9 (0.20)	1.0 (0.17)	0.4 (0.39)
Gestational age	2.8 (0.03)	2.1 (0.07)	0.2 (0.57)	1.8 (0.08)	1.6 (0.10)	0.0 (0.79)

Note: p values are indicated in parentheses.
[a] Covariates included gestational age, parent size measures and substance use measures for the birth weight, length and head circumference outcome measures and substance use for gestational age.
[b] These columns were reproduced from Table 2 for reference purposes.
[c] A missing data variable was used for 13 cases lacking Hct%. Missing data were related significantly to length such that smaller infants were more likely to lack Hct%.

the Brazelton Abnormal Reflexes Scale and the Graham/Rosenblith Neurological Soft Signs Scale. These were chosen because of existing reports of an association of polycythaemia and neurological sequelae, and because a significant association of these measures and cord PbB was detected in the Cleveland data (Ernhart *et al.*, 1986). This was noted in Table 1.

Before the tests of confounding for these variables are described, the rather unusual findings obtained are summarized. Each of these two measures, and also the Graham/Rosenblith Muscle Tonus Scale, was related to either maternal or cord PbB, but not both. (It should be noted that the correlation of maternal and cord PbB was 0.80.) To assess the joint effect of maternal and cord PbB in the published results, the sample was reduced to 132 paired cases. With this reduction, only the relationship of cord PbB and the Soft Signs Scale was statistically significant. When both maternal and cord PbB were entered into the model, the effect attributable to cord PbB increased, and the parameter for maternal PbB became negative. In other words, the Soft Signs Scale was related to that portion of the cord PbB variance that was not common to maternal PbB. This, of course, is statistical suppression. An *ad hoc* interpretation was made to the effect that the foetus under stress may tend to accumulate, or fail to excrete, lead and that the neurological indicators may reflect that stress. A modified replication is now being conducted by the authors of this study to test this possibility.

The possibility of a confound associated with elevated haematocrit levels was, thus, an important concern as this aspect of the results was explored more fully. The analyses bearing on the confounding are shown in Table 5. As was the case with the size and gestational age data, the use of the traditional Hct% adjustment decreased the effect size; for the Abnormal Reflexes Scale, the reduction was marked. The interesting models, however, are those in which both cord PbB and Hct% are entered as independent

Table 5 Analyses demonstrating the influence of Hct% on tests of the relationship of cord PbB and selected neurological outcomes, $n = 162$

| | Proportion of shared variance | | | |
| | | | Model including cord PbB and Hct% | |
Variable	Cord lead, not Hct% corrected	Cord lead, Hct% corrected	Cord PbB	Hct%
Abnormal reflexes	3.5 (0.02)	0.6 (0.31)	2.2 (0.06)	0.3 (0.74)
Neuro soft signs	4.4 (0.01)	2.7 (0.04)	4.2 (0.01)	0.1 (0.44)
Neuro soft signs, suppression model[a]	4.6 (0.01)	3.2 (0.03)	4.2 (0.01)	0.01 (0.90)

Notes: p values are indicated in parentheses.

Missing data variables were entered, as relevant, for missing Hct% (13 cases) and for missing maternal PbB (30 cases). Results for the missing data variable for Hct% indicated that the relationship of the Abnormal Reflexes and the Neurological Soft Signs with cord lead measures was slightly stronger for the neonates with missing Hct%.

Covariates included in all models were race, sex, gestational age, maternal AA/day and cigarettes per day.

[a] Maternal PbB included in models. Suppression was noted in each variation in that the PbB effect sizes were enhanced and the parameter estimates for maternal PbB were negative.

variables. As indicated, the cord PbB effect on Abnormal Reflexes was reduced somewhat and was no longer statistically significant with entry of Hct% into the model. The entry of Hct% in the models had no notable effect on the Neurological Soft Signs Scale, with or without the inclusion of maternal PbB.

This study was not designed to include a meticulous test of the general issue of haematocrit level and neonatal outcome. Neonatal blood samples were not drawn under a systematic protocol through the first days of life. Furthermore, an infant presenting polycythaemic symptomatology would have been considered for exchange transfusion and transfer to the intensive care unit. Since cases requiring intensive care were excluded, the range of the present study was restricted. With this exploratory analysis, the possibility of confounding by elevated Hct% was removed as a concern. The authors are now reasonably confident that the findings reported for the neurological examination of the neonate are not associated with haematocrit levels.

The most important result of these explorations in methodology is the emphasis on inclusion of optimal measures of crucial covariates. For size measures, these include parental size as well as maternal alcohol consumption and smoking. For a study of neonatal anomalies, an adequate measure of foetal alcohol exposure is indicated. For the measures studied, haematocrit correction reduced effect sizes. The authors hope to see similar analyses from the groups using this strategy. Although haematocrit level was related to cord PbB, it accounted for little of the association of cord PbB and the neurological status of the neonate. This was a matter of some concern, given the reported effects of polycythaemia.

Perhaps the single major inference to be drawn from the analyses reported herein is that the results reported and the inferences drawn are highly dependent on the choice of variables included in the analyses, the validity of the measures used (even those that are not our independent and dependent variables), and the adjustments made of research variables.

ACKNOWLEDGMENTS

This research was supported in part by Grant No. 12–69 from the March of Dimes Birth Defects Foundation, Grant No. LH–327 from the International Lead Zinc Research Organization, Grant No. AA06571 from the National Institute of Alcohol Abuse and Alcoholism, and Grant No. HD14883 from the National Institute of Child Health and Human Development. The assistance provided by Penny Erhard, BA, in the conduct of the blood analyses is gratefully acknowledged.

REFERENCES

Abel, E.L. (ed.) (1982). *Fetal Alcohol Syndrome.* (Boca Raton, FL: CRC Press)
Abel, E.L. (1983). *Marijuana, Tobacco, Alcohol and Reproduction.* (Boca Raton, FL: CRC Press)
Alexander, F.W. and Delves, H.T. (1981). Blood lead levels during pregnancy. *Int. Arch. Occup. Environ. Health,* **48**, 35–39
Allen, J.P. and Chilcote, R. (1979). Transient erythrocytosis during the neonatal period: Possible neurologic complications. *South. Med. J.,* **72**, 681–684

Angell, N.F. and Lavery, J.P. (1982). The relationship of blood lead levels to obstetric outcome. *Am. J. Obstet. Gynecol.*, **142**, 40–46

Bellinger, D., Leviton, A., Waternaux, C. and Allred, E. (1985). Methodological issues in modeling the relationship between low-level lead exposure and infant development: Examples from the Boston lead study. *Environ. Res.*, **38**, 119–129

Bellinger, D., Leviton, A., Needleman, H.L., Waternaux, C. and Rabinowitz, M. (1986). Low-level lead exposure and infant development in the first year. *Neurobehav. Toxicol. Teratol.*, **8**, 151–161

Black, V.D., Lubchenco, L.O., Luckey, D.W., Koops, B.L., McGuinness, G.A., Powell, D.P. and Tomlinson, A.L. (1982). Developmental and neurologic sequelae of neonatal hyperviscocity syndrome. *Pediatrics*, **69**, 426–431

Bogden, J.D., Thind, I.S., Louria, D.B. and Caterini, H. (1978). Maternal and cord blood metal concentrations and low birth weight – a case-control study. *Am. J. Clin. Nutr.*, **31**, 1181–1187

Bryce-Smith, D. (1986) Environmental chemical influences on behaviour and mentation. *Chem. Soc. Rev.*, **15**, 93–123

Chisolm, J.J. (1974). Lead in red blood cells and plasma. *J. Pediatr.*, **84**, 163–164

Clark, A.R.L. (1977). Placental transfer of lead and its effects on the newborn. *Postgrad. Med. J.*, **53**, 674–678

DeSilva, P.E. (1984). Blood lead levels and the haematocrit correction. *Ann. Occup. Hygiene*, **28**, 417–428

Dietrich, K.N., Krafft, K.M., Shukla, R., Bornschein, R.L. and Succop, P.A. (1987). The neurobehavioral effects of prenatal and early postnatal lead exposure. In Schroeder, S.R. (ed.) *Toxic Substances and Mental Retardation: Neurobehavioral Toxicology and Teratology.* (Washington, DC: AAMD Monograph Series)

Ernhart, C.B., Wolf, A.W., Sokol, R.J., Brittenham, G.M. and Erhard, P. (1985). Fetal lead exposure: Antenatal factors. *Environ. Res.*, **38**, 54–66

Ernhart, C.B., Wolf, A.W., Kennard, M.J., Erhard, P., Filipovich, H.F. and Sokol, R.J. (1986). Intrauterine exposure to low levels of lead: The status of the neonate. *Arch. Environ. Health*, **41**, 287–291

Ernhart, C.B., Sokol, R.J., Martier, S., Moron, P., Nadler, D., Ager, J.W. and Wolf, A. (1987). Alcohol teratogenicity in the human: A detailed assessment of specificity, critical period and threshold. *Am. J. Obstet. Gynecol.*, **156**, 33–39

Fahim, M.S., Fahim, Z. and Hall, D.G. (1976). Effects of subtoxic lead levels on pregnant women in the State of Missouri. *Res. Commun. Chem. Pathol. Pharmacol.*, **13**, 309–331

Gershanik, J.J., Brooks, G.G. and Little, J.A. (1974). Blood lead values in pregnant women and their offspring. *Am. J. Obstet. Gynecol.*, **119**, 508–511

Grandjean, P., Olsen, N.B. and Hollnagel, H. (1981). Influence of smoking and alcohol consumption on blood lead levels. *Int. Arch. Occup. Environ. Health.* **48**, 391–397

Gross, G.P., Hathaway, W.E. and McGaughey, H.R. (1973). Hyperviscosity in the neonate. *J. Pediatr.*, **82**, 1004–1012

Kochen, J.A. and Greener, Y. (1973). Levels of lead in blood and hematocrit: Implications for the evaluation of the newborn and anemic patient. *Pediatr. Res.*, **7**, 937–944

McMichael, A.J., Vimpani, G.V., Robertson, E.F., Baghurst, P.A. and Clark, P.D. (1986). The Port Pirie cohort study: maternal blood lead and pregnancy outcome. *J. Epidemiol. Commun. Health*, **40**, 18–25

Moore, M.R., Goldberg, A., Pocock, S.J., Meredith, A., Stewart, I.M., MacAnespie, H., Lees, R. and Low, A. (1982). Some studies of maternal and infant lead exposure in Glasgow. *Scott. Med. J.*, **27**, 113–122

Moore, M.R. and Bushnell, I.W.R. (1984). Lead and child development in Glasgow (Second Progress Report). Presented at the *Second International Conference on Prospective Studies of Lead*, April 9–11, Cincinnati, Ohio

Needleman, H.L., Rabinowitz, M., Leviton, A., Linn, S. and Schoenbaum, S. (1984). The relationship between prenatal exposure to lead and congenital anomalies. *J. Am. Med. Assoc.*, **251**, 2956–2959

Nordstrom, S., Beckman, L. and Nordenson, I. (1979). Occupational and environmental risks in and around a smelter in northern Sweden. VI: Congenital malformations. *Hereditas*, **90**, 297–302

Oski, F.A. and Naiman, J.L. (1972). *Hematologic Problems in the Newborn*, 2nd Edn. (Philadelphia:

W.B. Saunders)

Pocock, S.J., Shaper, A.G., Walker, M., Wale, C.J., Clayton, B., Delves, T., Lacey, R.F., Packham, R.F. and Powell, P. (1983). Effects of tap water lead, water hardness, alcohol, and cigarettes on blood lead concentrations. *J. Epidemiol. Commun. Health*, **37**, 1–7

Rajegowda, B.K., Glass, L. and Evans, H.E. (1972). Lead concentrations in the newborn infant. *J. Pediatr.*, **80**, 116–117

Roels, H., Hubermont, G., Buchet, J-P. and Lauwerys, R. (1978). Placental transfer of lead, mercury, cadmium, and carbon monoxide in women. III: Factors influencing the accumulation of heavy metals in the placenta and the relationship between metal concentration in the placenta and in maternal and cord blood. *Environ. Res.*, **16**, 236–247

Rom, W.N. (1976). Effects of lead on the female and reproduction: A review. *Mt. Sinai J. Med.*, **43**, 542–552

Rosen, J.F., Zarate-Salvador, C. and Trinidad, E.E. (1974). Plasma lead levels in normal and lead-intoxicated children. *J. Pediatr.*, **84**, 45–48

Schwartz, J., Angle, C. and Pitcher, H. (1986). Relationship between childhood blood lead levels and stature. *Pediatrics*, **77**, 281–288

Shohat, M., Merlob, P. and Reisner, S.H. (1984). Neonatal polycythemia: I. Early diagnosis and incidence relating to time of sampling. *Pediatrics*, **73**, 7–13

Sokol, R.J. (1981). Alcohol and abnormal outcomes of pregnancy. *Can. Med. Assoc. J.*, **125**, 143–148

Sokol, R.J., Martier, S. and Ernhart, C.B. (1985). Identification of alcohol abuse in the prenatal clinic. In *Early Identification of Alcohol Abuse*. NIAAA Research Monograph-17, NIAAA

Wesenberg, R.L. (1978). Neonatal "thick blood" syndrome. *Hosp. Pract.*, May, 137–145

Wibberley, D.G., Khera, A.K., Edwards, J.H. and Rushton, D.I. (1977). Lead levels in human placentae from normal and malformed births. *J. Med. Genet.*, **14**, 339–345

Wirth, F.H., Goldberg, K.E. and Lubchenco, L.O. (1979). Neonatal hyperviscosity: I. Incidence. *Pediatrics*, **63**, 833–836

4.6

A Prospective Study of the Results of Changes in Environmental Lead Exposure in Children in Glasgow

M. R. MOORE, I. W. R. BUSHNELL and SIR A. GOLDBERG

SUMMARY

Overexposure to lead in water supplies constitutes a major exposure vector to lead in the West of Scotland. Studies have linked this with various health effects including mental retardation, renal insufficiency and hypertension. Because of this we established a prospective investigation of mothers and children in Glasgow, who had been overexposed to lead. In the year following the start of the study the water acidity was reduced, with consequent reduction in plumbosolvency. The principal aim of the study was therefore altered to determine whether overexposure to lead prenatally and in early postnatal life has any long-term sequelae. Initially, we identified a stratified population of mothers, according to their blood lead concentrations, early in pregnancy. Their children have now been tested, using standard psychometric tests, at their first and second birthdays. The children's blood lead concentrations have been measured and tooth lead concentrations will be measured when collection, which is currently ongoing, is completed. Although there was evidence of overexposure to lead, stepwise linear regression analysis has failed to identify any of the lead-related factors as significant predictors of psychological function. Assessment of the home environment and birth weight proved to be reliable predictors of cognitive status.

From the outset of studies in Glasgow it was clear that potential problems existed with respect to the levels of environmental lead exposure (Goldberg, 1984). Our experience of this suggested that the problem was linked to soft plumbosolvent water supplies and lead plumbing, and consequent increases in blood lead concentration in the general population of the West of Scotland

(Beattie et al., 1972; Goldberg and Beattie, 1972; Moore, 1973; Addis and Moore, 1974; Moore et al., 1977). We (Moore et al., 1977) were also able to demonstrate that such a relationship between blood and water lead concentrations was nonlinear, following a cube root equation of the type:

$$\text{Blood lead} = a \cdot (\text{water lead})^{0.33} + b$$

Early studies indicated probable associations between decrement in intelligence and such lead exposure (Gibson et al., 1967; Beattie et al., 1975). In retrospect many of the investigations carried out at that time were naive in comparison with the sophistication of current analysis, but for the populations that we were dealing with, they pointed to the need for expert investigation of the role of lead in intelligence deficit. In view of the number and excellence of reviews presented recently, it is unnecessary to reiterate the current evidence for the association between lead exposure and neuropsychological deficit (EPA, 1986; Grant and Davis, and Smith, in this volume). It is sufficient to say that such a deficit exists. Our studies now try to look at the question beyond such an association, that is whether alteration, a decrease in exposure, can be linked with amelioration of the lead-related deficit.

The major problem that arose in the study was that, acting upon the available evidence, Strathclyde Water Board made the decision to carry out extensive water treatment aimed at diminishing water plumbosolvency. This treatment was singularly effective (Moore et al., 1981). Median blood lead concentrations of mothers in Glasgow fell dramatically between 1976 and 1980 (Richards and Moore, 1984). This included test groups for this study. In consequence, the initial aim of prospective assessment of continuous exposure to lead at about the same concentration throughout this period of study could not be achieved, and the final null hypothesis was that: 'Prenatal and perinatal overexposure to lead has no long-term sequelae.'

These previous studies showed that between 4% and 5% of the maternal population of Glasgow were overexposed to lead with resultant blood lead concentrations in excess of $30\mu g/dl$ (Moore et al., 1982a). This level of exposure was the highest in the United Kingdom and for populations not exposed to industrial lead emissions, probably the highest in Europe. In the following years we seized the opportunity of studying in greater depth the population of mothers and children in Glasgow who were identified as part of two major surveys – the Duplicate Diet Study and the Commission of European Communities Survey of Lead in the General Population (DOE/MAFF, 1982 – Lacey et al., 1985; EEC, 1977; DOE, 1981).

At this point in the investigations the children who have been identified in our study have reached the age of 7 years. Since we know that tooth lead concentrations may be related to early water lead exposure (Moore et al., 1978), we are continuing with tooth collection at this time as a means of assessing likely exposure to lead in the peri- and postnatal period.

MATERIALS AND METHODS

The design of these experiments has been described in detail previously (Moore et al., 1982b). This is a prospective study which is aimed at following a group of children from birth through to school age with regular testing at defined ages. Information has therefore been sought which will highlight the psychological functioning of the child at different ages, and which will adequately describe relevant environmental factors. The Duplicate Diet Study gave us an ideal opportunity to examine children in various categories of lead exposure. This study presented us with a population sample of 885 pregnant women for each of whom we have detailed records of blood and water lead levels from early in pregnancy. Attempts to recruit further numbers of mothers to the study proved to be unsuccessful because of the successes achieved in alteration to water plumbosolvency by calcium hydroxide addition. From the records of the Duplicate Diet Study, groups of women with high blood levels during pregnancy were identified together with matched control groups with lesser degrees of exposure. In the children examined as part of the Duplicate Diet Study, cord blood levels were measured and dietary lead concentrations measured in the tenth week of life. These showed a positive regression relationship equivalent to the cube root relationship found between blood and water lead. These studies have also established an inverse relationship between gestational age and lead exposure during pregnancy (Moore *et al.*, 1982a).

Subject selection

The study group consists of 151 subjects drawn from an initial selection of 885 families. All subjects were born in the United Kingdom and have parents who speak English as a first language. This sample has been divided into three groups on the basis of maternal blood lead analysis during pregnancy. Using this criterion three groups of women were identified with high lead exposure (blood lead $> 30\,\mu g/dl$), medium lead exposure ($15-25\,\mu g/dl$) and low lead exposure ($< 10\,\mu g/dl$). The blood lead analysis for all subjects has been coded and is unknown to any tester. Mothers in each of these groups, including two intermediate groups, volunteered to be included in the assessment programme. Matching of the families was carried out with respect to social class (using the Registrar General's Classification) and housing stock (from available records). This will avoid the effect of the known relationship between likelihood of exposure to lead and socioeconomic backgrounds conducive to lowered development.

Biochemical testing

Measurement of blood lead levels and other biological indices of lead exposure were carried out annually. These other biological indices are blood delta-aminolaevulinic acid concentrations, the activity of ALA dehydratase in blood, and erythrocyte protoporphyrin concentrations. In addition, deciduous tooth lead concentrations will be measured.

Paediatric assessment

All children have been checked for developmental milestones, for head circumference, weight and height. Checks have been made that childhood development is progressing normally, and that an allowance can be made for any non-lead-related change in development.

Psychological assessment

The programme for this has been designed to allow detailed individual testing with a wide range of measures. The battery of tests employed will subsequently be supplemented by follow-up reports from the school environment. Testing has taken place on the child's first and second birthday. This initial assessment has included both standardized and psychometric procedures and questionnaires. The questionnaires have provided information about clinical and socioeconomic factors, together with information about attitudes and relationships within the home setting. Statistics have been carried out using the BMDP programmes (University of California, 1977)

Assessment programme

The assessment of the children from each of these groups has been planned on a longitudinal basis during the first years of life. The programme will hopefully be extended, taking in, especially, early scholastic performance.

RESULTS AND DISCUSSION

The blood lead measures were assessed, and due to inconsistencies in measurement, only maternal blood lead during pregnancy (maternal PbB) and water lead levels during pregnancy were used as dependent variables. The mean values of these variables divided into the original three groupings are shown in Table 1, with the means of the available infant blood lead values at 1 year (infant PbB1) and at 2 years (infant PbB2). Pica in year 1 and year 2 was also measured.

There was a significant correlation between maternal PbB and water lead of $r = 0.49$. Although the year 1 and year 2 blood leads were not utilized in the multivariate analysis, due to incomplete records, inspection of the data

Table 1 Summary of lead values (μg/dl)

	Grouping		
Lead measures	Low	Medium	High
Maternal PbB	7.02	17.73	33.05
Water lead	40.00	120.00	475.00
Infant PbB1	9.83	13.62	22.40
Infant PbB2	13.85	15.79	19.08

which are available from 65% of the sample indicates the scale of the reduction in blood leads over the 2-year period, and supports the effectiveness of the water treatment scheme initiated on the basis of Moore *et al.*'s seminal work on water lead.

The main paediatric measures are summarized in Table 2, where it can be seen that the clearest difference between the groups was in terms of birth weight, with the high-lead group showing the lowest mean birth weight, unrelated to similar deficiencies in length or head circumference. None of the other measures clearly differentiated the groups.

A subset of possible predictor variables was then identified and this included home environment assessment score at year 1 (HOME1) and year 2 (HOME2), obstetric complication score, birth weight, birth order, socioeconomic class of the father in year 1 (SC1) and in year 2 (SC2). The dependent variables considered were Bayley mean score at year 1 and year 2, Bayley Mental Development Index (MDI) at year 1 and year 2 and the Bayley Psychomotor Development Index (PDI) at year 1 and year 2. The overall mean scores at year 1 and year 2 were significantly correlated ($r = 0.39$). The mean values for these dependent variables are set out in Table 3.

The regression selected was a stepwise linear regression in which the explanatory variables were brought into the regression equation in order of importance to the response variable, given the variables already entered, with the selection criterion being the F-to-enter value. For the first year data the stepwise regressions selected the same first three regressors (birth weight; SC1, HOME 1) and in the same order, with each of the three Bayley scores as response variable. A lead variable was selected as fourth-best predictor for each regression, water lead with Bayley mean score and PDI; and maternal PbB with Bayley MDI. The last four places had no systematic selection order across the regressions. A further analysis was used to compare all possible

Table 2 Summary of paediatric measures

Paediatric measures	Low	Medium	High
Obstetric complications score	3.6	3.47	3.45
Birth weight (kg)	3.51	3.43	3.32
Length (cm)	50.55	50.77	51.15
Head circumference (cm)	34.62	35.00	34.32
Apgar1	8.10	7.99	7.95
Apgar5	9.30	9.37	9.50

Table 3 Summary of psychometric measures

Psychometric measures: Bayley scores of infant development	Low	Medium	High
Mean: year 1	103.35	102.44	101.38
Mean: year 2	107.18	106.00	104.50
MDI: year 1	104.00	104.68	101.92
MDI: year 2	105.56	104.29	104.61
PDI: year 1	103.15	101.41	101.95
PDI: year 2	109.74	108.39	104.89

subsets of the explanatory variables and give relevant statistics for the five best subsets for every possible number of variables in a subset. The best subset was then selected based on several criteria: coefficient of determination (R^2), adjusted R^2 and Mallows C_p. The best subset included the three variables which dominated the stepwise linear regressions (birth weight, SC1, HOME 1) while the best subset including a lead variable was the second best with each response variable, including water lead with Bayley mean score and PDI score, and maternal blood lead with MDI.

With year 2 data for all three response variables, the home environment assessment was selected first and birth weight second. The first lead variable was selected third in each regression, pica in year 2 for Bayley mean score (year 2) and MDI, and maternal PbB with PDI. The fourth selected regressor in the first two cases was maternal PbB while in the third case it was pica in year 2. Fathers' social class in year 2 fell to sixth place in each regression compared with the second place standing of social class father (SC1) in the first year analysis. The best subset of regressors included HOME score in year 2 and birth weight, while the second-best subset included the lead variable which came third in the stepwise regression, and these subsets were nearly as good as the best subsets.

The conclusion that might be drawn is that response variables are adequately described without information from the lead variables, as the lead variables were not selected to the best subset of regressors in either year 1 or year 2. The fact that the selection order of the best regressors was identical for the three response variables at each year indicates that the explanatory variables have equivalent effects on both mental and psychomotor functioning. The decrease in the effectiveness of birth weight over the first 2 years was coupled with an increasing importance of home environment, effects which have been suggested before in the developmental literature.

Since birth weight was negatively and significantly correlated with all three lead variables, and as it was always selected before any of the lead indices, then the amount of new information held by the lead variables would be reduced once birth weight was selected into the regression equation. To liberate the lead variables from this handicap, the birth weight variable was removed for further stepwise and best subset regression. The explanatory variables were otherwise unchanged. Removing birth weight, however, did not significantly alter the importance of any of the remaining variables at year 1, although it did cause a noticeable improvement in the standing of the second-year pica score, which improved to second-best predictor behind HOME score in year 2 and was included in the second-best subset, HOME score in year 2 + pica in year 2, behind HOME score in year 2 itself. This may reflect the gradual increase in the importance of pica over the second year of life.

The data obtained from the Infant Behaviour Record were also assessed by comparing the performance of each child on each of the 30 items with the appropriate age norm and scoring performance as better than normal, normal, or worse than normal. A principal-components analysis of the three lead variables for each year (maternal PbB, water lead, pica in year 1 or 2) was then undertaken and the data transformed to give one measure of lead

376

for each year. The largest correlation between this lead value and the 30 Infant Behaviour Record items for year 1 was −0.26 with Object Orientation (1), followed by 0.24 with Object Orientation (2), 0.21 with Listening to Sounds and −0.19 with Looking at Sights. In year 2 the largest correlation was with Toys (0.16), followed by General Education (0.14), Judgement of Test (0.14) and Goal Directedness (−0.12). The inconsistencies of sign in these data, coupled with the lack of consistency between years 1 and 2, suggest that little confidence can be placed in these results.

CONCLUSIONS

It is clear from the review of the data from the first 2 years of this study that the response variables are ideally described without recourse to information from the lead variables, since these were not selected from the eight possible explanatory variables for the best subset of regressors in either year 1 or year 2. The best regressors were as expected, selected from home environment, socioeconomic factors and birth weight. This may have been the result of the sharp fall in the water supply lead exposure, which took place shortly after these children were born. This would suggest that prenatal and early postnatal exposure to lead is less critical than continuing exposure over a period of years into early childhood.

The importance of birth weight and home environment as predictors of cognitive outcome may, of course, be connected with lead exposure, since it could be argued that lead exposure *in utero* may have directly contributed to a reduction in growth rate and birth weight, with the consequence of slight neurological impairment. However, the failure of any lead variable to improve its standing as a predictor when birth weight was removed from the analysis does not support this interpretation. Another possibility is that lead exposure may affect the caretakers' competence to provide the most appropriate home environment for the child, and thus influence cognitive development in this indirect way. However, unless one were to argue that lead exposure had greater effects on adults than children, this does not seem to explain why lead did not seem to be operating directly on the child. It therefore seems to be safer to conclude that there is no firm evidence for either a direct or an indirect contribution of lead to decrements in cognitive development, at least from this data set.

In order to clarify the discrepancies between the results of this study and those of several other studies a further analysis of cumulative lead status, coupled with further psychometric assessment, is required. These aspects of this study are correctly being completed through deciduous tooth lead collection and a planned application of further psychological measures.

REFERENCES

Addis, G. and Moore, M. R. (1974) Lead levels in the water of suburban Glasgow. *Nature*, **252**, 120–121

Beattie, A. D., Moore, M. R., Devenay, W. T., Miller, A. R. and Goldberg, A. (1972)

Environmental lead pollution in an urban soft-water area. *Br. Med. J.*, **1**, 491–493

Beattie, A. D., Moore, M. R., Goldberg, A., Finlayson, M. J. W., Graham, J. F., Mackie, E. M., Main, J C., McLaren, D. A., Murdoch, R. M. and Stewart, G. T. (1975) Role of chronic low-level lead exposure in the aetiology of mental retardation. *Lancet*, **1**, 589–591

DOE: Department of the Environment (1981) *European Community Screening Programme For Lead – U.K. Results for 1979–1980.* HMSO Pollution Report No. 10

Department of the Environment (1983) *European Community Screening Programme For Lead – U.K. Results for 1981–1982.* HMSO Pollution Report No. 18

DOE/MAFF: Department of the Environment and Ministry of Agriculture, Fisheries and Food (1982) *The Glasgow Duplicate Diet Study – a joint survey.* HMSO Pollution Report No. 11

EEC: European Economic Community (1977) On biological screening of the population for lead. *Off. J. Eur. Commun.*, **20**, 10–17

Environmental Protection Agency (1986) *Air Quality Criteria For Lead*, Vols I–IV, and addendum. EPA 600/8-83/028. (Research Triangle Park, NC: EPA)

Gibson, S. L. M., Lam, C. N., McRae, W. M. and Goldberg, A. (1967) Blood lead levels in normal and mentally deficient children. *Arch. Dis. Child.*, **42**, 573

Goldberg, A. (1984) Why did Glasgow not consult Christison of Edinburgh in 1854. *Glasgow Med.*, **1**, 6–7

Goldberg, A. and Beattie, A. D. (1972) Studies in environmental lead pollution. *Health Bulletin*, **XXX**(3), 181

Lacey, R. F., Moore, M. R. and Richards, W. N. (1985) Lead in water, infant diet and blood – the Glasgow Duplicate Diet Study. *Sci. Total Env.*, **41**, 235–257

Moore, M. R. (1973). Plumbosolvency of waters. *Nature*, **243**, 222–223

Moore, M. R. (1980) Exposure to lead in childhood – the persisting effects. *Nature*, **283**, 334–335

Moore, M. R., Meredith, P. A., Campbell, B. C., Goldberg, A. and Pocock, S. J. (1977) Contribution of lead in drinking water to blood lead. *Lancet*, **2**, 661–662

Moore, M. R, Campbell, B. C., Meredith, P. A., Beattie, A. D., Goldberg, A. and Campbell, D. (1978) The association between lead concentrations in teeth and domestic water lead concentrations. *Clin. Chim. Acta*, **87**, 77–83

Moore, M. R., Goldberg, A., Meredith, P. A., Lees, R., Low, R. A. and Pocock, S. J. (1979) Contribution of drinking water lead to maternal blood lead concentrations. *Clin. Chim. Acta*, **95**, 129–133

Moore, M. R., Goldberg, A., Fyfe, W. M., Low, R. A. and Richards, W. N. (1981) Lead in water in Glasgow – a story of success. *Scot. Med. J.*, **26**, 354–355

Moore, M. R., Goldberg, A., Pocock, S. J., Meredith, P. A., Stewart, I. M., McAnespie, H., Lees, R. and Low, R. A. (1982a). Some studies of maternal and infant lead exposure in Glasgow. *Scot. Med. J.*, **27**, 113–122

Moore, M. R., Goldberg, A., Bushnell, I. W. R., Day, R. and Fyfe, W. M. (1982b) A prospective study of the neurological effects of lead in children. *Neurobehav. Toxicol. Teratol.*, **4**, 739–743

Richards, W. N. and Moore, M. R. (1984) Plumbosolvency in Scotland – the problem, remedial action taken and health benefits observed. *J. Am. Water Works Assoc.*, **76**, 60–67

University of California, Los Angeles (1977) *BMDP Bio-Medical Computer Programs.* (Los Angeles: University of California Press)

4.7
Environmental Lead, Reproduction and Infant Development

J. GRAZIANO, D. POPOVAC, M. MURPHY, A. MEHMETI,
J. KLINE, G. AHMEDI, P. SHROUT, Z. ZVICER, G. WASSERMAN,
E. GASHI, Z. STEIN, B. RAJOVIC, L. BELMONT, B. COLAKOVIC,
R. BOZOVIC, R. HAXHIU, L. RADOVIC, R. VLASKOVIC,
D. NENEZIC and N. LOIACONO

SUMMARY

This study is evaluating the relationship of chronic lead exposure to adverse pregnancy outcome and infant development. The study draws upon a unique community surrounding a lead smelter, refinery and battery plant in Titova Mitrovica, Yugoslavia. Control subjects are being studied in Pristina, a non-lead-exposed town 40 km to the south.

Recruitment of women at 12–20 weeks gestation terminated in January 1987, by which time approximately 1000 women from each town were entered into the study. Preliminary data from 456 women in Mitrovica and 650 women in Pristina indicate that, at midpregnancy, the blood lead (PbB) concentrations in Mitrovica ranged from 2–47 μg dl^{-1}, with a mean of 17.4 μg dl^{-1}. The major determinant of elevated PbB is geographic proximity to the lead industry. In Pristina, midpregnancy maternal PbB levels ranged from 1–23 μg dl^{-1}, with a mean of 5.4 μg dl^{-1}. Thus far, 207 pregnancies have come to term in Mitrovica and 268 in Pristina. There is a strong association between maternal PbB at delivery and umbilical cord PbB across a wide range of PbB levels; in Mitrovica, the mean cord PbB is 19.0 μg dl^{-1}, while in Pristina it is 5.4 μg dl^{-1}. The socioeconomic, ethnic, and maternal physical characteristics are quite comparable between the two towns, an important asset in a study of this type.

A study of infant development has been initiated in subsets of infants born to women in the pregnancy outcome study. In Mitrovica, infants with high, midrange and low cord PbB levels are being selected for follow up; thus far, the mean cord PbB values of these groups are 25.2,

17.3, and 11.2 μg dl^{-1}, respectively. In Pristina, a control group of infants matched with the Mitrovica high PbB group on SES has a mean cord PbB of 3.9 μg dl^{-1}. Another control group in Pristina, matched with the Mitrovica low PbB group on SES and cord PbB, has a mean cord PbB of 8.2 μg dl^{-1}.

The autonomous province of Kosovo, Yugoslavia, is a mountainous farm region in the process of industrialization because of its rich mineral resources. The city of Titova Mitrovica, approximately 40 km north of Pristina, the capital of the province, is the site of one of the largest lead smelters in Europe. Approximately 100 000 people are exposed to lead emissions from the smelter, of whom 60 000 live in the highly exposed city area which lies in a valley at the convergence of the Ibar and Sitnica rivers. In 1982, we reported an alarming prevalence of elevated blood lead (PbB) concentrations among children and adults in Mitrovica (Popovac et al., 1982). At that time, the mean air lead concentration, measured monthly at five locations in the town, ranged from 21.3 to 29.2 μg m^{-3}. In 1983, prior to the initiation of this study, a new filtration system went on line at the smelter; since that time, the mean air lead concentration has been reduced to 7.0 μg m^{-3}, still 10 times the allowable limit of 0.7 μg m^{-3} in Yugoslavia. Thus, elevated PbB remains a problem in Mitrovica.

After reviewing the literature concerning possible effects of lead on human pregnancy outcome (Graziano, et al., 1985), we became convinced of the need for specific effects to be explored in relation to precise measures of PbB during pregnancy. In particular, previous studies had generally failed to control adequately for known risk factors, such as maternal weight, height, parity, previous reproductive history, smoking and social class. The populations of Mitrovica and Pristina, with their comparable social structures but widely divergent ranges of PbB levels, provide an opportunity for such a study. For similar reasons, they also provide a unique opportunity for a prospective study regarding the influence of prenatal and postnatal lead exposure on infant development.

THE PREGNANCY OUTCOME STUDY

Recruitment of approximately 1000 pregnant women (12–20 weeks gestation) in each town began in May 1985 and terminated in January 1987. Since the study is ongoing, we provide in this report only descriptive data about those cases recruited and analysed to date, i.e. 456 women in Mitrovica and 650 women in Pristina. We will ultimately examine whether exposure to lead, assessed by PbB and erythrocyte protoporphyrin (EP) at midpregnancy and at term, is associated with an increased risk of the following selected adverse pregnancy outcomes: late spontaneous abortion and stillbirth, premature delivery, intrauterine growth retardation, and congenital malformations. The possible interaction between iron deficiency and lead toxicity will be examined utilizing concurrent measurements of serum ferritin and haemoglobin concentrations. Factors known to influence reproductive outcome, such as social class, past reproductive history and general health status, are being assessed through questionnaires. Fetal lead exposure will be determined by measurements of PbB and EP in umbilical cord blood; serum ferritin and haemoglobin concentrations are also being measured. The possible influence of exposure to other heavy metals will be examined by analysis of various elements in placental tissue obtained at delivery. Evaluation of the newborn infants includes gestational age assessment (Ballard et al., 1979) and a carefully structured physical examination for congenital malformations. Multivariate analyses of this data should ultimately reveal important information concerning the dose-response relationships between lead exposure and pregnancy outcomes.

Preliminary analyses of data from the midpregnancy interviews suggest that these two populations are similar with respect to parental age and education, maternal height and weight, gravidity, ethnicity and socioeconomic status. They are somewhat dissimilar with respect to the higher proportion of women in Pristina reporting smoking, any alcohol drinking and working (Table 1). Of these three characteristics, smoking is known to influence birth weight (Abel, 1980); findings for alcohol drinkers (Stein et al., 1983) and maternal occupation in relation to birth weight are inconsistent. The relationships of these factors and others to birth weight and late fetal death in the study pregnancies will be examined, and analytical adjustment will be made for their effects in assessing the influence of geographical location and PbB on the various pregnancy outcomes. The midpregnancy questionnaires have shown social characteristics to be similar with regard to socioeconomic status (Table 2).

The distribution of midpregnancy PbB levels in the two towns are illustrated graphically in Figure 1. Thus far, the mean PbB in Mitrovica is $17.4 \mu g \, dl^{-1}$ while the mean PbB in Pristina is $5.4 \mu g \, dl^{-1}$. The mean EP in Mitrovica is $49.8 \mu g \, dl^{-1}$, while that in Pristina is $32.5 \mu g \, dl^{-1}$; the mean serum ferritin concentrations are identical in the two towns, $19.8 \mu g \, dl^{-1}$.

Table 1 Sociodemographic characteristics and habits of the populations

	Titova Mitrovica	Pristina
Sample size	456	650
Maternal age (y)	26.3	26.9
Maternal education (y)	9.5	9.3
Paternal age (y)	30.6	30.7
Paternal education (y)	12.1	11.7
Maternal weight (kg)	66.7	66.8
Maternal height (cm)	163.2	166.1
Total number of pregnancies	3.3	3.3
Ethnicity: % Albanian	55.9	59.4
% Serbian	24.8	24.9
% Other	17.8	14.9
% No answer	1.5	0.7
% cigarette smokers	23.0	29.8
% women who drink any alcohol	5.7	9.5
% women with jobs	30.5	45.8

Table 2 Social characteristics of the populations

	Titova Mitrovica	Pristina
Sample size	456	650
Number of adults in home	4.5	4.4
Number of children in home	2.1	2.1
Number of rooms in home	3.4	3.2
Monthly family income (millions of old dinars)	7.0	7.1

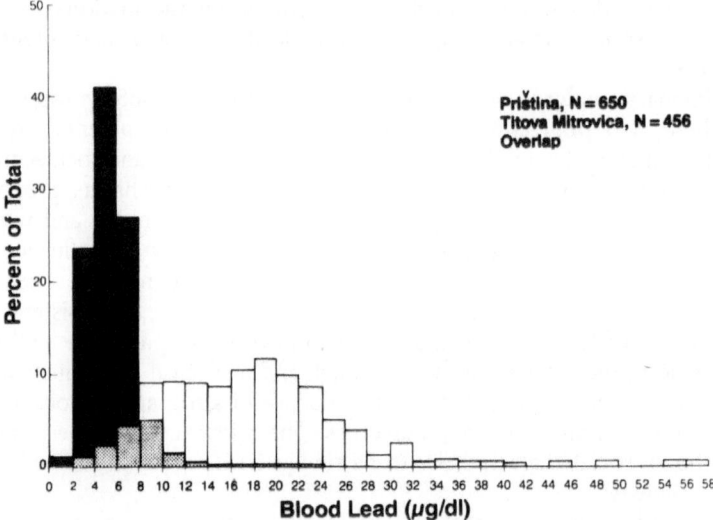

Figure 1 Frequency distribution of blood lead concentrations at midpregnancy

The first births to study participants occurred in October 1985. To date, PbB data have been compiled from 207 maternal/infant pairs in Mitrovica and 268 pairs in Pristina. In Mitrovica, thus far, the mean maternal PbB at term is $21.4\,\mu g\,dl^{-1}$, while the mean umbilical cord PbB is $19.0\,\mu g\,dl^{-1}$. In Pristina, the mean maternal PbB at term is $6.7\,\mu g\,dl^{-1}$, while the mean umbilical cord PbB is $5.4\,\mu g\,dl^{-1}$. The distributions of maternal PbB concentrations at term are illustrated in Figure 2, while the distributions of umbilical cord PbBs are illustrated in Figure 3.

While numerous other studies have described an association between maternal and fetal PbB levels (as reviewed by Bell and Thomas, 1980), none have involved a population with such a wide range of PbB levels. The placenta appears to be a very weak barrier to lead over a wide range of PbB, as evidenced by the strong association between maternal and umbilical cord PbB concentrations in Mitrovica shown in Figure 4 ($r = 0.86$; $p < 0.001$; slope $= 0.87$); once additional data are accumulated, we will determine whether the association involves non-linear as well as linear components. The average maternal midpregnancy PbB levels, maternal PbB levels at delivery, and umbilical cord PbB levels for those cases which have come to term are

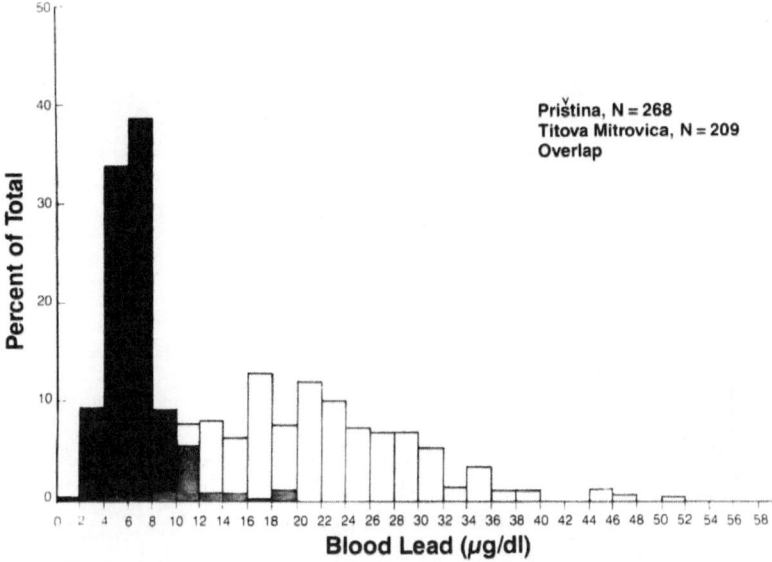

Figure 2 Frequency distribution of maternal blood lead concentrations at delivery

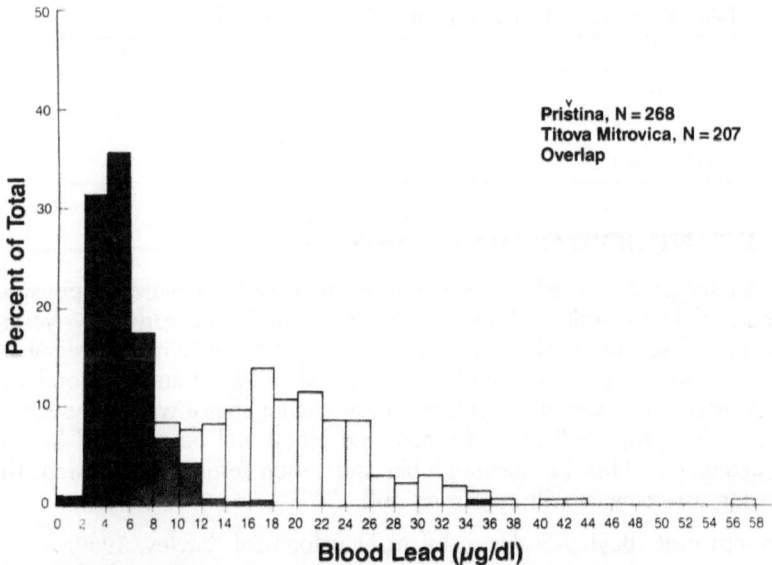

Figure 3 Frequency distribution of umbilical cord blood lead concentrations

presented in Table 3.

Thus, because of the wide range of PbB levels, the apparent lack of confounding by social class and the large number of women involved, this prospective study promises to answer many issues surrounding the possible influence of lead exposure on pregnancy outcome. It is still too early, however, for us to present any definitive data concerning pregnancy outcome.

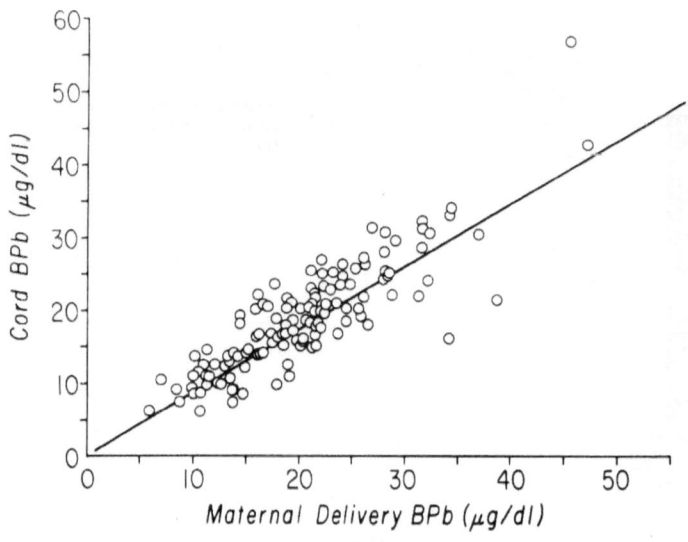

Figure 4 Maternal delivery PbB *vs* cord PbB in Titova Mitrovica

Table 3 Average PbB levels (μg dl^{-1}) for cases come to term

	Titova Mitrovica	Pristina
Sample size	207	268
Maternal midpregnancy	17.6	5.4
Maternal delivery	21.4	6.7
Umbilical cord	19.0	5.4

THE INFANT DEVELOPMENT STUDY

In order to assess the effects of environmental lead exposure on physical, behavioural and cognitive–linguistic development during early life, we are following subsets of infants born to women who participate in the pregnancy outcome study. The infants will be examined at 6, 12, 18 and 24 months of age. At each visit, weight, height, and head circumference will be measured; a paediatric history will be performed; and blood will be collected for the measurement of PbB, EP, haemoglobin and serum ferritin. In addition, the following assessments will be carried out:

6 month visit: Bayley Scales of Infant Development (Bayley, 1969)
               Bates Infant Characteristics Questionnaire (Bates *et al.*, 1979)
12 month visit: Bayley Scales of Infant Development
               Bates Infant Characteristics Questionnaire
18 month visit: Bayley Scales of Infant Development
               Memory for Locations Task (Kagan, 1981)
24 month visit: Bayley Scales of Infant Development
               Bates Infant Characteristics Questionnaire
               Memory for Locations Task
               Receptive Language Assessment (Hedrick *et al.*, 1984)

In Mitrovica, 384 infants will be selected on the basis of cord PbB. Three different groups will be formed as follows:

Group A: the 144 infants with the highest cord PbBs; infants with cord PbB levels of 20 μg dl^{-1} or more are eligible for entry into this group.

Group B: the 120 infants with the lowest cord PbBs; infants with cord PbB of $<15\,\mu$g dl^{-1} are eligible.

Group C: a random sample of 120 infants from the remaining births, with PbB levels of $>15\,\mu$g dl^{-1} and $<20\,\mu$g dl^{-1}.

In Pristina, 264 infants will be selected and assigned to two groups for comparative purposes, as follows:

Group D: 144 infants will be matched for SES to the 'high' cord PbB group noted above, i.e. Group A. The hypothesized effects of lead on mental development in the first years of life are likely to be seen in this comparison. It is likely that only minimal adjustment for SES will be required in the statistical analysis.

Group E: 120 infants will be matched to the above 'low' cord PbB group, i.e. Group B, for both SES and cord PbB. By virtue of their town of residence, it is likely that the PbB levels of infants in children in Group B will rise during the first two years of life, while those of Group E will not. Thus, this control group will enable us to attempt to distinguish prenatal from postnatal lead effects.

We have established that there is a strong association between parental education and other indicators of SES, such as family income, rooms/home, number of residents/home, etc. We have therefore used maternal and paternal education as the SES selection factors. In order to minimize loss to follow up, infants living more than 10 km from the hospital have been excluded in each town. Other exclusion criteria include: twins; major central nervous system defects; and chromosomal abnormalities or other conditions (e.g. microcephaly, hydrocephaly) likely to profoundly affect growth or mental development.

Thus far, 243 infants have been selected for follow up from births which occurred during the interval from October 1985 to March 1986. Of those, 150 have been evaluated at 6 months of age. The mean cord PbB levels and other characteristics of groups A–E are illustrated in Table 4.

CONCLUSION

In summary, we are studying the influence of Pb exposure on pregnancy outcome and infant development in two Yugoslavian populations with an exceptionally wide range of PbB levels. The socioeconomic characteristics of the two towns appear to be quite similar. Thus, in this study, lead exposure is not linked to a particular social class or ethnic group, an important limitation of many other previous or current studies. Because this study is still in the process of data collection, the full presentation of data and results concerning outcomes of interest must await completion of future statistical analyses.

Table 4   Mean cord PbB levels (μg dl^{-1}) and other characteristics of selected infants (all mean values)

	Group A (Titova Mitrovica)	Group B (Titova Mitrovica)	Group C (Titova Mitrovica)	Group D* (Pristina)	Group E† (Pristina)
PbB (μg dl^{-1})	25.2	11.2	17.3	3.9	8.2
Maternal education (y)	9.6	8.3	9.2	9.5	9.3
Paternal education (y)	11.1	12.2	12.0	11.3	11.3
Family income (10 dinars/month)	5.7	5.0	5.6	6.3	5.9
Birth weight (g)	3337	3295	3310	3232	3310

*matched to group A on SES
†matched to group B on SES and PbB

REFERENCES

Abel, E.L. (1980). Smoking during pregnancy: A review of effects on growth and development of offspring. *Hum. Biol.*, **52**, 593–625

Ballard, J.L., Novak, K.K. and Driver, M. (1979). A simplified score for assessment of fetal maturation of newly born infants. *J. Pediatr.*, **95**, 769–774

Bates, J.E., Freeland, C.A. and Lounsbury, M.L. (1979). Measurement of infant difficulties. *Child Develop.*, **50**, 794–803

Bayley, N. (1969). *Manual for the Bayley Scales of Infant Development*. (New York: Psychological Corporation)

Bell, J.U. and Thomas, J.A. (1980). Effects of lead on mammalian reproduction. In Singhal, R.L. and Thomas, J.A. (eds.) *Lead Toxicity*, pp. 169–186. (Baltimore: Urban & Schwartzenberg)

Graziano, J.H., Popovac, D., Murphy, M.J., Colakovic, B., Stein, Z., Mehmeti, A., Kline, J., Ahmedi, G., Rajovic, B., Gashi, E., Haxhiu, R., Radovic, L., Hoxha, I., Zvicer, Z., Popovac, R., Bozovic, R., Shrout, P. and Lolacono, N. (1985). Environmental lead and pregnancy outcome. *Proc. Fifth Int. Conf. Heavy Metals Environ. (Athens)*, **1**, 414–416

Hedrick, D.L., Prather, E.M. and Tobin, A.R. (1984). *The Sequenced Inventory of Communicative Development*, 2nd Edn. (Seattle: Seattle University Press)

Kagan, J. (1981). *The Second Year: The Emergence of Self-Awareness.* (Cambridge, MA: Harvard University Press)

Popovac, D., Graziano, J., Seaman, C., Kaul, B., Colakovic, B., Popovac, R., Osmani, I., Haxhiu, M., Begraca, M., Bozovic, Z. and Mikic, M. (1982). Elevated blood lead in a population near a lead smelter in Kosovo, Yugoslavia. *Arch. Environ. Health*, **37**, 19–23

Stein, Z. and Kline, J. (1983). Smoking, alcohol and reproduction. *Am. J. Public Health*, **73**, 1154–1156

4.8

Effects of Lead on Neurobehavioural Development in the First Thirty Days of Life

S. J. ROTHENBERG, L. SCHNAAS, C. J. N. MENDEZ and
H. HIDALGO

SUMMARY

Effects of maternal blood lead at 36 weeks and birth, and of umbilical cord lead, upon trend of development in the first 30 days of life, as measured by the Brazelton Neonatal Behavioural Assessment Scale, were assessed by multiple regression techniques. Much of the significant bivariate effect of cord lead upon abnormal reflex trend could be accounted for by control variables. However, the difference between maternal lead at birth and cord lead remained significant in the multivariate model, accounting for 6.2% additional variance in outcome. Change in maternal lead between 36 weeks and birth was a significant predictor of abnormal reflex trend and trend in regulation of states.

In the last few decades, a series of cross-sectional studies of childen chronically exposed to low levels of lead has documented a variety of problems, including attentional deficits, impaired school performance, slowed psychomotor performance and lowered IQ. While several studies have failed to detect such effects, the major issues discussed today are not whether low-level lead exposure can cause such damage, but rather at what levels and during what stages of development lead can produce these effects.

Cross-sectional studies suffer from many shortcomings. For instance, many rely on a single lead determination, often using blood lead measurements taken around the time of behavioural and neurological evaluation to estimate exposure. These measurements give little information about lead exposure preceding the sample by more than several weeks or months. Even purportedly time-integrated measures, such as tooth lead, cannot be used as reliable indicators of past patterns of exposure due to our limited knowledge of the dynamics of lead deposition in teeth with age. Furthermore, cross-sectional studies must often rely on retrospective techniques to assess the many other variables acting during the life of a child that can affect the outcome measures we wish to associate with lead. Faulty memories reduce the reliability of data collected in this way, and many potentially important variables just cannot be measured. Yet another issue refractory to adequate assessment by cross-sectional designs is the time course of effects of lead. As a result of the failure of cross-sectional study designs to assess effects of the history of lead exposure upon child development, to provide adequate control of confounding variables also affecting development, and to determine the permanence or reversibility of any lead effects, cross-sectional studies have now been largely abandoned in favour of prospective designs.

Prospective designs can repeatedly assess lead exposure, from or even before birth, to give a complete record of exposure during development. Development itself can be repeatedly measured from birth, and confounding variables can be analysed in a timely fashion under controlled conditions. Several prospective studies have shown that children are vulnerable to prenatal and perinatal lead exposure. Bellinger et al. (1984; 1986; this volume) have reported that umbilical cord lead levels as low as $10 \, \mu g \, dl^{-1}$ are associated with deficits in mental development up to two years of age. Dietrich et al. (1986; this volume) have found deficits in psychomotor performance of infants at 6 and 12 months of age associated with prenatal lead exposures of less than $9 \, \mu g \, dl^{-1}$. Ernhart et al. (1986) have shown abnormal reflexes and neurological soft signs in 48-hour-old babies associated with similarly low-umbilical cord PbB levels at birth.

Because blood lead levels greater than $10 \, \mu g \, dl^{-1}$ are found in a substantial percentage of the population of childbearing age in developing and developed countries, replication and extension of these findings are important. A recent study (Friberg and Vahter, 1983) showed that a sample of school teachers in Mexico City had mean blood lead levels exceeding $22 \, \mu g \, dl^{-1}$, the highest of a dozen major metropolitan areas throughout the world reported in the study. Umbilical cord blood lead levels of over 400 newborns in another study in Mexico City averaged $13.5 \, \mu g \, dl^{-1}$ (Montoya-Cabrera et al., 1981).

Mexico City occupies a high mountain valley of $10\,000 \, km^2$ area. The valley floor is at 2200 m above sea level and mountains up to 5200 m nearly completely surround the city. Approximately 20 million people share the valley with almost half the country's industrial and manufacturing capacity and with 3 to 4 million motor vehicles. Topography, high population, industrial and traffic densities, and frequent temperature inversions combine to produce high levels of atmospheric contamination. Although sources of lead have not been systematically studied, air pollution, secondary lead recovery, lead paint and gasoline, and the common use of low-temperature lead-glazed ceramics all contribute to the relatively high body burdens of lead measured in samples of Mexico City residents.

The pilot study of the Mexico City Prospective Lead Study, reported here, was designed primarily to train staff and to improve data collection and analysis systems for the more extensive prospective study to follow. To a

388

limited extent, however, we can use the data to expand on some of the findings alluded to above. We have sampled blood lead levels in a group of women at 36 weeks of pregnancy and at birth and, also, measured umbilical cord lead levels of their babies. We examine here the effects of lead exposure at these times upon behavioural and neurological development during the first 30 days of life. Of particular interest is the relative contribution of maternal prenatal and perinatal lead and the impact of perinatal lead of the baby upon early development.

METHODS

Subjects

Pregnant women visiting the out-patient clinic at the National Perinatology Institute or the General Hospital in Mexico City on or before their 36th week of pregnancy, as determined from the date of last menses, were contacted for inclusion in the pilot study. Those who met one or more of the following exclusion criteria were not included in the study:

(1) Consumption of one or more alcoholic drinks per day;
(2) Drug addiction or habitual use of prescribed, over-the-counter or folk medicines;
(3) Age under 17 or over 40 years;
(4) High blood pressure or kidney disease; or
(5) Psychoses.

The project director at each site interviewed each patient to explain the nature of the experiment and to obtain informed consent. A project social worker gathered data on: SES; nutritional habits; alcohol consumption, smoking and drug habits; history of past pregnancies; and so on. Additional information was obtained from hospital records.

Blood samples

A sample of blood up to 7 ml was obtained by venepuncture during the 36th week of pregnancy (M36). Samples were stored in a refrigerator at 4°C in Becton–Dickonson purple top Vacutainers with EDTA until analysis. Two sterile prepackaged alcohol wipes were used, each with a single wipe in the same direction, to clean the skin immediately before venepuncture.

At the moment of birth, an umbilical cord blood sample (UC) was drawn. A maternal blood sample (MB) was drawn within 30 minutes of delivery. These samples were stored as those above.

Birth record

A project physician attending the birth noted birth conditions, complications, physical measurements and 1- and 5-minute Apgar scores and also determined gestational age.

Brazelton Neurobehavioural Assessment Scale (NBAS)

At 48 hours after birth, psychologists certified in the use of the NBAS by the Child Development Unit of Children's Hospital, Boston, MA administered the NBAS to the infant in the hospital. The test was administered again in the subject's home at 15 and 30 days after birth.

The seven NBAS cluster scales were calculated from each NBAS protocol sheet. Examiners were not aware of the lead status of the infants they tested.

Blood lead analysis

Refrigerated Vacutainers were packed in foam and delivered by air courier for analysis by ESA Laboratories, Inc. (Bedford, MA) within 24 hours of packing. All analyses were performed in duplicate by anodic stripping voltammetry, using an ESA 3010A Trace Metals Analyzer. Empty Vacutainers from the same manufacturing lots were also sent as blanks.

Statistical analyses

The data were analysed in several stages. Descriptive statistics and bivariate correlations were calculated for independent, dependent and control variables. Control variables with significant bivariate correlations with outcome as measured by the NBAS scales were used in forward stepwise multiple regression analyses to determine the best joint predictors of the NBAS. After the best multiple regression model was constructed from the non-lead variables, lead measurements recorded at the three time points were added to the model to determine the relationship between each of the lead measurements and the adjusted NBAS scores. The overall plan of analysis follows Bellinger *et al.* (1984; this volume). Analyses were performed with SAS programs.

RESULTS

The sample was mostly young women at lower or middle socioeconomic levels with small families. Table 1 shows that the infants had slightly lower lead levels than the mothers. All but 8 infants had 5-minute Apgar scores of 9; none were lower than 6. All infants weighed more than 2.5 kg and had

Table 1 Characteristics of sample included in this study

Characteristics	Mean
Age of mother	25.3 y
Weight of child	3.13 kg
Gestational age	39.3 weeks
Blood lead of mothers at 36 weeks (M36)	$15.0\ \mu g\ dl^{-1}$
Blood lead of mothers at birth (MB)	$15.4\ \mu g\ dl^{-1}$
Blood lead of infants at birth (UC)	$13.8\ \mu g\ dl^{-1}$

gestational ages of 36 weeks or more.

The trend of the scores of each Brazelton scale from 48 hours to 30 days was calculated for each subject by using a linear regression analysis on the three test results obtained in the first month. For the reflex scale only, a positive trend indicates increasing abnormal reflexes. For all other scales, a positive trend indicates improvement in the scale factor. Pearson correlations of blood lead levels with trend of NBAS scales show a significant relationship between increasing abnormal reflexes and increasing UC lead levels. An even stronger correlation between increasing abnormal reflexes and lead levels can be seen in the difference score between maternal lead at birth and the umbilical cord lead. As the infant's lead level approaches and surpasses the mother's lead level at birth, abnormal reflexes increase. Regulation of states is significantly related to the change in maternal lead between 36 weeks and birth; the lower the lead level at 36 weeks of pregnancy relative to lead level at birth, the greater the improvement in range of states.

Table 3 shows significant bivariate correlations between physical outcome measures of the infant at birth and differences in lead levels between mother and child. All physical measures show a decrease as the umbilical cord lead level tends to exceed the maternal lead level. In contrast to the correlations of lead with NBAS trend, it is the difference between the maternal PbB level at 36 weeks and the infant's lead level which shows the most correlation with the physical size of the infant.

Since both the trend in NBAS scores and the physical size of the infant at birth may be mediated by factors other than lead, we calculated the associations between a number of variables known through prior research to affect

Table 2 Significant bivariate correlations of 30-day NBAS trend and lead measures

Maternal lead at 36 weeks (M36)	—
Maternal lead at birth (MB)	—
Umbilical cord lead (UC)	reflexes, 0.299**
M36 − MB	regulation of states, 0.378**
M36 − UC	—
MB − UC	reflexes, −0.451***

$^{*}p < 0.05$
$^{**}p < 0.01$

Table 3 Significant bivariate correlations among physical outcome measures for infant and lead levels†

Lead measure	Gestation age	Weight	Gestation age/weight
M36 − UC	—	0.289**	0.315**

Lead measure	Body length	Trunk length	Chest cir.	Head cir.
M36 − UC	0.257*	0.404**	0.337**	0.305**
MB − UC	0.289*	—	—	—

$^{*}p < 0.10$;
$^{**}p < 0.05$;
† lead variables not listed were not significant at $p < 0.10$

pregnancy outcome with our outcome variables. These measures included: alcohol consumption; smoking and drug use during and prior to the present pregnancy; socioeconomic variables; demographic variables; nutritional variables; and experiences during the present and prior pregnancies. All control variables significantly associated with the outcome variables at a probability of less than 0.10 were entered into a forward stepwise multiple regression against each outcome variable. All control variables originally entered into the model for each outcome measure were retained in the model, even if subsequent control variable entries reduced the significance of the prior entries. This conservative statistical procedure results in a model of the outcome measure with the least possible amount of unexplained variance. After constructing the least unexplained variance model for each outcome measure with the control variables, each of the lead measures were independently added to the model.

Table 4 shows that the two NBAS scales identified by the bivariate correlations as being significantly affected by lead still remained statistically significant in the multiple regression model. The difference in lead levels between mother and child at birth adds still further to the explanatory power of the models tested to predict change in reflexes over the first thirty days of life, accounting for an additional 6.2% of unexplained variance of trend in the model. Umbilical cord lead alone is no longer significantly associated with reflex trend, but a new lead measure, change in lead in the mother between 36 weeks of pregnancy and at delivery, becomes significant. This type of unmasking of effect in multiple regression models has been noted before in lead research and discussed at length (Bellinger et al., 1984; 1986; this volume). The association between trend of the regulation of states scale and the change in lead in the mother between 36 weeks of pregnancy and delivery also remains significant in the multiple regression model.

An identical strategy was followed for assessing the effect of lead on physical outcome variables in the presence of control variables. After constructing least unexplained variance models for physical outcome measures with the control variables, lead variables were separately entered into the model. Table 5 shows that infant's weight at birth, chest circumference and trunk length were all affected by lead even after control variables were taken into account. Additionally, umbilical cord lead alone, absent in the bivariate correlations, now shows some association with trunk length.

Table 4 Effect of addition of lead to the stepwise multiple regression model using prior entry of all control variables that have significant bivariate correlations with 30-day trend of NBAS[†]

NBAS scale	Lead measure	Subject n	F value	Additional percent of variance explained by lead	Probability
Reflex	M36 − MB	44	4.87	6.0	0.034
	MB − UC	44	5.08	6.2	0.030
Regulation of states	M36 − MB	44	5.54	8.5	0.025

[†] NBAS habituation scale not tested because of low number of subjects with complete data. All other variables not shown were not significant

Table 5 Effect of addition of lead to the stepwise multiple regression model using prior entry of all control variables that have significant bivariate correlations with physical outcome measures[†]

Physical outcome measure	Lead measure	Subject n	F value	Additional percent of variance explained by lead	Probability
Weight of baby	M36 − MB	51	4.45	7.9	0.040
	M36 − UC	51	4.61	8.2	0.037
Chest circumference	M36 − UC	51	3.93	5.1	0.054
Trunk length	UC	33	3.82	8.2	0.062
	M36 − UC	33	3.94	8.4	0.059

† Variables not shown were not significant at $p < 0.10$

DISCUSSION

One of the major shortcomings of this study is the small sample size. Because small sample size reduces the power of statistical tests, especially multivariate tests, a probability criterion of 0.10 has been selected for significance. Nonetheless, a considerable risk of failing to recognize a real effect of lead upon infant development still exists.

The failure to sustain the significant bivariate correlation of umbilical cord lead and abnormal reflex trend in the multivariate analysis parallels the experience of Ernhart et al. (1986), who also found a significant bivariate correlation of UC lead with NBAS abnormal reflexes. Using only maternal–infant paired data in the multivariate analysis, the authors report that the association was reduced to a non-significant level. However, their sample size was three times larger than that of the present study.

Another factor that might have been responsible for the reduction of UC lead effect upon reflexes in multivariate analysis in the present study was the use of the very conservative model. For example, retaining only the variables that remain significant in the model by backward elimination would leave more variance in reflex trend unaccounted for at the point of testing for the lead effect, and might preserve the significance of lead in the final model.

All the factors just discussed can act to reduce the effect of the other lead variables upon outcome as well. It is all the more remarkable, then, that the difference in lead level between mother and child at birth is still a significant predictor of abnormal reflex trend in the multivariate model. Typically, UC lead is 10–20% lower than maternal lead at birth (see Table 1). The present study indicates that there exists, in cases where UC lead approaches and exceeds maternal lead, a trend toward increasing abnormal reflexes in the first 30 days of life. This effect is apparently controlled by factors regulating UC lead and not by factors decreasing maternal lead at birth, as maternal lead shows no correlation with outcome, even in the bivariate tests.

Ernhart et al. (1986) have noted the same effect. They show a significant UC effect upon neurological soft signs, using the Graham–Rosenblith Scale in multivariate analyses, but no effect of maternal lead at birth. Since the correlation between maternal and UC lead was high, the authors suggested that a factor such as foetal stress could lead both to increased foetal accumulation of lead and to poor infant outcome. The pattern of results in the present study, where UC lead levels nearly equal to or higher than maternal lead levels are associated with poor outcome, could be similarly explained. If a factor such as foetal stress acted to increase foetal absorption of maternal lead, or to increase mobilization of stored foetal lead, or to decrease foetal elimination of lead, higher UC lead levels relative to maternal lead levels would be observed. If this same factor also acted independently of, or in concert with, UC lead levels to produce unfavourable infant outcome, the existing correlation between maternal–UC lead difference and outcome would be observed.

To the extent that this hypothesized factor acts independently of or interactively with elevated UC lead, several possibilities exist with regard to observed UC lead relationships with outcome. First, anything serving to raise UC lead relative to maternal lead, independently of the lead level of the mother or the infant, and which also unfavourably affects outcome, would tend to associate higher UC lead levels with poorer outcome. In this case, some portion of lead's observed contribution to negative outcome may then actually be due to the as-yet-unmeasured factor. Secondly, if this hypothesized factor acts only to alter foetal lead but does not itself affect outcome, then observed relationships between foetal lead and outcome are substantiated. However, this would increase the uncertainties in using maternal PbB levels during pregnancy to assess foetal exposures. Reanalysis of existing data sets could provide clues about the nature of the hypothesized factor and guide new studies designed to clarify these relationships.

ACKNOWLEDGMENTS

The following personnel served as collaborators in the study:

Selene Cansino-Ortiz, Mtra. en Psic.
Pilar de la Torre-Arribas
Estela Perroni-Hernandez, Mtra. en Psic.
Antonio Briseno-Sains, M.D.
Raul Garcia-Palacios, M.D.
Tomas Hernandez-Mejia, M.D.
Valentin Ibarra, M.D.
Pedro Ortega, M.D.
Francisco Casado-Aguilera, M.D.
Jorge Carrasco-Rendon, M.D.

This project was supported, in part, by grants from Consejo Nacional de Ciencia y Tecnologia (CONACYT) and the Milton Fund of Harvard University. Although the research described in this chapter has been funded wholly or in part by the Health Effects Research Laboratory, U.S. Environmental Protection Agency through Project No. CR813477 to McLean Hospital, it has not been subjected to the Agency's peer and policy review and therefore does not necessarily reflect the views of the Agency and no official endorsement should be inferred. We also thank the Instituto Mexicano

394

de Psiquiatria, McLean Hospital Corporation, and the Universidad Nacional Autonoma de Mexico for their material support of the project.

We thank the staffs of the Instituto Mexicano de Psiquiatria, Instituto Nacional de Perinatologia and the Hospital General de Mexico, Secretaria de Salud.

Dr John Creason and Dr David Svendsgaard provided invaluable statistical assistance and advice.

REFERENCES

Bellinger, D.C., Needleman, H.L., Leviton, A., Waternaux, C., Rabinowitz, M.B. and Lewis, M.L. (1984). Early sensory—motor development and pre-natal exposure to lead. *Neurobehav. Toxicol. Teratol.*, **6**, 387–402

Bellinger, D.C., Leviton, A., Needleman, H.L., Waternaux, C. and Rabinowitz, M. (1986). Low-level lead exposure and infant development in the first year. *Neurobehav. Toxicol. Teratol.*, **8**, 151–161

Bellinger, D.C., Leviton, A., Waternaux, C., Needleman, H. and Rabinowitz, M. (1988). Low-level lead exposure and early development in socioeconomically-advantaged urban infants. (This volume).

Dietrich, K.N., Krafft, K.M., Shukla, R., Bornschein, R.L. and Succop, R.A. (1986). The neurobehavioral effects of prenatal and early postnatal lead exposure. In Shroeder, S.R. (ed.) *Toxic Substances and Mental Retardation: Neurobehavioral Toxicology and Teratology.* (Washington, DC: AAMD)

Dietrich, K.N., Krafft, K.M., Bier, M., Berger, O., Succop, P.A. and Bornschein, R.L. (1988). Neurobehavioural effects of fetal lead exposure: the first year of life. (This volume).

Ernhart, C.B., Wolf, A.W., Kennard, M.J., Erhard, P., Filipovich, H.F. and Sokol, R.J. (1986). Intrauterine exposure to low levels of lead: the status of the neonate. *Arch. Environ. Health*, **41**, 287–291

Friberg, L. and Vahter, M. (1983). Assessment of exposure to lead and cadmium through biological monitoring: results of a UNEP/WHO global study. *Environ. Res.*, **30**, 95–128

Montoya-Cabrera, M.A., Maldono-Torres, L., Landazuri-Laris, P., Montes-Allende, F., Escobar-Marquez, R. and Margain-Compean, J.C. (1981). Lead determinations in the blood of the umbilical cord of normal neonates. *Arch. Invest. Med. (Mexico)*, **12**, 457–462

Section 5

ANIMAL STUDIES AND MECHANISMS

Introduction

Animal studies can potentially answer questions which are not answerable by studies of children (this was discussed in the review chapters). The papers in this section, relating to research on rats and monkeys, provide an indication of the range of areas which can be tackled in animal studies of the effects of low levels of lead.

Cory-Slechta discusses questions of critical periods of exposure, vulnerability, and the time course of toxicity, and proposes experimental strategies which must be adopted if animal studies are to contribute to our understanding of the effects of lead in humans. The research reported by Lilienthal *et al.* on rats and monkeys was designed to explore the origins of behavioural change by investigating possible target structures within the brain, and the persistence of lead effects after exposure has ceased. Rice also reports on the persistence of lead effects on the behaviour of monkeys, using operant conditioning techniques to investigate attention and memory, among other things.

Finally there are two papers which more directly investigate the possible mechanisms of action of lead in and around the brtain. Regan *et al.* have investigated the structuring of the brain in young rats exposed to lead, and Pelling ad colleagues have assessed the functioning of the blood—brain barrier in rats dosed with lead.

5.1
The Lessons of Lead for Behavioural Toxicology

D. A. CORY-SLECHTA

SUMMARY

Alternative strategies are needed if questions aroused by chronic low-level lead exposure in humans are to be effectively answered by experimental studies in animals. Studies embodying prolonged lead exposures, behavioural endpoints with closer correspondence to complex performance in humans, and longitudinal performance evaluation help to characterize the time course of toxicity and vulnerability throughout the life cycle. Individual differences in susceptibility, even in a homogeneous strain of animals, and shifts in behavioural response over time warrant more refined data analysis techniques and novel statistical approaches. Such alternative experimental strategies should help define risks more precisely and enhance our understanding of the specific behavioural processes or mechanisms responsive to lead and other environmental contaminants.

Although lead has been recognized as a neurotoxicant for centuries, unanswered questions regarding even its most basic effects still haunt us. For example, what are the behavioural consequences of exposure to lead, and how do they relate to exposure parameters? Are they reversible? What is the extent of vulnerability across the life span? From a policy perspective, these questions may be subsumed by a more general one: Who is at risk? From a scientific standpoint they highlight the puzzles of underlying mechanisms or processes, both neurological and behavioural. Viewed broadly, such queries pervade environmental health and toxicology, and in this context lead may function as a prototypical poison, especially in relation to behavioural toxicology.

Many experimental animal studies devoted to the behavioural toxicology of lead appeared between 1973 and 1979. Interest has since waned considerably, perhaps reflecting the frustrations experienced by many investigators in failing

399

to find consistent and reliable behavioural changes. Yet the need to answer the questions posed above remains a pressing one. Finding more effective ways to resolve them, however, requires us to re-examine the experimental strategies and issues featured in the lead literature. This paper describes some alternative strategies which have proven useful in the search for answers to such questions.

AGE CONSIDERATIONS

One such issue is age, which is of concern from at least two perspectives. The first is the life cycle stage at which exposure occurs. The predominant focus of experimental studies has been prenatal and neonatal lead treatment. Such exposure regimens, however, have little correspondence with the environmental lead exposures encountered by humans. The National Academy of Sciences (NAS, 1975) reported, for example, that the peak incidence of childhood lead encephalopathy and elevated lead burden occurs between 1 and 3 years of age, a stage of maturation far more advanced than that represented by prenatal or neonatal rodents. Dobbing (1981) has suggested that the newborn rat is equivalent to an 18-week-old fetus.

Human exposure is sustained over the life span, because lead is a ubiquitous environmental pollutant. Moreover, various components of the human central nervous system (CNS) continue to mature well into adolescence (Sands *et al.*, 1979). In experimental studies, however, lead exposure typically ends at birth or at weaning. Such considerations led us to design a treatment regimen in which exposure of the rat to lead begins at weaning and continues for long durations. Such studies have demonstrated that vulnerability of the rodent to lead extends well beyond the presumed critical exposure periods.

Actually, little, if any, experimental evidence documents the presumption that lead-induced behavioural changes are provoked only by exposures during the earliest stages of development. In fact for some behavioural endpoints the developmental period of exposure can be shown to be a relatively unimportant variable. A comparison of published studies based on fixed-interval (FI) schedule-controlled behaviour (see below) reveals that effects may be better related to lead body burden than to exposure period. Figure 1 shows the inverse-U-shaped function that results when maximal changes in FI performance are plotted against lead dose (see Cory-Slechta, 1984, 1986; Cory-Slechta and Weiss, 1985), even though such studies encompass different developmental exposure periods. A similar function emerges when FI effects are plotted against blood lead (PbB) level, another indicator of exposure. In all but one study (Barthalmus *et al.*, 1977), these effects were observed early in the course of training, suggesting that they reflect alterations in the acquisition of FI performance. Another message conveyed by Figure 1 is that the extent of a critical exposure period is dependent upon the behavioural endpoint evaluated. Thus there is no single answer to what constitutes the critical exposure period. Various classes of behaviour may be differentially sensitive to toxicants such as lead, during different developmental periods.

Health effects provoked by prolonged low-level lead exposure are the

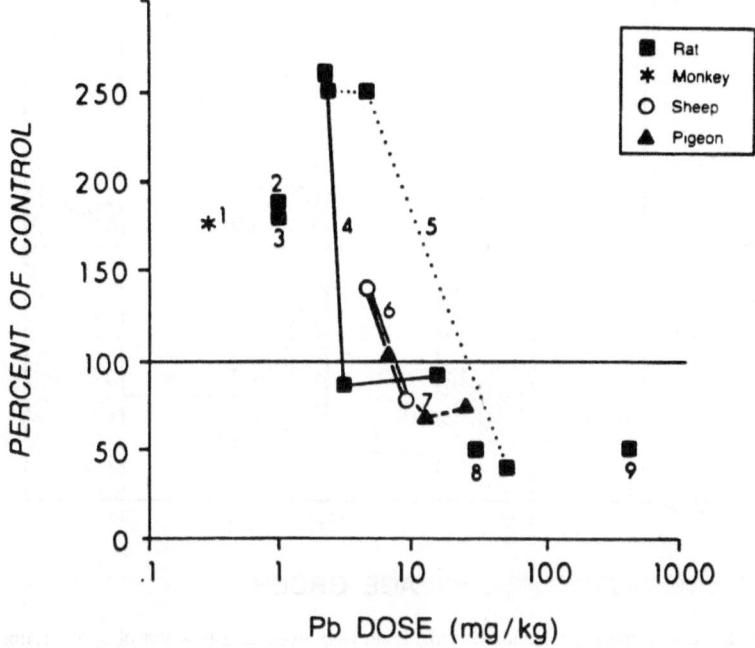

Figure 1   Dose–effect function for lead-induced changes in FI performance. The lead effect (response rate, IRT, or percentage of control reinforcers) was calculated as a percentage of the control group value for the sessions in which peak effects occurred and plotted as a function of the exposure dose (recalculated as mg/kg). Different symbols represent different experimental species. The different numbers represent the following studies: (1) Rice *et al.*, 1979; (2) Cory-Slechta *et al.*, 1985; (3) Cory-Slechta, unpublished data; (4) Cory-Slechta, *et al.*, 1983; (5) Cory-Slechta and Thompson, 1979; (6) Van Gelder *et al.*, 1973; (7) Barthalmus *et al.*, 1977; (8) Angell and Weiss, 1982; (9) Zenick *et al.*, 1979

current focus of human concern. Although childhood represents a period of dramatic physiological and behavioural development, adulthood should not be conceived of as a steady state. Multiple functional and structural changes occur during the life span and provoke questions about their relation to toxicity, especially the vulnerability of ageing organisms to lead. The ageing process introduces degenerative changes in virtually every organ and system, posing the likely possibility of enhanced susceptibility later in the life cycle. Schroeder and colleagues (1965), for example, reported shortened life span, cirrhosis of the liver, and alterations in the tissue distribution of rats fed 5 ppm lead in drinking water from weaning until death.

Ageing-associated events may alter toxicokinetics, as determined in a recent cross-sectional study from our laboratory (Cory-Slechta, in preparation). Groups of young (weanling), adult (8 months of age) and old rats (16 months of age) were exposed to 50 ppm lead acetate in drinking water for 8 months. Subsequent tissue lead determinations revealed an age-related shift in the distribution of lead, with a pronounced increase with age in both brain (Figure 2) and liver, but not in kidney. This effect may have resulted from the release

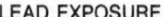

LEAD EXPOSURE

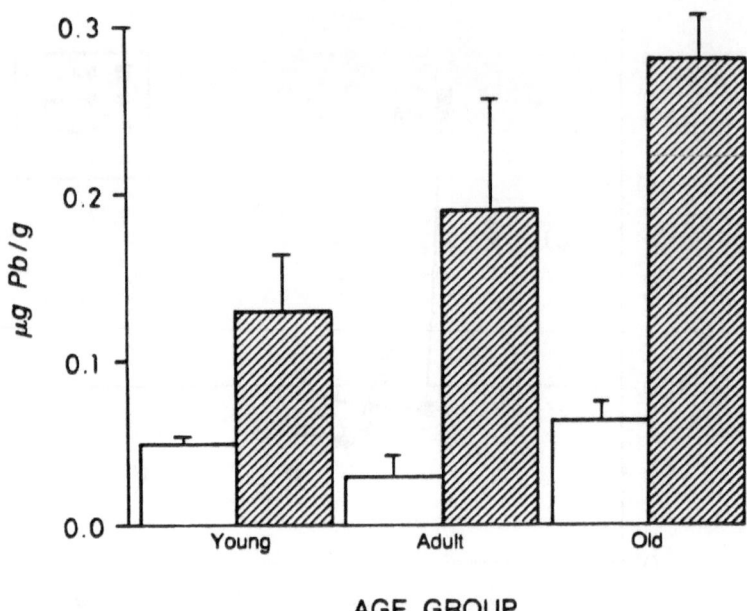

Figure 2 Group mean (± standard error) brain lead levels as a function of age. Groups of young (weanling), adult (8 months of age) and old (16 months of age) rats were exposed for 8 months to 50 ppm lead acetate in drinking water. Age-matched control groups are shown in open bars, lead-treated groups in dashed bars

of bone lead, because lead content in bone declined with age. The hypothesis that the ageing process might be accelerated by a toxicant was further substantiated by the increased incidence of morbidity and mortality in the old lead-exposed group relative to their non-treated counterparts. More work is urgently needed to evaluate susceptibility beyond the earliest stages of development, and the possibility of enhanced vulnerability with advancing age.

STRATEGIES FOR SELECTING BEHAVIOURAL ENDPOINTS

On what basis should an investigator select a behavioural endpoint? Many past studies have relied on some measure of motor activity (see Bornschein *et al.*, 1980). Their findings have proven to be remarkably inconsistent. Also, besides the lack of a reliable treatment effect, motor activity may have little correspondence with the more complex functions that are of primary concern in the human population. Intelligence tests, used extensively in studies of lead-exposed children, measure complex integrative functions and may even include sensory, perceptual and motor components.

Surprisingly, endpoints for which homologous or analogous behavioural assays exist for animals and humans have not been well exploited. Reaction time, for example, has been shown to increase in children as a function of PbB level (Needleman, 1985; Hunter *et al.*, 1985). A similar effect on reaction time was reported by Williamson and Teo (1986) in occupationally exposed workers. No parallel studies of lead effects on reaction time in experimental animals have been reported, although the techniques are easily implemented.

Performance maintained by schedules of reinforcement represents a class of complex learned or operant behaviour. In such cases a designated response may be rewarded either on the basis of time, number of responses, response topography, stimulus characteristics, or some combination of these. In the complex human environment, many different schedules, yielding many different consequences, tend to operate concurrently. These can be simplified in a laboratory setting. Typically, schedules of reinforcement yield quite stable patterns of behaviour over prolonged periods of time, making them ideal baselines for chronic toxicity studies.

Comparable behavioural performances in humans and many different species of experimental animals are produced by operant schedules of reinforcement under many circumstances (Kelleher and Morse, 1968). Furthermore, effects of CNS drugs on various schedules of reinforcement also exhibit species generality. One such example is the fixed-interval (FI) schedule, in which the first occurrence of a designated response after the lapse of a specified interval of time is reinforced (rewarded). Responses during the time interval itself have no programmed consequence.

As noted above, the performance of rats on the FI schedule is sensitive to chronic postweaning lead exposure (Cory-Slechta et al., 1983). Figure 3 plots group median overall response rates of lead-treated rats as a percentage of the corresponding control group value. In this study, exposure to lead began

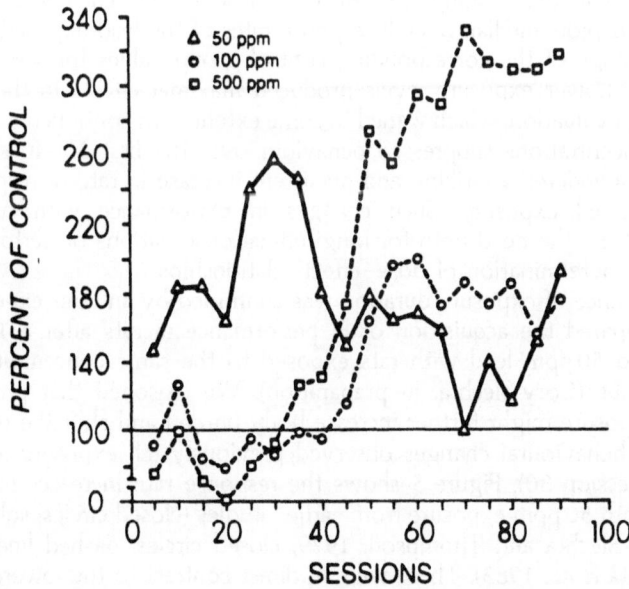

Figure 3 Group median overall response rates of lead-treated animals plotted as a percentage of the corresponding control values over 90 experimental sessions. Each data point represents a median value for five consecutive sessions (Cory-Slechta et al., 1983)

at weaning, and behavioural evaluation began when the rats reached 55 days of age. Lead exposure continued over the 90 experimental sessions (60 minutes a day, 5 days a week) shown. The lowest exposure level, 50 ppm, initially increased rates of responding (total number of responses divided by session time) to a median value greater than 250% of control, after which rates declined, but generally remained above control levels. In contrast, the two higher exposure concentrations, 100 and 500 ppm, initially decreased response rates by as much as 50%. This was followed, however, by a marked increase in response rate after 30–40 experimental sessions. Despite consistent findings of lead-induced changes in FI performance in experimental animals, and the well-documented species generality of the baseline behaviour, no comparable studies have been carried out in lead-exposed children or occupationally exposed workers. Again, such techniques are not difficult to implement.

ISSUES RELATED TO STUDY DESIGN

With the focus on prenatal and neonatal exposure protocols the influence of duration of lead exposure has received little experimental attention, despite its relationship to total body burden, and, consequently, to tissue dose. In our studies of chronic postweaning lead exposure and FI performance, however, duration of exposure can be shown to alter markedly the pattern of behavioural changes (Cory-Slechta et al., 1983; Cory-Slechta, in preparation). Figure 4, for example, summarizes the joint role of exposure concentration and duration in determining the effects of lead on FI schedule-controlled behaviour. It plots median overall response rates of the lead-exposed groups as a percentage of the corresponding control group values for sessions 30, 60 and 90. Lower exposure levels produced maximal effects in the earlier stages of FI evaluation, which waned to some extent with continued exposure. Higher concentrations suppressed behaviour over the first 30–40 sessions, but then engendered a striking and persistent increase in rate of responding with continued exposure. Such changes in performance with sustained exposure stress the need both for longitudinal observations of performance, and for the determination of dose–effect relationships.

The influence of exposure duration was confirmed by another experiment, which compared the acquisition of FI performance in rats after a 1-month exposure to 50 ppm lead with rats exposed to the same concentration for 8–11 months (Cory-Slechta, in preparation). We reasoned that prolonged 50 ppm exposure might further increase body burden and shift the resulting pattern of behavioural changes observed previously (cf. exposure levels in Figure 4, session 30). Figure 5 shows the response rate increases produced by a 1-month 50 ppm exposure from earlier studies (closed circles, solid lines; from Cory-Slechta and Thompson, 1979; closed circles, dashed lines; from Cory-Slechta et al., 1983). These were in direct contrast to the lowered rates observed when 8 or 11 months of exposure preceded behavioural testing (open symbols).

A too infrequently asked question, given its clinical relevance, stems from

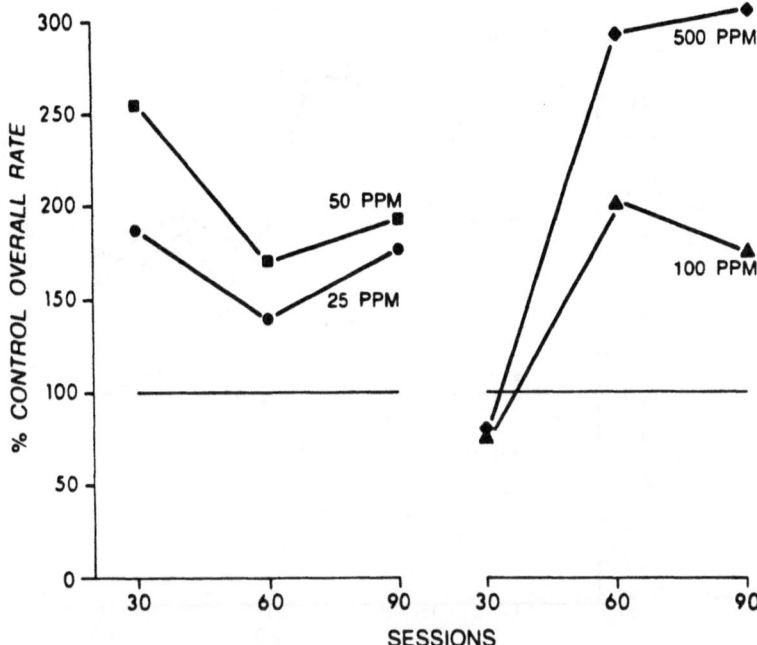

Figure 4 Changes in FI overall response rate as a function of the lead acetate exposure concentration and duration. Each data point represents the median value of the lead-treated group plotted as a percentage of the corresponding control group median (Cory-Slechta *et al.*, 1985)

the issue of reversibility of effects after lead exposure ends. There is no single answer to such a question, because reversibility presumably depends upon many factors, including exposure parameters, kinetics of elimination, age of exposure and age of the organism, etc. Reversibility must be examined under a variety of exposure and design conditions. In a previous study, for instance, we found that the response rate increases produced by a 50 ppm exposure declined to control levels within 30 additional sessions after lead exposure ended following session 30 (Cory-Slechta and Thompson, 1979).

Prolonged exposure to higher concentrations, however, produced little evidence for behavioural recovery, as illustrated in Figure 6. In this study (Cory-Slechta *et al.*, 1983), lead treatment of half of the animals in each exposure group ended after 90 experimental sessions; the other half (matched on the basis of response rate) remained on lead. At the time exposure ended, the response rates of all lead-treated groups were still elevated relative to controls, with the magnitude of the increase related to exposure concentration. Despite a marked decline in brain lead levels (e.g. from 1.38 ± 0.38 to 0.14 ± 0.15 $\mu g/g$ in the 500 ppm group), there was no corresponding decline in response rate in either the 100 or 500 ppm groups. Low-level effects (50 ppm) waned gradually, even with sustained exposure. The persistence of elevated response rates in the 100 and 500 ppm groups long past cessation of exposure demonstrates that the effects of the chronic treatment are not

405

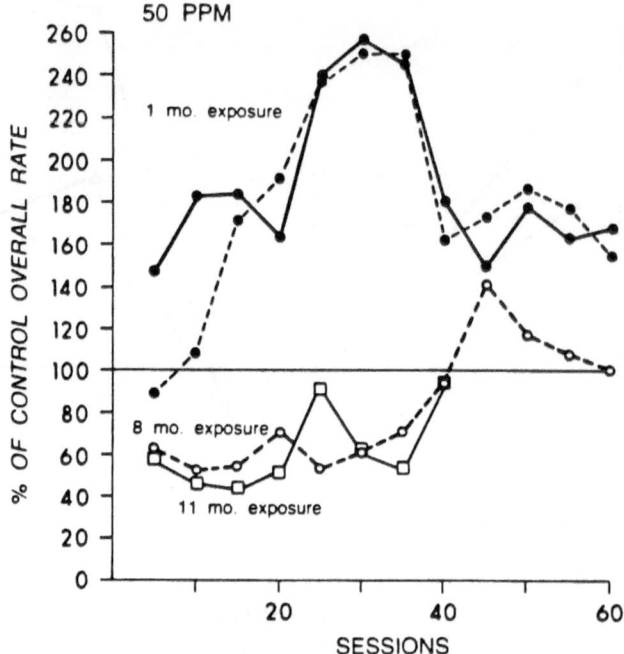

Figure 5 Group median overall response rates of 50 ppm lead-acetate treated rats given 1 (closed circles) or 8 (open circles) or 11 (open squares) months of exposure prior to evaluation of FI performance. Each data point represents a group median value over five sessions and is plotted as a percentage of the corresponding control group median value (Cory-Slechta, in preparation)

mediated by the acute daily exposure to lead.

Another method for assessing reversibility relies on the administration of chelating or complexing agents, such as calcium ethylenediamine tetra acetate (CaEDTA), that bind metals and enhance their urinary excretion. Several studies have reported improvements in IQ and function following chelation therapy in lead-exposed children (Bradley and Baumgartner,1958; Pueschel *et al.*, 1972; Albert *et al.*, 1974; Sachs *et al.*, 1978). While intuitively reasonable, most such studies suffer from the absence of a comparably treated control group. Improved scores in the chelated group could be attributed to added attention by parents and hospital staff associated with chelation treatment.

Such questions prompted us to determine if CaEDTA would reverse 50 ppm lead-induced increases in response rate on the FI schedule (Cory-Slechta, 1987). CaEDTA is currently the standard agent of choice for both diagnosis and therapy. It was hypothesized that FI response rates should decline faster following CaEDTA administration than after termination of lead exposure alone; however, this hypothesis was rejected. Although CaEDTA administration (75 or 150 mg/kg i.p. daily for 5 days) had no discernible effects in control animals, it actually exacerbated effects in lead-exposed rats (Figure 7), further increasing the proportion of short inter-response times (IRTs, or times

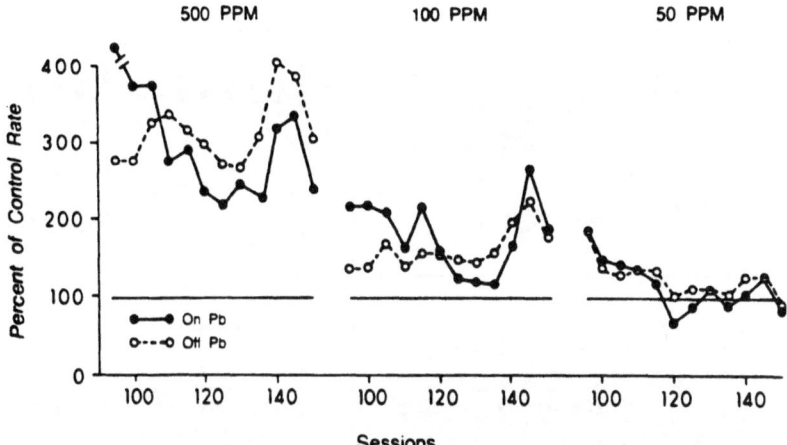

Figure 6 Changes in FI overall response rates following termination (open circles) or continuation (closed circles) of lead exposure after 90 FI experimental sessions. Each data point represents a group median value over five sessions and is plotted as a percentage of the corresponding control group median value over the sessions indicated. Lead acetate exposure concentrations are indicated above each set of curves (Cory-Slechta, in press)

between successive responses; typically the shorter the IRTs, the higher the rate of responding; see below) to 70–80% of the total IRTs, while lead-exposed saline-injected rats continued to exhibit a proportion of short IRTs generally below 60%.

These observations were undertaken in conjunction with an attempt to track the pattern of tissue lead mobilization over 5 days of CaEDTA administration, the standard therapy protocol, using the same doses as above. Different groups of animals were given different numbers of CaEDTA injections, and tissue lead determinations were carried out 24 h after the final injection. The findings from the behavioural study were consistent with the failure of CaEDTA administration to enhance the net loss of lead from brain (Figure 8). In fact, a single injection of CaEDTA (analogous to the CaEDTA mobilization test used diagnostically) actually increased brain lead content, an effect subsequently replicated in groups of animals exposed to 25 and 500 ppm lead acetate (Cory-Slechta and Weiss, submitted). Although CaEDTA clearly decreased total lead body burden, its ability, based on these studies, to directly counteract behavioural toxicity, seems dubious.

CONSIDERATIONS IN DATA ANALYSIS

Investigations of the neurobehavioural toxicity of lead may influence public policy. A 'significant' or a 'non-significant' effect (as defined statistically), can heavily influence such decisions. Most studies, however, rely on statistical procedures that focus on traditional measures such as means and standard deviations, a practice which ignores the frequently noted individual differences in susceptibility to lead (e.g. Rhavagan et al., 1980; Angell and Weiss, 1982;

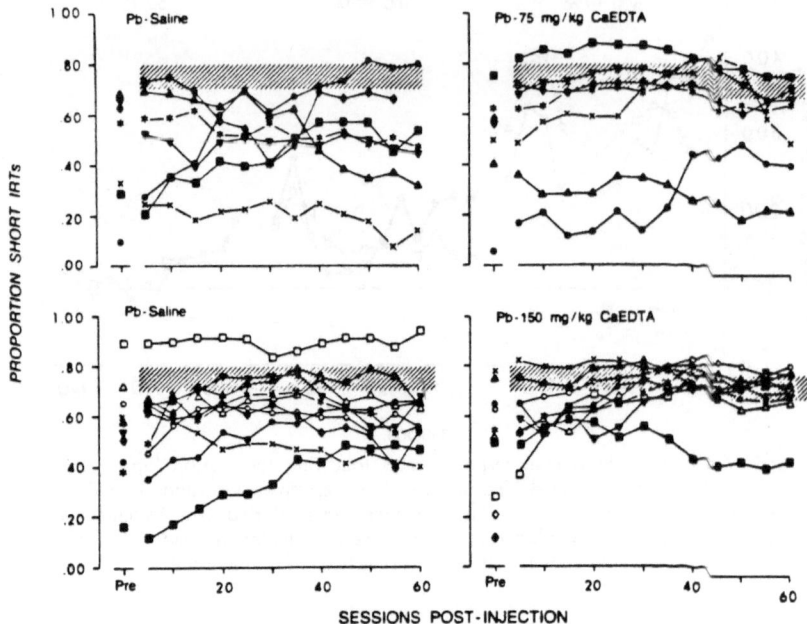

Figure 7 The proportion of short IRTs in 50 ppm lead-acetate treated rats following termination of lead exposure and five daily injections of saline (left panels) or 75 (top right) or 150 mg/kg (bottom right) CaEDTA administered i.p. Each curve represents an individual rat. The proportions of short IRTs for each rat prior to chelation are indicated in the 'Pre'-column. Each data point represents a median value for five sessions; changes in IRTs were evaluated for 60 sessions after chelation. The shaded area between 70 and 80% represents the typical upper boundary of short IRTs observed across various experiments

Rice *et al.*, 1979; Hastings *et al.*, 1979; Seppalainen *et al.*, 1975) and, in fact, conflicts with regulatory and legislative mandates to protect the most vulnerable individuals.

We have noted, repeatedly, wide individual variations in response. Figure 9, for example, shows overall response rates of individual control (top left) and lead-treated rats from the study summarized in Figure 3 (Cory-Slechta *et al.*, 1983). Each curve represents an individual animal, and each data point a median value for 10 sessions. Typically, control animals exhibit very stable patterns of performance on the FI schedule over the course of an experiment with response rates ranging from 5 to 25 responses per minute. An exceptional animal (one out of five or six) may exhibit a much higher, more erratic response rate. The range of response rates is actually very similar among groups, but the distribution of response rates in the lead-treated groups is almost a mirror-image of the controls: most treated animals exhibit the higher response rates, while a few parallel the more typical control performance. Additionally, among the treated animals exhibiting elevated response rates, the magnitude of the effect varies considerably. A comparison of the lead and control distributions suggests that one result of exposure is to shift performance towards the more extreme values of the distribution.

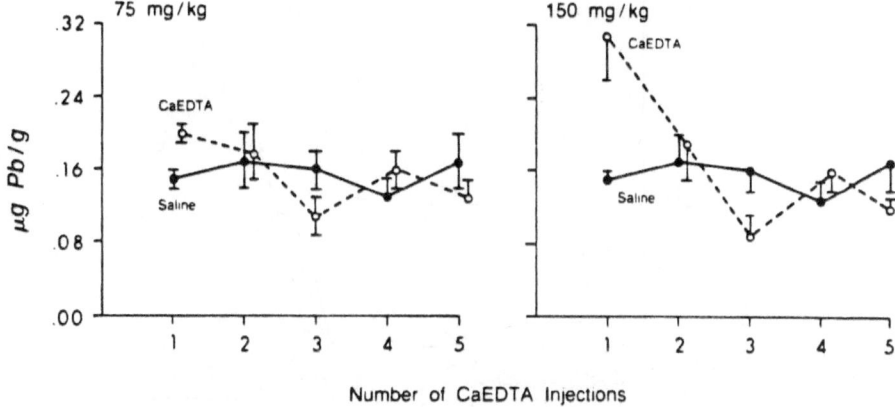

Figure 8 Changes in brain lead levels of rats treated with 75 (left) or 150 (right) mg/kg CaEDTA (open circle–dashed line) after a 3–4-month exposure to 50 ppm lead acetate. Data are compared to comparably lead-treated animals that received saline (closed circles–solid line). Different groups of animals received different numbers of injections; each data point shows the group mean and one standard error

Individual differences in vulnerability, as well as dose–response data, are important components of any risk analysis. Yet such information cannot easily be derived from studies which report only mean values. By examining individual performances it is easy to see that conventional statistical procedures will reflect only increased variability with lead exposure, but no significant main effect. Yet consistent distributions can be observed in all three treatment groups shown in Figure 9, as well as in different studies (e.g. Cory-Slechta and Thompson, 1979; Cory-Slechta et al., 1983, 1985). Consistency of findings across studies argues far more convincingly for reliability than does a single p-value.

Furthermore, longitudinal observations following lead exposure may reveal changing behavioural processes over time, as shown in Figures 3 and 4. Differences between lead-exposed and control animals over time might take several forms: for example, the two groups may attain the same level of performance, but do so at different rates; or they might exhibit differential trends in attaining a final performance. Longitudinal observations are frequently used to determine the time course of toxicity. Traditional statistical approaches, even repeated-measures analysis of variance, may not be appropriate or sensitive. We have approached this problem through polynominal fitting of each animal's performance over time, subjecting the resulting coefficients to randomization tests (Cox and Cory-Slechta, submitted). Such procedures take advantage of the ability of computer technology to press beyond classical statistical methods formulated in pre-computer days.

The ability to differentiate between lead-exposed and control animals may also be markedly influenced by the level of behavioural analysis. For example, overall response rate on the FI schedule represents an integrated measure of

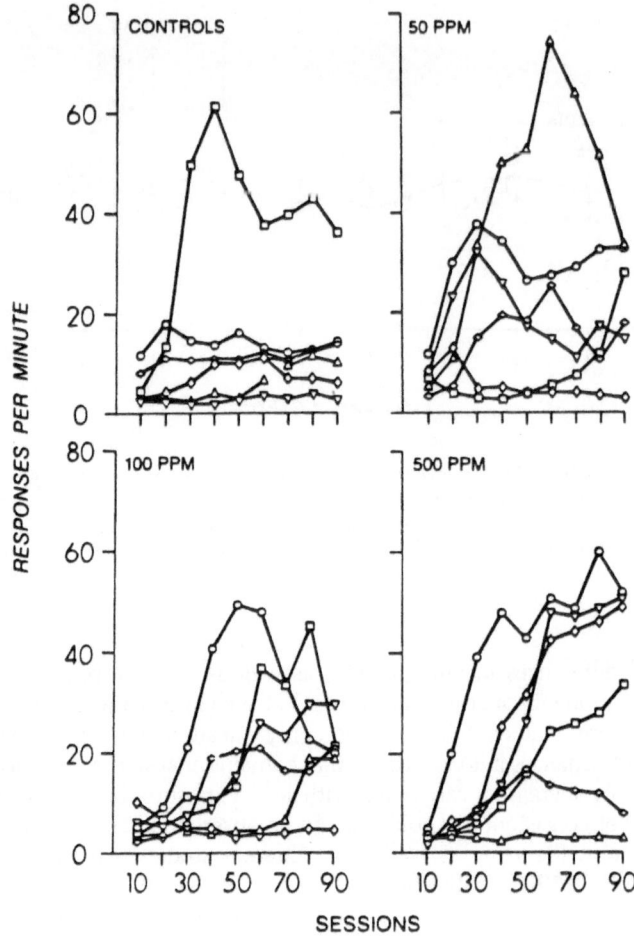

Figure 9 Individual overall response rates of control (top left) and lead-treated animals over the first 90 experimental sessions. Each curve represents an individual animal and each data point represents a median value calculated over 10 successive sessions (Cory-Slechta *et al.*, 1983)

performance that includes both the periods of responding and of pausing (Gentry *et al.*, 1982). When FI performance is decomposed into its component parts for a direct examination of how those aspects of performance are affected by lead, such a microanalysis of behaviour can serve two functions: (1) it can focus more specifically on that aspect most responsive to lead; and (2) it can suggest the behavioural mechanisms by which lead acts, and strategies for further experimental work.

A microanalysis of FI performance revealed, for example, that the time spent pausing by lead-treated rats after food delivery, or during the interval did not differ from controls. When the lead-exposed animals did begin to respond, however, they typically did so at a much higher rate than controls.

410

A similar effect was observed in monkeys exposed chronically to lead by Rice *et al.* (1979). Figure 10 shows the proportion of the successive responses separated by less than 1.0 s (i.e. short IRTs or inter-response times) of individual control (left) and 25-ppm lead-exposed rats (right) in two separate replications (Cory-Slechta *et al.*, 1985). This measure removes periods of pausing that distort overall response rate measures. Control animals show a proportion of short IRTs ranging from 0.2 to 0.6 of the total IRTs by the 40th experimental session. Again, the range observed in the lead-treated animals towards the higher proportion of short IRTs is readily apparent in both replications and is statistically reliable. Such a fine-grained analysis yields more consistent treatment effects as defined by the number of animals affected, the magnitude of the effect, and its sensitivity. The 25-ppm exposure level produced PbB values averaging only 15–20 μg/dl, levels observed in many suburban children and in a species often assumed to be more resistant than humans.

ACKNOWLEDGMENTS

My special thanks to Dr Bernard Weiss for his helpful comments on the manuscript. This work was supported in part by Grants ES-01247, ES-01248,

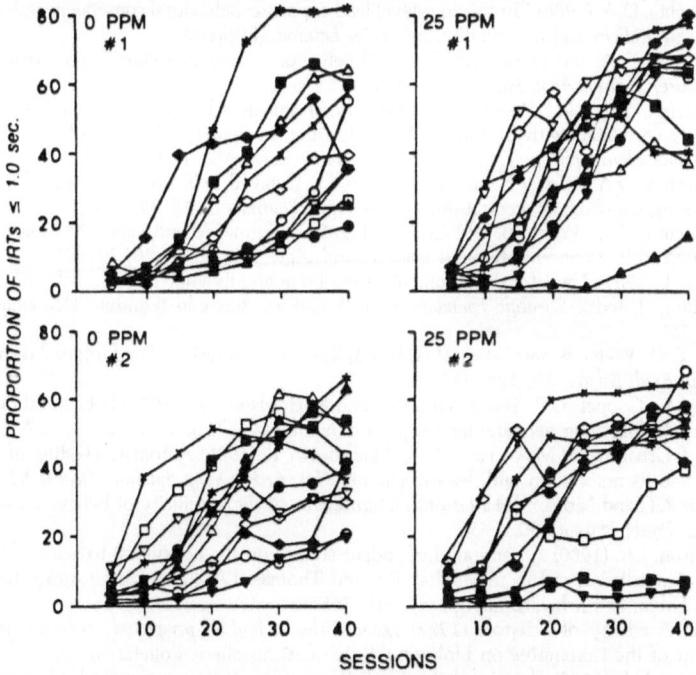

Figure 10 The proportion of IRTs $\leqslant 1.0$ s for individual control (left) and 25 ppm lead-acetate treated rats (right) over the first 40 experimental sessions on a fixed-interval food reinforcement schedule. The experiment was replicated twice. The results of the first replicate are shown in the top panels, the second replicate in the bottom panels. Each curve is from an individual rat, each data point represents a median value for five sessions (Cory-Slechta *et al.*, 1985)

ES-03054 and ES-01577 from the National Institute of Environmental Health Sciences (NIEHS)

REFERENCES

Albert, R.E., Shore, R.E., Sayers, A.J., Strehlow, C., Kniep, T.J., Pasternack, B.S., Friedhoff, A.J., Covan, F. and Cimino, J.A. (1974) Follow-up of children overexposed to lead. *Environ. Health Perspect.*, 33–39

Angell, N.F. and Weiss, B. (1982) Operant behavior of rats exposed to lead before or after weaning. *Toxicol. Appl. Pharmacol.*, **63**, 62–71

Barthalmus, G.T., Leander, J.D., McMillan, D.E., Mushak, P. and Krigman, M.R. (1977) Chronic effects of lead on schedule-controlled pigeon behavior. *Toxicol. Appl. Pharmacol.*, **42**, 271–284

Bornschein, R., Pearson, D. and Reiter, L. (1980) Behavioral effects of moderate lead exposure in children and animal models: Part 2, animal studies. *CRC Crit. Rev. Toxicol.*, **7**, 101–152

Bradley, J.E. and Baumgartner, R.J. (1958) Subsequent mental development of children with lead encephalopathy as related to type of treatment. *J. Ped.*, **53**, 311–315

Cory-Slechta, D.A. (1984) The behavioral toxicity of lead: problems and perspectives, in Thompson, T., Dews, P.B. and Barrett, J.E. (eds.), *Advances in Behavioral Pharmacology*, Vol. 4 (New York: Academic Press), pp. 211–255

Cory-Slechta, D.A. (1986) Vulnerability to lead at later developmental stages. In Krasnegor, N.A., Gray, D.B. and Thompson, T. (eds), *Developmental Behavioral Pharmacology*, Vol. 5: *Advances in Behavioral Pharmacology* (New Jersey: Lawrence Erlbaum), pp. 151–168

Cory-Slechta, D.A. (1988) Chronic low-level lead exposure: behavioral consequences, biological exposure indices and reversibility. *Sci. Total Environ.* (In press)

Cory-Slechta, D.A. and Thompson, T. (1979) Behavioral toxicity of chronic postweaning lead exposure. *Toxicol. Appl. Pharmacol.*, **47**, 151–159

Cory-Slechta, D.A. and Weiss, B. (1985) Alterations in schedule-controlled behaviour of rodents correlated with prolonged lead exposure, in Seiden, L.S. and Balster, R.L. (eds), *Behavioral Pharmacology, The Current Status* (New York: Alan R. Liss), pp. 487–502

Cory-Slechta, D.A., Weiss, B. and Cox, C. (1983) Delayed behavioral toxicity of lead with increasing exposure concentration. *Toxicol. Appl. Pharmacol.*, **71**, 342–352

Cory-Slechta, D.A., Weiss, B. and Cox, C. (1985) Performance and exposure indices in rats exposed to low concentrations of lead. *Toxicol. Appl. Pharmacol.*, **78**, 291–299

Dobbing, J. (1981) The later development of the brain and its vulnerability, in Davis, J.A. and Dobbing, J. (eds), *Scientific Foundations of Paediatrics*, 2nd edn (London: Heinemann), pp. 744–759

Gentry, G.D., Weiss, B. and Laties, V.G. (1983) The microanalysis of fixed-interval responding. *J. Exp. Anal. Behav.*, **39**, 327–343

Hastings, L., Cooper, G.P., Bornschein, R.L. and Michaelson, I.A. (1979) Behavioral deficits in adult rats following neonatal lead exposure. *Neurobehav. Toxicol. Teratol.*, **1**, 227–231

Hunter, J. Urbanowicz, M.A., Yule, W. and Lansdown, R. (1985) Automated testing of reaction time and its association with lead in children. *Int. Arch. Occup. Environ. Health*, **57**, 27–34

Kelleher, R.T. and Morse, W.H. (1968) Determinants of the specificity of behavioral effects of drugs. *Ergeb. Physiol.*, **60**, 1–56

Michaelson, I.A. (1980) An appraisal of rodent studies on the behavioral toxicity of lead: the role of nutritional status, in Singhal, R.L and Thomas, J.A. (eds), *Lead Toxicity* (Baltimore, MA: Urban and Schwarzenberg), pp. 301–365

National Academy of Sciences (1972) *Lead: Airborne lead in perspective.* (Washington, DC: Report of the Committee on Biologic Effects of Atmospheric Pollutants)

Needleman, H.L. (1985) The neurobehavioral effects of low-level exposure to lead in childhood. *Int. J. Mental Health*, **14**, 64–77

Pueschel, S.M., Kopito, L. and Schwachman, H. (1972) Children with an increased lead burden. A screening and follow-up study. *J. Am. Med. Assoc.*, **222**, 462–466

Rhagavan, S.R.V., Culver, B.D. and Gonick, H.C. (1980) Erythrocyte lead-binding protein after occupational exposure. I. Relationship to lead toxicity. *Environ. Res.*, **22**, 264–270

Rice, D.C., Gilbert, S.G. and Willes, R.F. (1979) Neonatal low-level lead exposure in monkeys:

locomotor activity, schedule-controlled behavior and the effects of amphetamine. *Toxicol. Appl. Pharmacol.*, **51**, 503–513

Sachs, H.K., Krall, V., McCaughran, D.A., Rozenfeld, I.H., Yongsmith, N., Crowe, G., Lazar, B.S., Lovar, N., O'Connell, L. and Rayson, B. (1978) IQ following treatment of lead poisoning: a patient–sibling comparison. *J. Ped.*, **93**, 428–431

Sands, J., Dobbing, J. and Gratrix, C.A. (1979) Cell number and cell size: organ growth and development and the control of catch-up growth in rats. *Lancet*, **2**, 503–505

Schroeder, H.A., Balassa, J.J. and Vinton, W.H. (1965) Chromium, cadmium and lead in rats: effects on life span, tumors and tissue levels, *J. Nutr.*, **86**, 51–66

Seppalainen, A.M., Tola, S., Hernberg, S. and Kock, B. (1975) Subclinical neuropathy at 'safe' levels of lead exposure. *Arch. Environ. Health*, **30**, 180–183

Williamson, A.M. and Teo, R.K.C. (1986) Neurobehavioral effects of occupational exposure to lead. *Br. J. Ind. Med.*, **43**, 374–380

Van Gelder, G.A., Carson, T., Smith, R.M. and Buck, W.B. (1973) Behavioral toxicologic assessment of the neurologic effect of lead in sheep. *Clin. Toxicol.*, **6**, 405–418

Zenick, H., Rodriquez, W., Ward, J. and Elkington, B. (1979) Deficits in fixed-interval performance following prenatal and postnatal lead exposure. *Dev. Psychbiol.*, **12**, 509–514

5.2
Neurobehavioural and Electrophysiological Effects of Lead in Rats and Monkeys

H. LILIENTHAL, C. MUNOZ, G. WINNEKE, C. LENAERTS and
R. HENNEKES

SUMMARY

The experiments reported here deal with three different topics: (1) the search for brain structures primarily involved in lead-induced neurobehavioural dysfunction, (2) the influence of the time span between indirect maternal exposure and age at behavioural testing in the rat, and (3) the role of lead in central and peripheral visual processes in monkeys. The results indicate that there are differences in the effects of lead exposure and hippocampal lesions, that permanent post-weaning lead exposure does not add to the neurobehavioural deficit due to indirect maternal exposure, and that in monkeys parameters of the visual evoked potentials and electroretinograms are altered by lead.

An increasing number of studies are dealing with the neurobehavioural deficit of asymptomatic children exposed to low levels of lead. However, the difficulties of relating the observed effects to lead, and of excluding confounding variables, are obvious. In order to establish a direct cause–effect relationship animal experiments have been carried out, and these have demonstrated lead-induced behavioural deficits. Until now, however, little has been known about the origin of the behavioural changes. Therefore, the first purpose of the present experiments was to examine which brain structures can account for the observed effects, and the second purpose was to investigate possible recovery after termination of the exposure.

Several lines of evidence suggest that the hippocampus may be the primary target for lead in the brain. Following the reports that lead preferentially accumulates in the hippocampus (Fjerdingstad et al., 1974; Danscher et al., 1976), there are many studies showing morphological alterations after lead exposure: there are reductions in the length and width of the hippocampus as well as in the length of the dentate gyrus and the mossy fibre pathway (Alfano et al., 1982). Dendritic branching and axonal development are impaired (Alfano and Petit, 1982). Number of glia cells per area in the stratum pyramidale and the numerical and areal density of profiles of mossy fibre buttons increased (Campbell et al., 1984). In infant rats lead exposure retarded the development of the neuropil within the hilus of the dentate gyrus and affected synaptogenesis in the mossy fibre zone (Cambell et al., 1982). Further studies demonstrated an interaction between lead and the hippocampal cholinergic system (Shih and Hanin, 1978; Alfano et al., 1983).

Moreover, there are similarities between the behavioural changes following lead exposure and those seen after hippocampal damage (Alfano and Petit, 1981). Therefore, a direct comparison between lesioned animals and lead-exposed ones is desirable. For this purpose ibotenic acid, an excitotoxin, was used to induce chemical lesions of intrinsic neurons to the hippocampus only, while fibres of passage and afferents were spared. Lesioned animals were compared with animals exposed to low levels of lead.

After examination of hippocampal damage chemical lesions of the amygdala were studied in looking for a model which resembled lead-induced behavioural alterations more closely than the first approach. The amygdala was chosen because accumulation of lead has also been reported for this region (Danscher et al., 1975). The second purpose of the present experiments was to examine the question of reversibility. There are several studies suggesting that the neurobehavioural deficit resulting from lead exposure may be long-lasting, or even irreversible, if exposure occurs during the early developmental stages of brain maturation (Bushnell and Bowman, 1979; Gross-Selbeck and Gross-Selbeck, 1981; Hastings et al., 1979). To answer this question visual discrimination and spatial learning were studied, and emphasis given to memory processes.

METHODS

Exposure regimen

Full details of the method are given elsewhere (Munoz et al., 1986). Briefly, female Wistar albino rats were given 0, 250, 750, or 2250 ppm lead acetate in the laboratory diet. Mating was 50 days after the start of exposure. After delivery half of the litters in each exposure group were switched to a control diet, while the other half was fed the same diet as the mothers. Thus there were two exposure models: indirect maternal only (M) and permanent (P), until the beginning of behavioural testing. For the behavioural part of the experiments only the offspring were used. Testing was carried out in completely blind fashion.

Surgery

For surgery 20 control females were anaesthetized at the age of 165 days with an intraperitoneal injection of 45 mg/kg of ketamine. Ibotenic acid (IBO) was stereotaxically injected into the dorsal hippocampi (10 μg IBO in 0.5 μl of phosphate buffer into each hemisphere). Ten additional females were treated alike without IBO injection (sham operation). For amygdala lesions 0.4 μg IBO in 0.4 μl phosphate buffer were stereotaxically injected into each side.

Radial arm maze

As spatial acquisition and retention is particularly sensitive to conventional lesions of the hippocampus (Olton *et al.*, 1979) the radial arm maze was chosen for the present experiments. For this task 10 female control rats and 10 female animals from each of the groups M 750 and P 750 were used. The apparatus was an automated eight-arm radial maze (RAM) modified after Walsh *et al.* (1982). At the end of each arm there was a swinging door giving access to a 45 mg food pellet. Time of alley entry was detected via Foto-Darlington transistors. Four pairs of these were placed at regular intervals in the midline along each alley, the first pair directly behind the entrance. Opening of the swinging door operated a microswitch. The apparatus was controlled by a microprocessor (AIM 65) and diffusely illuminated by a system of lamps above the device.

Fourteen days after surgery rats from all five groups were food-deprived to 85% of their free feeding weight. They were allowed to explore the maze for 10 min without pellet reward. Beginning the following day after, they were tested on two consecutive days. Rats had free access to all eight arms. A training session stopped when all rewards were taken or when 10 min had elapsed. Errors were defined as entry into a previously visited arm. Criterion of entrance was putting the head into an alley. Besides errors the following dependent variables were recorded: time to make eight correct choices, number of correct choices for the first eight trials, and days to criterion. The criterion for successful learning was to take all rewards on five consecutive days.

Four weeks after the end of the acquisition period (that is the original learning phase) successful animals were retested for retention of the task.

Visual discrimination learning

At age 100 days, 10 male rats from the groups O, M and P 250, and M and P 750 were food-deprived to 80% of their normal daily intake and trained in a modified Lashley jumping stand for visual discrimination learning (VDL) according to the standard procedure (Winneke *et al.*, 1977). The task was a difficult discrimination between two white circles differing in size painted on a black background. The criterion for successful learning was ten correct choices out of twelve on each of two consecutive days. Successful animals were retested for retention after 6 weeks of training-free interval. This experiment was repeated with animals from the same groups at an age of 400 days.

416

RESULTS

General observations and tissue lead levels

Except for the 2250 ppm group there were no differences in litter size and pup weight means. Body weights were reduced in the M/P 2250 ppm groups at the ages of 100, 250, and 400 days. For this reason 2250 ppm lead acetate is considered an overtly toxic dose. Blood and brain lead levels are given in Table 1. Blood and brain values of all permanently exposed groups are in the expected range, and the correspondence between the levels in these different targets is good. ALAD activity, as expected, is negatively correlated with blood lead levels. Maternally exposed groups are indistinguishable from controls for all available measures of internal exposure.

Radial arm maze

Histological examinations of lesioned animals indicated a complete bilateral depletion of granular and pyramidal cells in the dorsal hippocampi. Light microscopy failed to reveal neuronal depletion in any other region of the brain. There was no detectable damage in any region of the brain in lead-exposed animals.

Performance of the rats in the maze is given in Table 2. In IBO-lesioned animals exploratory activity was significantly increased on the pretraining day ($p < 0.05$, Mann-Whitney U-test). As control and sham-operated rats did not differ from each other their data were pooled. There was a tendency for control and IBO rats to make fewer errors in the first eight choices. Using a performance criterion of eight correct choices on five consecutive days there was a significant ($p < 0.05$, Mann-Whitney U-test) increase in terms of days to criterion in the lead-exposed groups. Correspondingly, the number of days missing rewards was significantly raised in these groups ($p < 0.05$, Mann-Whitney U-test). In terms of time to make eight correct choices, not shown in Table 2, there were significant main effects between groups according to ANOVA with repeated measures on the day factor ($p < 0.05$). Post hoc comparisons revealed significantly less time for IBO vs. controls and significantly more time for P 750 ppm vs. controls ($p < 0.05$, Tukey). Rats having reached criterion in the acquisition phase were tested for retention

Table 1 Measures of internal exposure: blood and brain lead levels and ALAD activity in red blood cells at the age of 100 days (means ± SD)

Groups	PbB (μg/100 ml)	Pb-Brain (μg/g)	ALAD (U/l)
Controls	< 1	< 0.03	5.67 ± 1.12
P 250	16.2 ± 3.7	0.122 ± 0.030	3.00 ± 0.83
P 750	31.5 ± 4.0	0.278 ± 0.025	2.01 ± 0.37
P 2250	63.0 ± 14.3	0.880 ± 0.195	1.60 ± 0.60
M 250	< 1	< 0.03	6.11 ± 1.76
M 750	< 1	< 0.03	5.24 ± 1.59
M 2250	< 1	< 0.03	5.91 ± 1.65

Table 2 Performance by control rats (Co), rats with maternal (M 750) and permanent (P 750) lead exposure, and rats with selective neuronal depletion in the dorsal hippocampus (IBO); original acquisition in the radial arm maze

Group	n	No. of rats reaching criterion	No. of days to reach criterion	No. of days missing rewards	No. of different arms in the first eight choices	No. of errors	No. of correct choices before first error
Co	19	19	7.1 ± 1.3	1.9 ± 0.8	5.9 ± 0.3	6.9 ± 0.9	5.2 ± 0.3
IBO	20	19	7.0 ± 1.2	1.6 ± 0.7	5.9 ± 0.1	6.4 ± 0.8	5.1 ± 0.3
M 750	10	6	10.7 ± 3.1†	3.7 ± 1.9*†	5.5 ± 0.6	7.1 ± 1.7	4.9 ± 0.4
P 750	10	8	10.2 ± 2.6†	4.0 ± 2.4*†	5.5 ± 0.5	7.2 ± 1.2	5.1 ± 0.5

The values reported are means ± 95% confidence intervals. *Significantly ($p < 0.05$) different from control values; † significantly ($p < 0.05$) different from IBO values

Table 3 Performance by control rats (Co), rats with maternal (M 750) and permanent (P 750) lead exposure, and rats with selective neuronal depletion in the dorsal hippocampus (IBO); retention in the radial arm maze

Group	n	No. of rats making eight correct choices · daily	No. of days missing rewards	No. of different arms in the first eight choices	No. of errors	No. of correct choices before first error
Co	19	13	0.4 ± 0.3	5.4 ± 0.7	7.9 ± 2.3	4.5 ± 0.6
IBO	19	9	0.9 ± 0.4*	5.2 ± 0.6	10.6 ± 2.3	4.8 ± 0.6
M 750	6	3	1.0 ± 0.9*	5.7 ± 0.7	7.3 ± 1.5	4.7 ± 1.3
P 750	8	2*	1.4 ± 0.7*	5.6 ± 0.6	9.3 ± 2.9	4.7 ± 0.9

The values reported are means ± confidence intervals. *Significantly ($p < 0.05$) different from Co values

after 4 weeks. More control rats completed the task (eight correct choices/day) than lead-exposed or IBO animals (see Table 3). Time to make eight correct choices during the 3 days, not given in Table 3, was not significantly different between groups. However, when this time measure was related to time to make eight correct choices in the acquisition phase the ratio was found to be significantly increased in all treated groups (lead-exposed vs. controls, $p < 0.05$, IBO vs. controls, $p < 0.002$).

The deficit induced by amygdala lesions at the age of 500 days was similar to that induced by lead, in that there was an increase in time to make eight correct choices in comparison to controls by either kind of treatment. Testing for retention also revealed similar behaviour between lead-exposed and lesioned animals. This outcome must be considered preliminary as the histological examination is not yet complete. In addition to the deficit exhibited by lesioned and lead-treated rats, and in contrast to all previous age points, there was a significant ($p < 0.05$) difference between permanently and maternally exposed rats at this age in the acquisition part.

Visual discrimination learning

In contrast to previous observations there were no group differences for errors in the acquisition phase of visual discrimination learning at the age of 100 days. After 6 weeks retention of the task was significantly impaired ($p < 0.01$; Figure 1) in all lead-exposed groups as compared to controls. There were no differences between maternally and permanently exposed animals

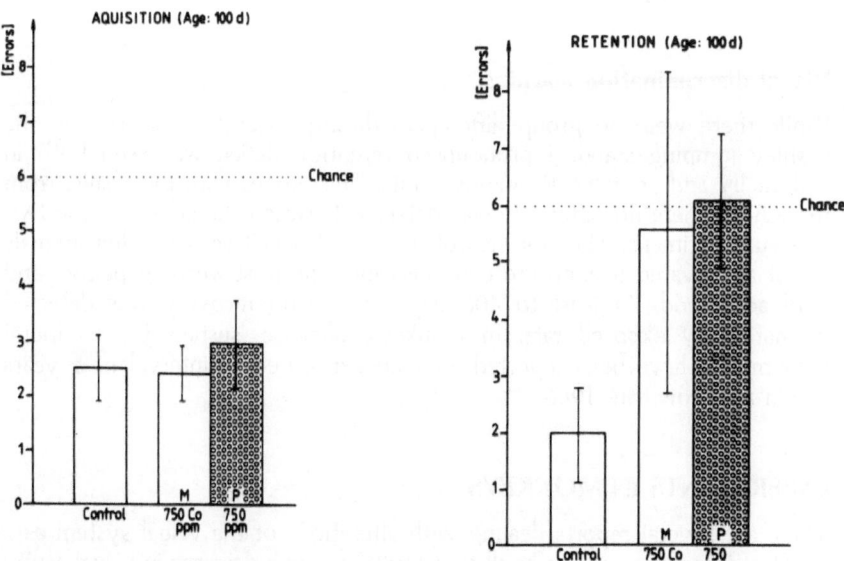

Figure 1 Visual discrimination, learning. Mean error scores ± confidence limits for control, maternal (750 Co) and permanent (750 ppm) lead-exposed rats. Both treated groups were significantly different ($p < 0.01$) from controls in the retention part

(see Figure 1). This outcome was replicated in animals at age 400 days. A significant retention deficit was also observed in animals having received 250 ppm lead acetate in their diet at this age.

DISCUSSION

Radial arm maze

The impaired performance of lead-exposed rats during acquisition of spatial learning agrees with former observations at much higher levels of exposure (Alfano and Petit, 1981). This lead-induced deficit does not resemble effects of chemical lesions of the hippocampus with ibotenic acid. Unlike lead-exposed animals, those with hippocampal depletion took less time than controls to make eight correct choices. Thus chemical lesions of the hippocampus, in contrast to mechanical ones, fail to impair spatial learning. This outcome is in accordance with previous results (Jarrard, 1983; Jarrard et al., 1984).

In the retention part of the experiment IBO-lesioned animals, as well as lead-exposed ones, are impaired, although only rats successful in the acquisition phase were used. Thus the behavioural profile obtained after chemical lesions of the hippocampus causing depletion of only intrinsic neurons is different from that seen after lead exposure. Therefore the hippocampus cannot be considered the sole target of lead, and examination of other brain regions is desirable. Recent data from chemical lesions of the amygdala show a greater similarity with lead-induced effects, in that both acquisition and retention were impaired by either kind of treatment.

Visual discrimination learning

While there were no group differences during acquisition of VDL in the Lashley jumping stand, a pronounced retention deficit was seen both in maternally and permanently exposed rats. This agrees with the results from the RAM where no difference was detected between the effects of the two exposure regimens. Thus the neurobehavioural deficit seen in adult animals is not aggravated if exposure continues into the post-weaning period, and until adulthood. At least to 400 days of age no recovery was detected in maternally exposed rats. In monkeys, likewise, sustained behavioural impairments have been reported after an exposure-free interval of 5 years (Levin and Bowman, 1986).

EXPERIMENTS IN MONKEYS

There are several reports dealing with alterations of the visual system as a result of lead exposure. Bushnell et al. (1977) found a decrease in visual acuity under scotopic conditions in monkeys. In rats visual evoked potentials are affected by lead, but the results are not consistent: latency increase (Fox et al., 1977) and decrease (Feeney et al., 1979), as well as amplitude decrement

420

(Winneke, 1979) have been reported. From *in vitro* experiments there is evidence that retinal function is influenced by lead (Fox and Sillman, 1979; Sillman *et al.*, 1984). The purpose of the present experiments was to investigate the visual evoked potential (VEP) and the electroretinogram (ERG) in lead-exposed monkeys, in order to assess central and peripheral aspects of visual information processing. The results reported here are still preliminary, since additional animals remain to be tested.

Methods

For details of the exposure regimen and internal exposure parameters see Lilienthal *et al.* (1986). For VEP measurements 10 male rhesus monkeys were used at the age of $7-7\frac{1}{4}$ years. They were pre- and postnatally exposed to 0 ($n = 3$), 350 ($n = 3$), or 600 ppm ($n = 4$) lead acetate in lab chow. Mean blood lead levels at the age of 3–4 years had been 9.5, 51.7, and 71.4 µg/100 g blood, respectively (Lilienthal *et al.*, 1986). Subjects for the ERG part of the study were 10 male and five female monkeys (controls: $n = 5$, 350 ppm: $n = 6$, 600 ppm: $n = 4$).

Visual evoked potentials

VEP responses were recorded to flash stimulation at a frequency of 1.5 Hz; 128 responses were averaged on a 1500 Digital EMG-System (DISA). The frequency range of the amplifier was 2 Hz–0.1 kHz. Needle electrodes were placed under the skin over the right striate cortex and on the midline of the frontal cortex for reference. Potentials were taken at two different background illumination conditions: bright (95 lux) vs. dark (0.02 lux). On a single session five VEPs were recorded under each condition and means taken across two different sessions. Pupil dilatation was achieved with one drop each of a 0.2% solution of tropicamide and of a 2% solution of phenylephrine. A half-circular arrangement of mirrors was placed in front of the monkey's head. The flash was behind and above the monkey's head, pointing to the mirror image of his face.

Electroretinograms

For ERG recordings ERG jets (Universo SA) were placed on the cornea of each eye. The cornea was desensitized with topical application of oxybuprocain (0.4%). The reference electrodes were positioned behind the supraorbitalic tori. The monkeys looked directly into the flash, which was at a distance of 60 cm. ERGs were taken during the course of dark adaptation. Responses to two single flashes were recorded at intervals of 4 min. For ERG measurements animals were sedated with an intramuscular (i.m.) injection of ketamine (10 mg/kg) and maintained on 1 mg/kg xylazine i.m. Pupil dilatation was achieved in the same way as for VEP recordings. Signals were bandpass filtered between 2 and 50 Hz.

In the fully dark-adapted eye oscillatory potentials (OP) were measured after the ERG records were finished. Sixteen responses were averaged. Stimulation frequency was 1 Hz. Filter setting of the amplifier was 0.1 kHz (lower) and 1 kHz (upper). Two OPs were taken from each eye. Between records there was a stimulus-free interval of 2 min.

Results

Visual evoked potentials
An example of VEP traces is given in Figure 2. Amplitude was defined as the overall amplitude of the signal. Under the dark background illuminance condition there was a dose-dependent decrease in amplitudes. The difference was significant for controls vs. 600 ppm animals ($p < 0.028$, Mann-Whitney U-test) and approaching significance for controls vs. 350 ppm ($p < 0.1$). With the bright background there was a significant decrease ($p < 0.05$) in amplitudes in the 350 ppm group when compared to controls and a marginally significant decrease for controls vs. 600 ppm ($p < 0.1$). Latencies of the VEP were defined as peak latencies of the latest peak in the first negative deflection of the signal. There was a significant increase in latencies for controls vs. 600 ppm ($p < 0.028$) under the dark background condition. With the bright background a dose-dependent increase in latencies was found. Differences were significant for controls vs. 350 ppm ($p < 0.05$) and for controls vs. 600 ppm ($p < 0.028$).

Electroretinograms
Figures 3 and 4 give examples of ERGs and OPs, respectively. ERG records were analysed by analysis of variance with repeated measures. Increases in amplitudes of the b-wave during the course of dark adaptation were more pronounced in lead-exposed animals than in controls ($p < 0.0521$); Table 4. Peak latencies of the b-wave, as well as OPs, were not affected by lead-exposure.

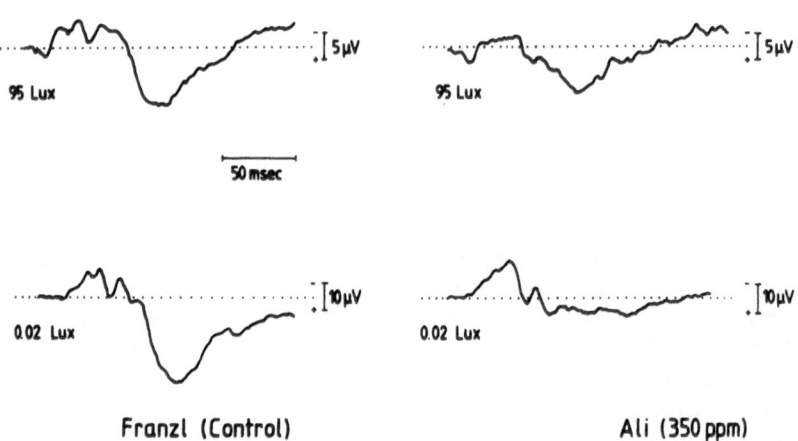

Figure 2 Examples of VEP traces of individual monkeys. Potentials were recorded under a bright (95 lux) and a dark (0.02 lux) background illuminance condition

422

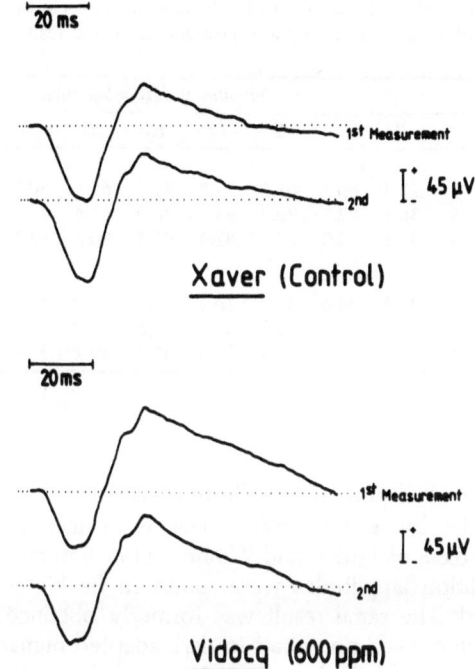

Figure 3 Examples of ERG traces of individual monkeys after 20 min of dark adaptation. Two potentials were recorded in response to two single flashes every 4 min. The cornea negative a-wave appears first, then the cornea positive b-wave

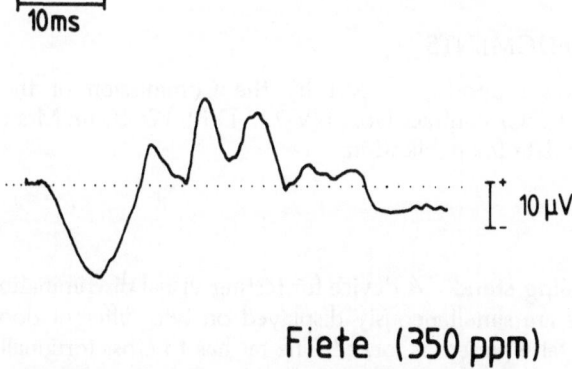

Figure 4 An example of oscillatory potentials (OP) which are bandpass filtered from the ERG. The OP was not found to be altered by lead treatment

Table 4 Latency and amplitude of the ERG b-wave: increases in amplitudes during the course of dark adaptation were more pronounced in the lead-exposed groups ($p = 0.52$)

Group	n	\multicolumn{9}{c}{Minutes of dark adaptation}
		0	4	8	12	16	20	24	28	32
Amplitude (μV)										
Control	5	27.4	60.2	68.8	71.5	71.8	68.1	50.3	54.1	52.4
350 ppm	5	38.1	72.7	79.9	83.4	78.9	82.4	84.8	84.7	80.9
600 ppm	4	32.8	72.0	87.2	87.4	92.3	90.8	92.3	83.1	76.6
Latency (ms)										
Control	5	24.8	33.6	34.7	36.4	37.7	39.0	39.6	40.3	40.6
350 ppm	5	24.6	32.2	34.1	36.1	37.6	37.9	39.3	39.8	40.5
600 ppm	4	25.4	33.1	35.4	36.8	38.2	39.1	39.9	39.9	40.2

Discussion

Findings in flash-evoked potentials indicate a decrease in amplitudes and an increase in latencies by lead exposure. This is in accordance with earlier observations by Fox *et al.* (1977) and Winneke (1979) in rats. Under the dark background condition amplitudes were found to be higher than with the bright background. The same result was formerly obtained by Perry *et al.* (1968) testing flash-evoked potentials in dark-adapted humans.

Increase in amplitude of the b-wave of the ERG during the course of dark adaptation was more pronounced in lead-exposed than in control monkeys. There is some evidence that the summed ERG arises primarily from the paramacular parts of the retina, in contrast to the VEP which is dominated by the response of the macular area (Spekreijse and Apkarian, 1986); however, the precise interrelationship of ERG and VEP findings, and the effects of lead on these different responses, remain to be determined.

ACKNOWLEDGMENTS

This work was supported in part by the Commission of the European Communities (CEC), contract No. ENV-733-D(B). We thank Mrs H. Krüll for preparing the data for publication.

GLOSSARY

Lashley jumping stand A device for testing visual discrimination learning. Two patterns are simultaneously displayed on two different doors and the one with the false pattern is locked. The rat has to cross (originally to jump) and pass through the door with the correct pattern to get a reward.

Stereotaxically A stereotax is a device in which the head of an animal is put in a frame with scales for the three dimensions. In this way one is enabled to insert the tip of an injection needle or electrode into distinct brain regions according to the coordinates reported in a brain atlas for a given species.

Macular The area of the macula lutea (yellow spot) on the retina. In primates this includes the fovea. It is the region where cones are most densely packed, and where the acuity is highest.

Paramacular The area on the retina surrounding the macula.

Scotopic Scotopic vision is the vision of the dark-adapted eye, in contrast to photopic vision when the eye is light-adapted.

REFERENCES

Alfano, D.P and Petit, T.L. (1981) Behavioral effects of postnatal lead exposure: possible relationship to hippocampal dysfunction. *Behav. Neural Biol.*, **32**, 319–333

Alfano, D.P. and Petit, T.L. (1982) Neonatal lead exposure alters the development of hippocampal dentate granule cells. *Exp. Neurol.*, **75**, 275–288

Alfano, D.P., LeBoutillier, J.C. and Petit, T.L. (1982) Hippocampal mossy fiber pathway development in normal and postnatally lead exposed rats. *Exp. Neurol.*, **75**, 308–319

Alfano, D.P., Petit, T.L. and LeBoutillier, J.C. (1983) Development and plasticity of the hippocampal cholinergic system in normal and early lead exposed rats. *Dev. Brain Res.*, **10**, 117–124

Bushnell, P.J., and Bowman, R.E. (1979) Persistence of impaired reversal learning in young monkeys exposed to low levels of dietary lead. *J. Toxicol. Env. Health*, **5**, 1015–1023

Bushnell, P.J., Bowman, R.E., Allen, J.R. and Marlar, R.J. (1977) Scotopic vision deficits in young monkeys exposed to lead. *Science*, **196**, 333–335

Campbell, J., Woolley, D.E., Vijayan, V.K. and Overmann, S.R. (1982) Morphometric effects of postnatal lead exposure on hippocampal development of the 15-day-old rat. *Dev. Brain Res.*, **3**, 595–612

Campbell, J., Overmann, S.R., Woolley, D.E. and Vijayan, V.K. (1984) Morphometric effects of preweaning lead exposure on the hippocampal formation of adult rats. *Neorotoxicology*, **5**, 125–148

Danscher, G., Hall, E., Fredens, K., Fjerdingstad, E. and Fjerdingstad, E.J. (1975) Heavy metals in the amygdala of the rat: zinc, lead and copper. *Brain Res.*, **94**, 167–172

Danscher, G., Fjerdingstad, E.J., Fjerdingstad, E. and Fredens, K. (1976) Heavy metal content in subdivisions of the rat hippocampus (zinc, lead and copper). *Brain Res.*, **112**, 442–446

Feeney, D.M., Longo, J.F., Cosden, M.A., Zenick, H. and Padich, R. (1979) Detection of the effects of lead exposure by visual evoked response latency. *Physiol. Psychol.*, **7**, 143–145

Fjerdingstad, E.J., Danscher, G. and Fjerdingstad, E. (1974) Hippocampus: selective concentration of lead in the normal rat brain. *Brain Res.*, **80**, 350–354

Fox, D.A. and Sillman, A.J. (1979) Heavy metals affect rod, but not cone, photoreceptors. *Science*, **206**, 78–80

Fox, D.A., Lewkowski, J.P. and Cooper, G.P. (1977) Acute and chronic effects of neonatal lead exposure on development of the visual evoked response in rats. *Toxicol. Appl. Pharmacol.*, **40**, 449–461

Gross-Selbeck, E. and Gross-Selbeck, M. (1981) Changes in operant behavior of rats exposed to lead at the accepted no-effect level. *Clin. Toxicol.*, **18**, 1247–1256

Hastings, L., Cooper, G.P., Bornschein, R.L. and Michealson, I.A. (1979) Behavioral deficits in adult rats following neonatal lead exposure. *Neurobehav. Toxicol.*, **1**, 227–231

Jarrard, L.E. (1983) Selective hippocampal lesions and behavior: effects of kainic acid lesions on performance of place and cue tasks. *Behav. Neurosci.*, **97**, 873–889

Jarrard, L.E., Okaichi, H., Steward, O. and Goldschmidt, R.B. (1984) On the role of the hippocampal connections in the performance of place and cue tasks: comparison to damage of the hippocampus. *Behav. Neurosci.*, **98**, 946–954

Levin, E.D. and Bowman, R.E. (1986) Long-term lead effects on the Hamilton search task and delayed spatial alternation in monkeys. *Neurobehav. Toxicol. Teratol.*, **8**, 219–224

Lilienthal, H., Winneke, G., Brockhaus, A. and Molik, B. (1986) Pre- and postnatal lead exposure in monkeys: effects on activity and learning set formation. *Neurobehav. Toxicol. Teratol.*, **8**, 265–272

Munoz, C., Garbe, K., Lilienthal, H. and Winneke, G. (1988) Significance of hippocampal dysfunction in low level lead exposure of rats. *Neurobehav. Toxicol. Teratol.*, **10**, 245–253

Olton, D.S., Becker, J.T. and Handelman, G.E. (1979) Hippocampus, space and memory. *Behav. Brain Sci.*, **2**, 313–365

Perry, N.W., Childers, D.G., Dawson, W.H. and Stewart, H.L. (1968) Dark-adapted visual evoked response. *76th Annual Convention of the American Psycological Association*, pp. 315–316

Shih, T.M. and Hanin, I. (1978) Effects of chronic lead exposure on levels of acetylcholine and choline and acetylcholine turnover rate in rat brain areas *in vivo*. *Psychopharmacology*, **58**, 263–269

Sillman, A.J., Bolnick, D.A., Bosetti, J.B., Haynes, L.W. and Walter, A.E. (1984) The effect of lead on photoreceptor response amplitude – Influence of the light stimulus. *Exp. Eye Res.*, **39**, 183–194

Spekreijse, H. and Apkarian, P. (1986) The use of a system analysis approach to electrodiagnostic (ERG and VEP) assessment. *Vision Res.*, **26**, 195–219

Walsh, T.J., Miller, D.B. and Dyer, R.S. (1982) Trimethyltin, a selective limbic system neurotoxicant, impairs radial arm maze performance. *Neurobehav. Toxicol. Teratol.*, **4**, 177–183

Winneke, G. (1979) Modification of visual evoked potentials in rats after longterm blood lead elevation. *Activ. Nerv. Sup.*, *(Praha)*, **21**, 282–284

Winneke, G., Brockhaus, A. and Baltissen, R. (1977) Neurobehavioral and systemic effects of longterm blood lead-elevation in rats. *Arch. Toxicol.*, **37**, 247–263

426

5.3
Behavioural Effects of Low-level Developmental Exposure to Lead in the Monkey

D. C. RICE

SUMMARY

Cynomolgus monkeys (*Macaca fascicularis*) dosed from birth onward with 0, 50, 100, or 500 µg/kg per day of lead had blood lead (PbB) levels of 3, 15, 25, or 55 µg/dl, respectively, before withdrawal of infant formula at 200 days of age, and later steady-state PbB levels of 3, 11, 13 or 33 µg/dl. Beginning at age 3 years these monkeys began performance on behavioural tasks designed to assess types of deficits found in children with moderate body burdens of lead, including various forms of intellectual impairment, distractibility and short attention span, and hyperactivity. The first task used here was an intermittent schedule of reinforcement, the fixed interval (FI), which required the monkey to make one response after a specified time had elapsed in order to receive a fruit juice reward. Although responding before the specified time had no consequences, monkeys (as well as other animals and humans) typically respond throughout the interval. Thus, this schedule is capable of measuring the ongoing activity of the monkey. Treated monkeys made more responses under these conditions than did control monkeys, and the effect was dose-related. Moreover, response rates for treated monkeys were more variable, both between days and even across a 50-min session, than for the control animals.

Following FI schedule testing, each monkey was tested on another intermittent schedule, the DRL (differential reinforcement of low rate), which assessed the monkey's ability to inhibit responding. This required the monkey to wait at least 30 s before responding in order to receive a reward. Although the lead-treated monkeys were able to learn the task, they did so at a slower rate than controls and were more variable in their performance from day to day than the controls (similar to the FI results).

Short-term memory and attention were measured by two techniques: (1) delayed matching to sample, which required the monkey to remember a stimulus and signal this by choosing the correct stimulus out of three samples; and (2) a test of spatial memory, which required the monkey simply to alternate responses between two buttons, with a delay interposed between responses. On both tasks, treated monkeys were markedly deficient compared to controls.

The final task measured the monkeys' ability to adapt to changes in the behavioural requirements of their environment. Each monkey was required to learn a series of discrimination tasks and, once learned, to learn the exact opposite task; that is, the correct answer became the incorrect, and vice-versa. Again, treated monkeys were impaired relative to controls in regard to such reversal behaviour.

These results collectively provide strong evidence for developmental exposure to lead causing behavioural impairment in the monkey, even at PbB levels near the current average for children in the United States and below presently accepted US criteria for undue risk of lead toxicity.

It has become increasingly apparent that body burdens of lead common in children living in industrialized nations result in unequivocal behavioural changes, several types of which are predictable. In the Needleman *et al.* (1979) study, it was reported that children with moderate lead body burdens suffered an IQ deficit compared to children with lower body burdens, as well as increased distractibility, decreased attention span, and difficulty in following directions. Subsequently, a number of studies have reported virtually identical findings (Winneke *et al.*, 1983; Yule *et al.*, 1981). These studies collectively strongly support the notion that lead exposure during early development has profound effects on behaviour in children.

The monkey is often the best animal model with which to characterize effects on nervous system development produced by toxicants. Like humans, monkeys have a long period of gestation, infancy, and sexual immaturity during which they continue to develop. This long period of vulnerability allows both investigation of critical variables concerning sensitive periods of exposure and testing of the organism over a period of years before adulthood is reached. The monkey's nervous system is very similar to the human and often responds to toxic insult in a similar manner. The monkey's behavioural repertoire, both spontaneous and conditioned, is also more like that of the human than is that of other laboratory species. The sensory systems of monkeys are also like those of humans, whereas those of other species may be so dissimilar as to render them inappropriate as models for sensory system testing.

A variety of operant conditioning techniques have been used to assess nervous system damage produced by exposure to lead in the monkey. Several classes of tests are proving to be sensitive in detecting behavioural impairment produced by toxicants (Laties, 1978), tests that are drawn largely from the fields of behavioural pharmacology, experimental psychology, and the neurosciences. Intermittent schedules of reinforcement offer a powerful tool for studying the effects of toxicants and have proven to be sensitive indicators of low-level lead exposure in both rodents and monkeys (Rice and Gilbert, 1985; Cory-Slechta *et al.*, 1983; Angell and Weiss, 1982; Rice *et al.*, 1979). Tests of cognitive processes have also revealed impairment produced by lead exposure in the monkey (Rice, 1984a, 1985a, b; Levin and Bowman, 1983; Rice and Willes, 1979; Bushnell and Bowman, 1979a, b), as might be expected from reports of intellectual impairment and distractibility in children exposed to lead.

In the present study, monkeys were tested by using a minicomputer for experimental control and data acquisition. This obviates the need for subject–experimenter interaction during behavioural testing, simplifies testing of many monkeys at once, and allows more sophisticated data collection and analysis than is possible with other types of behavioural testing equipment.

SUBJECTS AND TOXICANT EXPOSURE

Infant monkeys (*Macaca fascicularis*) separated from their mothers at birth were reared in a primate nursery (Willes *et al.*, 1977). The infant monkeys were able to see and hear other monkeys at all times and, beginning at 3 weeks of age, were exercised in large cages with their peers. This regimen allowed them to develop normally both socially and intellectually (Harlow *et al.*, 1971). The monkeys were dosed orally 7 or (later in the study) 5 days per week. Infants were dosed by syringe, and older monkeys voluntarily consumed gelatin capsules containing the dose. Food consumption, weight gain, routine haematology, blood biochemistry, and clinical neurological status did not differ between control and treated monkeys.

Monkeys were exposed to lead from day 1 of life onward, at doses equivalent to 0, 50, 100 or 500 μg/kg per day. For all treated groups, blood lead (PbB) levels peaked by 100 days of age and decreased to a steady level after withdrawal from infant formula at 200 days of age (Willes *et al.*, 1980) (Table 1). The highest dose of lead resulted in both peak and steady-state blood levels considered to be deleterious to children by criteria of the United States Environmental Protection Agency (1984) and Centers for Disease Control (1985). Both agencies regard a blood concentration for an individual child of 25 μg/dl without elevation of erythrocyte protoporphyrin (EP) concentration to be safe. This presumably allows an adequate margin of safety

Table 1 Blood lead and EP concentrations early in life (peak) and at steady-state conditions

Lead dose (μg/kg per day)	Blood level mean $\pm$ SE (μg/100 ml whole blood)		EP mean $\pm$ SE (μg/100 ml whole blood)	
	Peak	Steady state	Peak	Steady state
0 (control)	2.2 $\pm$ 0.4	3.4 $\pm$ 0.8	19.9 $\pm$ 2.7	30.9 $\pm$ 4.8
50	15.4 $\pm$ 1.7*	10.9 $\pm$ 0.7*	53.5 $\pm$ 14.2	15.9 $\pm$ 3.1
100	25.4 $\pm$ 2.0*	13.1 $\pm$ 1.4*	72.1 $\pm$ 18.3	15.8 $\pm$ 5.2
500	53.4 $\pm$ 6.7*	32.8 $\pm$ 5.5*	222.9 $\pm$ 32.2*	151.7 $\pm$ 24.1*

* Significantly different from control ($p < 0.01$) using modified Dunnett's procedures (log scale)

against adverse health effects, including behavioural impairment. Accordingly, in this study, PbB levels of monkeys in both of the lower dose groups were always within the limits presently established for safety and, in fact, are found routinely in the general human population (Mahaffey et al., 1982). In contrast, the PbB levels of control monkeys were below those of most people in industrialized countries (i.e. $< 5 \mu g/dl$). EP levels were significantly higher than control values only for the highest dose group, both for peak and steady-state conditions. A significant linear log dose—response relationship was observed at the time of peak PbB concentrations, although the lower two lead dose groups were not different from control. These data are in good agreement with those for children. EP elevation in children occurs at PbB levels between 15 and 20 $\mu g/dl$ (Cavalleri et al., 1981; Piomelli et al., 1982; Hernberg, 1980). However, EP may not be a very good predictor of PbB level for an individual child; elevated PbB levels often occur in the absence of detectable EP elevation (Bush et al., 1982).

The above monkeys have thus far been tested on a variety of behavioural tasks beginning as juveniles (2.5–3.0 years of age) and continuing through young adulthood (7.0–8.0 years of age). Such tests have included measures of activity, learning, short-term memory, and adaptability.

MEASURES OF 'ACTIVITY'

Fixed interval performance

The effect of lead has been examined on an intermittent schedule of reinforcement, the fixed interval (FI) schedule (Rice et al., 1979; Rice, 1984b). Activity measures are most often made on a particular activity (e.g., locomotion or rearing behaviour), while the organism is engaging in a variety of other behaviours at the same time. Such methods are bound to be both variable and imprecise. One advantage of studying an intermittent schedule is that the activity to be performed by the animal is specified by the investigator. In the present experiment the monkey was required to press a lever once after 8 min had elapsed in order to receive a fruit juice reward. Responding earlier than 8 min had no scheduled consequences. Although only one response is required for reinforcement, FI performance is characterized by responding throughout most of the interval. The rate and pattern of responses are characteristic of the individual, since they are not specified by the FI schedule. The performance of normal animals, as well as the effects of many psychoactive agents, have been well characterized for this schedule.

One way of examining characteristics of the rate and pattern of responding is to compile histograms of the time between successive responses during a session. For example, the interresponse time (IRT) distributions for control and monkeys exposed to 500 $\mu g/kg$ per day of lead (the highest dose group) is depicted in Figure 1. All of the treated monkeys had a greater absolute number of responses than did the control animals, with three of the four lead-exposed monkeys having a distribution skewed towards very short times between successive responses. Thus, three of the treated monkeys were different from control in a manner similar to each other, while the fourth was

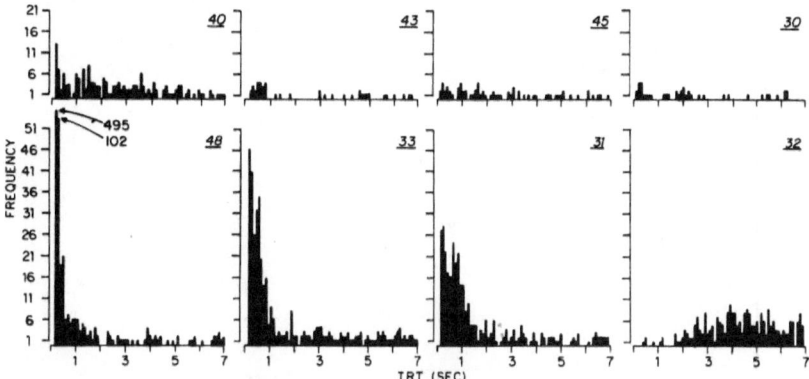

Figure 1 IRT absolute frequency distribution for one session of a fixed interval schedule for control (top) and monkeys exposed to 500 μg/kg per day of lead (bottom). The divisions along the abscissa represent classes of time between successive responses, in 100 ms increments. The lead-treated monkeys in general had a much higher absolute frequency of IRTs and a distribution skewed towards shorter IRTs

different from all others. This is an indication of the variability of response between treated animals, although at this dose the performance of all the monkeys may be considered to be affected by lead exposure.

A summary measure that may be derived from this kind of analysis is the median IRT, which reflects the number of responses emitted but omits much information concerning the pattern of response. On this measure there is a wide range of values for the control monkeys (Figure 2). This is typical of FI performance, since the reinforcement density does not depend on rate of response, within reasonable limits. With increasing lead dose the number of monkeys with longer median IRTs decreased, as did the average median IRT for the group. Thus, exposure to lead may shift the behaviour of the animal towards more activity.

Differential reinforcement of low rates (DRL)

Immediately following testing under the FI schedule, the lower dose groups (50 and 100 μg/kg per day and their controls) were tested under a DRL schedule (Rice and Gilbert, 1985), to determine whether the lead-exposed monkeys would be able to inhibit responding if required. In this schedule the monkey was required to withhold responding for at least 30 s. The first response made after 30 s had elapsed was reinforced. Responding before that time reset the contingency, and the monkey had to wait another 30 s for an opportunity for reinforcement. The terminal schedule was preceded by several training sessions in which the length of the waiting period was increased from 5 to 30 s.

During the initial sessions, lead exposure resulted in a decrease in the

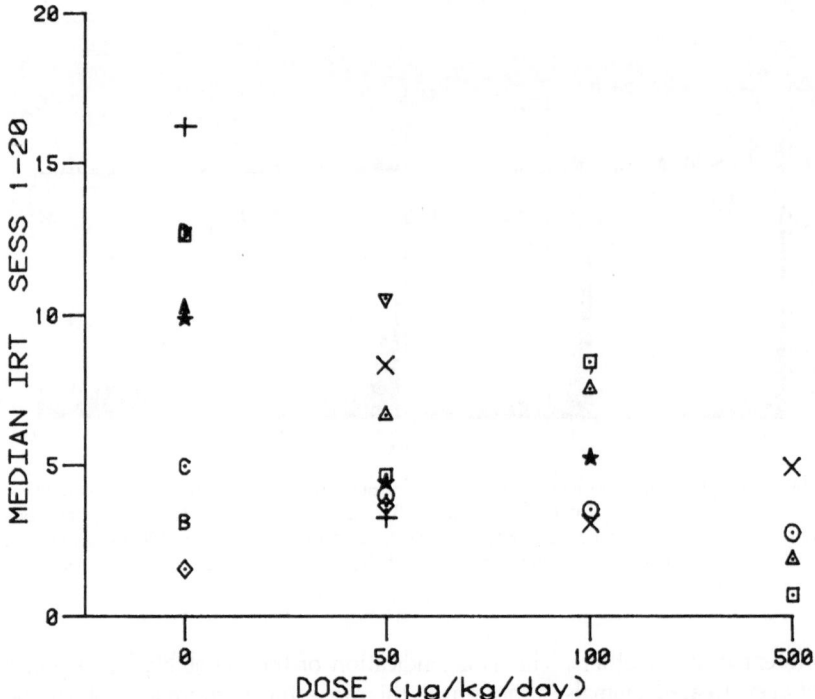

Figure 2 Median IRT for Sessions 1–20 of a fixed-interval schedule for monkeys exposed to 0, 50, 100 or 500 µg/kg per day of lead from birth (randomization test, $p = 0.05$, 0.08, 0.018 for 0 versus three dose groups, respectively). Each symbol represents an individual monkey

ability to adapt to the contingencies of the DRL. For example, the difference in number of reinforcements between Session 1 and Session 2 (both DRL 5 s) decreased with increasing lead body burden, indicating less improvement in performance in lead-treated monkeys (Figure 3). Similarly, a comparison of the first five to the second five DRL 30 s sessions revealed that increasing lead dose resulted in a dose-related impaired ability to 'learn' the DRL.

The treated monkeys also displayed more variability in their performance from day to day than did control monkeys. For example, there was a dose-related increase in variability for number of reinforcements per session over the last 10 sessions (Figure 4). This was true even though the number of reinforcements *per se* did not differ between groups. This reflects a more inconsistent performance of the treated monkeys.

COGNITIVE SKILLS

Discrimination reversal

A paradigm that examines a different set of behavioural skills was examined in monkeys from all the dose groups. This experiment was designed to test

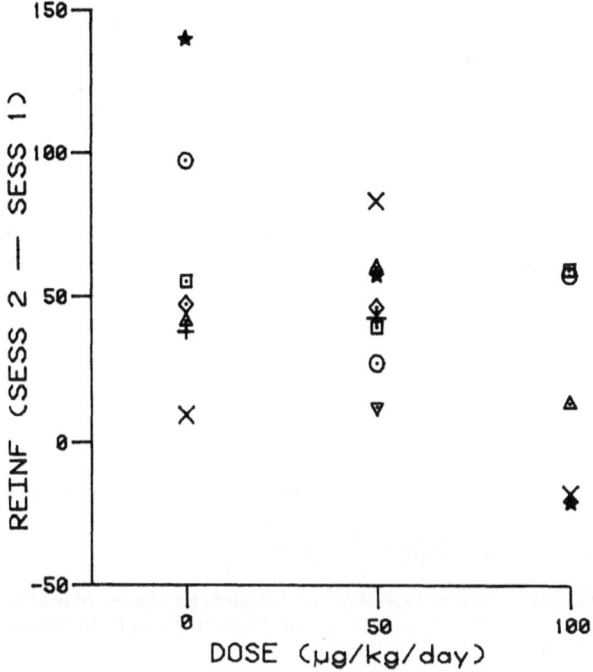

Figure 3 Difference in number of reinforcements between Session 1 and Session 2 on a DRL schedule for monkeys exposed to 0, 50, or 100 µg/kg per day of lead from birth (linear trend analysis, $p = 0.023$). Symbols as in Figure 2

the monkey's ability to adapt to a change in the effect its own behaviour produced in its environment, specifically, the ability of the monkey to respond in a manner opposite to a previously learned response. The performances of the 500 µg/kg per day group and its controls were examined before the lower dose groups were tested (Rice and Willes, 1979). The monkey faced two food wells, one covered with a cube and the other with a tetrahedron. Only the well under the cube contained a raisin, and the monkey learned to knock the cube off either well to get the raisin. When each monkey made at least nine correct choices out of 10 trials, the raisin was placed under the tetrahedron instead of the cube, and the monkey had to learn to respond to the formerly incorrect stimulus. A series of 20 such reversals was performed. At two points in the experiment the monkey was given extra trials between reversals to see if the performance of the lead-treated and control monkeys was disrupted differentially, as had been observed in rhesus monkeys at higher lead body burdens (Bushnell and Bowman, 1979a). The lead-treated monkeys made more errors per reversal, although their learning curves over successive reversals paralleled those of the controls (Figure 5). Lead-treated and control monkeys were disrupted to the same extent by the first series of 150 extra trials. The second series of 500 extra trials disrupted the performance of both sets of animals. These results suggest that the lead-treated monkeys had a more difficult time adapting their behaviour to new circumstances than

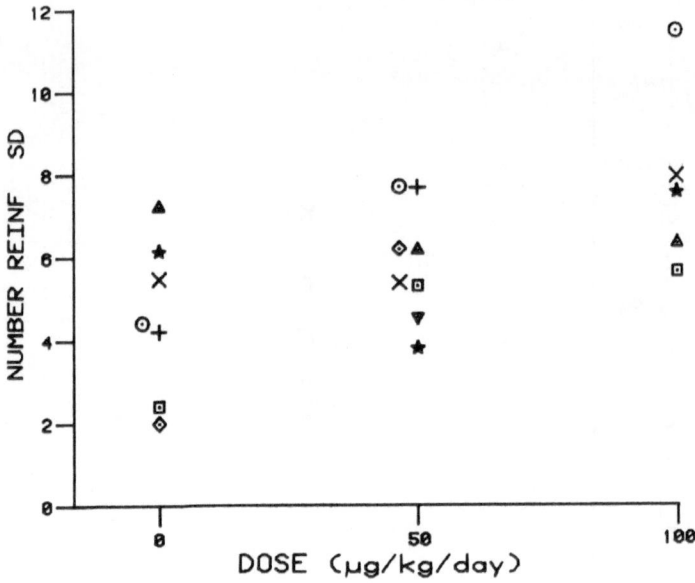

Figure 4 Variability of performance (standard deviation) for number of reinforcements over the last 10 sessions of a DRL 30 s schedule of reinforcement (linear trend analysis, $p = 0.003$). Symbols as in Figure 2

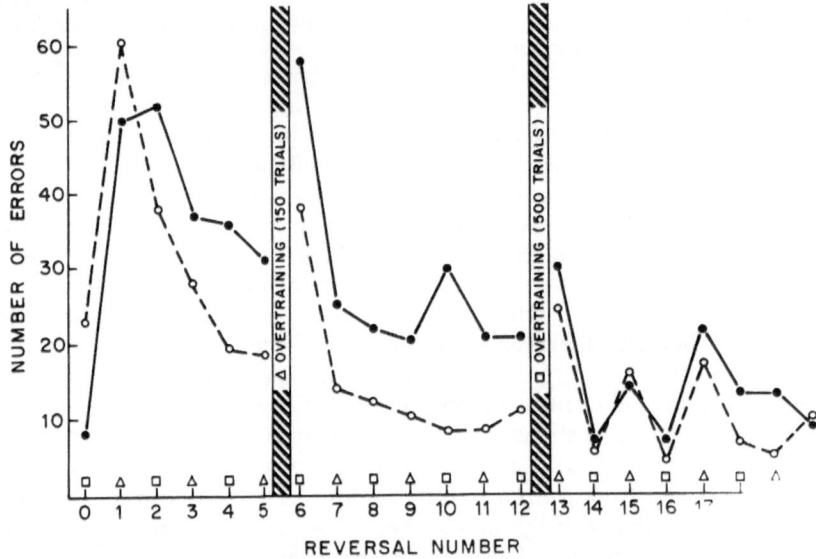

Figure 5 Mean number of unsuccessful trials to reversal criterion on a form discrimination task. Ordinate represents the mean number of trials for control (unfilled circles) and monkeys dosed with 500 μg/kg per day lead (filled circles) to satisfy the requirement of acquisition for each reversal. Striped bars represent the points in the experiment where monkeys were given extra trials before the next reversal. Treated monkeys made statistically more errors than controls before the second set of extra trials (ANOVA, $p < 0.05$)

434

did controls, and persevered in behaviours that were no longer appropriate to a changed environment.

A similar experiment was performed with the lower dose groups and their controls, utilizing a computer for stimulus display as well as experimental control and data acquisition (Rice, 1985a). The monkey faced a panel on which were two clear response discs and a tube for delivery of apple juice. The discs could be backlit with either a square or a triangle, and either a red or green surround. For the first task of the experiment one disc was backlit with the square and the other with the triangle, both with a red surround; the position at which they appeared was chosen randomly from trial to trial. The monkey was required to respond on the disc displaying the square in order to receive a small amount of apple juice. When the monkey had learned the task to a criterion of at least 9 out of 10 correct, the previously correct stimulus became the incorrect one, for a total of 15 reversals. After completion of this task the monkeys were tested on a colour discrimination with irrelevant forms. In addition to the cross and triangle, there was a red background on one disc and a green background on the other. Positions of forms and colours were displayed independently of each other. The monkey was required to attend to the colours and ignore the forms. Fifteen reversals were completed by each monkey. For both tasks there were treated monkeys that made more errors over the series of reversals than controls (Figure 6). An important aspect of these results is the presence of individual differences within the treated groups. Some animals were clearly different from controls, while others were not. This may be a typical effect of neurotoxicants at near-threshold levels.

Matching to sample

Short-term memory function was examined in monkeys exposed to the highest dose of lead (500 μg/kg per day) and their controls (Rice, 1984a). The ability to remember both spatial and non-spatial information was tested. For the non-spatial paradigm the monkey was required to press a disc that was lit with one of three colours a specified number of times, which turned off the light. After a specified delay period (varying from 0 s to several minutes), three test discs were lit, each with one of the three colours. The monkey pressed the disc corresponding to the colour that had appeared on the sample disc to receive a fruit juice reward. For the spatial matching to sample, one of the three test discs was lit. The monkey responded on this disc a specified number of times, which turned off the light. After a predetermined delay of variable duration, all three test discs were lit and the monkey responded on the previously lit disc to be reinforced. Performance on the non-spatial task was examined twice, with the spatial task interposed between. Each monkey was tested at increasing delay values until it reached a delay value at which it responded at a chance level.

The treated monkeys were impaired relative to controls on both the spatial and non-spatial matching tasks, even though they learned the matching tasks as readily as controls and performed as well at 0 s delay. For example, the

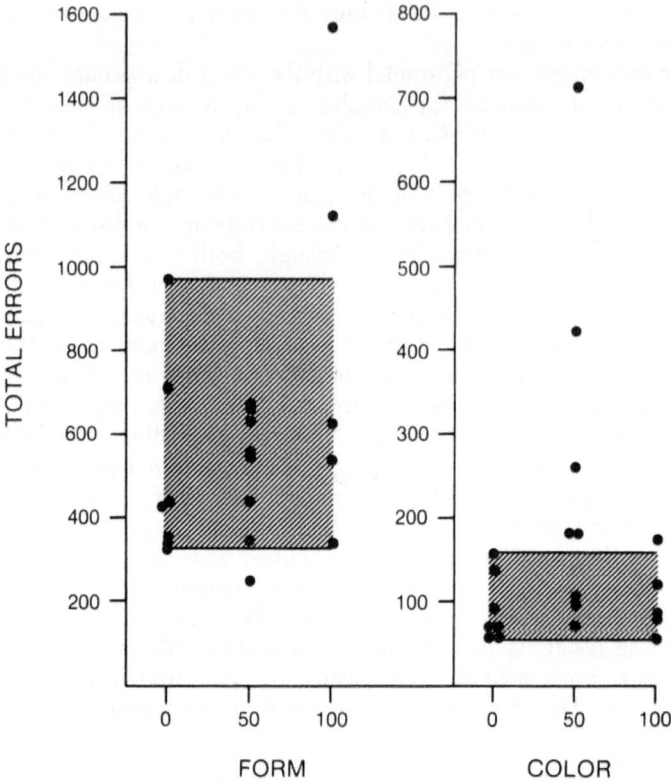

Figure 6 Total errors over the acquisition and 15 reversals of a form discrimination and colour discrimination with irrelevant cues for monkeys dosed with 0, 50, or 100 μg/kg per day of lead from birth (form discrimination, 0 versus 100, $p = 0.037$; colour discrimination, 0 versus 50, $p = 0.011$; 0 versus 100, $p = 0.08$ randomization test)

control monkeys were able to remember the stimulus to be matched longer than treated monkeys; that is, their performance decreased to chance levels at a longer delay value than that of treated monkeys (Figure 7). In addition, the number of errors over the course of delay values completed by all monkeys was significantly greater for lead-exposed monkeys ($p = 0.014$). An extremely interesting aspect of these results was that the errors made by the treated monkeys were due to interference from responses made on previous trials ($p = 0.029$), i.e., by responding on the lever and/or colour that had been correctly chosen on the previous trial. This suggests that an attentional deficit may be a component of the short-term memory deficit disclosed by this experiment.

Delayed alternation

The spatial memory of the lower dose groups (50 and 100 μg/kg per day) was tested by a different procedure, delayed alternation. In this task the

436

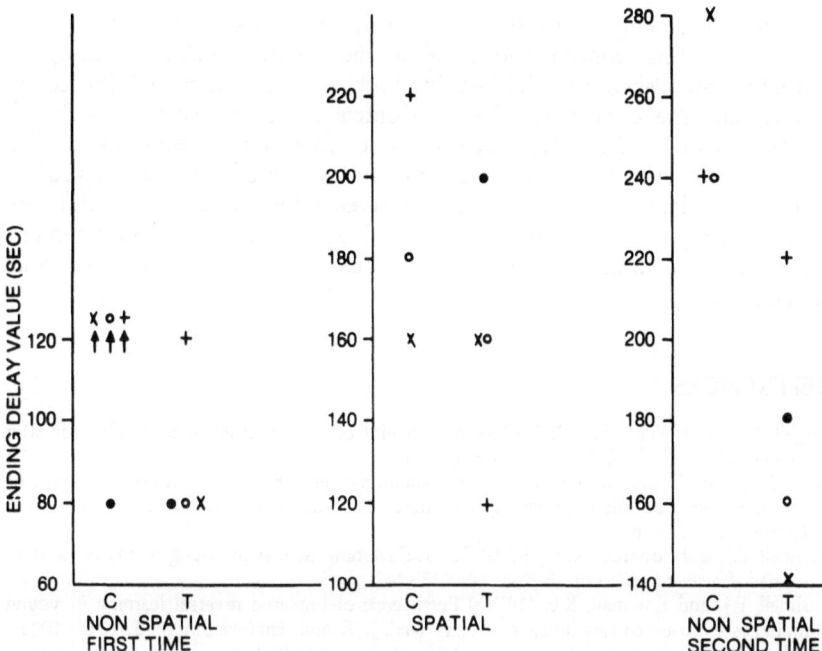

Figure 7 Ending delay value for variable-delay schedule for control (C) and monkeys exposed to 500 μg/kg per day of lead (T). For the non-spatial (first time), three control monkeys were performing above chance at 120 s but were not tested further, because all the treated monkeys were performing at chance levels (randomization test, $p = 0.033$, 0.20, and 0.029 for the three tasks, respectively)

monkey was required to alternate responses between two discs; each alternation was rewarded with a small amount of juice. After each monkey had learned the task, a delay was instituted between trials. The initial delay was very short and was increased in steps to 15 s by the end of the experiment. The most profound effect was at the longest delay, at which some of the treated monkeys failed to switch between discs, but rather responded on only one disc, in some cases for hours at a time (Rice, 1985b). Such behaviour was exhibited by all but one of the higher dose group and by 25% of the lower dose group. This represents a profound deficit on a behavioural task that proved extremely simple for the control monkeys. Moreover, these monkeys were no longer juveniles at the time of testing, but adults. This suggests that monkeys do not recover from the effects of developmental lead exposure.

SUMMARY AND CONCLUSIONS

We have found the monkey to be an extremely useful animal model with which to explore the effects of lead (as well as other neurotoxic agents) on the developing organism. The use of sophisticated behavioural methodology has allowed detection of clear, dose-related deficits as a result of lead exposure on tests of activity, attention and memory, distractibility and adaptability. In fact, deficits analogous to those observed in children were observed in monkeys at PbB concentrations below the criterion value ($\leqslant 25\ \mu g/dl$) currently established for children by both the Environmental Protection Agency and the Centers for Disease Control as being associated with risk for lead toxicity. Moreover, deficits were observed in monkeys at PbB concentrations near the mean for children in the United States at the present time. These data, especially when considered with the data from children, provide strong evidence that developmental exposure to lead at body burdens considered the norm in industrialized society may result in intellectual impairment.

REFERENCES

Angell, N.F. and Weiss, B. (1982) Operant behavior of rats exposed to lead before or after weaning. *Toxicol. Appl. Pharmacol.*, **63**, 62–71

Bush, B., Doran, D. and Jackson, K. (1982) Evaluation of erythrocyte protoporphyrin and zinc protoporphyrin as micro screening procedures for lead poisoning detection. *Ann. Clin. Biochem.*, **19**, 71–76

Bushnell, P.J. and Bowman, R.E. (1979a) Reversal learning deficits in young monkeys exposed to lead. *Pharmacol. Biochem. Behav.*, **10**, 733–742

Bushnell, P.J. and Bowman, R.E. (1979b) Persistence of impaired reversal learning in young monkeys exposed to low levels of dietary lead. *J. Toxicol. Environ. Health*, **5**, 1015–1023

Cavalleri, A., Baruffini, A., Minoia, C. and Bianco, L. (1981) Biologic response of children to low levels of inorganic lead, *Environ. Res.*, **25**, 415–423

Centers for Disease Control (1985) Preventing lead poisoning in young children – United States. *Morbidity and Mortality Weekly Report*, **34**, 66–73

Cory-Slechta, D.A., Weiss, B. and Cox, C. (1983) Delayed behavioral toxicity of lead with increasing lead exposure. *Toxicol. Appl. Pharmacol.*, **71**, 342–352

Harlow, H.F., Harlow, M.K., Schiltz, K.A. and Mohr, D.J. (1971) The effect of early adverse and enriched environments on the learning ability of rhesus monkeys, in Jarrard, L.E. (ed), *Cognitive Processes of Nonhuman Primates*, pp. 121–149 (New York: Academic Press)

Hernberg, S. (1980) Biochemical and clinical effects and responses as indicated by lead concentration, in Singhal, R. and Thomas, J. (eds), *Lead Toxicity*, pp. 367–399 (Baltimore: Urban & Schwartzenberg)

Laties, V.G. (1978) How operant conditioning can contribute to behavioral toxicology. *Environ. Health Perspect.*, **26**, 29–35

Levin, E.D. and Bowman, R.E. (1983) The effect of pre- and post-natal lead exposure on Hamilton search task in monkeys. *Neurobehav. Toxicol. Teratol.*, **5**, 391–394

Mahaffey, K., Annest, J., Roberts, J. and Murphy, R. (1982) National estimates of blood lead levels: United States, 1976–1980. *N. Engl. J. Med.*, **307**, 573–579

Needleman, H.L., Gunnoe, C., Leviton, A., Reed, R., Peresie, H., Maher, C. and Barrett, P. (1979) Deficits in psychologic and classroom performance of children with elevated dentine lead levels. *N. Engl. J. Med.*, **300**, 689–695

Piomelli, S., Seaman, C., Zullow, D., Curran, A. and Davidow, B. (1982) Threshold for lead damage to heme synthesis in urban children, *Proc. Natl. Acad. Sci. USA*, **79**, 3335–3339

Rice, D.C. (1984a) Behavioral deficit (delayed matching to sample) in monkeys exposed from birth to low levels of lead. *Toxicol. Appl. Pharmacol.*, **75**, 337–345

Rice, D.C. (1984b) Effect of lead on schedule-controlled behavior in the monkey, in Seiden, L.S. and Balster, R.L. (eds), *Behavioral Pharmacology: The Current Status*, pp. 473–486 (New York: Alan R. Liss)

Rice, D.C. (1985a) Chronic low-lead exposure from birth produces deficits in discrimination reversal in monkeys. *Toxicol. Appl. Pharmacol.*, **77**, 201–210

Rice, D.C. (1985b). Behavioral toxicity in monkeys exposed to low levels of lead from birth. *Toxicologist*, **5**, 23

Rice, D.C. and Gilbert, S.G. (1985). Low lead exposure from birth produces behavioral toxicity

(DRL) in monkeys. *Toxicol. Appl. Pharmacol.*, **80**, 421–426

Rice, D.C. and Willes, R.W. (1979). Neonatal low-level lead exposure in monkeys: effect on two-choice non-spatial form discrimination. *J. Environ. Pathol. Toxicol.*, **2**, 1195–1203

Rice, D.C., Gilbert, S.G. and Willes, R.W. (1979) Neonatal low-level lead exposure in monkeys: locomotor activity, schedule-controlled behavior, and the effects of amphetamine. *Toxicol. Appl. Pharmacol.*, **51**, 503–513

US Environmental Protection Agency (1984) Regulation of fuel and fuel additives; lead phase down. *Fed. Regist.*, **49**(150), 31032–31050

Willes, R., Kressler, P. and Truelove, J. (1977). Nursery rearing of infant monkeys (*Macaca fascicularis*) for toxicity studies. *Lab. Animal Sci.*, **27**, 90–98

Willes, R.F., Rice, D.C. and Truelove, J.F. (1980). Chronic effects of lead in nonhuman primates, in Singahl, R.L. and Thomas, J.A. (eds), *Lead Toxicity*, pp. 213–240 (Baltimore: Urban & Schwartzenberg)

Winneke, G., Kramer, V., Brockhaus, A., Ewers, U., Kujanek, G., Lechner, H. and Janke, W. (1983) Neuropsychological studies in children with elevated tooth-lead concentration. *Int. Arch. Environ. Health*, **51**, 231–252

Yule, W., Lansdown, R., Millar, I.B. and Urbanowicz, M.A. (1981) The relationship between blood lead concentrations, intelligence, and attainment in a school population: a pilot study. *Dev. Med. Child. Neurol.*, **23**, 567–576

5.4

The Effects of Chronic Low-level Lead Exposure on the Early Structuring of the Central Nervous System

C. M. REGAN*, G. R. COOKMAN, G. J. KEANE, W. KING and
S. E. HEMMENS

SUMMARY

Chronic low-level lead exposure has been demonstrated to inhibit neural cell acquisition and impair early postnatal structuring of the central nervous system. Lead was demonstrated to have an anti-mitotic action both *in vitro* and *in vivo*, although the latter was confined to the cerebellum at blood lead threshold values of 30–40 μg/dl. Low-level lead exposure more potently affected *in vivo* cell positioning and fibre outgrowth, as judged by the impaired developmental desialylation of the D2-CAM/N-CAM protein, and these effects were seen at blood lead threshold values of 20–30 μg/dl. This inhibition of normal D2-CAM/N-CAM desialylation is attributed to improper guidance of neuronal cells and their fibres, as lead is demonstrated to specifically induce precocious differentiation of the glial cells.

Chronic low-level lead exposure (< 45 μg lead/dl blood) has repeatedly been demonstrated to impair the early neural development of children (Needleman *et al.*, 1979; Yule *et al.*, 1981; Winneke *et al.*, 1982, 1983); however, as yet the significance of the confounding variables in these studies remains to be resolved (Rutter, 1980; Yule, 1986). Consequently it is necessary to identify a molecular basis by which relevant, subclinical blood lead levels may impair the structuring of the central nervous system and lead to neurobehavioural deficits.

*To whom all correspondence should be addressed

Using rodent models similar to that originally described by Pentschew and Garro (1966) many workers have demonstrated neurobehavioural deficits to occur with a no-effect threshold of approximately 20-30 μg lead/dl blood (Cory-Slechta and Thompson, 1979; Gross-Selbeck and Gross-Selbeck, 1981; Taylor et al., 1982; Winneke et al., 1977). Furthermore these studies have demonstrated that neural deficits may be induced by exposure to lead in the prenatal (Bull et al., 1983), postnatal (Gross-Selbeck and Gross-Selbeck, 1981) and postweaning (Corey-Slechta and Thompson, 1979) periods of development. Thus it is reasonable to suggest that chronic low-level lead exposure may impair early structuring and subsequent modification of the neuronal circuitry as synaptic modelling is known to be associated with the acquisition of learned behaviour (Wenzel et al., 1977) and synaptic deficits have been demonstrated in lead-exposed animals (Averill and Needleman, 1980; McCauley et al., 1982).

In order to understand how lead-induced neurobehavioural deficits may arise we have studied lead's action in the postnatally developing brain, and particularly in the cerebellum, as this is completely formed after birth and the periods representative of cell acquisition, migration and fibre outgrowth and synapse formation have been well documented (Jacobson, 1978). The effect of chronic low-level lead exposure on the development of this brain area was monitored using a variety of techniques. Cell acquisition was measured by the rate of [^{3}H]thymidine incorporation, and cell positioning and synaptic elaboration were monitored using a developmentally regulated protein, D2-CAM/N-CAM, which is believed to regulate these events (Meier et al., 1984; Edelman, 1985). Using this approach we have identified a glial-dependent mechanism which could account for the impaired structuring of the central nervous system which is associated with chronic low-level lead exposure.

CELL DIVISION

The effect of lead on the *in vitro* rate of [^{3}H]thymidine incorporation

The anti-mitotic action of acute lead exposure was assessed using actively dividing neuroblastoma (Neuro-2A) and glioma (C$_6$) cell lines as previously described (Regan, 1985). The effect of increasing, serial concentrations of lead chloride on the mitotic index of C$_6$ and Neuro-2A cells is demonstrated in Table 1. The IC$_{50}$ values for glioma and neuroblastoma cells were found to be 3×10^{-5} and 10^{-4} mol/l PbCl$_2$, respectively. When compared to the glioma, the mitotic rate of the neuroblastoma cell line appeared to be more sensitive to lead insult at concentrations ranging from 10^{-7} to 10^{-9} mol/l PbCl$_2$, and this was consistently depressed by about 20% of the rate observed in the control cells. In a similar concentration range the mitotic rate of the glioma cell line appeared to be slightly stimulated when compared to that of the control. Although this effect was not statistically significant ($p > 0.05$), it was a constant finding in each individual experiment performed. At higher concentrations (10^{-5} to 10^{-3} mol/l), the glioma cell line was found to be more sensitive to lead insult than that of the neuroblastoma. This is clearly seen at 10^{-4} mol/l PbCl$_2$, at which the mitotic index of the glioma is inhibited

Table 1 The effect of increasing concentrations of lead chloride on the incorporation of [^{3}H]thymidine into actively dividing neuroblastoma (Neuro-2A) and glioma (C$_6$) cells

	Percentage control value	
PbCl$_2$ (mol/l)	Neuro-2A	C$_6$
10^{-9}	88 ± 6	97 ± 7
10^{-8}	90 ± 6	104 ± 4
10^{-6}	82 ± 8	99 ± 9
10^{-7}	64 ± 8	87 ± 5
10^{-5}	66 ± 11	64 ± 14
10^{-4}	48 ± 12	11 ± 3
10^{-3}	12 ± 3	2 ± 1

All values are expressed as the mean ± SEM ($n = 3$)

by 90%, and that of the neuroblastoma by 50%. These effects could not be attributed to cell death as all cells appeared viable by visual inspection. Furthermore, inhibition of [^{3}H]thymidine incorporation could not be attributed to a blockade of nucleoside uptake as a 15 min pre-exposure of cells to lead chloride had no effect on this parameter. Although these values are in excess of those representative of chronic low-level lead exposure they demonstrate that lead can affect mitotic index, and that neuroblastoma mitotic rate may be inhibited by about 20–30% with lead levels equivalent to 0.3–30 µg/dl blood.

Thus lead chloride appears to inhibit cell division in both neuroblastoma and glioma, and no recovery of mitotic rate was noted in these cell lines when exposed to lead for periods of up to 30 days (data not shown).

The effect of lead on the *in vivo* rate of [^{3}H]thymidine incorporation

The *in vivo* effect of chronic lead exposure on the acquisition of neural cells in the developing rat brain was assessed by measuring the rate of [^{3}H]thymidine incorporation into DNA. Wistar rats were used throughout the entire study and were maintained at 20°C and in a 12 h light/dark cycle. The animals had *ad libitum* access to food and water at all times. The pups were exposed to lead from their time of conception to the required postnatal period via their dams, who had *ad libitum* access to drinking water containing 400 mg PbCl$_2$/l. Food and water intake was constantly monitored over exposure periods, and no difference in food and water intake was observed between control and lead-exposed animals.

Litters (culled to eight at birth) from control and lead-exposed groups were killed on postnatal days 4, 8, 12, 16 and 20. One hour prior to sacrifice, pups received an intraperitoneal injection of 20 µCi [^{3}H]thymidine (sp. act. 20 Ci/mmol) per 100 g body weight. The litters were sacrificed by decapitation and the individual brains were rapidly removed, weighed and microdissected into the appropriate regions. Blood samples were also collected in heparinized tubes (50 µl heparin/ml blood) and stored at −20°C until required. The individual brain regions were homogenized in 0.32 mol/l sucrose containing phenylmethylsulphonyl fluoride (PMSF; 0.1 mmol/l) and aprotinin (25 KIE/ml), sonicated and stored at $-20°C$. Subsequently the dissected and homogenized brain areas were added to an equal volume of 7.5% perchloric acid (PCA) in order to precipitate the DNA. The precipitated material was gathered by centrifugation (12,000 g x 2 min), the supernatant was retained and the pellets were solubilized overnight in Soluene-350. Both pellet and supernatant were counted by liquid scintillation spectrophotometry and the results were expressed as relative specific activity (RSA), which is acid insoluble cpm/acid soluble cpm/organ.

Blood lead levels were determined using an electrothermal atomic absorption technique. The atomic absorption spectrometer (Perkin-Elmer 2380) was equipped with a hollow cathode lead lamp and a deuterium background corrector. A Perkin-Elmer HGA 400 hollow graphite atomizer with a pyrolytically coated graphite tube was used. Sonicated blood samples were diluted five-fold with 0.1% aq. Triton-X-100 solution and 20 μl aliquots were automatically delivered to the argon-purged graphite tube. The furnace was programmed to dry the aliquots at $100°C$ (10 s) and $120°C$ (5 s), char them at $530°C$ (5 s) and atomize them at $2300°C$ (1 s). Absorption of the atomized samples was measured at 283.3 nm. Blood samples with known lead concentrations were used for calibration.

Using these procedures, the postnatal blood levels of pups from dams exposed to lead at time of conception were found to be markedly elevated (45 μg lead/dl blood) between postnatal days 4–8 (Table 2). This corresponds with periods of extensive cell acquisition, particularly in the cerebellum which is completely formed postnatally (Jacobson, 1978). Subsequently the blood lead levels dramatically declined to 20 μg/dl by day 12 and then slowly increased to 40 μg/dl at time of weaning (day 20).

Administration of [³H]thymidine to postnatally developing pups resulted in the incorporation of labelled precursor into PCA-precipitable DNA. In both the cerebrum and the cerebellum of control animals the incorporation of [³H]thymidine increased between days 4 and 8, a time coincident with cell acquisition. Thereafter, incorporation remained constant with a relative specific activity of 1–1.25 at all time points examined. This is shown for the cerebellum in Figure 1. Lead was found to have no effect on [³H]thymidine incorporation in the postnatally developing cerebrum of pups exposed from time of

Table 2 Postnatal blood lead levels compared in pups exposed to lead from conception and birth

Postnatal day	Postconception 400 mg/l	Postnatal	
		200 mg/l	400 mg/l
4	45 ± 7	8 ± 3	8 ± 1
8	39 ± 5	6 ± 2	17 ± 1
12	20 ± 2	11 ± 1	18 ± 1
16	26 ± 3	17 ± 2	17 ± 1
20	39 ± 3	29 ± 6	40 ± 10

All values are rounded to the nearest μg/dl and are the mean ± SEM ($n > 3$). The control values averaged 3 μg/dl and never exceeded 6 μg/dl

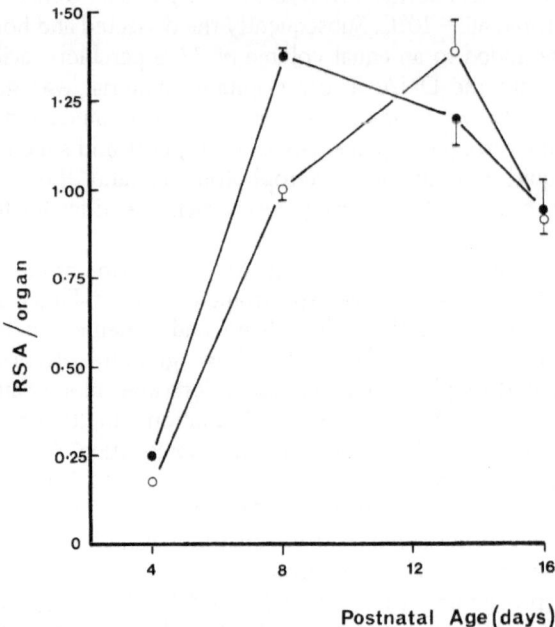

Figure 1   The effect of prenatal lead exposure on the incorporation of [³H]thymidine in the cerebellum. All values are expressed as the relative specific activity per organ and are the mean ± SEM of the number of animals in each litter. The open circles represent the control values

conception. In contrast, [³H]thymidine incorporation in the cerebellum of prenatally exposed animals was significantly higher than that in the corresponding control animals at postnatal day 8 when the mitotic rate could be expected to be highest (Figure 1). This also corresponds to the period of increased blood lead levels, as demonstrated in Table 2.

Although chronic low-level lead exposure was found to have no effect on *in vivo* cell acquisition in the cerebrum, an increase in cerebellar [³H]thymidine incorporation was noted on postnatal day 8. This apparent increase is not interpreted as a stimulation of DNA synthesis, but rather a slowing of cell acquisition as this process is complete by day 8 during normal development. Thus it seems that *in vivo* cell acquisition will be slowed at blood lead levels equivalent to approximately 40 μg/dl, and this would have the consequence of impairing the temporal orchestration of neural development. In this regard it is of interest that the cerebellum has been reported to accumulate higher lead levels than the cortex (Sandstrom *et al.*, 1983). These findings also indicate that lead induced anti-mitotic action may be specifically directed to neurons as cell acquisition in the cortex during postnatal development is mainly confined to glia (Jacobson, 1978) and this is in agreement with the *in vitro* studies.

CELL MIGRATION AND SYNAPTIC FORMATION

In order to understand the mechanisms underlying possible lead-induced synaptic and neurobehavioural deficits it is necessary to study its effects on the developmentally regulated neuronal glycoconjugates which are believed to be involved in the early structuring of the central nervous system. The neural cell adhesion molecule (D2-CAM/N-CAM) is composed of three immunologically related cell surface glycoproteins (Choung and Edelman, 1984; Sheehan et al., 1986) which are believed to be intimately involved in the temporal orchestration of cell movement, fibre outgrowth and adhesion in the developing brain (Edelman, 1985). D2-CAM/N-CAM is believed to control cell movement (Burskirk et al., 1980) and fibre outgrowth (Rutishauser et al., 1978) by regulating the strength of cell–cell adhesion by a homophilic binding mechanism, the strength of which is inversely proportional to the amount of sialic acid on each molecule (Brackenbury et al., 1977; Hoffman and Edelman, 1983). This mechanism is best observed in vivo in the cerebellum (Meier et al., 1984; Choung and Edelman, 1984) which is completely formed postnatally and in which the major epochs of neural development have best been demonstrated (Jacobson, 1978). Here the sialic acid-rich form of D2-CAM/N-CAM is expressed at times coincident with cell acquisition and fibre outgrowth and the sialic acid-poor form only becomes predominant with synaptogenesis and the final structuring of the central nervous system. Furthermore this conversion from sialic acid-rich to sialic acid-poor forms of D2-CAM/N-CAM has been shown to be inhibited in the granuloprival mouse mutant staggerer (sg/sg) in which failure in synaptic structuring in the cerebellum is known to occur (Edelman and Choung, 1982).

The effect of lead on in vivo D2-CAM/N-CAM expression

The animal model used was as previously described, but with the exception that the pups were exposed to lead from time of birth. D2-CAM/N-CAM expression was analysed by rocket immunoelectrophoresis (Bjerrum and Bøg-Hansen, 1976) in 1% agarose (Miles Laboratories) gels using a Tris-barbital buffer (73 mmol/l Tris. HCl, 24 mmol/l barbital, 2 mmol/l NaN_3, pH 8.6) containing 0.6% Triton-X-100. The running buffer was the same but Triton-X-100 was omitted. The precipitating gel contained anti-BPM (30 μl/cm^2), a neuron-specific antiserum which predominantly recognizes D2-CAM/N-CAM in Triton-solubilized whole brain homogenates (Meier et al., 1982). Furthermore, this antiserum has a differential affinity for sialic acid-rich and sialic acid-poor forms of D2-CAM/N-CAM (Meier et al., 1984) and has previously been used in rocket immunoelectrophoresis to discriminate between these forms (Sheehan et al., 1986). The samples were prepared by solubilizing the homogenates at 0°C in 15 mmol/l sodium phosphate, pH 8.5, containing 15 mmol/l EDTA, 3% Triton-X-100, 100 μmol/l PMSF and aprotinin (100 KIU/ml). After 4 h the solution was clarified by centrifugation (12,000 g, 10 min) and the supernatants (10–20 μg) were immunoelectrophoresed into the antibody-containing gel at 2 V/cm^2 on a water-cooled plate for a 16 h period. The gels were dried and stained as previously described (Weeke,

445

1973). The peak heights were measured from the front of the wells and were defined in arbitrary units (a.u.), one a.u. being equivalent to $1 \, mm/\mu g$ protein. Protein was estimated according to the procedure of Lowry et al. (1951) and the correct amount of Triton-X-100 was included in all bovine serum albumin standards.

Blood lead levels of exposed animals are shown in Table 2, and these correspond to the postnatal periods of D2-CAM/N-CAM desialylation (postnatal days 12–20) (Meier et al., 1984). Chronic exposure to 200 mg $PbCl_2/l$ drinking water resulted in a slow increase in pup blood lead levels to $40 \, \mu g/dl$ at postnatal day 20, a period coincident with weaning, and at which time the pups would have direct access to their drinking water. Chronic exposure to 400 mg $PbCl_2/l$ drinking water did not further elevate blood lead levels between postnatal days 12 and 20, although that of their dams was doubled (data not shown). Thus it appears that blood lead levels between postnatal days 12 and 16 rarely exceed $20 \, \mu g/dl$ and that this is independent of postconception or postnatal exposure protocols. Similar findings have been reported (Bull et al., 1983; McCauley et al., 1982; Bailey and Kitchen, 1985) but, as yet, the pharmacokinetic mechanism(s) underlying these observations remain to be demonstrated.

D2-CAM/N-CAM sialylation state was monitored by rocket immunoelectrophoresis during the postnatal development of the cerebellum in both control and lead exposed animals (Table 3). In control animals the faster-moving form of D2-CAM/N-CAM, which is sialic acid-rich, developmentally decreased at times coincident with synapse formation, as has been previously demonstrated (Meier et al., 1974). This is in contrast to that observed in animals chronically exposed to 200 mg $PbCl_2/l$ drinking water, where the sialic acid-rich form of D2-CAM/N-CAM steadily decreased until postnatal day 16, whereupon its conversion to the sialic acid-poor form was significantly impaired ($p < 0.05$). Furthermore, this blockade only occurred when blood lead levels exceeded $20 \, \mu g/dl$, and it is of interest to note that this has previously been suggested to be the threshold level above which lead induces neurobehavioural deficits (Winneke, 1986). A similar effect was also observed in animals chronically exposed to 400 mg $PbCl_2/l$ drinking water. Furthermore no lead-induced alteration in immunoprecipitate formation was evident with material derived from animals which had been chronically exposed to either 200 or 400 mg $PbCl_2/l$ drinking water.

Table 3 D2-CAM/N-CAM desialylation in the cerebella of control and lead-exposed animals as demonstrated by the disappearance of the sialic acid-rich form

Postnatal day	Blood lead levels ($\mu g/dl$)		D2-CAM/N-CAM (a.u.)	
	Control	Exposed	Control	Exposed
+8	6.15 ± 2.1	8.15 ± 2.6	1.72 ± 0.08	1.73 ± 0.08
12	<2	12.43 ± 0.9	1.44 ± 0.10	1.52 ± 0.09
16	5.77 ± 0.6	24.45 ± 2.7	1.19 ± 0.04	1.22 ± 0.06
20	7.28 ± 1.0	43.09 ± 7.9	1.03 ± 0.05	$1.23 \pm 0.07^*$

All values are the mean $\pm$ SEM ($n > 3$). D2-CAM/N-CAM values are in arbitrary units (a.u.) and those marked with an asterisk are significantly different from the control ($p < 0.05$)

The orderly structuring of the CNS has previously been demonstrated to be dependent on the normal functioning of D2-CAM/N-CAM (Buskirk et al., 1980) and more specifically its conversion from the embryonic to adult form has been shown to be severely impaired in a mouse cerebellar mutant with extensive connection deficits (Edelman and Choung, 1982). Thus, from the studies reported here it is reasonable to assume that chronic low-level lead exposure has the potential to interfere with the proper structuring of the central nervous system as this also has the capability to block D2-CAM/N-CAM desialylation. This failure potentially will lead to incorrect cell–cell interaction at critical developmental times, and result in reduced synaptic elaboration and possible cell death. This effect is not only localized in the cerebellum, as we have also demonstrated D2-CAM/N-CAM desialylation to be similarly blocked in whole-brain synaptosomal preparations derived from lead-exposed animals (data not shown).

The effect of lead on in vitro fibre outgrowth

As the blockade of D2-CAM/N-CAM desialylation during development may reflect reduced synaptic elaboration it was necessary to establish if this could be accounted for by impaired fibre outgrowth. To explore this possibility, spinal cord explants ($0.5 mm^2$) from 8-day-old chick embryos were grown on collagen substrates (Elsdale and Bard, 1972) in the presence and absence of lead. The explants were allowed to adhere to the moist collagen (0.5 cm apart) for 30 min before the addition of the culture medium, which was composed of Dulbecco's modified Eagle's medium containing 10% foetal calf serum and 100 μg/ml gentamicin. Lead was then added to a series of explants at final concentrations ranging from 10^{-6} to 10^{-4} mol/l $PbCl_2$. The explants were maintained at $37°C$ in a humidified atmosphere containing 9% CO_2 in air and cytosine arabinoside (10 μmol/l) was added after 18 h to prevent non-neuronal proliferation and outgrowth. The explants were analysed for fibre outgrowth after 48 h.

As can be seen from Figure 2, lead had no effect on fibre outgrowth and this exceeded 500 μm at all concentrations examined. Furthermore no evidence of necrosis was apparent in the explants. Thus lead does not appear to affect fibre outgrowth and the blockade of D2-CAM/N-CAM desialylation may therefore arise from an inability of the fibres to locate their target cell.

Lead-induced differentiation of glial cells in vitro and in vivo

During early development glial–neuronal interactions have been suggested to be critically important for neurons and their fibres to locate their eventual positions (Rakic and Sidman, 1971). Thus precocious differentiation of guiding glia could perturb synaptic elaboration and account for inhibition of D2-CAM/N-CAM desialylation. The possibility of lead mediating this effect was prompted by observations on the morphology of the neuroblastoma and glioma cell lines after mitotic inhibition by $PbCl_2$. The effect of a 3-day chronic lead exposure on the morphology of the Neuro-2A cell line is shown

447

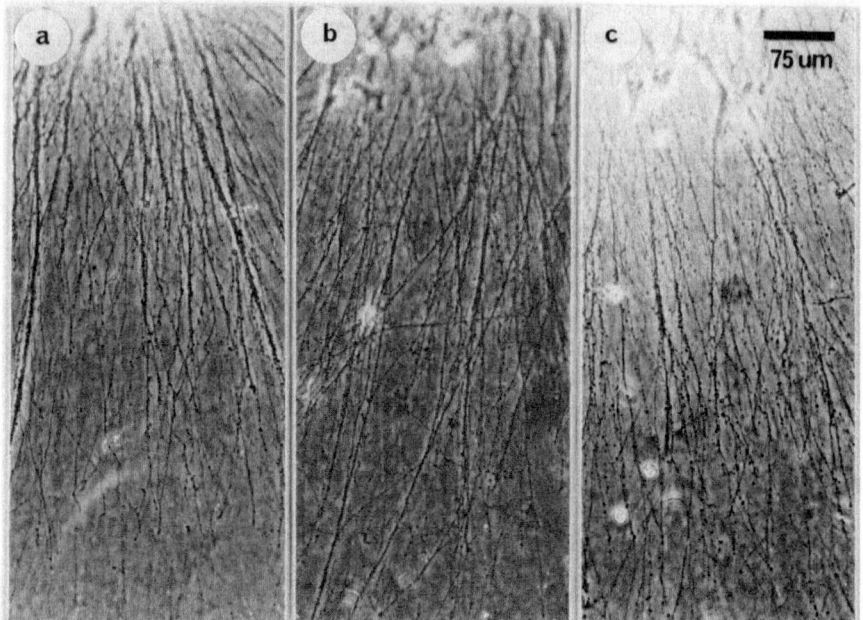

Figure 2 Fibre outgrowth in control explants (a) and those cultured in the presence of 10^{-6} mol/l (b) and 10^{-4} mol/l (c) PbCl$_2$

in Figure 3B. In all cases the cells appeared viable, and no obvious effect on fibre outgrowth or cell substratum adhesivity was apparent. The only marked feature was a decrease in cell number, and this is to be expected with increasing lead concentrations. In contrast, the glial cells (C$_6$) showed extensive morphological change. The control cells (Figure 3C) showed a typical fibroblastoid morphology with cell length being approximately twice the width. However exposure to 10^{-5} mol/l PbCl$_2$ for 3 days brought about a dramatic change in the morphology of these cells (Figure 3D). They became extremely elongated with fibre outgrowths of up to 200 μm in length. Furthermore structures resembling glial end-feet were apparent at the fibre tips. Similar effects were also noted at concentrations as low as 10^{-6} mol/l PbCl$_2$ (data not shown).

This effect was further demonstrated *in vivo* by using the glial-specific enzyme glutamine synthetase (Norenberg and Martinez-Hernandez, 1979) which is known to be developmentally regulated (Phelan and Regan, 1982). Pups were postnatally exposed to lead via their dams, whose drinking water contained 400 mg PbCl$_2$/l. The brain tissue homogenates were prepared as previously described, and glutamine synthetase activity was estimated according to the procedure of Kirk (1965). Over the time period examined, glutamine synthetase activity was found to be significantly ($p < 0.01$) increased during the early phases of development in lead-exposed animals (Figure 4) although this returned to the normal value by day 20.

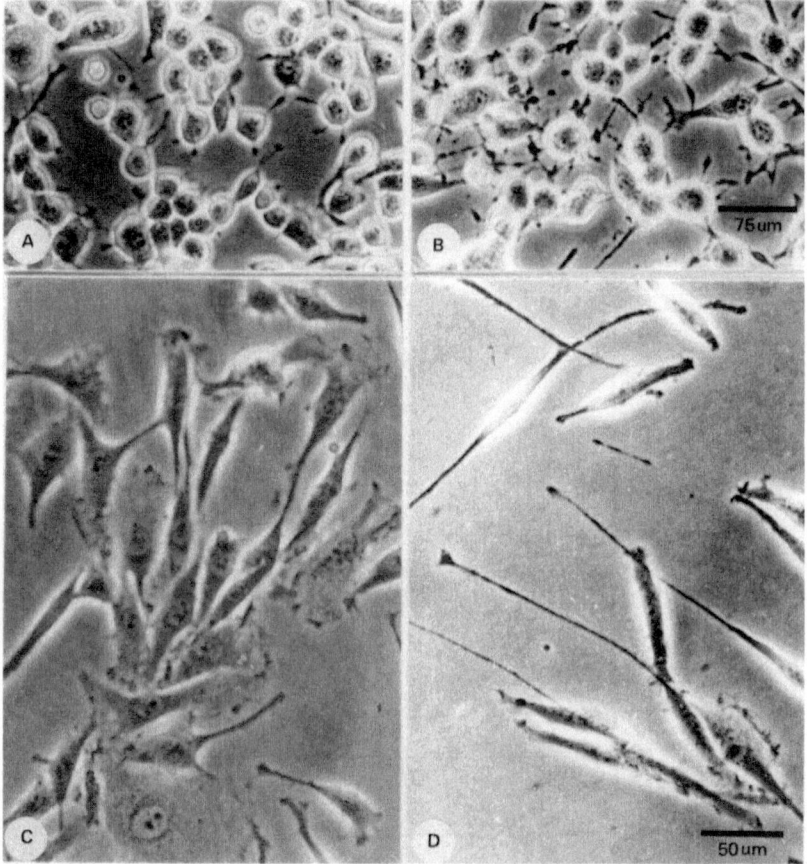

Figure 3 The effect of lead exposure on neuroblastoma (Neuro-2A) and glioma (C$_6$) cell lines. The final concentration of PbCl$_2$ in the medium was 10^{-5} M (**B** and **D**) and the control cells are shown in **A** and **C**

Thus it appears that lead is capable of precociously inducing morphological and biochemical differentiation in glia both *in vitro* and *in vivo*. It is tempting to speculate that the expression of the component(s) which interact with, and guide, the neuronal fibres may also be reduced or absent from glia in a temporally advanced state of differentiation. This would have the consequence of impairing fibre outgrowth, and presumably result in an inhibition of D2-CAM/N-CAM desialylation.

CONCLUSIONS

These findings clearly demonstrate that chronic low-level lead exposure is capable of impairing the early structuring of the central nervous sytem. The

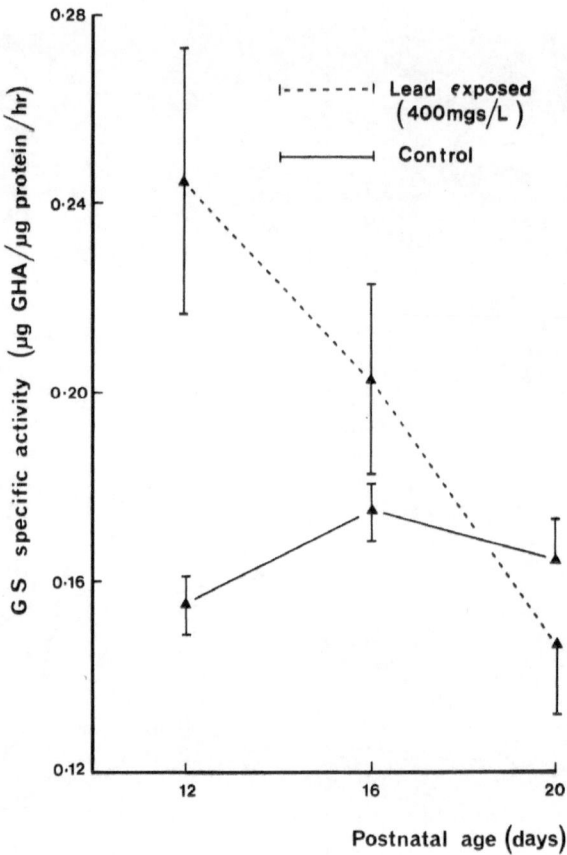

Figure 4 The effect of postnatal lead exposure on glutamine synthetase activity in the cerebral cortex. Similar results were found for the cerebellum

three major epochs of development — cell acquisition, fibre outgrowth and synapse formation — are susceptible to varying extents and this is dependent on blood lead levels.

Neuronal cell mitotic rate could be depressed but not inhibited with blood lead threshold values of approximately 30–40 μg/dl. This also appears to be dependent on the preferential accumulation of lead into defined areas such as the cerebellum. In contrast glial cell mitotic rate was only affected by relatively high blood lead level equivalents.

Low-level lead exposure more potently affected cell positioning and fibre outgrowth, as judged by the impaired developmental expression of the D2-CAM/N-CAM protein, and these effects were seen at blood lead threshold values of 20–30 μg/dl. Furthermore, these observations would explain the reduced synaptic elaboration (Averill and Needleman, 1980; McCauley et al., 1982) and neurobehavioural deficits (Needleman et al., 1979; Yule et al., 1981; Winneke et al., 1982, 1983) associated with lead exposure. Normal D2-CAM/N-CAM desialylation appears to be dependent on the fibres reaching their correct location, but no specific effect of lead on *in vitro* fibre outgrowth could be demonstrated. As lead could be shown to be capable of precociously inducing differentiation in glia, it is possible that impaired fibre guidance by these cells gives rise to a blocked D2-CAM/N-CAM desialylation.

ACKNOWLEDGMENTS

The technical assistance of Patricia Bonnar and David O'Gara of the State Laboratory is gratefully appreciated, as is the assistance of Ms Naomi FitzGerald and Mr Roddy Monks in the preparation of this manuscript. This work was supported by the Commission of the European Communities, Grant No. ENV-820-EIR.

REFERENCES

Averill, D. R. and Needleman, H. L. (1980) Neonatal lead exposure retards cortical synaptogenesis in the rat. In Needleman, H. (ed.), *Low Level Lead Exposure: the Clinical Implications of Current Research*, pp. 201–210 (New York: Raven Press)

Bailey, C. and Kitchen, I. (1985) Ontogenesis of proenkephalin products in rat striatum and the inhibitory effects of low level lead exposure. *Dev. Brain Res.*, **22**, 75–79

Bjerrum, O. J. and Bøg-Hansen, T. C. (1976) Immunochemical gel precipitation in membrane studies. In Maddy, A. H. (ed.), *Biochemical Analysis of Membrane*, pp. 378–427. (London: Chapman & Hall)

Brackenbury, R., Thiery, J.-P., Rutishauser, U. and Edelman, G. M. (1977) Adhesion among neural cells of the chick embryo. I. An immunological assay for molecules involved in cell–cell binding. *J. Biol. Chem.*, **253**, 7314–7318

Buskirk, D. R., Thiery, J.-P., Rutishauser, U. and Edelman, G. M. (1980) Antibodies to a neural cell adhesion molecule disrupt histogenesis in cultured chick retinae. *Nature*, **285**, 488–489

Bull, R. J., McCauley, P. T., Taylor, D. H. and Croften, K. M. (1983) The effects of lead on the developing central nervous system of the rat. *Neurotoxicology*, **4**, 1–18

Choung, C.-M. and Edelman, G. M. (1984). Alterations in neural cell adhesion molecules during development of different regions of the nervous system. *J. Neurosci.*, **4**, 2354–2368

Cory-Slechta, D. A. and Thompson, T. (1979) Behavioural toxicity of chronic post weaning lead exposure in the rat. *Toxicol. Appl. Pharmacol.*, **47**, 151–159

Edelman, G. M. (1985) Cell adhesion and the molecular processes of morphogenesis. *Ann. Rev. Biochem.*, **54**, 135–169

Edelman, G. M. and Chuong, C.-M. (1982) Embryonic to adult conversion of neural cell adhesion molecules in normal and staggerer mice. *Proc. Natl. Acad. Sci.*, **79**, 7036–740

Elsdale, T. and Bard, J. (1972) Collagen substrata for studies of cell behaviour. *J. Cell Biol.*, **54**, 626–637

Gross-Selbeck, E. and Gross-Selbeck, M. (1981) Changes in operant behaviour of rats exposed to lead at the accepted no-effect level. *Clin. Toxicol.*, **18**, 1247–1256

Hoffman, S. and Edelman, G. M (1983) Kinetics of homophilic binding by embryonic and adult forms of the neural cell adhesion molecule. *Proc. Natl. Acad. Sci. USA*, **89**, 5762–5766

Jacobson, M. (1978) *Developmental Neurobiology*, 2nd edn (New York and London: Plenum)

Kirk, D. L. (1965). The role of RNA synthesis in the production of glutamine synthetase by developing chick neural retina. *Proc. Natl. Acad. Sci. USA*, **54**, 1345–1353

Lowry, O. H., Rosebrough, N. J., Farr, A. L. and Randall, R. J. (1951) Protein measurement with the Folin reagent. *J. Biol. Chem.*, **193**, 265–275

McCauley, P. T., Bull, R. J., Tonti, A. P., Lutkenhoff, S. D., Meister, M. V., Doerger, J. U. and Stober, J. A. (1982) The effect of prenatal and postnatal lead exposure on neonatal synaptogenesis in rat cerebral cortex. *J. Toxicol. Env. Health*, **10**, 639–651

Meier, E., Regan, C., Balazs, R. and Wilkin, G. P. (1982) Specific recognition of the neuronal cell surface by an antiserum raised against a plasma membrane preparation of immature rat cerebellum. *Neurochem. Res.*, **7**, 1031–1043

Meier, E., Regan, C. M. and Balazs, R. (1984) Changes in the expression of a neuronal surface protein during development of cerebellar neurones *in vivo* and in culture. *J. Neurochem.*, **43**, 1328–1334

Needleman, H. L., Gunnoe, C., Leviton, A., Reed, M., Peresie, H., Maher, C. and Barrett, P. (1979) Deficits in psychological and classroom performance of children with elevated dentine lead levels. *N. Engl. J. Med.*, **300**, 689–695

Norenberg, M. D. and Martinez-Hernandez, A. (1979) Fine structural localization of glutamine synthetase in astrocytes of rat brain. *Brain Res.*, **161**, 303–310

Pentschew, A. and Garro, F. (1966) Lead encephalomyelopathy of the suckling rat and its implications on the porphyrinopathic nervous diseases. *Acta Neuropathol.*, **6**, 266–278

Phelan, P. and Regan, C. M. (1982) Developmental expression of glutamine synthetase activity in rat brain. *Ir. J. Med. Sci.*, **151**, 403–404

Rakic, P. and Sidman, R. L. (1971) Guidance of neurons migrating to the foetal monkey neocortex. *Brain Res.*, **33**, 471–476

Regan, C. M. (1985) Therapeutic levels of sodium valproate inhibits mitotic indices in cells of neural origin. *Brain Res.*, **347**, 394–398

Rutishauser, U., Gall, W. E. and Edelman, G. M. (1978) Adhesion among neural cells of the chick embryo. IV. Role of the cell surface molecule CAM in the formation of neurite bundles in cultures of spinal ganglia. *J. Cell Biol.*, **79**, 382–393

Rutter, M. (1980) Raised lead levels and impaired cognitive/behavioural functioning: a review of the evidence. *Dev. Med. Child. Neurol.*, **22** (Suppl. 42), 1–26

Sheehan, M. C., Halpin, C. I., Regan, C. M., Moran, N. M. and Kilty, C. G. (1986) Purification and characterisation of the D2 cell adhesion protein: analysis of the postnatally regulated polymorphic forms and their cellular distribution. *Neurochem. Res.*, **11**, 1343–1356

Sundstrom, R., Conrad, N. G. and Sourander, P. (1983). Low dose lead encephalopathy in the suckling rat. *Acta Neuropathol.*, **60**, 1–8

Taylor, D. H., Noland, E. A. Brubaker, C. M., Croften, K. M. and Bull, R. J. (1982) Low level lead (Pb) exposure produces learning deficits in young rat pups. *Neurobehav. Toxicol. Teratol.*, **4**, 311–314

Weeke, B. (1973) A manual of quantitative immunoelectrophoresis. Methods and applications. 1. General remarks and principles, equipment, reagents and procedures. *Scand. J. Immunol.*, **2** (Suppl. 1), 15–35

Wenzel, J., Kammerer, E., Joschko, R., Joschko, M., Kaufmann, W., Kirsche, W. and Matthies, H. (1977) The influence of a learning experience on synaptosomes in the rat hippocampus. *Z. Mikrosk.-Anat. Forsch., Leipzig*, **91**, 57–73

Winneke, G. (1986) Animal studies. In Lansdown, R. and Yule, W. (eds), *The Lead Debate: the Environment, Toxicology and Child Health*, pp. 217–234 (London: Croom Helm)

Winneke, G., Brockhaus, A. and Baltissen, R. (1977) Neurobehavioural and systemic effects of longterm blood lead-elevation in rats. I. Discrimination learning and open field behaviour. *Arch. Toxicol.*, **37**, 247–263

Winneke, G., Hrdina, K.-G. and Brockhaus, A. (1982) Neuropsychological studies in children with elevated tooth-lead concentrations. I. Pilot study. *Int. Arch. Occup. Env. Health*, **51**, 169–183

Winneke, G., Kramer, U., Brockhaus, A., Ewers, U., Kujanek, G., Lechner, H. and Janke, W. (1983) Neuropsychological studies in children with elevated tooth-lead concentrations. II. Extended study. *Int. Arch. Occup. Env. Health*, **51**, 231–252

Yule, W. (1986) Methodological and statistical issues. In Lansdowne, R. and Yule, W. (eds), *The Lead Debate: The Environment, Toxicology and Child Health*, pp. 193–216 (London: Croom Helm)

Yule, W., Lansdown, R., Millar, I. B. and Urbanowicz, M.A. (1981) The relationship between blood lead concentrations, intelligence and attainment in a school population: a pilot study. *Dev. Med. Child. Neurol.*, **23**, 567–576

5.5
Studies on Lead and Blood–Brain Barrier Function in the Developing Rat

D. PELLING, R. J. HARGREAVES and S. R. MOORHOUSE

SUMMARY

Blood–brain barrier function was assessed in two lead exposure models using 19–21-day-old rats. In animals receiving lead via the milk, blood lead ranged between 20 and 90 μg/dl without affecting growth. Cerebrovascular permeability (PS-product) was increased to basic and neutral amino acids and thiamine in certain regions of the cerebral hemisphere. Regional permeability to mannitol was unchanged. These alterations may have been due to tissue repair processes or to delayed maturation. In animals infused with lead to maintain steady plasma levels up to 764 μg/dl, blood–brain barrier integrity was unaffected but regional glucose uptake was inhibited.

In the brain, adjoining capillary endothelial cells lack the intercellular clefts and the fenestrae characteristic of these cells in other tissues, and the continuous membrane barrier so formed restricts the movement of proteins, ions and hydrophilic non-electrolytes between blood and brain. However, the transcellular flux of nutrients essential for normal brain metabolism is facilitated by specific carrier-mediated transport systems (for review see Bradbury, 1985). Thus the cerebral capillary endothelium, which constitutes the blood–brain barrier, serves both a protective function and a homeostatic role in maintaining the nutrient environment of the brain.

There is considerable neuropathological evidence that the brain microvasculature is a primary target for lead in the central nervous system (CNS) (reviewed by Winder et al., 1983). Relatively high blood lead levels are associated with extensive capillary breakdown, haemorrhage and oedema, and these changes are more frequently encountered in the young than in the adult. Although there is no evidence of gross structural damage to the capillary endothelium with low-level lead exposure, it is possible that a subtle functional deficit, particularly during the vulnerable period of postnatal brain growth, could seriously affect brain development and maturation. At this time the endothelial transport systems are geared to the increased metabolic demands of the CNS for essential nutrients from the circulation (Pratt, 1979; Braun et al., 1980; Cremer and Cunningham, 1981).

There have been relatively few reports on the functional integrity of the developing blood–brain barrier at blood lead levels below those associated with gross microvascular lesions and their sequelae. Lorenzo and Gewirtz (1977) found a marked reduction in the transfer of the essential amino acid tryptophan into the developing rabbit brain. In contrast, Lefauconnier et al. (1980) were unable to demonstrate altered transport of several important nutrients into the suckling rat brain, and Michaelson and Bradbury (1982) found no effect on choline and tyrosine transport at 8–10 weeks in rats exposed to low-level lead from birth. In these studies blood–brain barrier function was assessed in a single gross brain sample, and it is possible that alterations localized to critical brain regions may not have been detected. Moreover, the blood lead levels in the studies of Lorenzo and Gewirtz (1977) and Lefauconnier et al. (1980), although below the threshold for encephalopathy, were within the range associated with malnutrition (Michaelson, 1980; Carmichael et al., 1981), an established cause of pathological changes in the developing brain (Balázs et al., 1979).

In the present study the effect of lead on nutrient supply to discrete regions of the brain has been investigated in 3-week-old rats. To control for potential nutritional effects of lead two types of exposure model were investigated. A chronic model was used, in which rats received lead via the milk throughout the suckling period. This treatment regime produced blood lead concentrations in the neonates within the range 20–90 μg/dl, levels below those associated with clinical lead poisoning in children (Winder et al., 1983). Secondly, an acute exposure model was set up in which plasma lead levels were raised and held steady by intravenous infusion. In both models cerebrovascular integrity was assessed using [^{14}C]D-mannitol as a diffusion marker, and carrier-mediated transport function was evaluated from measurements of regional brain uptake rates of selected essential substrates.

EXPERIMENTAL

Models of lead exposure

To prepare animals for the chronic exposure model, pregnant Ola:Sprague-Dawley rats were fed breeding diet (No. 3, SDS Ltd, Essex; lead content < 1.6 mg/kg) and tap water. Within 12 h of parturition 0.1% lead acetate (547 mg lead/l), or deionized water (control) containing < 1 mg lead/l, were substituted for the drinking water. Litters were culled to nine pups. Fluid and food intake were depressed in some dams when they were introduced to lead, but providing the taste aversion was overcome within 2–3 days, pup growth was unaffected (Figure 1). Litters from dams showing a persistent reduction in fluid intake were not used. Blood–brain barrier integrity and transport function were assessed in the suckling rats at 19–21 days postpartum.

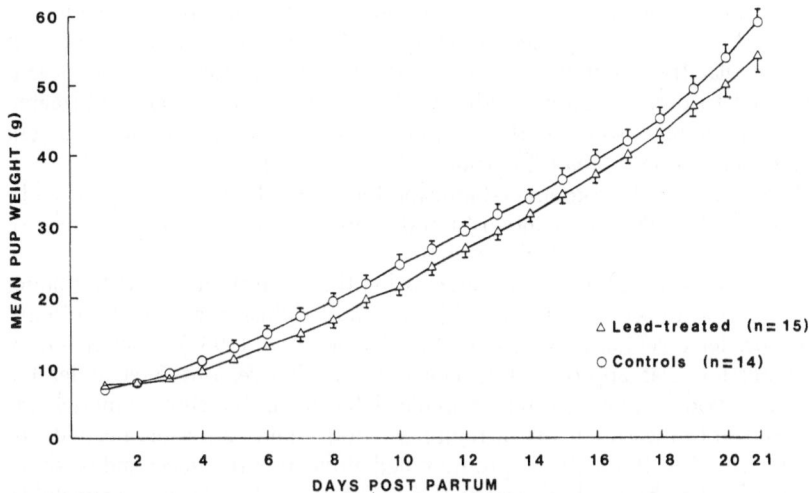

Figure 1 Mean pup weight for control litters and litters of rats exposed to lead in the drinking water at 547 mg/l. Values are means and SE for the number of litters shown (*n*)

Untreated animals of this age range were also used in the acute exposure model. They were anaesthetized with pentobarbitone Na (40 mg/kg i.p.) and steady levels of lead were maintained in the circulating plasma for a 20 min period by programmed iv infusion (Pratt, 1985) of lead acetate in saline (pH 5.4). The total volume of solution infused did not exceed 150 μl. Animals were not heparinized, to avoid interaction with lead (Bradbury and Deane, 1986).

Measurements

Regional brain uptake of all substrates except glucose and the diffusion marker mannitol were determined by the *in situ* brain perfusion method of Takasato *et al.* (1984), with minor modifications for use in small animals. The oxygenated bicarbonate-buffered electrolyte was infused at 5.42×10^{-2} ml/s. This rate was found by calibrating 21-day-old rats to provide a perfusion pressure of 130–160 mmHg and thereby minimizing collateral arterial supply and the risk of cerebrovascular injury (Takasato *et al.*, 1984). Perfusion produced no change in gross EEG tracing recorded from the cerebral hemisphere.

The following substrates were used to assess blood–brain barrier transport systems: L-lysine and L-histidine (basic and neutral amino acid systems, respectively), adenine (purine base), thiamine (vitamin), choline (amine), pyruvate (monocarboxylic acid) and 3-hydroxybutyrate (ketone body). Tracer levels of the ^{14}C-labelled substrates (Amersham International plc) were added to the perfusate at 0.3–1.2 μCi/ml together with [^{3}H]inulin at 1.0 μCi/ml as intravascular marker. Following a net perfusion time of 18.5 s, the animal was decapitated. The brain was rapidly removed, sliced into 2 mm coronal sections and quick-frozen on solid CO_2. Each slice was dissected on a freezing

455

microscope stage to obtain samples of discrete regions localized by the brain atlas of Pellegrino et al. (1979). The samples were weighed and solubilized, and dual-label counting used to correct tissue substrate radioactivity for intravascular tracer content. Uptake of [^{14}C]diazepam (Takasato et al., 1984) was used to derive regional perfusate flow data in control and lead-treated pups. These data were used to express substrate uptake as an apparent permeability-surface area (PS)-product (Crone, 1963).

The steady-state programmed infusion technique (Pratt, 1985) was used to assess blood–brain barrier integrity and to measure regional brain uptake of glucose in both lead exposure models.

Cerebrovascular integrity was assessed in the acute studies by determining regional transfer constants for [^{14}C]D-mannitol diffusion across the blood–brain barrier essentially as described by Daniel et al. (1985). Since mannitol accumulation was approximately linear in all CNS regions over at least a 15 min period (Figure 2), cerebrovascular integrity in the chronic model was assessed from measurements of regional blood–brain barrier permeability to [^{14}C]D-mannitol after a 10 min programmed infusion of the tracer and washout of blood from the cerebral vessels (Daniel et al., 1974). Barrier permeability to mannitol was expressed as an apparent PS-product (see Table 2). Regional blood-to-brain glucose transfer was measured in both exposure models at endogenous plasma glucose levels using methods detailed in Cunningham et al. (1986). To permit a direct comparison between lead-treated and control animal data, regional kinetic constants for glucose transport determined in age-matched suckling rats (Moorhouse, Hargreaves and Pelling, unpublished data) were used to adjust control glucose uptakes to values corresponding to the mean plasma glucose levels in the lead-treated groups.

Data were analysed by ANOVA using the GENSTAT program (Alvey et al., 1982).

Lead in whole blood and plasma was measured by graphite furnace atomic absorption spectrophotometry (Perkin-Elmer 2380 and HGA 400) using the method of Fernandez and Hilligoss (1982). Standards and blanks were matrix-matched with test samples. Analyses on each batch of lead drinking solution were within 3% of the nominal value. Laboratory analytical quality was monitored by the UK External Quality Assurance Scheme (UKEQAS).

RESULTS

Acute exposure model

The range of raised plasma lead levels examined was 240 to 764 μg/dl. During the lead infusions, arterial blood gases and pH did not differ significantly from pre-infusion values.

Mannitol accumulated linearly from 3 to 15 min in 10 CNS regions sampled from both lead-infused and control saline-infused rats (e.g. Figure 2). Examples of the apparent transfer constants (K_d) for mannitol diffusion, given by the slopes of the regression lines, are shown in Figure 3. This measure of regional blood–brain barrier permeability was unaltered even in the higher ranges of circulating plasma lead.

456

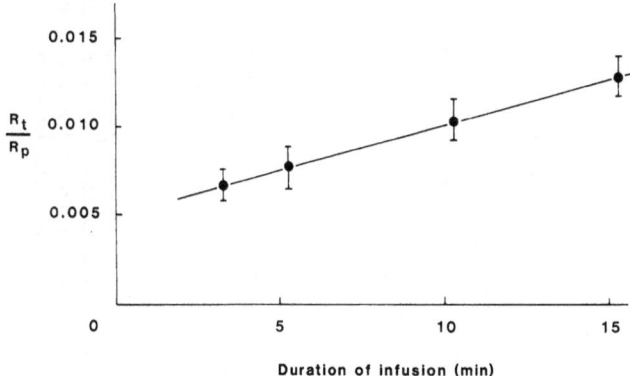

Figure 2 The accumulation with time of [^{14}C]D-mannitol in the occipital cortex of 19–21-day-old anaesthetized rats. Each point is the mean ($\pm$ SE) of five to eight experiments in which the tracer was maintained constant in the plasma. The ratio R_t/R_p is the radioactivity in the tissue (dpm/g) at the end of the experiment divided by the mean radioactivity in the plasma (dpm/ml) during the experiment. The slope of the regression line represents the apparent transfer constant (k_d) for mannitol diffusion (0.58 $\pm$ 0.10 μl/min/g tissue)

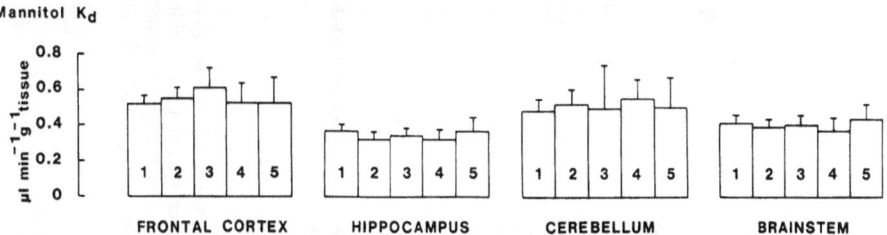

Figure 3 Apparent transfer constants (k_d) for [^{14}C]D-mannitol diffusion into four brain regions of 19–21-day-old rats exposed to various steady plasma lead concentrations. Column **1**: control (30 rats); **2**: lead-infused (20 rats). Remaining columns show the lead-infused rats divided into three arbitrarily chosen concentration ranges, **3**: 340–400 μg/dl (six rats); **4**: 470–550 μg/dl (eight rats); **5**: 600–670 μg/dl (six rats). Values are means $\pm$ SE

Over all CNS regions glucose uptake was significantly reduced by intravenous infusion of lead in each of three concentration ranges ($p < 0.001$, Figure 4). The statistical analysis did not reveal any dose-related trend or any specific regional effect of treatment. There was significant interregional variation of glucose uptake ($p < 0.001$) in both lead-treated and control groups.

Chronic exposure model

Blood and plasma lead levels measured in the 19–21-day-old animals, and in pups taken at 7 and 14 days, are shown in Table 1. At 19–21 days, the whole-blood lead levels were in the range 20–90 μg/dl and only at this time were plasma lead levels above the detection limit of 2 μg/dl.

Following surgical preparation for *in situ* brain perfusion, arterial pO_2, pCO_2

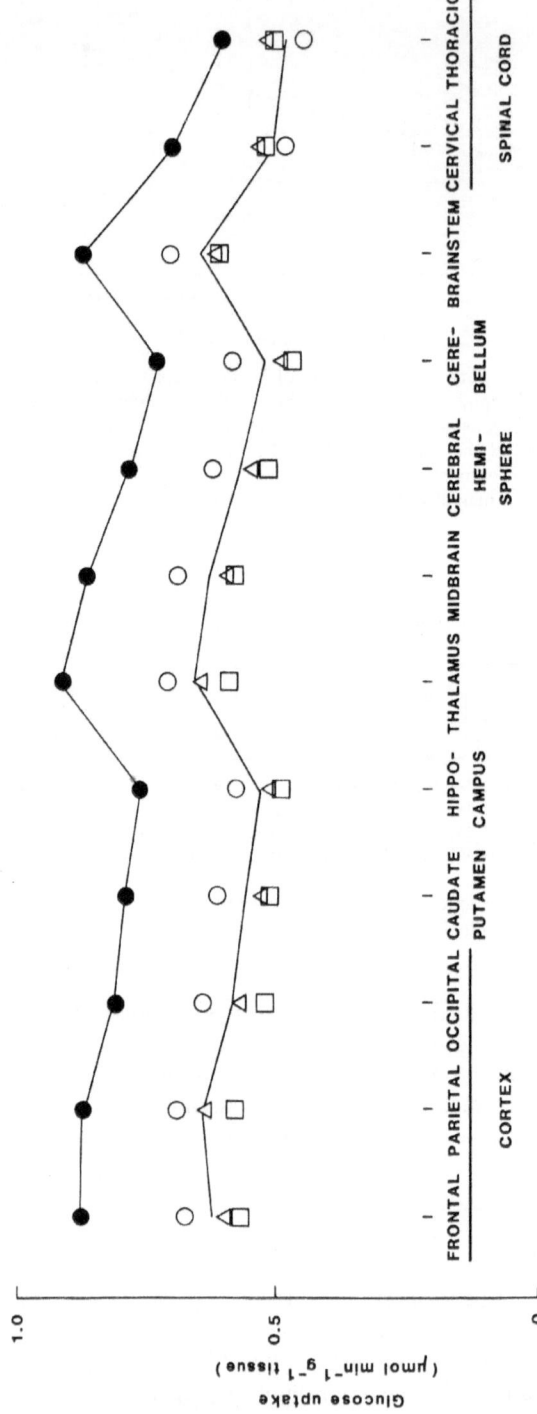

Figure 4 Effects of acutely raised plasma lead on the uptake of glucose by various regions of the CNS. Solid circles represent the grand mean regional uptake for control animals (see text for derivation). Open symbols represent glucose uptake in the group of lead-infused rats divided into sets whose plasma lead was maintained steady within three arbitrarily selected concentration ranges: circles, 240–400; triangles, 530–660; squares, 722–764 µg lead/dl. The lines through the grand mean of each group show the pattern of interregional variation which was significant by ANOVA in both ($p < 0.001$). Overall differences between the lead-treated and control animals were also significant ($p < 0.001$)

Table 1 Blood and plasma lead concentrations in control suckling rats and rats exposed to lead via the milk (chronic exposure model)

	Age/(days)	Control		Lead-treated	
		n	μg Pb/dl	n	μg Pb/dl
Whole blood	7	5	< 2	10	54 $\pm$ 4
	14	11	2.5 $\pm$ 1.7	17	43 $\pm$ 1
	19–21	60	6.0 $\pm$ 0.6	70	51 $\pm$ 2
Plasma	7	4	< 2	7	< 2
	14	11	< 2	17	< 2
	19–21	12	< 2	13	5.6 $\pm$ 1.4

Values are means $\pm$ standard error for the number (n) of animals shown. Detection limit 2 μg/dl

and pH were similar in lead-treated and control animals. Intravascular volumes as defined by the inulin space in corresponding brain regions did not differ significantly in the two groups (Table 2). The values are similar to those reported for saline-perfused brains of 250–350 g rats (Takasato et al., 1984).

With two substrates, lysine and thiamine, analysis of variance showed a significant ($p < 0.05$) increase in mean PS-product across all brain regions of the lead-treated rats compared with that of the respective controls, and with histidine there was a significant ($p = 0.05$) treatment/region interaction (Table 3). Taking lead-treated and control animals together, region-to-region differences were highly significant with most substrates except lysine (Table 3).

Testing for differences at a regional level using least significant difference criteria showed a significant elevation of PS-product in the frontal cortical region in lead-treated animals for lysine, histidine and thiamine. With thiamine, and to a lesser extent lysine, smaller increases were also apparent in other regions (Table 2).

Cerebrovascular permeability to [^{14}C]D-mannitol was not significantly different from control in forebrain regions of chronic lead-treated rats (Table 2). PS values in the hindbrain were also similar in the two groups; e.g. mean ($\pm$ SE) in the cerebellum was 1.92 $\pm$ 0.07 and 2.07 $\pm$ 0.10, and in the brainstem 1.90 $\pm$ 0.07 and 1.93 $\pm$ 0.05 x 10^{-5}/s in control and lead-treated rats, respectively.

Regional blood-to-brain transfer of glucose was not altered by chronic lead treatment. Table 2 shows mean values for regions of the cerebral hemisphere of control and lead-treated rats. Similar results were obtained in the hindbrain; e.g. mean uptake ($\pm$ SE) in cerebellum was 0.85 $\pm$ 0.05 and 0.82 $\pm$ 0.04, and in the brainstem 1.03 $\pm$ 0.05 and 1.00 $\pm$ 0.05 μmol/min/g wet tissue in control and lead-treated rats, respectively.

DISCUSSION

Lead-induced encephalopathy in the young rat generally occurs at blood levels of about 500 μg/dl and above, whereas 100 μg/dl is regarded as an

Table 2 Regional brain intravascular volumes and uptake data for various substances in 19–21-day-old control rats and rats exposed to lead via the milk throughout suckling (chronic exposure model)

Substrate	Treatment group	n	Frontal cortex	Parietal cortex	Occipital cortex	Caudate-putamen	Hippo-campus	Thalamus	SED
Lysine[a]	Control	6	0.649	0.859	0.838	0.777	0.855	0.826	
$(s^{-1} \times 10^2)$	Lead	6	1.005***	1.047*	0.941	1.002*	0.934	0.966	0.0855
Histidine[a]	Control	6	0.662	1.110	0.966	0.935	1.042	1.026	
$(s^{-1} \times 10^2)$	Lead	7	0.976**	1.075	1.094	1.005	1.034	1.041	0.0914
Adenine[a]	Control	6	0.192	0.215	0.194	0.182	0.196	0.196	
$(s^{-1} \times 10^{-2})$	Lead	6	0.220	0.224	0.237	0.195	0.190	0.220	0.0160
Thiamine[a]	Control	6	1.163	1.460	1.191	0.852	1.001	0.917	
$(s^{-1} \times 10^4)$	Lead	6	1.751**	1.548	1.678*	1.359*	1.427*	1.384*	0.1984
Choline[a]	Control	7	0.176	0.215	0.182	0.218	0.178	0.213	
$(s^{-1} \times 10^4)$	Lead	7	0.152	0.179	0.168	0.194	0.159	0.209	0.0206
Pyruvate[a]	Control	8	1.077	1.100	0.963	0.835	0.802	0.933	
$(s^{-1} \times 10^2)$	Lead	8	1.137	1.308	1.072	0.944	0.929	1.065	0.1809
3- hydroxybutyrate[a]	Control	8	0.363	0.388	0.365	0.376	0.327	0.352	
$(s^{-1} \times 10^2)$	Lead	8	0.308	0.320	0.317	0.302	0.272	0.265	0.0353
Glucose[b]	Control	6	1.08	1.06	0.97	0.96	0.89	1.07	
$(\mu mol/min/g)$	Lead	7	1.03	1.03	0.93	0.91	0.86	1.04	0.0734
Mannitol[c]	Control	6	2.10	1.95	2.13	1.63	1.65	1.78	
$(s^{-1} \times 10^5)$	Lead	6	2.32	2.05	2.25	1.65	1.72	1.73	0.0012
Intravascular[d] volume	Control	38	9.2 ± 0.4	8.2 ± 0.3	8.6 ± 0.3	6.5 ± 0.4	8.1 ± 0.4	7.0 ± 0.5	
$(ml/g \times 10^3)$	Lead	35	8.6 ± 0.3	8.3 ± 0.3	8.8 ± 0.4	6.3 ± 0.4	8.0 ± 0.3	6.7 ± 0.4	

[a] PS-products were determined by in situ brain perfusion (Takasato et al., 1984)

[b] Uptakes determined in vivo by programmed intravenous infusion. Control glucose uptakes adjusted (see methods) to values corresponding to the mean plasma glucose in the lead-treated rats (8.7 mmol/l)

[c] PS-product was determined from the ratio of tissue to mean plasma tracer concentrations divided by the duration of mannitol infusion (600 s). Significance of differences at regional level were determined by least significant difference criteria using the standard error of differences of means for treatment/region interaction (SED): *$p < 0.05$, **$p < 0.01$, ***$p < 0.001$

[d] Space determined by in situ brain perfusion using [³H]inulin added to the perfusion fluid, means ± SE

Caption for Chapter 5.5

Table 3 Summary of F-ratio probability from ANOVA applied to regional brain PS-product for various substrates in lead-treated and control 19–21-day-old rats

	Source of variation		
Substrate	Treatment	Region	Treatment/region
Lysine	0.009	0.288	0.091
Histidine	0.142	<0.001	0.050
Adenine	0.052	0.032	0.288
Thiamine	0.014	<0.001	0.263
Choline	0.259	<0.001	0.755
Pyruvate	0.451	<0.001	0.927
3- Hydroxybutyrate	0.061	<0.001	0.587

ANOVA was carried out using the GENSTAT statistical program (Alvey *et al.*, 1982)

approximate threshold for this disorder in children (Winder *et al.*, 1983). However, regimes that produce blood lead levels as low as 20 µg/dl without overt toxicity have been associated with impaired learning performance in the rat (Winneke, 1986). Thus, although the rat may be less susceptible to lead-induced encephalopathy, there is a rationale for proposing a neurophysiological impairment in this species at blood lead levels comparable to those of asymptomatic infant populations exposed to lead in the environment.

The chronic exposure regime used in the present study produced blood lead concentrations in the subclinical range (20–90 µg/dl), and these levels were present during most of the 3-week suckling period. Mannitol uptake provided a quantitative regional index of blood–brain barrier integrity in this model, and avoided the subjectivity associated with dye extravasation methods. The data showed that the barrier remained 'intact' after this regime; increased 'leakiness' did not appear to explain the increased uptake of some substrates in certain brain regions. Moreover, a similar change in uptake of all the substrates would be expected with a generalized increase in barrier permeability. These observations at 19–21 days do not preclude a transient increase in barrier permeability at an earlier stage, as has been demonstrated using Evans blue-albumin (Sundström *et al.*, 1985), albeit at higher exposure levels (i.e. blood lead > 300 µg/dl).

There was no evidence of impaired transport of tracer quantities of nutrient substrates in the chronic exposure model. This supports earlier observations in whole brain (Lefauconnier *et al.*, 1980; Michaelson and Bradbury, 1982). The instances of increased uptake in some regions may reflect direct interference by lead at the level of the endothelial cell, or be due to selective alterations in cerebral metabolism resulting from changes in tissue demand. Lead is known to accumulate in capillary endothelial cells of the brain (Thomas *et al.*, 1973; Silbergeld *et al.*, 1980) and there is experimental evidence to suggest that another heavy metal compound (methylmercury) may increase transport by membrane effects (Hargreaves *et al.*, 1986). However, it seems unlikely that such a mechanism was operative here, unless there were large interregional differences in capillary endothelial sensitivity to the phenomenon. Evidence from studies on some essential substrates (ketone bodies, glucose and amino acids) indicates a close coupling between cerebral metabolism and transport at the blood–brain barrier (Pardridge, 1983, for review). Thus the observed increases in PS-product may reflect lead-induced differences in region-specific demand for these substances. Cortical regions, notably the frontal cortex, showed the most significant differences. The changes may represent a biochemical lesion or altered substrate utilization associated with repair processes, although to our knowledge the frontal cortex has not been identified histopathologically as a target for lead. If not attributable to these processes, it is conceivable that the lead treatment delayed maturation in the developing brain by a mechanism unrelated to the nutritional status of the animals. Brain uptake rates of many amino acids and other essential substrates are high soon after birth, and fall progressively during the first few weeks of life (Baños et al., 1978; Cornford et al., 1982; Lefauconnier and Trouvé, 1983). These changes are thought to signify a fall-off in tissue demand as maturation proceeds. Thus a lead-induced delay in maturation might, in susceptible regions, extend the period during which tissue substrate requirements remain high.

In the acute studies elevated lead levels were maintained constant in the plasma by programmed infusion. Based on estimates of the binding of lead to albumin (Simons, 1986), it is unlikely that the formation of insoluble lead salts in the circulation would be a significant consideration over the range of lead levels used (see also Aungst et al., 1981; Bradbury and Dean, 1986).

The regional blood-to-brain transfer constants for mannitol found in control animals (Figure 3) were comparable to those reported for the adult rat (Daniel et al., 1985), and confirm previous observations in whole brain (Saunders, 1977; Braun et al., 1980), that the restrictive properties of the blood–brain barrier are present at an early stage of development. The changes in cerebrovascular permeability reported with chronic exposure to high circulating lead levels were not reproduced in these acute experiments. No significant increases in barrier permeability were evident in any CNS regions, including the cerebellum, which has been shown to be particularly susceptible to elevated lead levels in the suckling rat (Pentschew and Garro, 1966; Goldstein et al., 1974). Thus, although lead is taken up rapidly by the endothelial cells (Thomas et al., 1973), the present findings suggest that timing and duration of exposure may be important factors in the pathogenesis of lead encephalopathy.

Although inhibition of glucose transport following lead treatment has been demonstrated in vitro using isolated rat brain microvessels (Kolber et al., 1980) and cultured endothelial cells (Maxwell et al., 1986), this was not substantiated in vivo using chronic low-level exposure by the present study, nor by others (Lefauconnier et al., 1980) in whole brain. However, a significant inhibition was evident in all CNS regions after acute high-level exposure. This latter finding accords with results obtained with another heavy metal (mercury) after brief perfusion of cerebral vessels with mercuric ions (Steinwall, 1968; Pardridge, 1976). Both lead and mercury have appreciable affinity for sulphydryl groups (Passow et al., 1961), which are essential constituents of the membrane proteins associated with nutrient transport (Orlowski, 1976; Hervonen and Steinwall, 1984; Abbot et al., 1986). The inhibition of glucose uptake in suckling rats was not seen in adult rats following acute high-level lead exposure (unpublished observations). This difference may be due to an age-related difference in the functional state of the hexose transport system.

Kinetic studies of glucose transport at the blood–brain barrier (Daniel et al., 1978; Cremer et al., 1979) have shown that transport capacity is significantly lower in the suckling rat compared to the mature animal. Because of this limited capacity, the activity of the hexose transport system in neonates may be relatively easily depressed by acute exposure to high levels of lead.

ACKNOWLEDGMENTS

We thank Mrs Susanne Carden, Mrs Brenda Eley and Mrs Victoria Lee for competent technical assistance. The lead analyses were conducted by Mr P. Drewitt. This work was supported by the Commission of the European Communities, Environmental Research Programme, Contract No. ENV-781-UK.

REFERENCES

Abbot, R. E., Schachter, D., Batt, E. R. and Flamm, M. (1986) Sulfhydryl substituents of the human erythrocyte hexose transport mechanism. Am. J. Physiol., 250, C853–860

Alvey, N., Galway, N. and Lane, P. (1982) An Introduction to GENSTAT (London: Academic Press)

Aungst, B. J., Dolce, J. A. and Fung, H. L. (1981). The effect of dose on the disposition of lead in rats after intravenous and oral administration. Toxicol. Appl. Pharmacol., 61, 48–57

Balazs, R., Lewis, P. D. and Patel, A. J (1979) Nutritional deficiencies and brain development. In Falkner, F. and Tanner, J. M. (eds), Human Growth, vol. 3 (London: Bailliere Tindall)

Baños, G., Daniel, P. M. and Pratt, O. E. (1978). The effect of age upon the entry of some amino acids into the brain, and their incorporation into cerebral proteins. Dev. Med. Child Neurol., 20, 335–346

Bradbury, M. W. B. (1985) The blood–brain barrier. Transport across the cerebral endothelium. Circ. Res., 57, 213–222

Bradbury, M. W. B. and Deane, R. (1986) Rate of uptake of lead-203 into brain and other soft tissues of the rat at constant radiotracer levels in plasma. Ann. N.Y. Acad. Sci., 481, 142–160

Braun, L. D., Cornford, E. M. and Oldendorf, W. H. (1980) Newborn rabbit blood–brain barrier is selectively permeable and differs substantially from the adult. J. Neurochem., 34, 147–152

Carmichael, N. G., Winder, C. and Lewis, P. D. (1981) Dose response relationships during perinatal lead administration in the rat: a model for the study of lead effects on brain development. Toxicology, 21, 117–128

Cornford, E. M., Braun, L. D. and Oldendorf, W. H. (1982) Developmental modulations of blood–brain barrier permeability as an indicator of changing nutritional requirements in the brain. Ped. Res., 16, 324–328

Cremer, J. E. and Cunningham, V. J. (1981) Properties of transport processes of the blood–brain barrier during development. In Kovách, A. G. B., Hamar, J. and Szabó, L. (eds), Advances in Physiological Science, vol. 7: Cardiovascular Physiology, Microcirculation and Capillary Exchange (London: Pergamon Press)

Cremer, J. E., Cunningham, V. J., Pardridge, W. M., Braun, L. D. and Oldendorf, W. H. (1979) Kinetics of blood–brain barrier transport of pyruvate, lactate and glucose in suckling, weanling and adult rats. J. Neurochem., 33, 439–445

Crone, C. (1963) The permeability of capillaries in various organs as determined by use of the 'Indicator Diffusion' Method. Acta Physiol. Scand., 58, 292–305

Cunningham, V. J., Hargreaves, R. J., Pelling, D. and Moorhouse, S. R. (1986) Regional blood–brain glucose transfer in the rat: a novel double-membrane kinetic analysis. J. Cerebral Blood Flow Metab., 6, 305–314

Daniel, P. M., Lam, D. K. C. and Pratt, O. E. (1985) Comparison of the vascular permeability of the brain and spinal cord to mannitol and inulin in rats. *J. Neurochem.*, **45**, 647–649

Daniel, P. M., Love, E. R., Moorhouse, S. R., Pratt, O. E. and Wilson, P. A. (1974) A method for rapidly washing the blood out of an organ or tissue of the anaesthetized living animal. *J. Physiol.*, **237**, 11p–12p

Daniel, P. M., Love, E. R. and Pratt, O. E. (1978) The effect of age upon the influx of glucose into the brain. *J. Physiol.*, **274**, 141–148

Fernandez, F. J. and Hilligoss, D. (1982) An improved graphite furnace method for the determination of lead in blood using matrix modification and the L'vov platform. *Atomic Spectrosc.*, **3**, 130–131

Goldstein, G. W., Asbury, A. K. and Diamond, I. (1974) Pathogenesis of lead encephalopathy. Uptake of lead and reaction of brain capillaries. *Arch. Neurol.*, **31**, 382–389

Hargreaves, R. J., Moorhouse, S. R., Gangolli, S. D. and Pelling, D. (1986) The effects of methylmercury on glucose transport, glucose metabolism and blood flow in the central nervous system of the rat. In Suckling, A. J., Rumsby, M. G. and Bradbury, M. W. B. (eds), *The Blood–Brain Barrier in Health and Disease* (Chichester: Ellis Horwood)

Hervonen, H. and Steinwall, O. (1984) Endothelial surface sulfhydryl-groups in blood–brain barrier transport of nutrients. *Acta Physiol. Scand.*, **121**, 343–351

Kolber, A. R., Krigman, M. R. and Morell, P. (1980) The effect of *in vitro* and *in vivo* lead intoxication on monosaccharide transport in isolated rat brain microvessels. *Brain Res.*, **192**, 513–521

Lefauconnier, J. M., Lavielle, E., Terrien, N., Bernard, G. and Fournier, E. (1980) Effect of various lead doses on some cerebral capillary functions in the suckling rat. *Toxicol. Appl. Pharmacol.*, **55**, 467–476

Lefauconnier, J. M. and Trouvé, R. (1983) Developmental changes in the pattern of amino acid transport at the blood–brain barrier in rats. *Dev. Brain Res.*, **6**, 175–182

Lorenzo, A. V. and Gewirtz, M. (1977) Inhibition of [^{14}C]tryptophan transport into brain of lead exposed neonatal rabbits. *Brain Res.*, **132**, 386–392

Maxwell, K., Vinters, H. V., Berliner, J. A., Bready, J. V. and Cancilla, P. A. (1986) Effect of inorganic lead on some functions of the cerebral microvessel endothelium. *Toxicol. Appl. Pharmacol.*, **84**, 389–399

Michaelson, I. A. (1980) An appraisal of rodent studies on the behavioural toxicity of lead: the role of nutritional status. In Singhal, R. L. and Thomas, J. A. (eds), *Lead Toxicity* (Baltimore: Urban & Schwarzenborg)

Michaelson, I. A. and Bradbury, M. (1982) Effect of early inorganic lead exposure on rat blood–brain barrier permeability to tyrosine or choline. *Biochem. Pharmacol.*, **31**, 1881–1885

Orlowski, M. (1976) Possible role of glutathione in transport processes. In Levi, G., Battistin, L. and Lajtha, A. (eds), *Transport Phenomena in the Nervous System; Physiological and Pathological Aspects* (New York and London: Plenum Press)

Pardridge, W. M. (1976) Inorganic mercury: selective effects on blood–brain barrier transport systems. *J. Neurochem.*, **27**, 333–335

Pardridge, W. M. (1983) Brain metabolism: a perspective from the blood–brain barrier. *Physiol. Rev.*, **63**, 1481–1535

Passow, H., Rothstein, A. and Clarkson, T. W. (1961) General pharmacology of the heavy metals. *Pharmacol. Rev.*, **13**, 183–224

Pellegrino, L. J., Pellegrino, A. S. and Cushman, A. J. (1979) *A Stereotaxic Atlas of the Rat Brain* (New York: Plenum Press)

Pentschew, A. and Garro, F. (1966) Lead encephalo-myelopathy of the suckling rat and its implications on the porphyrinopathic nervous diseases. *Acta Neuropathol. (Berlin)*, **6**, 266–278

Pratt, O. E. (1979) Adequate nutrition of the developing brain. In Korobkin, R. and Guilleminault, C. (eds), *Advances in Perinatal Neurology*, vol. I (New York: Spectrum)

Pratt, O. E. (1985) Continuous-injection methods for the measurement of flux across the blood–brain barrier. The steady-state, initial-rate method. In Marks, N. and Rodnight, R. (eds), *Research Methods in Neurochemistry*, vol. 6 (New York–London: Plenum Press)

Saunders, N. R. (1977) Ontogeny of the blood–brain barrier. *Exp. Eye Res.*, (Suppl.), 523–550

Silbergeld, E. K., Wolinsky, J. S. and Goldstein, G. W. (1980) Electron probe microanalysis of isolated brain capillaries poisoned with lead. *Brain Res.*, **189**, 369–376

Simons, T. J. B. (1986) Passive transport and binding of lead by human red blood cells. *J.*

Physiol., **378**, 267–286

Steinwall, O. (1968) Transport inhibition phenomena in unilateral chemical injury of blood–brain barrier. *Prog. Brain Res.*, **29**, 357–364

Sundström, R., Müntzing, K., Kalimo, H. and Sourander, P. (1985) Changes in the integrity of the blood–brain barrier in suckling rats with low dose lead encephalopathy. *Acta Neuropathol.*, **68**, 1–9

Takasato, Y., Rapoport, S. I. and Smith, Q. R. (1984) An *in situ* brain perfusion technique to study cerebrovascular transport in the rat. *Am. J. Physiol.*, **247**, H484–H493

Thomas, J. A., Dallenbach, F. D. and Thomas, M. (1973) The distribution of radioactive lead (^{210}Pb) in the cerebellum of developing rats. *J. Pathol.*, **109**, 45–50

Winder, C., Garten, L. L. and Lewis, P. D. (1983) The morphological effects of lead on the developing central nervous system. *Neuropathol. Appl. Neurobiol.*, **9**, 87–108

Winneke, G. (1986) Animal studies. In Lansdown, R. and Yule, W. (eds), *The Lead Debate: the environment, toxicology and child health* (London–Sydney: Croom Helm)

Section 6

EXTENDED ABSTRACTS OF POSTERS

6.1

Low-Level Lead Exposure and Intelligence in the Early Preschool Years

C. B. ERNHART and M. MORROW-TLUCAK

SUMMARY

Two hypotheses were tested: (a) that cognitive development is negatively related to measures of current and/or prior lead exposure and (b) that lead level is related negatively to prior measures of cognitive development and/or positively to prior measures of psychomotor maturity. Blood lead (PbB) was measured at ages 6 months, 2 years and 3 years. These PbB measures were related to developmental measures at ages 6 months, 1 year, 2 years, and 3 years. With statistical control of confounding, associations of PbB and concurrent and later development were attenuated and not statistically significant. Similarly, PbB was not related significantly to prior measures of cognitive development or psychomotor acceleration. The relationship of PbB and developmental status in the early preschool years appeared to be a function of the dependence of each on the quality of the caretaking environment.

The period of infancy and the early preschool years is a time of increased risk for lead exposure because of metabolic factors and the exploratory and mouthing behaviour of young children. Questions asked in this study were (a) whether developmental status at this age is related to concurrent or prior low-level lead exposure and (b) whether child characteristics, i.e. slower mental development and/or advanced psychomotor development, are related to increased risk of later lead exposure.

Results from several cohort studies are now available. Bellinger *et al.* (1986) failed to find any relation, for middle-class infants, of 6-month and 12-month blood lead levels (PbB) and the Mental Development Index (MDI) of the Bayley Scales of Infant Development. Dietrich *et al.* (in press) reported a significant relationship of 3-month, but not 6-month, PbB with 6-month MDI for 27 white but not for 158 black infants. They also reported a positive relation of 6-month PbB and the Bayley Psychomotor Index (PDI). Vimpani *et al.* (1987) found 6-month (but not 15-month or 2-year) PbB to be related to 2-year MDI.

The present report relates 6-month, 2-year, and 3-year PbB to the MDI and PDI at 6 months, the MDI at 1 and 2 years, and the Stanford–Binet (S–B) Scale at 3 years.

METHOD

Description of sample

All children in the cohort being studied came from disadvantaged families. Half of the mothers were identified as alcoholic. 39% of the mothers were black. The mean maternal Peabody Picture Vocabulary Test (revised version score) (PPVT-R IQ) was 73 compared with an expected mean of 100. The data being reported are for the 247 children for whom at least one PbB sample was available.

Data collection

The Bayley Scales, the Stanford–Binet Intelligence Scale (S-B IQ) and the Home Observation for the Measurement of the Environment (HOME) Inventory were administered in the homes by trained examiners blinded to lead level. Staff members drawing venous blood samples were trained in paediatric blood collection. PbB levels were determined by atomic absorption spectrophotometry using a graphite furnace and matrix modification to control chemical interference.

Data analysis

Multiple regression was used with entry of a set of covariates selected *a priori* on the basis of a plausible relationship with preschool intelligence. These were sex, age at testing, race, birth order, maternal PPVT-R, parental education, maternal attitude towards child-rearing, and, for ages 1, 2 and 3 years, the HOME Inventory. Alpha was set at 0.01 to minimize studywise error but testwise *p* values for each analysis are provided.

RESULTS

Descriptive statistics

Descriptive statistics are given in Table 1. PbB increased from age 6 months to 2 years and remained stable to age 3 years. At 6 months the highest PbB was 24 µg/dl whole blood. At 2 years, seven children had PbB levels that exceeded 30 µg/dl and at 3 years eight children exceeded this figure. The

Table 1 Descriptive statistics, blood lead level (PbB) and developmental tests

		PbB			Development measure			
Age	n	$\bar{x}$	S.D.	r with race	Test	$\bar{x}$	S.D.	r with race
6 months	146	10.05	3.28	0.01	Bayley MDI	110.24	18.18	−0.21**
					Bayley PDI	111.61	14.10	0.01
1 year	131				Bayley MDI	110.33	15.33	−0.11
2 years	165	16.74	6.50	0.29**	Bayley MDI	100.33	16.51	−0.19*
3 years	167	16.95	6.49	0.25**	S-B IQ	88.27	15.59	−0.31**

* $p < 0.05$; ** $p < 0.01$, two-tailed tests

correlation of 2-year and 3-year PbB was 0.66; the correlations of each with 6-month PbB were, respectively, 0.30 and 0.34.

Relation of PbB and developmental measures

As shown in Table 2, 6-month PbB was not related significantly to any outcome measure, with or without consideration of the covariate set. The concurrent analyses for ages 2 and 3 years, and the prospective analysis of age 2-year PbB and 3-year S-B IQ were statistically significant in the initial correlations. In each case, however, the effect was greatly diminished and did not approach statistical significance with control of confounding variables. There was no significant interaction of PbB and race.

Obtained effect sizes were extremely small. Power analysis was used for the analysis of 2-year PbB and 3-year S-B IQ. With alpha = 0.01, $n = 153$, and the covariate variance 0.31, the power to detect an increment in variance of 5% or greater is 77%, and the power for an increment of 6% or greater is 87%.

Relation of individual characteristics and later lead level

As shown in Table 3, with control of confounding variables, none of the MDI assessments of early development was related significantly to the later PbB measure. The covariates that contributed most strongly to the models were the HOME (total), race, maternal PPVT-R, and parent education.

The converse question, i.e. whether children advanced in psychomotor development would have higher lead levels, was also assessed. The correlations of 6-month PDI with PbB at 6 months, 2 years, and 3 years were 0.06, −0.07, and −0.02, respectively.

DISCUSSION

Major finding

The results do not support the hypothesis that low-level lead burden in the early years is related to psychological deficit. Six-month PbB did not correlate

Table 2 The relationship of PbB with the Bayley MDI and Stanford–Binet developmental measures

PbB	Developmental measure	n	Simple correlation		Regression model					
					Covariates		Increment due to PbB		Increment due to race by PbB interaction	
			r	p*	Variance	p	Variance	p	Variance	p
6 months	6 month MDI	146	−0.09	0.29	0.18	0.000	0.01	0.31	0.01	0.34
	1 year MDI	131	0.08	0.40	0.14	0.02	0.01	0.25	0.00	0.51
	2 year MDI	126	−0.03	0.74	0.30	0.000	0.00	0.95	0.00	0.63
	3 year S-B IQ	126	−0.04	0.65	0.29	0.000	0.00	0.49	0.00	0.87
2 years	2 year MDI	165	−0.25	0.000	0.32	0.000	0.00	0.95	0.01	0.07
	3 year S-B IQ	153	−0.31	0.000	0.31	0.000	0.01	0.29	0.00	0.32
3 years	3 year S-B IQ	167	−0.27	0.000	0.36	0.000	0.00	0.98	0.01	0.08

* Two-tailed statistical test

Table 3 The predictive relationship of early preschool developmental measures and later lead level

| MDI | PbB as outcome measure | n | Simple correlation | | Regression model | | | |
| | | | | | Covariates | | Increment due to MDI | |
			r	p*	Variance	p	Variance	p
6 months	2 year	150	−0.24	0.004	0.32	0.000	0.003	0.47
	3 year	153	−0.10	0.20	0.28	0.000	0.001	0.61
1 year	2 year	156	−0.10	0.22	0.30	0.000	0.002	0.50
	3 year	156	−0.10	0.24	0.23	0.000	0.001	0.62
2 year	3 year	157	−0.17	0.04	0.23	0.000	0.009	0.19

* Probabilities are two-tailed

significantly with any developmental measure. The correlations relating 2-year and 3-year PbB to concurrent and ensuing developmental measures (MDI and S-B IQ) can be accounted for through common cause, i.e. the influence of the caretaking environment, and are fully attenuated with statistical control of confounding.

Secondary findings

Race
Like ours, the children of the Dietrich *et al.* study were disadvantaged urban American children. Although our 6-month PbB levels were higher than theirs at 3 and 6 months, and we had a larger proportion of white children (61% as opposed to 15%), we failed to replicate their finding of a race-by-PbB interaction, i.e. a PbB effect observed only for white children.

Individual characteristics and lead level
One explanation of an association of lead level and mental retardation is that elevations in lead level might be secondary to lower intelligence, i.e. that less intelligent children would be more prone to pica or mouthing behaviour with resulting increased lead ingestion. Our data, for the ranges of intelligence sampled, do not support this interpretation. Another characteristic suggested as causing elevated lead level is advanced mobility in infancy resulting in greater access to dust or other lead-bearing material. This was the explanation of a positive relationship of 6-month PDI and 6-month PbB in the Dietrich *et al.* report. We did not replicate this finding.

CONCLUSIONS

The results of the various analyses of this study indicate that the association of lead level and cognitive development, suggested by simple correlations, may be mediated by the quality of the child-rearing environment which is related strongly to lead level and to the cognitive outcome measures. Further tests of the research hypotheses will be made when these PbB data are related to the intelligence test (Wechsler Preschool and Primary Scale of Intelligence) being administered before school entry. We are now analysing other preschool age outcome measures.

ACKNOWLEDGMENTS

This research was supported in part by Grant No. LH-327 from the International Lead Zinc Research Organization, Grant No. 12-69 from the March of Dimes Birth Defects Foundation, Grant No. AA06571 from the National Institute of Alcohol Abuse and Alcoholism, and Grant No. HD14883 from the National Institute of Child Health and Human Development. The assistance provided by Penny Erhard, B.A. in the conduct of the blood analyses, is gratefully acknowledged.

REFERENCES

Bellinger, D., Leviton, A., Needleman, H.L., Waternaux, C. and Rabinowitz, M. (1986) Low-level lead exposure and infant development in the first year. *Neurobehav. Toxicol. Teratol.*, **8**, 151–161

Dietrich, K.N., Krafft, K.M., Shukla, R., Bornschein, R.L. and Succop, P.A. (in press) The neurobehavioral effects of prenatal and early postnatal lead exposure. In Schroeder, S.R. (ed.) *Toxic Substances and Mental Retardation: Neurobehavioral Toxicology and Teratology* (Washington, DC: AAMD Monograph Series)

Vimpani, G.V., Wigg, N.R., Robertson, E.F., McMichael, A.J., Baghurst, P.A. and Roberts, R.J. (1987) The Port Pirie cohort study: blood lead concentration and childhood developmental assessment. In Goldwater, L.J., Wysocki, L.M. and Volpe R.A. (eds), *Lead Environmental Health: the current issues* (Durham, NC: Duke University Press)

6.2

Which Measures of Lead Burden Best Predict a Child's 2-Year Mental Development?

M. RABINOWITZ, D. BELLINGER and A. LEVITON

We have collected much, often redundant, data, and are now able to examine them systematically to determine which measures are the most useful in predicting a child's mental development. We really do not know how or when low levels of lead contamination disturb brain development. Thus, without imposing any prior restrictions, we should evaluate many measures of lead burden. In the absence of an assay for the bioactive species (ionic?) of lead at the target organ (brain) at the critical time(s), blood lead measurements (which are mostly erythrocyte bound lead, and which represent a very small fraction of the body's total lead level) were used to assess the child's body burden.

We constructed 12 different, simple ways to consider a child's internal lead burden (Table 1). Given our ignorance of lead's toxicokinetics, each way

Table 1 Spearman correlations (r) between 12 different measures of lead body burden and the difference between observed and expected 24-month mental development index

No.	Measure of body burden	r	n	p
1	Cord Blood Lead	−0.20	182	0.008
2	Mean Blood Lead (0 → 24 months)	−0.03	182	0.7
3	Mean Blood Lead (6 → 24)	0.02	182	0.7
4	Peak Blood Lead (0 → 24)	−0.05	182	0.5
5	24 Month Blood Lead	0.03	180	0.7
6	Mean of Blood Lead 18 & 24	0.07	182	0.4
7	Cummulative Positive Increments of Blood Lead (all ages)	−0.03	182	0.7
8	Positive Increment (0 → 6)	0.13	182	0.09
9	Mean EP (6 → 24)	0.04	182	0.6
10	Peak EP (6 → 24)	0.05	182	0.5
11	EP at 24 months	−0.01	179	0.9
12	Environmental Lead Exposure	−0.06	182	0.4

offered some biological plausibility. The first, only cord blood, was chosen because the infant may be especially vulnerable to lead at that time. The second and third models represent averages of the child's lead exposure up to the time that the outcome is measured. The fourth considers only the peak value whenever it occurred, which would be the best if the dose–response relationship to lead is very steep, giving a good fit if children were insensitive to lead variations in a low range, but responded more if lead values reached some higher value.

The fifth and sixth represent lead burdens nearly contemporaneous with the outcome. These would be the best models if the effects of lead were prompt and reversible. If the blood lead measurements are noisy and subject to fluctuations, averaging the two (model 6) would give a better estimate of body burden. The seventh and eighth, which consider only positive increments in blood lead, would fit well if the child responds to additional lead exposure, having become accustomed to or tolerant of a steady dose. In this case the response to lead would depend more on the rate of change of exposure rather than the absolute level of exposure.

The ninth through eleventh ways utilize erythrocytic protoporphyrin (EP), and offer several possible advantages. Not only does blood EP integrate lead exposure over a longer time than does blood lead, but EP also provides information about a child's biochemical reaction to a given blood lead dose, which may be idiosyncratic. Also, if EP itself is a toxic intermediary in lead's neurotoxicity, EP values might correlate better with Mental Development Index scores than do lead.

Lastly, blood lead concentrations may be a sufficiently poor marker of brain lead burden that environmental levels may be a better predictor. Thus, the twelfth measure of lead burden did not include blood data at all, but rather used a summary measure of environmental exposure.

Of the several ways we used the blood lead data, only one achieved statistical significance: umbilical cord blood lead levels. That measure was highly statistically significant. For these children the subsequent measurements, including protoporphyrin, provided little predictive power.

Another inference from our data is that to protect children from the harmful effects of lead, attention should be paid to the exposure of the pregnant and pre-pregnant woman.

6.3

Recent Observations Concerning the Relationship of Blood Lead to Erythrocytic Protoporphyrin

P. A. SUCCOP, P. B. HAMMOND, R. L. BORNSCHEIN,
S. B. RODA and R. D. GREENLAND

SUMMARY

Blood lead concentration (PbB) and erythrocytic protoporphyrin concentration (EP) are both used as indices of lead exposure in children and in occupationally exposed adults. In a previous study we reported dose–effect and dose–response relationships, in EP vs. PbB (Hammond et $al.$, 1985). In the present study we report the influence of age on the threshold for an EP response to PbB, as well as on the slope of the dose–effect interaction. In the age range 12–30 months the threshold for effect of PbB on EP falls progressively, while the magnitude of the dose–effect increases with age. The rate of decline in the threshold for ln EP and the rate of increase for ln EP·PbB^{-1} are linearly related to age.

BACKGROUND

The determination of erythrocytic protoporphyrin (EP) has been used extensively as a screening device to identify children with possible excessive lead exposure. The value of this procedure has diminished somewhat in recent years, for two reasons which are interdependent. On the one hand, the general perception of what constitutes excessive lead exposure has shifted downward. Thus, at one time the lower limit of excessive lead exposure was considered to be at a blood lead concentration (PbB) of 40 μg/dl (NAS–NRC, 1972). It is now widely believed that a PbB of 40 carries with it a high risk for subtle neurological damage in infants and young children, and that even PbBs in the range of 10–20, at least during intrauterine life, can result in postnatal

477

neurological deficits (Bellinger *et al.*, 1986; Dietrich *et al.*, 1986). In this same interval during which our range of concerns regarding PbBs have slipped well below 40 μg/dl, we have also been able to specify the approximate threshold for sensitivity of EP to elevated lead. Thus, two recent studies have shown that below a PbB of approximately 15–20 μg/dl there is no perceptible relationship to EP in young children (Piomelli *et al.*, 1982; Hammond *et al.*, 1985). The sensitivity of EP analyses therefore falls short of current needs.

In spite of the above qualifications regarding the utility of EP for screening purposes, it remains an important index of lead exposure, particularly in long-term prospective studies of the adverse effects of lead. This is so because considerable uncertainty exists as to whether PbB or EP is the better index of adverse effects of lead exposure. Hammond *et al.* (1980) found that PbB was significantly correlated with renal manifestations of toxicity in lead-exposed workers whereas EP was not. Quite the opposite was reported by Lilis *et al.* (1977). Similar disagreement exists concerning neurological manifestations of occupational lead exposure. Two reports suggest that PbB correlates better with frequency of signs and symptoms than EP in lead-exposed workers (Hammond *et al.*, 1980; Spivey *et al.*, 1979) while a third study reports the opposite (Valciukas *et al.*, 1978).

In our current prospective study of the health effects of lead in children, PbBs of many of the subjects rise well above 20 μg/dl for extended periods of time. Thus the opportunity exists to compare the utility of PbB and EP as exposure indices of neurobehavioural effects of lead exposure. The present report is an extension of one previously published concerning dose–effect and dose–response relationships of PbB to EP (Hammond *et al.*, 1985). The major objective of the present report is to establish whether the relationships between PbB and EP are influenced by the age of the subjects under study. Any significant influence of age on the relationship between EP and PbB would be of importance to those using EP as a surrogate for PbB in lead screening programmes, and for research purposes.

METHODS

The subjects in the present study were monitored continuously from birth as to PbB and EP, with determination of both being made at birth, at 10 days of age and at 3-month intervals thereafter. Recruitment of subjects into the study has been over a period of almost 5 years, with the last subject being entered on 9 December 1985. Thus, the number of subjects for which data are reported decreases progressively with increasing age.

Blood samples were obtained by venepuncture where possible, and by heel-stick or finger-stick as necessary. Analysis for PbB was by anodic stripping voltametry and EP was determined by an extraction method (Chisolm and Brown, 1975). Proficiency for measurement of both PbB and EP was monitored continuously as described earlier (Hammond *et al.*, 1985). Dose–effect analyses were made utilizing logarithmic transformation of EP data. The intersection (join point) of the regression lines for PbB-related rises in EP with the non-PbB-related EP was estimated as described earlier

(Hammond *et al.*, 1985). As in the earlier report, all PbBs and EPs were corrected for variations in haematocrit, and are expressed as micrograms per decilitre of whole blood.

RESULTS AND DISCUSSION

Data concerning the influence of age on the relationships between PbB and EP are summarized in Table 1. In the regression and hockey-stick analyses, EP values were converted to ln EP in order to achieve linearity of interactions with PbB. Although PbB and EP were also measured at 10 days and at 3, 6, and 9 months, at these ages the hockey-stick model was not found to significantly explain the PbB:EP relationship. Evidently the variability in EP is not significantly related to lead levels until 1 year of age. Therefore these earlier data are not presented.

Beginning at 12 months of age two clear age-related changes occur. First, background EP (unrelated to PbB) decreases progressively (Figure 1), and the threshold for an effect of PbB on EP increases progressively in linear fashion (Figure 2). At the same time, however, the impact of PbB on EP for children with PbBs greater than this threshold becomes progressively stronger; that is, β_1 increases progressively, with no sign of levelling off by 30 months (Figure 3).

The significance of the shifting response of EP to PbB is that small changes in EP (upward or downward) portend substantially greater changes in PbB in very young children, as compared with older ones. By way of illustration, a rise of EP from 30 to 40 μg/dl would be associated, on average, with a rise in PbB of 10.3 μg/dl at 12 months. This same modest rise in EP would be associated with a rise in PbB of only 5.9 μg/dl at 30 months of age (Figure 4).

On the other hand, small increases in PbB are associated with greater increases in EP in children at 30 months than at 12 months. It is not clear why the EP response to increasing PbB is greater at 30 months than at 12

Table 1 Hockey-stick regression: ln EP on PbB

Age (months)	n	$\alpha_0 \pm SE$	$\beta_0 \pm SE$	$\beta_1 \pm SE$	ΔR^2	R^2	Join point
12	258	3.37 ± 0.03	3.01 ± 0.12	0.028 ± 0.005	0.016*	0.17	12.91
15	242	3.31 ± 0.03	2.88 ± 0.10	0.032 ± 0.004	0.004	0.32	13.69
18	217	3.29 ± 0.03	2.80 ± 0.11	0.033 ± 0.004	0.019*	0.38	14.71
21	200	3.25 ± 0.03	2.65 ± 0.12	0.039 ± 0.004	0.026*	0.43	15.45
24	176	3.14 ± 0.04	2.61 ± 0.11	0.036 ± 0.004	0.023*	0.39	14.67
27	158	3.12 ± 0.04	2.33 ± 0.17	0.047 ± 0.006	0.040*	0.44	16.62
30	147	3.11 ± 0.03	2.21 ± 0.30	0.049 ± 0.011	0.036*	0.34	18.25

R^2 = the total effect of the hockey-stick regression models. All R^2 are significant at $p < 0.05$. α_0 = average background level of EP at PbB levels below threshold, as ln EP (μg/dl), β_1 = slope for increase in ln EP vs. PbB for children above threshold PbBs. β_0 = calculated intercept of ln EP at PbB = 0 for EPs above threshold, extrapolated from the equation: ln EP = $\beta_0 + \beta_1$ PbB. ΔR^2 = contribution of hockey-stick analysis to R^2. Asterisks indicate significant contributions at $p < 0.05$. Join point = threshold for effect (μg/dl). SE = standard error of estimate

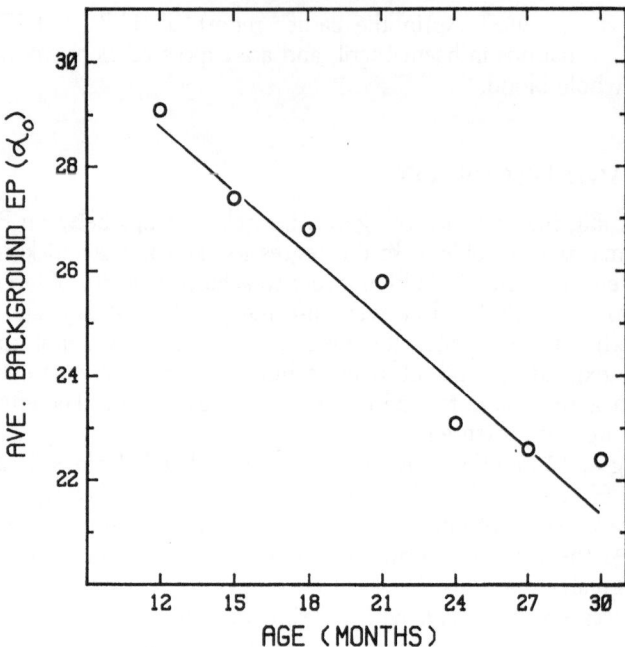

Figure 1 The influence of age on average background EP (α_0) in young children. Data are derived from Table 1

months. The only other study reporting age-related differences in the relationship of EP to PbB compared children, 18–60 months old, to adults (Lamola *et al.*, 1975). In this study the effect of age was the reverse of what we are observing. PbB was actually substantially lower in the adults than in the children. Thus, the increasing response of EP to PbB we see is most likely of a transient nature when viewed over the longer span ranging from infancy to adulthood.

In childhood lead screening programmes EP is used to identify children who may have elevated PbBs. Until recently the guidelines of the US Centers for Disease Control (CDC) suggested that any EP of 50 μg/dl or above triggers a PbB determination. The cutoff of 50 was recommended in order to identify children with PbBs of 30 μg/dl and greater. A new cutoff of EP = 35 μg/dl has recently been recommended. This was done because the PbB level of public health concern is now felt to be well below 30 μg/dl. It was estimated that EP = 35 is associated with PbB = 25. Since the correspondence between EP and PbB is imprecise, some children with EP = 35 will prove to have PbB < 25 (false positives) and some children with EP < 35 would prove to have PbB $\geqslant$ 25 (false negatives). Since both EP and PbB were determined in all children in the present study, it was possible to examine the frequency of the false positives (PbBs < 25 at EPs $\geqslant$ 35 or $\geqslant$ 50) and false negatives (PbBs $\geqslant$ 25 at EPs < 35 or < 50). The results of this analysis are summarized in Table 2. The sensitivity of EP = 35 as a cutoff for detecting children with PbBs $\geqslant$ 25 is somewhat greater than for EP = 50, especially in

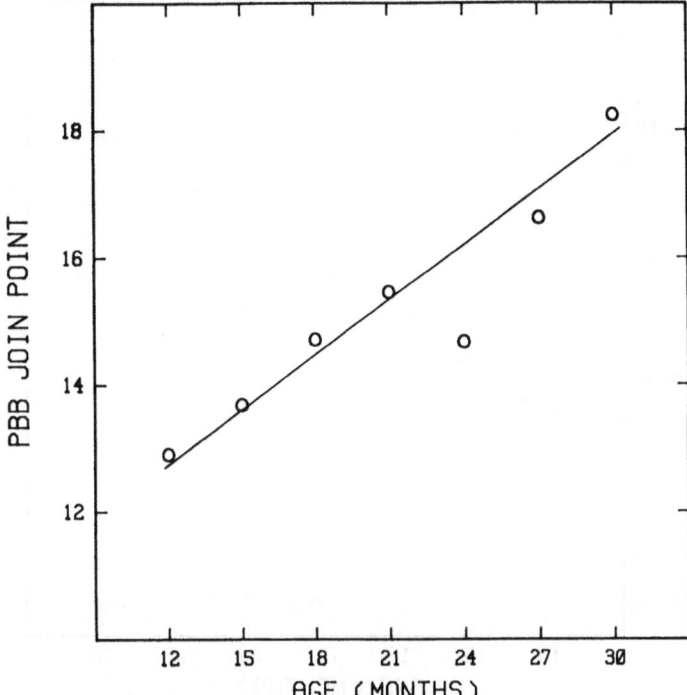

Figure 2   The influence of subject age on the threshold (join point) for a significant interaction between PbB and EP. Data are derived from Table 1

the younger children. Thus, for example, it is estimated that only 4% of children with PbB $\geq$ 25 would be missed (false negative) using a cutoff of EP = 35, whereas 8% would be missed using the EP cutoff of 50. By contrast, a substantially greater number of children would prove to have PbBs < 25 (false positives) using an EP cutoff of 35 as compared to using a cutoff of 50. The obvious advantage of the lower EP cutoff in avoiding false negatives must be balanced against its disadvantage, which is that it materially increases the number of PbB determinations which would result in order to identify children with elevated PbBs.

PbB has long been used as the standard index of dose in estimating dose–effect and dose–response relationships. Some would argue that it is perhaps less valid than certain other measurements which reflect in quantitative fashion the bioavailable fraction of PbB, much as erythrocyte cholinesterase inhibition reflects the toxic impact of exposure to organophosphate insecticides. Indeed, it has been reported that inhibition of erythrocyte membrane Na, K-ATPase activity is better correlated with lead toxicity than erythrocyte lead concentration (Raghavan *et al.*, 1981). This was attributed to the fact that the subjects had variable concentrations of a low molecular weight lead binding protein which influenced the bioavailable fraction of PbB. It is possible that EP reflects bioavailable lead in a similar fashion.

In our current study the opportunity exists to test the hypothesis that EP

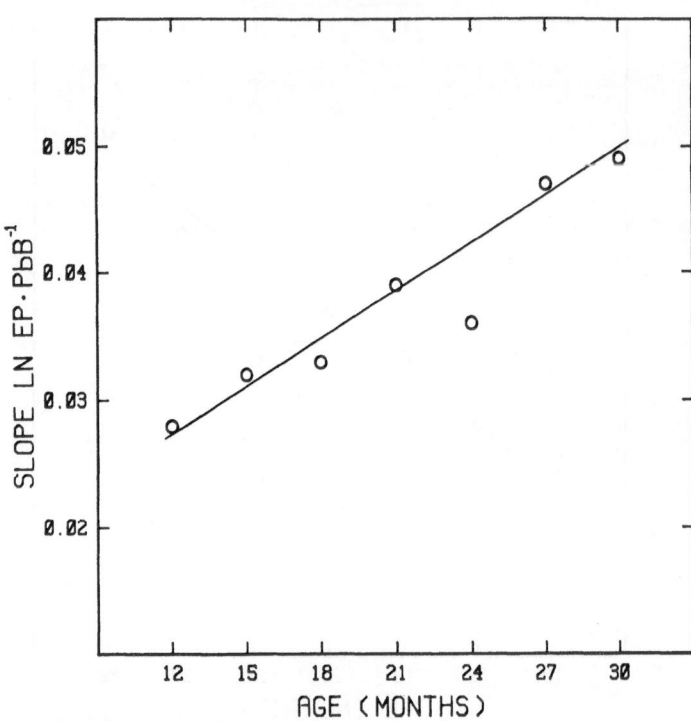

Figure 3 The influence of subject age on steepness of rise in EP in relation to PbB (slope). Data are derived from Table 1

Table 2 Probability of missing children with PbB $\geq 25\ \mu g/dl$ (false negative) and of finding PbB to be 25 (false positive) using EP ≥ 35 and $50\ \mu g/dl$ as the cutoffs

Age (months)	False negative (%)		False positive (%)	
	EP = 35	EP = 50	EP = 35	EP = 50
12	4	8	75	65
15	4	8	63	43
18	5	8	54	16
21	6	9	50	28
24	7	8	45	19
27	8	11	35	10
30	6	8	38	18

is a better index of certain health effects of lead in children than PbB. In spite of the high correlation between ln EP and PbB observed in large samples, we have observed striking differences in the EP/PbB relationship among subjects. For illustrative purposes two subjects were selected who had strikingly similar PbB profiles but very different EP profiles (Table 3). EP values for Subject A were much greater than for Subject B, and tracked the changing PbB profile over time. For Subject B, EPs not only were consistently very low, but also did not vary systematically with PbB. The reason for the difference in the

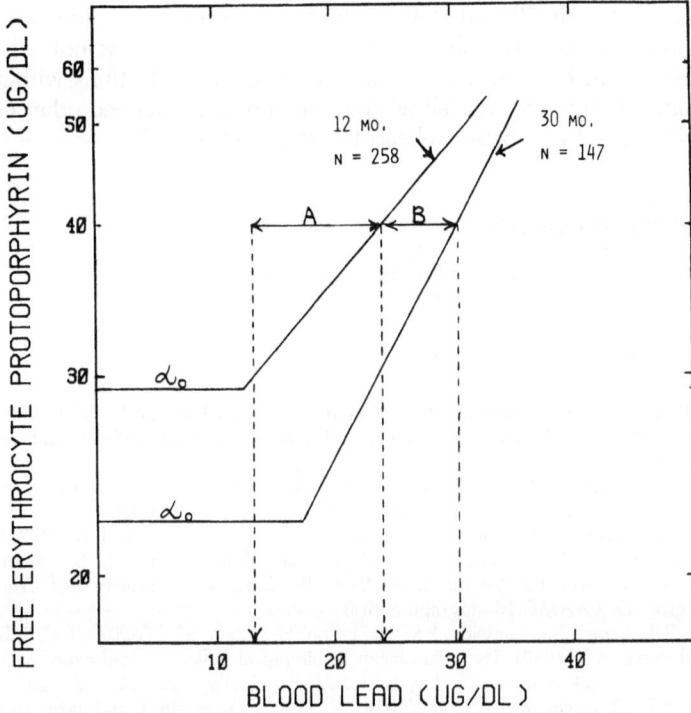

Figure 4   The average rise in PbB associated with a rise in EP of 10 μg/dl from 30 to 40 in children 12 months of age (PbB interval A) as contrasted to the average rise in children 30 months of age (PbB interval B). α_0 represents the EP level below which an interaction with PbB is not evident

Table 3   Contrasting variations in EP associated with PbB

Age (months)	Subject A*		Subject B*	
	PbB	EP	PbB	EP
9	15	19	14	—
12	34	46	30	13
15	40	111	22	—
18	43	215	43	25
21	33	166	39	19
24	35	111	33	32
27	36	93	—	—
30	43	130	43	15
33	38	116	40	26
x̄	38	123	36	22

* Neither of these subjects exhibited any evidence of iron deficiency

relationship between EP and PbB as illustrated here is not known at the present time. In this particular case, however, iron status was not a factor. Both subjects had haematocrits and haemoglobin concentrations within the normal range. Only time will tell whether neurobehavioural and other health effects will prove to be better related to EP or to PbB.

ACKNOWLEDGMENTS

This work was supported by USPHS Grant ES-01566.

REFERENCES

Bellinger, P., Leviton, A., Needleman, H.L., Waternaux, C. and Rabinowitz, M. (1986) Low-level lead exposure and infant development in the first year. *Neurobehav. Toxicol. Teratol.,* **8**, 151–161

Chisolm, J.J. and Brown, P. (1975) Micro-scale photofluorometric determination of free erythrocyte porphyrin (protoporphyrin IX). *Clin. Chem.,* **21**, 1669–1682

Dietrich, K.N., Krafft, K.M., Shukla, R., Bornschein, R.L. and Succop, P.A. (1986) The neurobehavioral effects of prenatal and early postnatal lead exposure. In Schroeder, S.R. (ed.), *Toxic Substances and Mental Retardation: Neurobehavioral Toxicology and Teratology* (Washington, DC: AAMD Monograph Series)

Hammond, P.B., Lerner, S.J., Gartside, P.S., Hanenson, J.B., Roda, S.B., Foulkes, E.C., Johnson, D.R. and Pesce, A.J. (1980). The relationship of biological indices of lead exposure to the health status of workers in a secondary lead smelter. *J. Occup. Med.,* **22**, 475–484

Hammond, P.B., Bornschein, R.L. and Succop, P. (1985) Dose–effect and dose–response relationships of blood lead to erythrocytic protoporphyrin in young children. *Environ. Res.,* **38**, 187–196

Lamola, A.A., Joselow, M. and Yamane, T. (1975) Zinc protoporphyrin (ZPp): a simple, sensitive fluorometric screening test for lead poisoning. *Clin. Chem.,* **21**, 93–97

Lilis, R., Fischbein, A., Diamond, S., Anderson, H.A., Selikoff, J.J., Blumberg and W.E., Eisinger, J. (1977) Lead effects among secondary lead smelter workers with blood lead levels below 80 μg/100 ml. *Arch. Environ. Health,* **32**, 256–266

NAS–NRC (1972) *Airborne Lead in Perspective* (Washington, DC: National Academy of Sciences)

Piomelli, S., Seaman, C., Zullow, D., Curran, A. and Davidow, B. (1982) Threshold for lead damage in heme synthesis in urban children. *Proc. Natl. Acad. Sci. USA,* **79**, 3335–3339

Raghavan, S.R.V., Culver, B.D. and Gonick, H.C. (1981) Erythrocyte lead-binding protein after occupational exposure. II. Influence on lead inhibition of membrane Na$^+$,K$^+$-adenosinetriphosphatase. *J. Toxicol. Environ. Health,* **7**, 561–568

Spivey, G.H., Brown, C.P., Baloh, R.W., Campion, D.S., Valentine, J.L., Massey, F.J., Browdy, B.L. and Culver, B.P. (1979) Subclinical effects of chronic increased lead absorption – a prospective study. 1. Study design and analysis of symptoms. *J. Occup. Med.,* **21**, 423–429

Valciukas, J.A., Lilis, R., Eisinger, J., Blumberg, W.E., Fischbein, A. and Selikoff, F.J. (1978) Behavioral indicators of lead neurotoxicity: results of a clinical field survey. *Int. Arch. Occup. Environ. Health,* **41**, 217–236

Section 7
Summary of Workshop Discussions, and Future Directions

The last sessions of the workshop were specifically devoted to discussions with all the invited speakers and representatives participating. There were four separate sessions under different headings: design and statistics, outcome measures, exposure assessment, and animal studies. These topics were chosen during the meeting as a result of the interest, and in some cases controversy, that had been apparent in these areas, and they also provided convenient headings under which to discuss future directions. The four sessions were summarized by Professor Yule who acted as rapporteur.

This last section of this book, which has drawn on Professor Yule's notes, is in part a report of the discussions which took place, but also incorporates the Editors' views on future directions more generally. The session headings have been used for the first part of this chapter.

DESIGN AND STATISTICS

It may be that epidemiological studies will never fully resolve the question of the degree to which lead at low dose affects the neurobehavioural development of children: epidemiological studies cannot ultimately answer questions of causality. Their value is limited when studying small, but important, environmental factors, in the presence of strong confounding factors, and this is particularly relevant if the sample size is small. This should not obscure the advances which have been made in design, methodology and in statistical techniques as a result of experience from epidemiological studies carried out over the last ten years.

In that time a number of problems in this area have been identified and have been the topic of much discussion and occasionally heated debate; as a result acceptable solutions to many of these problems have emerged.

There has been criticism of the use of probability values, and particularly the rigid adherence to $p < 0.05$ as a criterion for the inclusion or exclusion of variables, or to label a result as significant or not. This has resulted in whole study findings being labelled simply as positive or negative according to which side of the 0.05 level the results have fallen. It is now clear that the greater use of estimation methods such as confidence intervals is appropriate. These provide more information, and enable comparisons in terms of the size of any effects found, to be made between studies.

In study design, the problems of small numbers of subjects and large numbers of potential covariates indicate the need for realistic power estimates, in order to ensure that the numbers are sufficient to enable a deficit to be detected.

The nature of the test batteries, comprising a large number of tests, has demonstrated the problems of multiple non-independent outcomes. In some cases, the analyses have been carried out as if the tests were all independent, and with a large number of exploratory analyses in a search for significant results. Since significance is determined on the basis of probabilities these 'fishing expeditions', as they have been called, are bound to produce some spurious results. It is now clear that it is essential to have a predetermined analysis policy and plan, and for analyses to be carried out in accordance with this. In addition, the potential confounders should be defined on the basis of prior hypothesis of their association with the outcome, and not only because of their identified statistical association. This will have the effect of reducing bias in multivariate analysis with confounders.

A predefined analysis plan would include strategies for the examination of interactions, and for subgroup analyses to be carried out. The danger of searching for interactions and for subgroups with significant results is removed if the analysis plan specifies which interactions are thought to be important, and which subgroups are thought relevant to the hypothesis in question. This does not mean that these analyses cannot be exploratory, but it does mean that the analyses are limited, and planned in advance, rather than being data-driven. The prior planning also implies that the study has been designed to be large enough to allow for subgroup analyses.

The debate on the correct approach to the control of covariates in multivariate analyses has been heated at times. Statistical techniques have come a long way since the days of agricultural trials relating the results from one plot to the results from another. The very complex social/environmental data sets produced from this sort of research challenge existing statistics to the limit. The debate has centered on whether in regression procedures all variables should be entered into the model and eliminated in a backwards fashion, that is backwards regression, or whether the variables should be entered sequentially in terms of the size of their independent contribution to the explained variance, that is, forwards regression. At the same time there has been disagreement on the appropriate treatment of the variable of interest. Should the lead variable be forced into the model first, or last, or allowed to enter unforced? (Some investigators consider that all potential confounders should be included in the model at all times.) New techniques of regression and an increase in the sample size have largely taken the heat out of the argument. Techniques of optimal regression, described elsewhere (Pocock, Ashby and Smith, this volume) allow for an optimal set of confounders to be used in any analyses. With a general increase in the size of studies, it has also been demonstrated that the precise choice of statistical technique is unimportant. If the sample is large enough for all confounders to get an equal chance, the results are very similar whether forwards, backwards, or optimal regression techniques are employed.

The new statistical techniques, which can include confounders of marginal significance, cannot deal with the problem of collinearity between lead measures and outcomes. This has to be done at the design stage, in the variable specification. It is clear that variables which are hypothesized to be associated with body lead level should not be included, but it may be desirable to specify an acceptable level of collinearity, or rather a level beyond which collinearity is unacceptable. A further problem which the new statistical techniques do not help to resolve, is that of validity versus goodness of fit. If an important variable such as pica is not selected for optimization should it be included? This sort of decision is correctly made at the design stage, as part of the analysis plan. The availability of optimizing techniques should not lead to the conclusion that goodness of fit equals validity.

Comparisons of results across studies have been made by means of meta-analyses. These are relatively new techniques which have been designed largely for use on the results of experimental studies. In the present context they may be useful, but they do have several limitations. Like all cumulating techniques there have to be decisions about the criteria for inclusion or exclusion of studies, so meta-analyses are not necessarily objective or value-free. Studies must be checked for heterogeneity, and where this is present the results cannot simply be combined. In particular this applies to the differential treatment of confounders, or differences in confounders controlled in different studies.

Studies should be weighted by size, and the whole study data should be included. Most meta-analyses carried out to date have pooled the results of several studies and calculated a global probability value. It may be more informative to make a standardized comparison of the magnitude of the association (and the standard error). One possible way of doing this is to regress the outcome score on the lead measure (and confounders) for each study, and to calculate and plot an estimated change in outcome (and the 95% confidence limits) per doubling of the lead variable. This would provide a graphic display of the comparability (or lack of it) of results obtained from different studies.

Progress has been such that the stage of posing hypotheses for scientific purposes is past, and the value of further epidemiological studies to replicate previous studies is limited. Alternative research models which might illuminate the relationship between lead, social factors relating to disadvantage, and outcomes need to be explored. For example if groups of children can be identified where the relationship between social variables and uptake of lead differs from the normal pattern (which may be the case in the advantaged sample studied by Bellinger et al.) this would offer new possibilities for investigation.

If it were possible to identify another marker of disadvantage, for example some benign constituent of dust and dirt, another approach would be to carry out a similar study, using this marker as the independent variable. If similar results were obtained we would be none the wiser: the results could be due to lead (which would be correlated with the new marker) or to underlying social factors. If, on the other hand, the result was different, and the outcomes were not associated with the marker (after appropriate controls), this would provide evidence that lead, and not uncontrolled social factors, was the cause of the differences found.

Another more theoretical approach would involve hypothetical modelling to investigate the effect of different inter-correlations between social variables, lead measures and outcomes.

OUTCOME MEASURES

Theory-based selection of tests

The test batteries employed in lead studies have tended to be large and comprehensive, and have been described as following the blunderbuss approach; that is, if you do not really know what effect you are looking for, try to cover everything. This is time-consuming and clearly not efficient in terms of resources. A more recent criticism is that there has been an overemphasis on IQ measures. Since most test batteries include many other tests, this criticism may be more directed at the end point of the research, and the reporting of results, and may simply reflect that it is in tests of intelligence that lead-associated performance differences are most reliably noted. A justification for the continuing use of IQ tests is that they provide a broadly comparable indication of the magnitude of any effects found. The emphasis on tests such as intelligence tests which have a functional significance reinforces a black box approach, and highlights the division between such tests and those which provide information on mechanisms of operation or the primary processes involved. In general, functionally important measures involve the performance of complex, multi-skill tasks, and while these can indicate that there are lead-related differences, they provide no information on the specific processes or mechanisms which might be implicated. It clearly was important for studies to ascertain whether lead-associated deficits in performance were of functional significance, but now it seems to be more relevant to explain why they exist. For example, do deficits in attention, or in learning or in retention (or in all of these primary skills) underlie the deficits found in an intelligence test? Different research studies have included more specific tests with the aim of testing specific functions, such as memory or attention, or behavioural differences (e.g. Smith *et al.*, 1983; Harvey *et al.*, 1984) but not enough studies have done this, in a systematic enough way, for it to have produced useful results. What is needed is a body of knowledge, similar to that which relates to intelligence tests, relating to other more specific areas of functioning. This will only be available when tests of specific functions are used by many different groups of researchers, in different situations, but under standardized conditions.

More importantly, the selection of areas of functioning to be investigated should be guided by theory. Tests should be selected, not because they are there, or because someone else has used them before and found an association with lead, but on the basis of a theoretical model of the effects of lead. A number of different fields of work, for example, clinical and research experience drawn from clinical conditions, the findings from animal studies, and work relating to mechanisms of lead effect, will act to guide a theoretical selection of tests or areas of functioning to focus on.

Research work into clinical conditions such as attention deficit disorder has investigated performance of tasks such as serial and choice reaction time tests, and the relation of these to other areas of psychometric functioning. Information from tests to assess the effects of mild head trauma and other brain disorders, and tests and investigations used in demyelinating conditions, could also be studied to see what information they provide on the relationship of known functional deficit to test results.

In addition, knowledge from tests used in other areas of pure psychology, such as in research on spatial abilities, has not been utilized in guiding the choice of tests. It is true that much of the research relates to unstandardized, one-off tests, but there are tests such as rod-and-frame and visual rotation paradigms for which there is an extensive body of information, which has yet to be tapped in lead studies.

It is quite apparent from the papers in this volume (e.g. Cory-Slechta; Rice; Lilienthal et al.) that animal studies can also provide information on the selection of appropriate outcomes, and the types of tests which should be used in studies of children. Because of the difficulty of assessing complex multifactorial skills such as intelligence in animals, the majority of tests used have concentrated on assessing a single skill, and have provided more information on which processes or functions are likely to be affected. This information has not yet been used in designing test batteries for children. It is also likely (although this needs to be ascertained) that the number of other non-lead influences on a primary skill, such as long-term memory, is smaller than the number of influences on a more complex skill, such as reading.

As well as suggesting which primary skills might be investigated, the tests which have been used in animal studies suggest that, to some extent, the skills investigated in children by currently used test batteries are being assessed in the wrong way. The evidence from animal studies indicates that the complexity of the task is important, as there are several examples of occasions where an effect is apparent in a complex task (for example, discrimination reversal learning) but not in a simpler version of the same task (discrimination learning). Similarly, lead-associated deficits in performance have been found when animals have been required to solve a series of problems, although there were no apparent differences in the animals' ability to solve a single problem. This suggests that concept formation, or the ability to generalize from one situation to another, might be an area to assess, and this has not so far been done. Other results from animal studies suggest that it is long-term retention, that is retention over a period of days or weeks, rather than learning or short-term memory which should be assessed.

In general, the evidence from animal studies suggests that more attention should be paid to the nature of the task the child is required to do in a test situation, and that as well as recording an outcome score in terms of correct responses, other measures of performance such as incorrect responses, false positives, speed of response, and trials to criterion should be recorded. For example, lead-related differences in behavioural reactivity, which has been implicated in animal studies, may be unnoticed and unrecorded in a test where the only results recorded relate to the correctness or incorrectness of the response. Animal studies also indicate that the tasks should be designed so that they require the child's performance to be stretched to the limit. Test batteries are often designed to provide as much interest and stimulation for the child as is possible in the circumstances. In fact it may be more productive to require the child to do long boring tests, like continuous performance tests, in order to show an effect.

Another approach to the theory-guided selection of outcome measures would utilize information from biological research carried out both *in vitro* and *in vivo* into the mechanisms of operation of lead in the brain and other neural tissues. A knowledge of how lead is likely to operate in the brain, on a cellular level, and in terms of parts of the brain which might be targetted by lead, would suggest which functions are most likely to be affected at low levels of exposure, and therefore which skills should be assessed. Some recent research (Markovac and Goldstein, 1988) shows evidence of the effects of lead, at levels similar to those found in environmentally exposed children, on a regulatory enzyme which is critical to the control of cellular signal transduction in the brain. Biological evidence such as this on the mechanisms which would explain lead neurotoxicity would inform the choice of outcome measures. Other research, as yet fairly inconclusive, has investigated whether parts of the brain, such as the hippocampus, may be targetted by lead. Information of this sort would suggest types of behavioural processes worth investigating in children.

Finally, in terms of the sources of information which could, and should, be used in selecting an appropriate battery of tests, the results of previous research with children should not be forgotten. There are some tests, for example, the Bender Gestalt test, and the Wiener Reaction Time device, which do seem to show an association with lead more consistently than most others. A theoretical approach to test-selection would use this information to investigate further the components of performance in these tasks.

Variables which affect performance on outcome measures

Lead studies have been at the basis of the creation of a whole new field of research – that of behavioural toxicology. The problems relating to suitable outcome measures to assess the influence of one single variable on child development, amid the multitude of other interacting factors, have become apparent from efforts to interpret the results of lead studies, but they are not unique to them. They highlight the need for a much greater knowledge on the parameters of the outcome measures used.

Currently used psychometric measures have a number of major limitations in lead studies where it is the interpretation of the cause of any difference in performance found which is important. Measures of intelligence and academic achievement are known to be strongly related to a number of social factors. The interpretation of the behavioural results is hampered because information

490

on known influences is not collected or controlled. The interpretation of results relating to more specific skills is also made difficult because there is not enough information on the (non-lead) variables which are relevant to explain differences in performance.

There is a need for the development of predictive, stable and repeatable measures, which have known validity in terms of their functional significance to children, and more importantly, can be shown to have greater independence from the social influences which are related to lead uptake. It is likely that these measures will be highly specific, and that will be a further advantage, as discussed above, in identifying the nature of any deficit caused by lead.

There is a move in this direction with the work of Yule et al. (this volume) in developing automated methods for administering learning, attention and vigilance tests, and assessing the stability of these measures. Much more is needed, particularly with respect to the greater social independence of the measures, and knowledge of parameters underlying performance in specific skills. Once suitable measures are developed there is a need to standardize their administration to a level compatible with testing in a research context.

The prospective studies pose particular problems in the selection of appropriate outcome measures. What is needed are comparable tests which can be administered at a number of different points in time, and which have high predictive significance. Apparent effects or differences in performance found at one age which are not evident at a later age are probably of no great functional significance, unless they are responsible for other differences in performance at a later date. The question of the persistence of any kind of effects noted in infancy is important, as are later effects which may be attributable to earlier developmental delays. The most commonly used assessments for young children, the Bayley Developmental Scales, were not designed to predict future intellectual status. Not surprisingly they do not have a high predictive significance in relation to later intelligence scores (Lee, 1979), and there is some evidence that the predictive significance varies between different groups (Goffeney et al., 1971). This makes it difficult to interpret the importance of any differences in performance found. The lack of predictive significance may also explain inconsistencies between the early results obtained from developmental scales and later results obtained from IQ tests (e.g. Bellinger et al., 1987). The relationship of developmental differences on scales such as the Bayley to later intellectual differences will become clearer soon, and at the same time there will also be an opportunity to compare the results of the longitudinal prospective studies with those of cross-sectional studies.

The prospective studies are already beginning to answer questions on the significance of neonatal exposure to lead, and of effects on development noted in infancy, for children of school age, and more information will be available in the next few years as more of the prospective studies progress to that stage. This does not obviate the need for reliable, repeatable, and predictive tests for use in the infant stages. The work of Fagan (1984) in the USA in developing infant tests which are claimed to have greater social independence and better predictive validity for later intellect is one example of an outcome measure which should be investigated as an alternative to currently used measures.

The relationship between lead and outcomes may vary with dose, age at exposure and developmental level at exposure. If any or all of these are so, then the outcome measures which are appropriate in one situation will not be the same as those applicable in another situation. It is not implausible to hypothesize that the effects of lead observed are determined at least partly by the developmental stage of the child at exposure. At higher levels of lead exposure it is possible (and there is some evidence for this from animal studies at higher levels of lead) that early exposure to lead occurring at a time of maximum neuronal development causes irreversible structural changes (for example, reduced neuronal outgrowth, resulting in fewer synaptic connections) whereas later exposure causes chemical or neuro-endocrine change, which may be reversible. If this were the case, the effects of lead would be different depending on the age at exposure.

Quality control of test procedures

The need for stringent quality control procedures has long been recognized in chemical pathology, so measures of the exposure to lead, whether it is blood or teeth, are likely to be analysed in conditions where quality control is of paramount importance. A description of the quality control procedures employed, and the outcome of these, will usually be reported as part of the results. This has not been the case with psychometric testing. There is clear evidence of poor test quality in the past: in one study one tester produced IQ scores which were an average of 15 points lower than the others (Gregory et al., 1976). More often the data relating to training, reliability trials and inter-tester differences are not presented. A recent re-examination of over 450 WISC and WISC-R intelligence scores carried out for research purposes (though not in a lead study) showed that there were errors in the calculation of the scores in nearly a quarter of the tests (Beasley et al., 1988). This sort of laxity, if it was common to several testers, would not necessarily be apparent from reliability trials or an examination of inter-tester differences.

In order to demonstrate the reliability of psychometric data from within a study, stringent checks on the quality of psychometric testing are needed. This implies more time spent on training, the need for inter-tester reliability trials, and reporting of the results of these, as well as an examination of tester differences when testing has been completed. A video recording of the administration of the whole test battery should be made for reference purposes. Since testing may go on for a period of several years (and this is particularly relevant to the longitudinal prospective studies) it would be better to schedule retraining periods, and to make random checks on test quality throughout the test period. This could be done by means of video recordings made at intervals during the test period. As well as checks on test administration, a proportion of the tests should be rescored by a second person to check for errors.

Studies which are following a common protocol would benefit from inter-study collaboration on test procedures. At the least this could be done by the exchange of video recordings of testing sessions, but it would be better to exchange observers, and for the testers to receive training with other groups. This would also enable better between-study comparisons of findings, as one potential source of disparity in the findings, that of differences in the test procedures, would be removed.

Several of the suggestions for changes in the outcome measures or test administration have implications for the funding of studies. If we are to improve the quality of the outcomes obtained, the selection, and the development and standardization of new assessments, where suitable ones do not exist, are time-consuming processes, and therefore cost money. Similarly the more checks and quality control procedures built into testing the longer it will take. It must, however, be seen as a false economy to regard these as peripheral activities. They should be seen as necessary and integral parts of the research study, and this should be apparent in the research design.

EXPOSURE ASSESSMENT

There is a continuing need to estimate body burdens of lead in order to monitor exposure levels. In order to relate lead levels to neurobehavioural outcomes, the critical index is the amount of lead to which the brain has been exposed. Since exposures at different ages and developmental stages may have different outcomes, the ideal measure would be something that reflected the lead level in the brain at a critical point in time. Such a measure is not available, so researchers have used blood, shed deciduous teeth, or hair, as indicators of body lead burden. All these provide an imperfect estimate, but the question is which is the best measure under which circumstances? To add to the complications, it is possible that different estimates of body lead may relate to different outcomes. Hair has generally not proved to be a suitable measure, so the choice is between blood, or some blood constituent such as A-LAD or protoporphyrin, or shed teeth.

The cross-sectional studies, carried out at one point in time, have tended to use a single measure of exposure, with a few studies utilizing a second subsidiary measure, usually on a subgroup of children rather than on the whole sample. This has provided evidence relating both blood and tooth lead measures to outcomes, and some independent information on the validity of both measures in reflecting lead exposure, but relatively little comparative evidence on the relationship of the two measures, and on the nature and time scale of their association with lead exposure.

The prospective studies which are in progress are obtaining serial estimations of blood lead, and in many cases are collecting, or plan to collect, teeth as well. This will provide more information on the relationship of the different measures, and the pattern over time and different developmental stages. At the same time, since several of the prospective studies are investigating the potential sources of lead, such as dirt and dust, to which the child is exposed, it is expected that this will produce a great deal of information relating sources and habits associated with intake, to body burden.

Early results show that children's blood lead levels are not very stable over the first few years of life, although whether they fall or rise may be a feature of the general environmental levels as well as the individual habits and environment of the child. There is some indication that cord blood levels (providing an indication of the lead to which the fetus has been exposed) are more relevant to outcomes several years later, than blood lead levels obtained postnatally. The results from those studies which have investigated sources of lead show that dust and dirt are significant contributors to the body lead burdens in young children.

In some ways blood lead is a less problematic measure, as there is general agreement on the practices of collection and techniques of analysis of samples for lead. It was agreed that where it is possible to obtain them, venous blood samples were preferable to capillary samples. The need for careful and thorough cleansing of the skin to avoid surface contamination was also agreed, and this was particularly relevant for capillary samples.

There was much less agreement with respect to tooth lead measures. Teeth act as integrators of lead exposure over long periods so they offer the opportunity to assess past exposure in a way which blood lead measures cannot. There was little consensus between different research groups on which tooth, and which part of the tooth, to analyse. At present there is insufficient information on the kinetics of lead in the tooth, so that there is no way of distinguishing peak or point exposures from chronic or steady high exposures, nor of identifying the period in the past when peak exposures occurred. The anatomy of a tooth reveals that it is a complex set of tissues, with different uptakes of lead by its different parts. There is some evidence that lead is laid down in the tooth in a systematic way, like the growth rings of a tree, but, to date, analyses have been confined to rather gross partitions of tooth material. The circumpulpal dentine appears to be the most dynamic part of the tooth, but this may mean that it reflects more recent exposure, and is a worse integrator of past exposure than the whole tooth.

The value of whole tooth analyses was put in doubt by the observations of variation in lead content between different teeth from the same child. Recent studies have provided more information on the pattern of differences in tooth lead measurements with the type of tooth, which suggests that the differences are systematic, and therefore a standardized or corrected tooth lead measurement can be calculated for any tooth. Examination of variables associated with whole tooth lead content has resulted in an equation including position in mouth, jaw, weight of the tooth, and age at tooth shedding, to predict the estimated lead concentration for a standardized tooth (Paterson et al., 1988).

The importance of consensus in terminology was highlighted by a misunderstanding of the analytical procedures employed, because of a differential use of the labels, primary, secondary and circumpulpal dentine, by different research groups. This indicated one area where improvements in inter-study communication could be made with ease. Exchange of personnel between study groups to observe analytical procedures, or a video-recording to demonstrate the process, would resolve such differences. The latter procedure would also provide a record which could be kept for reference purposes.

Unlike psychometric outcome measures, the need for quality control procedures in the analysis of biological materials has long been recognized, and the assurance of quality of analytical procedures is high. It was clear from discussions, however, that there were some areas within the analytical process, such as in physically cutting teeth for analysis, where there was room for variation and error, and which were not usually covered by the quality control procedures.

At the present time, relationships between exposures to lead and body burden, as measured by either blood or teeth, and relationships between lead and outcomes, are investigated by comparing groups of children. Another approach to provide information on the kinetics of lead in the body and the mechanisms of operation would be to investigate individual differences in metabolism and susceptibility to lead.

It should be noted that the discussions had concentrated almost exclusively on total lead burden, which is mainly inorganic lead, but this ignores the contribution made by organic lead.

ANIMAL STUDIES

Many of the questions which are being tackled in studies of children can also be investigated in studies of animals. Information on dose–response relationships, the persistence or reversibility of effects, and periods of critical exposure can be obtained from animal work. Animal studies are of value because they are experimental in design, and therefore the exposure of the animal to lead and the time course of the exposure can be experimentally manipulated. A further major advantage is that they allow differentiation between biological and behavioural effects.

The difficulty of separating out one single influence on child development has been described. This does not apply in animal studies, where the experimental design means that other variables can be kept constant while lead exposure is varied, thus any effects in performance noted can be attributed to lead with a high degree of certainty. (This is not necessarily the case at higher doses of lead, where taste aversion may result in animals eating or drinking less, and performance differences may be due to nutritional differences.)

Research with animals can make a valuable contribution to two of the areas discussed earlier: outcome measures and exposure assessment. It can indicate which outcome measures are most sensitive to lead effects and which outcomes are insensitive, provide information on the types of processes involved, and inform the choice of outcome measures for studies of children; it also provides an opportunity to study the kinetics of lead in relation to the measures of body lead burden most frequently obtained in studies of humans. The effect of chelation therapy on lead levels in the brain, and the relation of these to levels of lead in blood and bone, is another area where animal work can inform studies of children. The limitations of extrapolation from animal data to studies of humans are addressed in the review section of this book. While it is unlikely that the rat provides an adequate model of

495

the kinetics of lead in humans, or the relation of lead levels in the blood to tissue levels, this is not necessarily so for primates. It is nevertheless informative to investigate the ratio of blood/brain lead levels across species, and changes in the ratio with exposure levels and age. The possibility of changes in the mechanisms of lead effect at the different ages, and at different developmental levels, which were discussed under the heading of outcome measures, can be explored in animal studies.

Since lead exposure is manipulated in studies of animals, the effects of changes in exposure can be investigated. For example, the question of the persistence of effects after lead exposure has ceased can be examined. This is directly relevant to studies of children in situations where the early exposure is high, and is then reduced. Animal studies indicate that although the initial blood lead levels of dosed animals are indistinguishable from those of control animals, effects in some areas of functioning can be demonstrated several years later. More work to clarify the extent and nature of critical periods for lead exposure is needed. Parallel biochemical work on the persistence of lead in neural tissues, and on changes in neural tissue or neuroendocrine mechanisms as a result of exposure at different critical periods, will begin to provide information on why these effects are observed.

A variety of experimental paradigms are available and used in animal studies, and it is clear that some of these, such as those assessing learning, concept formation, or retention, are readily transferable to studies of children. Yet this has not been done. It is possible that this is simply due to a lack of familiarity with the techniques and details of animal work on the part of researchers with children. It may also demonstrate a lack of confidence to move away from the traditional and well-used techniques and tests, and to implement new methods and procedures.

FUTURE PERSPECTIVES

Scientific research tends to proceed within the confines of a discipline, and often there is little communication between different disciplines even where there is overlap in the area of interest. This workshop is unusual in that research relating to the mechanisms of lead effect, and to effects on animals, has been presented and discussed alongside research relating to the effects of lead on children. While this volume reflects that, what it may not reflect so clearly is the learning experience which many of the participants of the workshop will have gone through. It was perhaps necessary for the animal experimenters (who were in the minority) to explain their techniques in more detail than they might have been accustomed to, and there were no doubt moments of misunderstanding due to ignorance of techniques and working practices in an unfamiliar field. Despite this, the overwhelming impression was that there is an immense amount that could be learned from a fuller knowledge of work in related fields, and that the benefits of greater collaboration would be enormous. The possibility of direct collaboration in designing joint research studies, and of schemes such as sponsorships to train experimenters in the techniques of behavioural pharmacology, would seem to offer a practical way forward.

There are a number of directions where future research on children is indicated, both in order to aid the interpretation of data already gathered in epidemiological studies, and to provide additional information on the relationship of lead to functioning in children.

Most current epidemiological research has been based on replication from other studies investigating children. The search for 'effects' has become the motivating force, with the result that studies often appear to lack a valid model to explain these effects. Equally there needs to be a model to explain differences in body lead burden in different children from similar environments, and some of the prospective studies have now developed sophisticated models to do this.

From a psychological point of view, research studies need to be based on a model which is designed to test specific hypotheses about functions affected, and will provide a consistent explanation of effects noted. A model which is based on a functional approach to the mechanisms of lead effects will also reduce the possibility that any effects found are social in origin. Apart from IQ and reading tests, there is little consistency in the reports of where effects are found, but this partly reflects the somewhat random selection of areas of functioning which are studied, and differences in the nature of the task used to assess the same skill.

From a neurological point of view, what is needed in the future is increased co-ordination or theoretical interchange between the different fields of lead research. There is now a substantial data base as a result of epidemiological, neurochemical, neurological, EEG, and animal behavioural work, but rather little co-ordination between these fields. The existing data would provide a conceptually sound base for the development of hypotheses linking knowledge from these fields, to be generated and tested in epidemiological studies.

Research with children, on animals and on mechanisms has now progressed to a stage where an integrated model of the effects of lead, which is consistent with current knowledge from biochemical, animal, neurophysiological and psychological research, is needed to direct future research along convergent lines, towards a common goal of understanding the effects of lead in the brain.

In the ten years since the results of the first epidemiological studies of the effects of low levels of lead were published, enormous progress has been made in almost all aspects of the research: in study design, in the statistical techniques employed, in the outcome measures assessed, and in the measures of exposure. As a result of this we know a great deal more about the effects of low levels of environmental lead on developing children than we did a decade ago. The fact that there is still a lot that we do not know should not blind us to the achievements and progress that has been made.

These achievements do not relate only to the field of lead research. The problems of investigating one single influence on child development are also applicable to other toxins, and in a wider medical context. Research into the effects on the child of maternal alcohol consumption in pregnancy, changes in obstetric practice, and glue sniffing, to pick a diverse selection, have all gained from the experience of research carried out to investigate the effects of lead. The field of behavioural toxicology in general has benefited greatly from the substantial advances which have been made in the study of the neurobehavioural effects of lead. There is a continuing need to disseminate not only the results of research, but also of the debate and discussions which have surrounded them, for it is in this way that the methodologies of behavioural toxicology will progress. This workshop has shown the value of the exchange of information between disciplines. What is needed now is an interdisciplinary sharing of skills, so that there is a real pooling of experience in designing future research studies in this and related fields.

References

Beasley, M.G., Lobasher, M., Henley, S. and Smith, I. (1988). Errors in computation of WISC and WISC-R intelligence quotients from raw scores. *J. Child Psychol. Psychiatry*, **29**, 101–104

Bellinger, D., Sloman, J., Leviton, A., Waternaux, C., Needleman, H. and Rabinowitz, M. (1987). Low-level lead exposure and child development: assessment at age 5 of a cohort followed from birth. Paper presented at the Sixth International Conference on Heavy Metals, New Orleans, September, 1987

Fagan, J.F. (1984). The relationship of novelty preferences during infancy to later intelligence and later recognition memory. *Intelligence*, **8**, 339–346

Gregory, R.J., Lehman, R.E. and Mohan, P.J. (1976). Intelligence test results for children with and without undue lead absorption. Idaho Department of Health and Welfare, Division of Health, State House, Boise, Idaho 83720, USA

Goffeney, B., Henderson, N.B. and Bother, B.V. (1971). Negro–white, male–female 8-month developmental scores compared with 7-year WISC and Bender test scores. *Child Devel.* **42**, 595–604

Harvey, P.G., Hamlin, M.W., Kumar, R. and Delves, H.T. (1984). Blood lead, behaviour and intelligence test performance in preschool children. *Science Total Environ.*, **40**, 45–60

Lee, P.C. (1979). A review of the literature concerning the reliability and validity of the Bayley Scales of Infant Development. Unpublished MSc thesis. Department of Psychology, La Crosse College of Education, University of Wisconsin, USA

Markovac, J. and Goldstein, G.W. (1988). Picomolar concentrations of lead stimulate brain protein kinase C. *Nature*, **334**, 71–73

Paterson, L.J., Raab, G.M., Hunter, R., Laxen, D., Fulton, M., Fell, G.S., Halls, D.J. and Sutcliffe, P. (1988). Factors influencing lead concentrations in shed deciduous teeth. *Science Total Environ.* (in press)

Smith, M., Delves, T., Lansdown, R., Clayton, B. and Graham, P. (1983). The effects of lead exposure on urban children: the Institute of Child Health/Southampton study. *Devel. Med. Child Neurol.* Supplement **47**

Alphabetical List of Participants

Principal authors of chapters in this book are indicated by the chapter number(s) in parentheses after the name.

Dr J. M. Anto
Institute de la Salud Publicca
Placa de Lesseps No.1
Barcelona 08023
Spain

Dr P. A. Baghurst
CSIRO
Division of Human Nutrition
Kintore Avenue
Adelaide, South Australia 5000
Australia

Prof. D. Barltrop
Westminster Medical School
Westminster Children's Hospital
Department of Child Health
Vincent Square
London, SW1P 2NS
UK

Dr D. Bellinger (4.4)
Children's Hospital
300 Longwood Avenue
Boston, MA 02115
USA

Dr R. Bornschein (4.1)
University of Cincinnati
Kettering Laboratory
Cincinnati, OH 45267
USA

Dr P. Bourdeau
Director
Directorate General for Science, Research
  and Development
Commission of European Communities
Rue de la Loi 200
B-1049 Brussels
Belgium

Prof. R. Cluydts (3.8)
Department of Psychology
Human Psychophysiology
Pleinlaan 2
1050 Brussels
Belgium

Dr D. A. Cory-Slechta (5.1)
Environmental Health Sciences Centre
University of Rochester
School of Medicine
Rochester, NY 14642
USA

Dr K. N. Dietrich (4.2)
Institute of Environmental Health
University of Cincinnati
College of Medicine
Cincinnati, OH 45267-0056
USA

Dr C. Ernhart (4.5, 6.1)
Cleveland Metropolitan General Hospital
Department of Psychiatry
Case Western Reserve University
Cleveland, OH 44109
USA

Dr G. Fell
University Department of Pathological
  Biochemistry
The Royal Infirmary
Castle Street
Glasgow, G4 0SF
UK

Dr G. I. Forbes
Scottish Home and Health Department
St. Andrew's House
Edinburgh, EH1
UK

Dr M. Fulton
Department of Community Medicine
Medical School
Teviot Place
Edinburgh, EH8 9AG
UK

Prof. M. Garraway
Department of Community Medicine
Medical School
Teviot Place
Edinburgh, EH8 9AG
UK

Prof. Sir Abraham Goldberg
University Department of Medicine
Western Infirmary
Glasgow, G11 6NT
UK

Prof. P. Grandjean
Indelukket 47
2900 Hellerup
Denmark

Dr L. D. Grant (1.2)
Director
Environmental Criteria and Assessment
    Office
US Environmental Protection Agency
MD-52
Research Triangle Park, NC 27711
USA

Dr J. Graziano (4.7)
Department of Pediatrics
Columbia College of Physicians and
    Surgeons
630 West 168 Street
New York, NY 10032
USA

Dr N. P. Hajjar
Dynamac Corporation
11140 Rockville Pike
Rockville, MD 20850
USA

Dr P. B. Hammond
University of Cincinnati
Institute of Environmental Health
Cincinnati, OH 45267
USA

Dr E. Hansen
Institute of Toxicology
National Food Agency
19 Mørkhøj Bygade
DK-2860 Søbors
Denmark

Dr O. N. Hansen (3.7)
Institute of Psychology
University of Aarhus
Asylvej 4
DK-8240 Risskov
Denmark

Dr P. Harvey (3.4)
Lancaster Street Clinic
90 Lancaster Street
Birmingham, B4 6AR
UK

Dr A. Hatzakis (3.5)
Department of Forensic Medicine and
    Toxicology
M. Asias Ave-Goudi
Athens
Greece

Prof. G. Kazantzis (2.1)
London School of Hygiene and Tropical
    Medicine
Keppel Street
London, WC1E 7HT
UK

Prof. A. Lafontaine
95 Boulevard Brand-Whitlock
1050 Brussels
Belgium

Dr D. Laxen
Air Pollution Group
Scientific Services Branch
Greater London Council
County Hall
London, SE1 7PB
UK

Dr H. Lilienthal (5.2)
Medical Institute of Environmental Hygiene
Curlittstr. 53
D-4000 Dusseldorf
FRG

Dr T. Lyngbye
Institute of Psychiatric Demography
Psychiatric Hospital in Aarhus
8240 Risskov
Denmark

Dr W. McBride (3.9)
Foundation 41
The Women's Hospital
365 Crown Street
Surry Hills 20202
Sydney, New South Wales 2010
Australia

500

Prof. L. Manzo
University of Pavia
Piazza Botta 10
Department of Pharmacology
I-2700 Pavia
Italy

Dr G. K. Mathew
DHSS
Hannibal House
Room 908
Elephant and Castle
London, SE1 6TE
UK

Dr M. R. Moore (4.6)
University Department of Medicine
Western Infirmary
Glasgow, G11 6NT
UK

Dr S. R. Moorhouse
The British Industrial Biological Research
    Association
Woodmansterne Road
Carshalton
Surrey, SM5 4DS
UK

Mr D. Muddiman
Institute of Psychiatry
DeCrespigny Park
Denmark Hill
London, SE5 8AF
UK

Dr M. Murphy
Department of Pediatrics
Columbia College of Physicians and
    Surgeons
630 West 168th Street
New York, NY 10032
USA

Dr P. Mushak (2.2)
Department of Pathology
University of North Carolina at Chapel Hill
Chapel Hill, NC 27514
USA

Dr H. L. Needleman (3.13)
Children's Hospital of Pittsburgh
Pittsburgh, PA 15213
USA

Dr H. Neus
Freie Und Hansestadt Hamburg
Gesundheitsbehorde
Postfach 25 24
2000 Hamburg 13
FRG

Dr V. O'Gorman
National Board for Science and Technology
Shelbourne Road
Dublin 4
Republic of Ireland

Dr D. Otto (3.12)
US Environmental Protection Agency
Clinical Studies Division
MD-58
Research Triangle Park, NC 27711
USA

Dr D. Pelling (5.5)
The British Industrial Biological Research
    Association
Woodmansterne Road
Carshalton
Surrey, SM5 4DS
UK

Prof. S. J. Pocock (3.1)
Department of Clinical Epidemiology and
    General Practice
Royal Free Hospital School of Medicine
Rowland Hill Street
London, NW3 2PF
UK

Dr D. Popovac
60/4 Pristina
1132 Belgrade
Yugoslavia

Dr R. D. Putnam
Consultant-Environmental Health
International Lead Zinc Research
    Organisation Inc.
292 Madison Avenue
New York, NY 10017
USA

Mr M. J. Quinn
Department of the Environment
Romney House
43 Marsham Street
London, SW1P 3PY
UK

Mrs G. Raab (3.3)
Medical Statistics Unit
Medical School, Teriot Place
Edinburgh, EH8 9AG
UK

Dr M. Rabinowitz (6.2)
Marine Biological Laboratory
Woods Hole, MA 02543
USA

Dr C. Regan (5.4)
University College Dublin
Department of Pharmacology
Belfield
Dublin 4
Republic of Ireland

Dr D. C. Rice (5.3)
Toxicology Research Division
Health and Welfare Canada
Tunney's Pasture
Ottawa, Ontario K1A OL2
Canada

Mr C. L. Robson
Department of the Environment
Chief Scientist Group
Room A 318
Romney House
43 Marsham Street
London, SW1P 3PY
UK

Dr S. Rothenberg (4.8)
Departamento de Neurobiología del
  Desarrollo
Instituto Nacional de Perinatología
Montes Urales Sur 800, Col. Lomas de
  Virreyes
CP 11000, México DF
Mexico

Dr E. Sabbioni
Nuclear Chemistry Division
CEC Joint Research Centre
Ispra Establishment
Ispra, Varese
Italy

Dr S. R. Schroeder (3.2)
The Nisonger Center
The Ohio State University
1581 Dodd Drive
Columbus, OH 43210-1205
USA

Dr de Shouwer
Ministry of Public Health and Family
Esplanade 7, Cité Administrative del 'Etat
1010 Brussels
Belgium

Dr D. Simms
Department of the Environment
A3 28 Romney House
43 Marsham Street
London, SW1P 3PY
UK

Mrs G. A. Smart
Food Science Division
Ministry of Agriculture, Fisheries and Food
Room 452
Great Westminster House
Horseferry Road
London SW1
UK

Dr M. Smith (1.1)
Department of Child Psychiatry
Institute of Child Health
Hospital for Sick Children
Great Ormond Street
London, WC1N 1EH
UK

Dr A. I. Sors
Commission of the European Communities
Directorate-General for Science, Research
  and Development
Environment Research Programme
Rue de la Loi 200
B-1049 Brussels
Belgium

Dr P. A. Succop (6.3)
University of Cincinnati
Kettering Laboratory
Cincinnati, OH 45267
USA

Dr S. Tarkowski
WHO
Regional Office for Europe
Scherfigsvej 8
DK2100 Copenhagen Ø
Denmark

Dr J. A. F. Thomas
Department of the Environment
Romney House
43 Marsham Street
London, SW1P 3PY
UK

Dr G. Thomson
Education Department
University of Edinburgh
10 Buccleuch Place
Edinburgh
UK

Dr Tonini
Department of Internal Medicine
University Pavia Medical School
Piazza Botta 10
27100 Pavia
Italy

Dr G. Vimpani (4.3)
Department of Paediatrics
Flinders Medical Centre
Bedford Park
South Australia, 5042
Australia

Prof. G. Vivoli (3.6)
Universita di Modena
Facolta di Medicina e Chirurgia
Cattedra d'Igiene
I-41100 Modena
Italy

Dr G. Winneke (3.10)
Medical Institute of Environmental Hygiene
University of Dusseldorf
Hennekamp 50
D-4000 Dusseldorf
FRG

Prof. W. Yule (3.11)
Institute of Psychiatry
De Crespigny Park
Denmark Hill
London, SE5 8AF
UK

Index